ORTHOPAEDIC SURGERY ESSENTIALS

PEDIATRICS

ORTHOPAEDIC SURGERY ESSENTIALS

PEDIATRICS

ORTHOPAEDIC SURGERY ESSENTIALS

Pediatrics
Kathryn E. Cramer, MD
Susan A. Scherl, MD

Foot and Ankle
David B. Thordarson, MD

Spine
Christopher Bono, MD
Steven R. Garfin, MD

Sports and Medicine
Anthony Schepsis, MD
Brian Busconi, MD

Oncology and Basic Science
Carol Morris, MD (Tentative)

Adult Reconstruction
Daniel J. Berry, MD

Hand and Wrist
James R. Doyle, MD

Trauma
Charles Court-Brown, MD
Margaret McQueen, MD
Paul Tornetta III, MD

ORTHOPAEDIC SURGERY ESSENTIALS

PEDIATRICS

Series Editors

PAUL TORNETTA III, MD
Professor
Department of Orthopaedic Surgery
Boston University School of Medicine;
Director of Orthopaedic Trauma
Boston University Medical Center
Boston, Massachusetts

THOMAS A. EINHORN, MD
Professor and Chairman
Department of Orthopaedic Surgery
Boston University School of Medicine
Boston, Massachusetts

Book Editors

KATHRYN E. CRAMER, MD
Associate Professor
Department of Orthopaedics
Wayne State University;
Department of Orthopaedics
Children's Hospital of Michigan
Detroit, Michigan

SUSAN A. SCHERL, MD
Assistant Professor
Department of Orthopaedic Surgery and Rehabilitation
The University of Nebraska;
Children's Hospital
Omaha, Nebraska

LIPPINCOTT WILLIAMS & WILKINS
A **Wolters Kluwer** Company
Philadelphia • Baltimore • New York • London
Buenos Aires • Hong Kong • Sydney • Tokyo

Acquisitions Editor: Robert Hurley
Developmental Editor: Grace R. Caputo
Production Editor: Rakesh Rampertab
Manufacturing Manager: Colin Warnock
Cover Designer: Karen Quigley
Compositor: Lippincott Williams & Wilkins Desktop Division
Printer: Edwards Brothers, Inc.

530 Walnut Street
Philadelphia, PA 19106 USA
LWW.com

Printed in the USA

Library of Congress Cataloging-in-Publication Data
Pediatrics / Kathryn E. Cramer, Susan A. Scherl (eds).—1st ed. p.; cm.—(Orthopaedic surgery essentials)
Includes bibliographical references and index.
ISBN 0-7817-4436-9
1. Pediatrics. I. Cramer, Kathryn E. II. Scherl, Susan A. III. Series.
[DNLM: 1. Orthopedics—Child. 2. Orthopedics—Infant. 3. Lower Extremity Deformities, Congenital—surgery. WS 270 P3711 2003]
RD732.3.C48P432 2003
618.92′7—dc22

2003058837

10 9 8 7 6 5 4 3 2 1

To those who have inspired and motivated us over the years: our patients and their families who allow us the privilege of caring for them, the medical students and residents who continually challenge and questions us, and the faculty and mentors who have encouraged and supported us along the way in our great adventure

—KEC

To my parents, Burton A. Scherl, MD, and Shelah B. Scherl, my first and best teachers

—SAS

CONTENTS

SECTION I: OUTPATIENT CLINIC

SECTION II: EMERGENCY DEPARTMENT

SECTION III: SPECIALTY CLINICS

SECTION IV: BACKGROUND

CONTRIBUTING AUTHORS

Edward Abraham, MD
Professor and Head
Department of Orthopaedics
University of Illinois
Chicago, Illinois

Gurpal S. Ahluwalia, MD
Children's Medical Center of Dayton
Dayton, Ohio

Michael Craig Ain, MD
Assistant Professor of
Orthopaedic Surgery
Johns Hopkins Hospital
Baltimore, Maryland

Michael Albert, MD
Director of Orthopaedics
Children's Medical Center of Dayton
Dayton, Ohio

Benjamin A. Alman, MD, FRCSC
Canadian Research Chair
Orthopaedic Surgery and Development Biology
Hospital for Sick Children
Toronto, Ontario, Canada

Richard D. Beauchamp, MD, FRCSC
Children's and Women's Health Centre of British Columbia
Vancouver, British Columbia
Canada

Robert J. Bielski, MD
Assistant Professor
Department of Orthopaedic Surgery and Rehabilitation
Loyola University
Maywood, Illinois

Roderick Birnie, MD
Assistant Professor of Orthopaedic Surgery
University of Chicago Hospitals
Chicago, Illinois

Robert D. Blasier, MD
Chief of Orthopaedic Trauma
Department Orthopaedic Surgery
Arkansas Children's Hospital
Little Rock, Arkansas

Suzanne Bowyer, MD
Professor of Pediatrics
Department of Pediatrics
Indiana University School of Medicine
Indianapolis, Indiana

Lorin M. Brown, MD
Assistant Clinical Professor of Orthopedic Surgery
Department of Surgery
Children's Memorial Hospital
Chicago, Illinois

Julie Buch, MD
Clinical Assistant Professor of Anesthesiology
Wayne State University
Department of Anesthesia;
Children's Hospital of Michigan
Detroit, Michigan

Michael T. Busch, MD
Surgical Director of Sports Medicine
Pediatric Orthopaedic Surgery
Children's Healthcare of Atlanta
Atlanta, Georgia

Brian T. Carney, MD
Shriners Hospital for Children
Lexington, Kentucky

Gail S. Chorney, MD
Assistant Professor
Department of Orthopedic Surgery
NYU-Hospital for Joint Diseases
New York, New York

Mark D. Clary, CO
Orthotics and Prosthetics Center
Physical Medicine and Rehabilitation
University Hospital
Ann Arbor, Michigan

Clifford L. Craig, MD
Clinical Associate Professor
Department of Orthopaedic Surgery
University of Michigan
Ann Arbor, Michigan

Kathryn E. Cramer, MD
Associate Professor
Department of Orthopaedics
Wayne State University;
Department of Orthopaedics
Children's Hospital of Michigan
Detroit, Michigan

Russell J. Crider, MD
Associate Clinical Professor of Orthopedics
New York University
New York, New York

Eliana Delgado, MD
Associate Clinical Professor of Pediatric Orthopaedic Surgery
University of California, San Francisco
San Francisco, California

Luciano Dias, MD
Chief
Orthopaedic Section
Children's Memorial Hospital
Chicago, Illinois

John P. Dormans, MD
Chief of Orthopaedic Surgery
Children's Hospital of Philadelphia
Philadelphia, Pennsylvania

Twee T. Do, MD
Associate Professor
Department of Pediatric Orthopaedics
Cinicinnati Children's Hospital Medical Center
Cincinnati, Ohio

David Emery, MB, BS, FRCS
Consultant Children's Orthopaedic Surgeon
Department of Orthopaedics
University Hospital of North Staffordshire
Stoke on Trent, Staffordshire, United Kingdom

Howard R. Epps, MD
Fondren Orthopedic Group, LLP
Texas Orthopaedic Hospital
Houston, Texas

Bulent Erol, MD
Attending Surgeon
Pediatric Orthopaedic Surgery
Children's Hospital of Philadelphia
Philadelphia, Pennsylvania

John M. Flynn, MD
Orthopaedic Surgeon
Division of Orthopaedic Surgery
Children's Hospital of Philadelphia
Philadelphia, Pennlylvania

Theodore J. Ganley, MD
Orthopaedic Director of Sports Medicine
Children's Hospital of Philadelphia
Philadelphia, Pennsylvania

Evan Geller, MD
Section Chief
Nuclear Medicine and Mesculoskeletal Imaging
Department of Radiology
St. Christopher's Hospital for Children
Philadelphia, Pennsylvania

Bruce Gillingham, CAPT, MC, USN
Director of Surgical Services
Naval Medical Center, San Diego
San Diego, California

Daniel W. Green, MD, MS, FACS
Assistant Attending Surgeon
Department of Pediatric Orthopaedic Surgery
Hospital for Special Surgery
New York, New York

Jan S. Grudziak, MD, PhD
Department of Orthopaedic Surgery
Children's Hospital of Pittsburgh
Pittsburgh, Pennsylvania

Kenneth Guidera, MD
Shriners Hospital
Tampa, Florida

Lawrence L. Haber, MD
Director of Pediatric Orthopaedics
Tod Children's Hospital
Youngstown, Ohio

Reggie C. Hamdy, MD
Assistant Chief of Staff
Shriners Hospital for Children
Montreal, Quebec, Canada

William L. Hennrikus, MD
Director of Sports Medicine
Children's Hospital of Central California
Madera, California

Robert Neil Hensinger, MD
Chairman
Department of Orthopaedic Surgery
University of Michigan Health System
Ann Arbor, Michigan

Martin J. Herman, MD
St. Christopher's Hospital for Children
Orthopedic Center for Children
Philadelphia, Pennsylvania

Sevan Hopyan, MD, PhD
Postgraduate Trainee
Division of Orthopaedics
Department of Surgery
University of Toronto
Toronto, Ontario, Canada

Brian L. Hotchkiss, MD
Private Practice
Grand Rapids, Michigan

B. David Horn, MD
Assistant Surgeon
Division of Orthopaedic Surgery
Children's Hospital of Philadelphia
Philadelphia, Pennsylvania

Andrew W. Howard, MD, MSc, FRCSC
Consulting Staff, Orthopaedics
Department of Surgery
Hospital for Sick Children
Toronto, Ontario, Canada

Jevere Howell, BS
Medical Student
University of Pennsylvania School of Medicine
Philadelphia, Pennsylvania

Robert P. Huang, MD
Orthopaedic Surgeon
Department of Pediatric Orthopaedics
Shriners Hospital for Children
Houston, Texas

Kosmos J. Kayes, MD
Assistant Professor of Orthopaedic Surgery
Department of Orthopaedic Surgery
Indiana University School of Medicine
Indianapolis, Indiana

Thomas F. Kling, Jr., MD
Professor of Orthopaedic Surgery
Department of Orthopaedic Surgery
Indiana University School of Medicine
Indianapolis, Indiana

D. Raymond Knapp Jr., MD
Pediatric Orthopaedic Surgeon
Pediatric Orthopaedic Division
Nemours Children's Clinic—Orlando
Orlando, Florida

Arabella I. Leet, MD
Assistant Professor
Department of Orthopaedic Surgery
Johns Hopkins University
Baltimore, Maryland

Laura M. Lemke, MD
Pediatric Orthopaedic Surgeon
Fox Valley Orthopaedic Institute
Geneva, Illinois

Julia E. Lou, BA
Clinical Research Coordinator
Division of Orthopaedic Surgery
Children's Hospital of Philadelphia
Philadelphia, Pennsylvania

David W. Manning, MD
Assistant Professor of Orthopaedic Surgery
University of Chicago Hospitals
Chicago, Illinois

David L. Marshall, MD
Medical Director
Sports Medicine Program
Children's Hospital of Atlanta
Atlanta, Georgia

Keith H. May, DPT, ATC, CSCS
Physical Therapist/Athletic Trainer
Department of Sports Medicine
Children's Healthcare of Atlanta
Atlanta, Georgia

James F. Mooney III, MD
Chief
Department of Orthopaedic Surgery
Children's Hospital of Michigan
Detroit, Michigan

George S. Naseef III, MD
Chief Orthopaedic Resident
Department of Orthopaedic Surgeons
Union Memorial Hospital
Baltimore, Maryland

Eloy Ochoa, MD
Orthopaedic Surgeon
Department of Orthopaedics
Naval Hospital Corpus Christi
Corpus Christi, Texas

Nicole Parent, CO, OTR
Certified Orthotist
Orthotics and Prosthetics
University of Michigan
Ann Arbor, Michigan

Bruce Pawel, MD
Assistant Professor of Pathology and Laboratory Medicine
Division of Pathology
Children's Hospital of Philadelphia
Philadelphia, Pennsylvania

Craig S. Phillips, MD
Assistant Professor of Orthopaedic Surgery
University of Chicago Hospitals
Chicago, Illinois

William A. Phillips, MD
Orthopaedic Surgery
Baylor College of Medicine
Houston, Texas

Juan A. Realyvasquez, MD
Department of Orthopaedics
St. Christopher's Hospital for Children
Philadelphia, Pennsylvania

Jeffrey R. Sawyer, MD
Assistant Professor of Orthopaedic Surgery
Rush-Presbyterian-St. Luke's Medical Center
Chicago, Illinois

Susan A. Scherl, MD
Assistant Professor
Department of Orthopaedic Surgery and Rehabilitation
The University of Nebraska;
Children's Hospital
Omaha, Nebraska

Michael Schreck, DPM
Foot and Ankle of West Georgia
Columbus, Georgia

Richard M. Schwend, MD
Chief
Division of Pediatric Orthopaedics
University of New Mexico
Carrie Tingley Hospital
Albuquerque, New Mexico

Jon R. Shereck, MD
Chief Resident
Department of Orthopaedic Surgery
Wilford Hall Medical Center
Lackland Air Force Base, Lackland, Texas

Eric Shirley, MD
Department of Orthopaedic Surgery
Johns Hopkins University
Baltimore, Maryland

David Skaggs, MD
Vice Chief
Department of Orthopaedic Surgery
Children's Hospital of Los Angeles
Los Angeles, California

Joshua T. Snyder, MD
Resident
Department of Orthopedic Surgery
Loyola University Medical Center
Maywood, Illinois

Lisa J. States, MD
Chief of Nuclear Medical
Department of Medical Imaging
A.I. DuPont Hospital for Children
Wilmington, Delaware

Stephen Karl Storer, MD
Pediatric Orthopaedic Fellow
Orthopaedic Center
Los Angeles Children's Hospital
Los Angeles, California

Christopher Sullivan, MD
Assistant Professor of Orthopaedic Surgery
University of Chicago Hospitals
Chicago, Illinois

George H. Thompson, MD
Director
Department of Pediatric Orthopaedics
Rainbow Babies and Children's Hospital
Cleveland, Ohio

Sovarinth Tun, MD
Private Practice
Chicago, Illinois

Michael Vitale, MD, MPH
Attending Surgeon
Division of Pediatric Orthopaedic Surgery
Children's Hospital of New York
New York, New York

Andrew M. Wainwright, FRCS
Nuffield Orthopaedic Centre
Windmill Road
Headington, Oxford, United Kingdom

Jeffrey Warman, MD
Pediatric Orthopaedic Associates
San Antonio, Texas

Lawrence Wells, MD
Department of Orthopaedics/Pediatrics
Children's Hospital of Philadelphia
Philadelphia, Pennsylvania

Barbara J. Wolfson, MD, FACR
Department of Radiology
St. Christopher's Hospital for Children
Philadelphia, Pennsylvania

Cemil Yildiz, MD
Assistant Professor
Department of Orthopaedic Surgery
Gulhane Military Medical Academy
Etlik, Ankara, Turkey

Maria Markakis Zestos, MD
Chief of Anesthesia
Children's Hospital of Michigan
Detroit, Michigan

SERIES PREFACE

Most of the available resources in orthopaedic surgery are very good, but they either present information exhaustively—so the reader has to wade through too many details to find what he or she seeks—or assume too much knowledge, making the content difficult to understand. Moreover, as residency training has advanced, it has become more focused on the individual subspecialties. Our goal was to create a series at the basic level that residents could read completely during a subspecialty rotation to obtain the essential information necessary for a general understanding of the field. Once they have survived those trials, we hope that the *Orthopaedic Surgery Essentials* books will serve as a touchstone for future learning and review.

Each volume is to be a manageable size that can be read during a resident's tour. As a series, they will have a consistent style and template, with the authors' voices heard throughout. Content will be presented more visually than in most books on orthopaedic surgery, with a liberal use of tables, boxes, bulleted lists, and algorithms to aid in quick review. Each topic will be covered by one or more authorities, and each volume will be edited by experts in the broader field.

But most importantly, each volume—*Pediatrics, Spine, Sports Medicine*, and so on—will focus on the requisite knowledge in orthopaedics. Having the essential information presented in one user-friendly source will provide the reader with easy access to the basic knowledge needed in the field, and mastering this content will give him or her an excellent foundation for additional information from comprehensive references, atlases, journals, and on-line resources.

We would like to thank the editors and contributors who have generously shared their knowledge. We hope that the reader will take the opportunity of telling us what works and does not work.

—Paul Tornetta III, MD

PREFACE

One's first rotation through pediatric orthopaedics can be a bit like a visit to a foreign country—certain things are familiar, but there are also new sights, unfamiliar terrain, and a language and culture to learn. Think of this book as a travel guide: It's been designed to provide you with useful information, point you in the right direction, and whet your appetite for further exploration on your own.

In other words, *Orthopaedic Surgery Essentials: Pediatrics* is not meant to be an exhaustive, encyclopedic compendium on the topic, nor does it include much in the way of technical surgical detail. Many other texts and atlases exist to fill those niches. Instead, it is meant to provide the first-time or sometime pediatric orthopaedic visitor with essential information so that he or she will be able to easily and confidently evaluate and initiate treatment on a pediatric patient with a given orthopaedic disorder, as well as provide the patient, family, and primary care or emergency physician with answers to their questions.

The text has been designed to be easily read cover to cover in the course of a 1- or 2-month rotation, or to be used as a quick reference immediately before evaluation of a patient in the emergency department, on the wards, or in the clinic. To facilitate this last use, the table of contents has been arranged to reflect the venue in which the various disorders are usually first encountered.

Finally, we hope that *OSE: Pediatrics* conveys, at least on some level, the enthusiasm that virtually all pediatric orthopaedists (and certainly all of the contributors to this book) have for our field. While we realize that most orthopaedic residents won't go on to a career in pediatrics, we hope that this book plays a role in making your mandatory tour through our territory fun and exciting. We truly believe that we do have the best job in the world, and we feel fortunate to be able to share that with you in this volume.

ACKNOWLEDGMENTS

First, I would like to thank the contributors to this book, all of whom generously donated their time and effort, and most of whom even met all the deadlines.

I'm grateful to Paul Tornetta III, MD, and Robert Hurley, for offering me the opportunity to work on this project; Kathy Cramer, MD, for being such a wonderful friend and coeditor; and especially Grace Caputo for guiding Kathy and me through the process of creating a book.

I need to acknowledge the support of my partners and staff, former and present, who enabled me to dedicate the necessary time to this project. Teaching medical students and residents adds an irreplaceable dimension to the practice of medicine; one truly learns as much as one teaches, and I've been honored to participate in the education of many wonderful people.

Finally, I wish to acknowledge my patients and their families. It is a joy, a privilege, and a challenge participating in their care.

—Susan A. Scherl, MD

I heartily thank Marilyn Dupell—who really kept me focused and organized during editing, and who was the *only* one on my end to have a good handle about what was going on! And thanks to my partners who always tolerate my extra projects with humor and grace.

—Kathryn E. Cramer, MD

THE PEDIATRIC ORTHOPAEDIC EXAMINATION

BRIAN T. CARNEY

In 1992, in his address as First Vice President to the American Academy of Orthopaedic Surgeons, Hensinger spoke of the responsibilities of orthopaedists to society. He noted that Hippocrates provided the initial ethical principle for us to be honest, truthful, and to have a scientific approach to patient care: to "do no harm." Hensinger challenged us to aspire to the highest level of knowledge, education, and research: to "do good." Caring for children provides an opportunity to have an impact not only on their lives but also on the members of their immediate family and society at large.

The orthopaedic care of the child begins with your examination. The pediatric orthopaedic examination is a tool in evidence-based medicine. If your examination is associated with human research, then appropriate protection of privacy and informed consent are needed. The recording of information and measurements will both contribute to the care and satisfaction of individual children and their families, as well as provide a record for review. As such, your examination is part of a medicolegal document. This chapter provides suggestions for the pediatric orthopaedic examination. Specific examination techniques are covered in the chapters that follow.

DEVELOPMENT

Children are unique and should not be thought of as small adults. The growth and development from infancy to maturity constitutes a significant difference relative to adults and among children themselves. Growth should be considered in both your diagnosis and treatment. Developmental milestones can be screened by the Denver Developmental Screening Test (DDST). The DDST is a standardized device used to assess the development of preschool children (Table 1-1).

Bleck has outlined prognostic indicators for walking in children with the developmental delay seen in cerebral palsy. Primitive reflexes that persist longer than 3 months of age may indicate a fixed motor–brain defect (Fig. 1-1). Testing is done after 12 months of age. If no abnormal responses are seen, there is a good prognosis that the child will walk. If two or more abnormal responses are present, there is a poor prognosis that the child will walk.

THE PROCESS

Covey notes that one of the seven habits of highly successful people is to begin with an end in mind. The goal of the pediatric orthopaedist is to arrive with a diagnosis. DeGowin and DeGowin have likened the physician to a detective. You have to gather information regarding a specific problem (history) and confirm or disprove your case (diagnosis) by the evidence (examination).

First Impressions

You only get one opportunity to make a first impression. The dynamics of dependence requires your interaction with at least two individuals, the child and the parent. For consistency, "parent" and "family" will be used when referring to the child's caregivers—mother, father, relative, or guardian. When you first meet the child and family, greet and identify all individuals in the examination room. Identify yourself, your role, and what you will be doing. Offer a form of greeting such as a handshake to include the child. Do what is natural for you. Wearing a white coat may create anxiety and complicate your evaluation of the child. Most children have some anxiety, possibly reinforced by the parent, about a visit to the doctor, and the formality of a white coat may exacerbate this anxiety. The parent may claim your white coat is making the situation difficult. Removing your coat later may not resolve that difficulty.

TABLE 1-1 DENVER DEVELOPMENTAL SCREENING TEST

Developmental Milestone	Age of Achievement by 90% of Children[a]
Rolling over	5 mo
Sitting without support	8 mo
Pulling self up to stand	10 mo
Walking well	15 mo
Hopping on one foot	5 yr

[a]Failure on an item achieved by 90% of children should be considered a "delay."

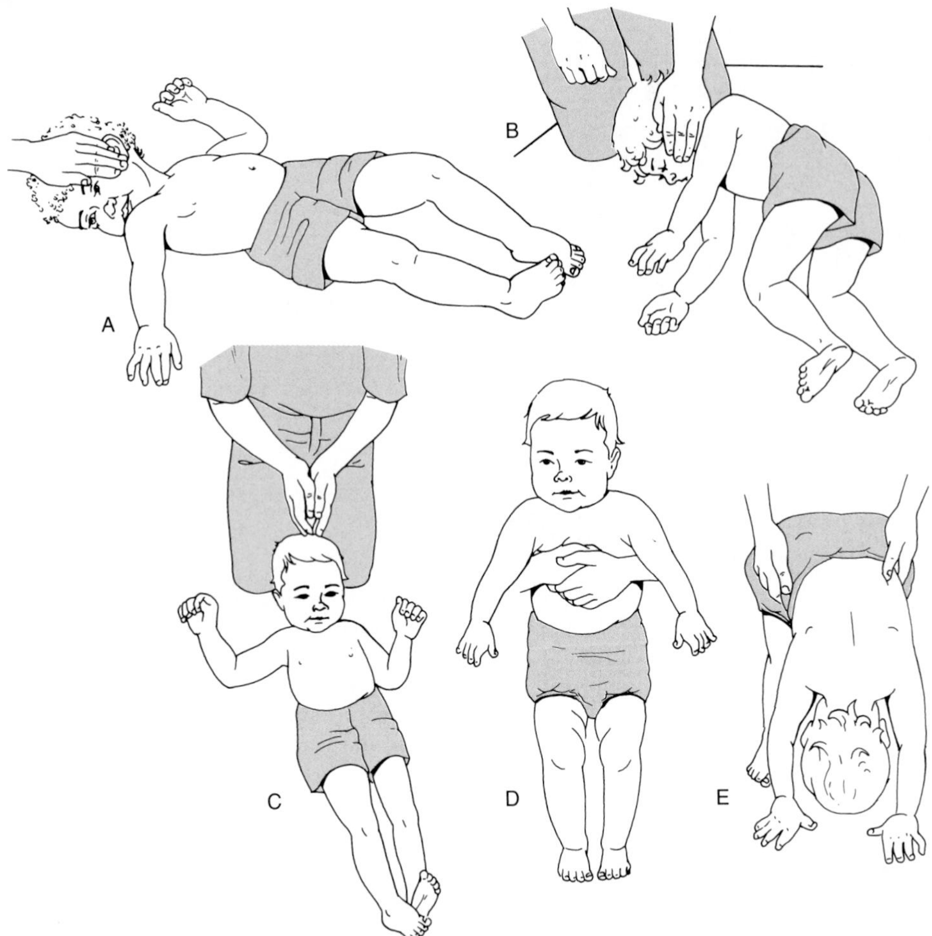

Figure 1-1 Testing for cerebral palsy-associated developmental delays. (**A**) The asymmetric tonic neck reflex is positive when a fencing posture—flexion of the limbs on the skull side and extension of the limbs on the face side—is assumed on turning the head sharply to one side. This is abnormal after 12 months of age. (**B**) The neck-righting reflex is positive when the body can be log-rolled by turning only the head. This response is abnormal after 12 months of age. (**C**) The Moro reflex is positive when there is abduction of the upper limbs followed by an embrace in response to a loud noise, such as a clap of the hands, or to jarring of the table. This is also abnormal after 12 months of age. (**D**): Extensor thrust is elicited by holding the child upright by the axillae and lowering the feet to the floor or a table surface. Progressive extension of the lower limbs and trunk is abnormal at any age. (**E**) The protective parachute reaction involves lowering the supine child to the table. Automatic hand placement should be present by at least 15 months of age. Hand withdrawal is never normal. (Adapted from Bleck EE. Cerebral palsy. In: Staheli LT. Pediatric orthopaedic secrets. Philadelphia: Hanley & Belfus, 1998:348–358.)

Interview

Be sensitive to the child and parent. Consider excusing all but the child and his or her primary caregiver(s) from the examination room (i.e., siblings and other relatives or friends brought along for moral support). Take the family's concerns seriously and listen carefully. Medical evaluation is sought for a problem that needs to be defined. Common concerns include pain, deformity, clumsiness, weakness, and stiffness. The history of present illness provides the background. Try to obtain the chief complaint directly from a school-age child or adolescent and verify the information with the parent. The complaint needs to be well-defined (described) including who has the concern and why. Symptoms can usually be dated to when something was first thought to be wrong or different. Follow the history of present illness in a clear, chronologic fashion. Note onset, setting in which the problem developed, and treatment. Symptoms should be related to location, severity, timing (onset, duration, frequency), and what aggravates or remits. Many symptoms are related to use/overuse/abuse, movement, or injury.

The birth and family history are important in the evaluation of the child:

- Birth history: inquiries of prenatal maternal bleeding, infection, medications, trauma
- Childbirth delivery information: presentation, type of delivery, difficulty of delivery, infant distress
- Neonatal information: Apgar scores, need for oxygen/ventilator support, duration of hospitalization
- Family history: inquiries about the presence of scoliosis, clubfoot, hip dysplasia, skeletal dysplasia, and neuromuscular disorders, as well as similar presentation of the chief complaint.

The effects of previous treatment may affect expectations. Alternative treatments may have been received. Often, the information will not be volunteered so you must ask about dietary, herbal, energy, or manipulative interventions.

Examination

Respect modesty while still performing an adequate examination. Shorts and T-shirts appear to be comfortable for children of all ages and should be readily available. Never miss an opportunity to examine the child without actually touching. Examine younger children in while on their parent's lap. If the parent/caregiver is absent, have a professional present to observe and chaperone. Observe action such as gait, mobility, arm swing/preference, guarding, climbing, and playing. Perform your examination without appearing to do so. Make your first touch innocuous and nonthreatening in areas you know do not hurt. If there is resistance, the parent should realize the difficulty you are facing and observe that any negative response is not due to pain. By examining the normal, asymptomatic limb first, you will have a comparison. Minimize discomfort without compromising purpose. If you are unable to examine, then ask the parent to palpate and perform motion while you observe. Recognize, and have the parent acknowledge, when you are unable to get an adequate examination. Do not presume a finding or give up out of frustration.

Closure

Avoid criticizing others and any previous care received. Try to agree as much as possible with the parents regarding their observations when discussing findings. Appear calm and unhurried, even if that is not the case. Take the time to sit down and discuss the results of the examination with the child and parent. If the parents are rushed, they will feel that you have not devoted the appropriate time or concern. When the problem is complex and needs more time, you can inform the parents that you will consult with others before you can provide a definitive answer or plan. Set a specific time for follow-up. Oftentimes the understanding of the parents may be lacking and additional visits will be helpful.

PHYSICAL EXAMINATION

Hoppenfeld has organized the physical examination into inspection, palpation, range of motion, neurologic examination, special tests, and examination of related areas.

Palpate bony landmarks, particularly relative to tenderness. Recognize and record deformity and measure with a goniometer. Deformity is described as the relationship of the distal segment relative to the proximal. Determine whether the deformity is bone, joint, or soft tissue. Can the deformity be passively corrected or is it fixed? Is there associated spasm or tenderness to palpation?

Specific joint range of motions and some primary motor muscles/nerves are recorded (Table 1-2). Muscle strength should be graded (Table 1-3). Peripheral pulses and digital capillary refill should be noted.

Neurologic

Test light touch with a cotton tissue or wisp. If abnormal, then note the demarcation between intact and altered sensation. Limb tightness can represent contracture or tone abnormalities. Spastically is a velocity-dependent change in tone. With fast stretch there is greater resistance than with slow stretch. The up-going plantar response (Babinski sign) can be normal in 10% of neonates and persist up to 2 years of age. Three to six beats of ankle clonus can be found in normal individuals, but sustained ankle clonus suggests severe central nervous system disease. Abdominal reflexes are stimulated by gently stroking the abdomen in a lateral-to-medial direction toward the umbilicus. The reflexes should be present bilaterally. Unilateral absence is usually associated with some corticospinal impairment. In children with cerebral palsy, muscle control rather than strength is assessed because of the inability for selective motor control. If you find mild spasticity in one limb and are not sure whether there is hemiplegia, ask the child to run in the hallway. If there is hemiplegia, one upper limb will have a flexed posture when running.

Laxity

Joint hyperlaxity is described by the presence of five features:

1. Metacarpophalangeal dorsiflexion greater than 90 degrees
2. Elbow recurvatum more than 10 degrees
3. Maximum wrist palmar flexion so that the thumb touches the volar forearm
4. Knee recurvatum more than 10 degrees
5. Ankle dorsiflexion greater than 60 degrees.

Clicks are usually innocuous and related to laxity. They are not infrequent in children and little is required except to discourage a voluntary component. Ligament tears are demonstrated by joint space opening and graded as interstitial (I), partial (II), or complete (III).

Newborn Screen

The newborn screen should include assessment of spontaneous and stimulated movement. Spine and skin should be inspected. Foot position and flexibility should be noted. An algorithm has been developed for foot deformi-

TABLE 1-2 JOINT MOTION AND PRIMARY MOTOR MUSCLE, NERVE, AND ROOT

Joint/Motion	Degrees	Muscle	Nerve	Root
Shoulder				
Abduction	180	Middle portion of the deltoid	Axillary	C5+C6
		Supraspinatus	Suprascapular	C5+C6
Adduction	45	Pectoralis major	Medial and lateral anterior thoracic	C5+C6+C7+C8+T1
		Latissimus dorsi	Thoracodorsal	C6+C7+C8
Flexion	90	Anterior portion of the deltoid	Axillary	C7
		Coracobrachialis	Musculocutaneous	C5+C6
Extension	45	Latissimus dorsi	Thoracodorsal	C6+C7+C8
		Teres major	Lower subscapular	C5+C6
		Posterior portion of the deltoid	Axillary	C5+C6
Internal rotation	55	Subscapularis	Upper and lower subscapular	C5+C6
		Pectoralis major	Medial and lateral anterior thoracic	C5+C6+C7+C8+T1
		Latissimus dorsi	Thoracodorsal	C6+C7+C8
		Teres major	Lower subscapular	C5+C6
External rotation	40–45	Infraspinatus	Suprascapular	C5+C6
		Teres minor	Branch of the axillary	C5
Elbow				
Flexion	135+	Brachialis	Musculocutaneous	C5+C6
		Biceps when forearm supinated	Musculocutaneous	C5+C6
Extension	0–5	Triceps	Radial	C7
Supination	90	Biceps	Musculocutaneous	C5+C6
		Supinator	Radial	C6
Pronation	90	Pronator teres	Median	C6
		Pronator quadratus	Anterior interosseous branch of median	C8-T1
Wrist				
Flexion	80	Flexor carpi radialis	Median	C7
		Flexor carpi ulnaris	Ulnar	C8
Extension	70	Extensor carpi radialis longus	Radial	C6
		Extensor carpi radialis brevis	Radial	C6
		Extensor carpi ulnaris	Radial	C7
Ulnar deviation	30			
Radial deviation	20			
Finger MCP				
Flexion	90	Medial two lumbricals	Ulnar	C8
		Lateral two lumbricals	Median	C7
Extension	30–45	Extensor digitorum communis, extensor indicis, extensor digiti minimi	Radial	C7
Abduction	20	Dorsal interossei	Ulnar	C8+T1
		Abductor digiti minimi	Ulnar	C8+T1
Adduction		Palmar interossei	Ulnar	C8+T1
Finger PIP				
Flexion	100	Flexor digitorum superficialis	Median	C7+C8+T1
Extension	0	Extensor digitorum communis, extensor indicis, extensor digiti minimis	Radial	C7
Finger DIP				
Flexion	90	Flexor digitorum profundus	Ulnar; anterior interosseous of median	C8+T1
Extension	20	Extensor digitorum communis, extensor indicis, extensor digiti minimi	Radial	C7
Thumb				
Palmar abduction	70	Abductor pollicis longus	Radial	C7
		Abductor pollicis brevis	Median	C6+C7
Dorsal adduction	0	Adductor pollicis	Ulnar	C8

(continued)

TABLE 1-2 (continued)

Joint/Motion	Degrees	Muscle	Nerve	Root
Thumb MCP				
Flexion	50	Flexor pollicis brevis—medial	Ulnar	C8
		Flexor pollicis brevis—lateral	Median	C6+C7
Extension	0	Extensor pollicis brevis	Radial	C7
Thumb IP				
Flexion	90	Flexor pollicis longus	Median	C8+T1
Extension	20	Extensor pollicis longus	Radial	C7
Hip				
Flexion	120	Iliopsoas	Femoral	L1+L2+L3
Extension	30	Gluteus maximus	Inferior gluteal	S1
Abduction	45–50	Gluteus medius	Superior gluteal	L5
Adduction	20–30	Adductor longus	Obturator	L2+L3+L4
Internal rotation	35			
External rotation	45			
Knee				
Flexion	135	Semimembranosus, semitendinosus, biceps femoris	Tibial portion of sciatic	L5+S1
Extension	0	Quadriceps	Femoral	L2+L3+L4
Internal rotation	10			
External rotation	10			
Ankle				
Dorsiflexion	20	Tibialis anterior, extensor hallucis longus, extensor digitorum longus	Deep peroneal	L4+L5
Plantarflexion	50	Peroneus longus and brevis	Superficial peronea	S1
		Gastrocnemius soleus, flexor hallucis longus, flexor digitorum longus, tibialis posterior	Tibial	L5+S1+S2
Subtalar				
Inversion	5			
Eversion	5			
Forefoot				
Adduction	20			
Abduction	10			
First MTP				
Flexion	45			
Extension	70–90			

DIP, distal interphalangeal; IP, interphalangeal; MCP, metacarpophalangeal; MTP, metatarsophalangeal; PIP, proximal interphalangeal.

TABLE 1-3 GRADING OF MUSCLE STRENGTH

Grade	Strength	Description
5	Normal	Complete ROM against gravity with full resistance
4	Good	Complete ROM against gravity with some resistance
3	Fair	Complete ROM against gravity
2	Poor	Complete ROM with gravity eliminated
1	Trace	Evidence of slight contractility; no joint motion
0	Zero	No evidence of contractility

ROM, range of motion.

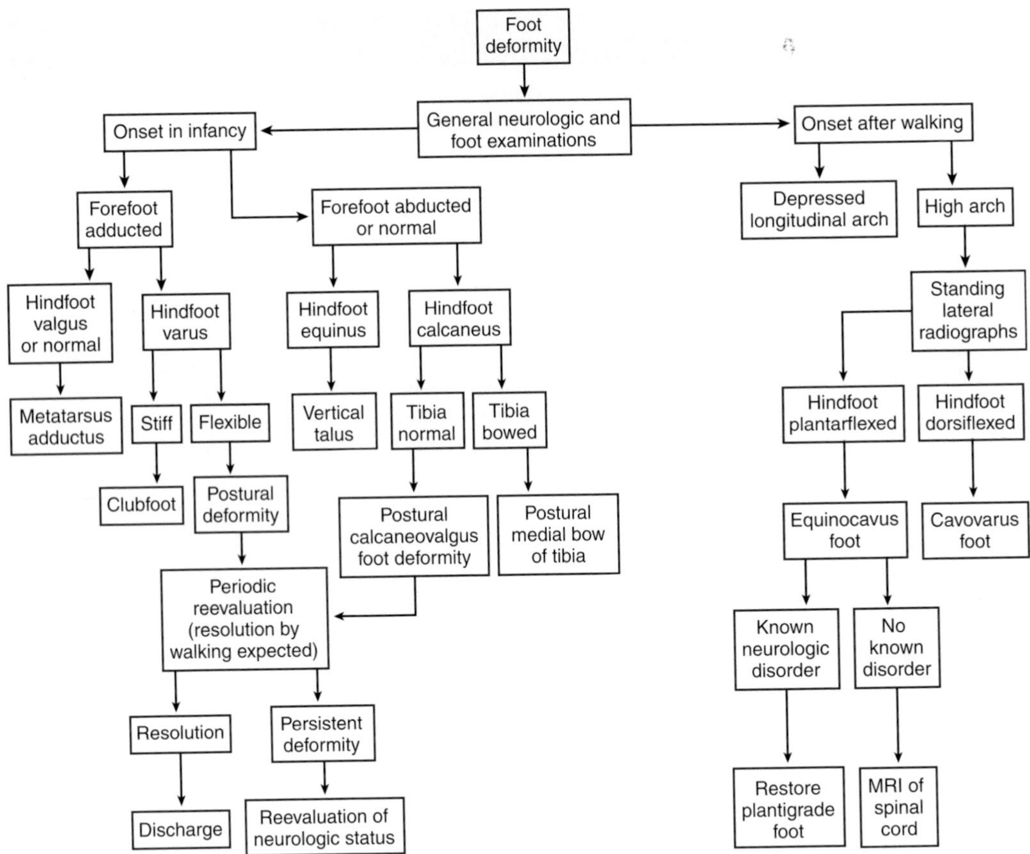

Algorithm 1-1 Assessment of foot deformity. (Adapted from Birch JG. Foot deformity. In: Bucholz RW, ed. Orthopaedic decision making, 2nd ed. St Louis: Mosby-Year Book, 1996:242.)

ties (Algorithm 1-1). Note whether the forefoot is adducted. If the forefoot is adducted, then note whether the hindfoot is in varus (clubfoot) or not (metatarsus adductus). If the forefoot is abducted, then note whether the hindfoot is in equinus (vertical talus) or not. If the hindfoot is in calcaneus, then note whether tibial bowing is present or not (postural calcaneovalgus). Hip instability signs should be assessed by the Barlow (positive, meaning a reduced hip that is dislocatable) and Ortolani maneuvers (positive, meaning a dislocated hip that is reducible).

Angular Deformity

An algorithm has been developed for angular deformity (Algorithm 1-2). Most angular deformities in the lower extremities are in the knee region. Children should be assessed relative to age. Varus deformity (bowleg) is normal between birth and 18 months of age. Varus deformity that persists after the age of 18 months is asymmetric or is associated with injury or infection and requires further evaluation. Findings of poor general health, short stature, and multiple long bone or joint deformities suggest metabolic disease or dysplasia. Children between 18 months and 6 years of age typically show symmetric genu valgum (knock-knee). The knock-knee is maximal at 3 to 4 years of age and assumes the average mature alignment of slight genu valgum by 6 to 7 years of age. If the knock-knee is asymmetric, worsens after 4 years of age, or is excessive after 7 years of age, then further evaluation is indicated.

Torsional Deformity

An algorithm has been developed for management of torsional problems (Algorithm 1-3). Torsional problems, in-toeing and out-toeing, often concern parents and frequently prompt evaluation. The lower limb rotates medially during the seventh fetal week to bring the great toe to midline. With growth, femoral anteversion

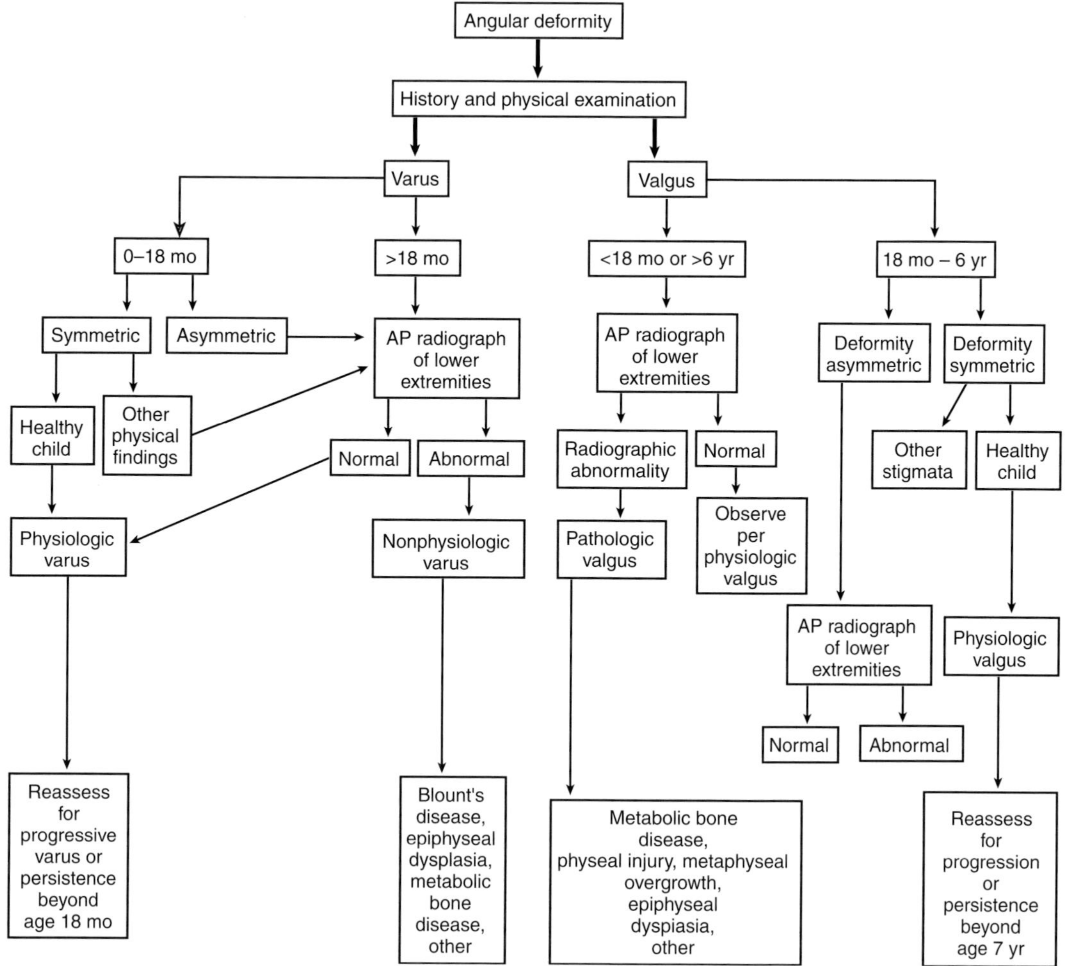

Algorithm 1-2 Assessment of angular deformity. (Adapted from Birch JG. Angular deformity. In: Bucholz RW, ed. Orthopaedic decision making, 2nd ed. St Louis: Mosby-Year Book, 1996:334.)

decreases from 30 degrees at birth to 10 degrees at maturity and the tibia laterally rotates from 5 degrees medial at birth to 15 degrees lateral at maturity. Lower extremity rotational alignment includes assessment of walking (foot progression), lateral border of the foot (adducted in metatarsus adductus), the thigh–foot angle (tibial torsion), and hip range of motion.

Scoliosis Screening

Screening for scoliosis includes observation of shoulder heights and belt line for asymmetry. The iliac crests can be palpated and visually assessed regarding possible limb length discrepancy. Minor degrees of body side differences are not unusual. The forward bend test is performed looking for a thoracic/rib or lumbar prominence. A scoliometer records asymmetry and can be used for screening.

PEARLS

- Ask about activities the child enjoys.
- Avoid threatening words like *hurt, cut,* and *break.*
- Pain is significant in children, especially if it interferes with play or sleep.
- Muscle pulls are uncommon in children.
- Check the hip when a child complains of knee or thigh pain.
- If hip examination and motion are not completely normal, obtain radiographs.
- Asymmetric hip motion needs further evaluation.
- Check the spine and perform a neurologic examination with foot deformities, especially unilateral.
- Check the abdominal reflex in spinal deformity.
- Treat others as you would like to be treated.

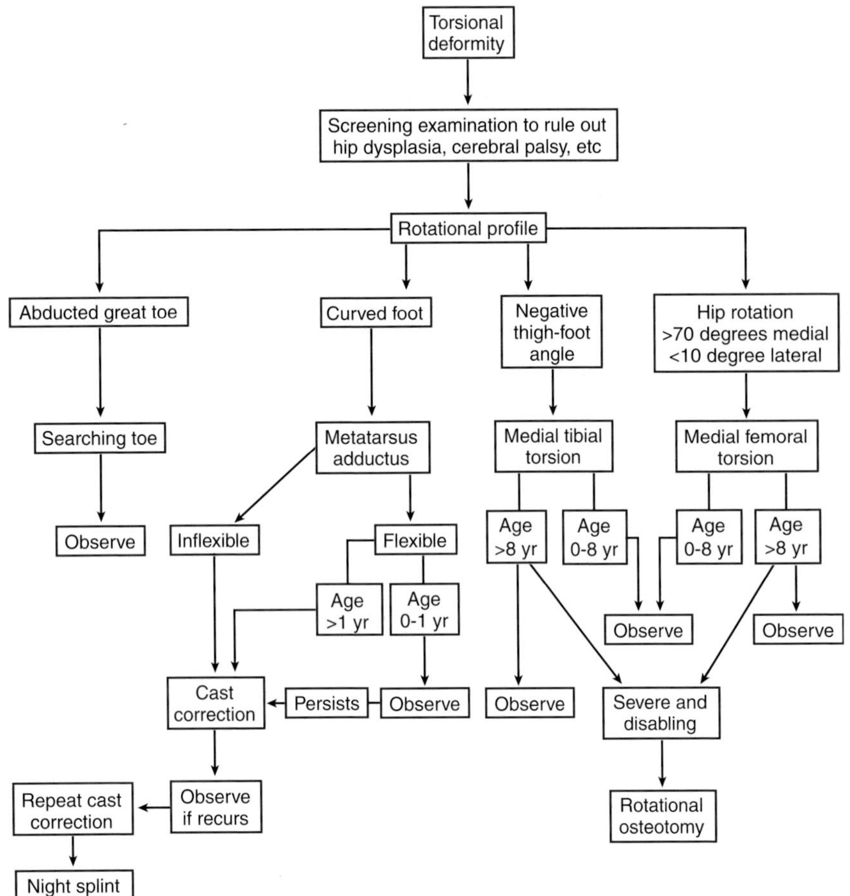

Algorithm 1-3 Assessment of torsional deformity. (Adapted from Staheli LT. Fundamentals of pediatric orthopaedics. New York: Raven Press, 1992:4–5.)

SUMMARY

The orthopaedic care of the child begins with your examination. Be thorough, be complete, and be focused. Start with the end in mind. Aspire to be the best you can be and to do good for the children you treat and their families. This chapter provides suggestions for the pediatric orthopaedic examination. The diagnostic chapters that follow will cover examination techniques, workup, and treatment of specific pediatric orthopaedic disorders.

SUGGESTED READING

Birch JG. Angular deformity. In: Bucholz RW, ed. Orthopaedic decision making, 2nd ed. St. Louis: Mosby-Year Book, 1996:334.

Birch JG. Foot deformity. In: Bucholz RW, ed. Orthopaedic decision making, 2nd ed. St. Louis: Mosby-Year Book, 1996:242.

Bleck E. Orthopaedic management in cerebral palsy. Clin Dev Med 1987:99–100.

Covey S. The seven habits of highly successful people. New York: Simon & Schuster, 1990.

DeGowin EL, DeGowin RL. Bedside diagnostic examination, 3rd ed. New York: Macmillan, 1976.

Hensinger R. Rhetoric and reality. J Bone Joint Surg 1992;74A; 463.

Herring JA. The orthopaedic examination: a comprehensive overview. In: Tachdjian's pediatric orthopaedics, 3rd ed. Vol 1. Philadelphia: WB Saunders, 2001:25.

Hoppenfeld S. Physical examination of the spine and extremities. Norwalk, CT: Appleton-Century-Crofts, 1976.

Staheli LT. Fundamentals of pediatric orthopaedics. New York: Raven Press, 1992:4-5.

Swaiman KF. Neurologic examination after the newborn period until two years of age. In: Pediatric neurology: principles and practice, 2nd ed. Vol 1. St Louis: Mosby, 1993:43.

ROTATIONAL DEFORMITIES OF THE LOWER EXTREMITIES

JAN S. GRUDZIAK
PATRICK BOSCH

Rotational deformity of the lower extremities is a common presenting complaint of children in a pediatric orthopedic office. The vast majority of deformities are a normal variation and resolve spontaneously. However, parental concern is high, especially among those who recall the use of splints and orthotics that "cured" a similar deformity in a relative in the past. A complete physical assessment of the rotational profile and ruling out more serious diagnoses is only the first step. Parental education and reassurance are necessary. In rare cases of severe or persistent deformity, surgical intervention is warranted.

NATURAL HISTORY

The lower extremity rotational alignment of a child changes significantly as the child grows. In general, intrauterine molding causes a lateral contracture of the soft tissues about the hip and internal rotation about the tibia and foot. As the hip soft tissue contracture resolves, for the most part the femoral anteversion determines an internal rotation at the hip. At birth, the femoral anteversion is around 30 degrees; it gradually decreases to 10 degrees by maturity. Similarly, the tibia is most internally rotated in a newborn child. It will also gradually externally rotate as the child matures, from about 5 degrees of internal rotation to 10 degrees of external rotation by 8 years of age. Despite wide individual variation, an understanding of these general trends is important in following the natural history of most rotational deformities.

PATHOPHYSIOLOGY

Patients present with either an *in-toeing* or *out-toeing* gait. The deformity can occur at one anatomic level, or a combination of levels. Rotation within two standard deviations (SD) from an average value at a given anatomic level is termed *version*. Outside of 2 SD, the rotational alignment is defined as pathologic and called *torsion*. Most cases of torsion represent the extremes of natural variability, without a clear cause other than heredity. Intrauterine forces may play a role in some cases of tibial torsion, particularly those associated with metatarsus adductus. In both cases the in-toeing will usually resolve spontaneously. Some other conditions can present as *in-toeing* and *out-toeing*. Cerebral palsy and tibia vara (Blount's disease) can present with associated increased tibial torsion. Slipped capital femoral epiphysis should be suspected in an obese adolescent presenting with *out-toeing*.

DIAGNOSIS

Examination of a child's gait and rotational profile is the key to evaluating *in-toeing* and *out-toeing*. The elements of the rotational profile are:

- Foot progression angle
- Hip rotation
- Thigh–foot angle
- Tibial torsion
- Foot morphology

The *foot progression angle* (Fig. 2-1) is the angle between the long axis of the foot and a line of the direction of gait. Generally, the foot is slightly externally rotated, about 5 to 10 degrees. By convention, external rotation is recorded as a positive value, and internal rotation as a negative angle. The foot progression angle is the summation of rotational alignment of the limb. The remainder of the exam attempts to identify the level of pathology. For hip rotation and thigh–foot angle exam the child is positioned prone on the exam table. The tibial torsion and foot morphology could be assessed in this same position or with the child sitting on the edge of the examination table.

Hip rotation depends on the amount of femoral anteversion. The femoral anteversion angle is created between the long axis of the femoral neck and a line drawn through the medial and lateral condyles of the femur (Fig. 2-2). The amount of rotation is assessed by measuring the

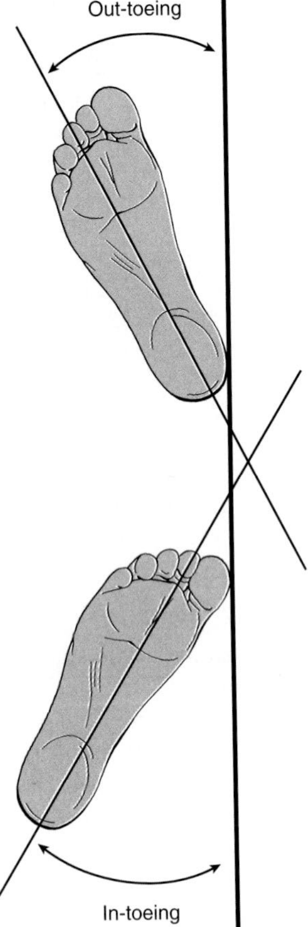

Figure 2-1 The foot progression angle is the angle between the long axis of the foot and the direction of gait.

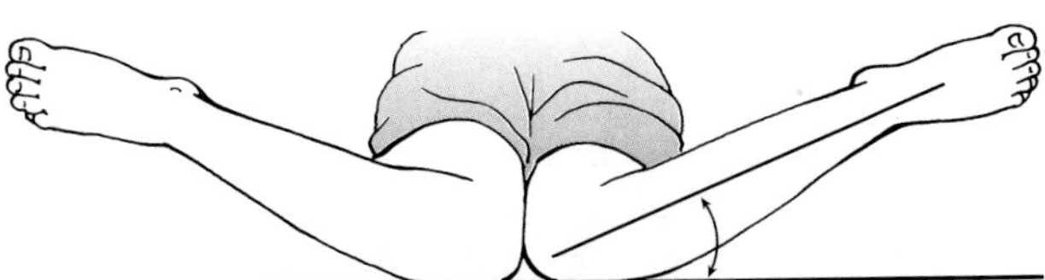

Figure 2-3 With the patient lying supine on the examination table, hip rotation is assessed by measuring the angle between the table and the lower legs.

angle between the exam table and lower legs with bent knees at a right angle (Fig. 2-3). The amount of internal rotation decreases as a child's anteversion decreases with age. Concomitantly, the external rotation improves. However, children with abnormally increased anteversion, or femoral torsion, may continue to have abnormal internal rotation and might lack external rotation. Femoral torsion usually begins to be noticeable in a child as the lateral soft tissue contracture resolves after 2 or 3 years. Internal rotation approaching 90 degrees and external rotation less than 15 degrees are abnormal. These are children frequently described as sitting comfortably with their legs in a "W" or "TV" position. Unusual gait patterns identified in these children have been described as "eggbeater" gait. Patellar tracking problems can result, particularly when associated with increased compensatory external tibial torsion.

Tibial torsion can be estimated by examining the thigh–foot angle. The angle formed between the thigh and the long axis of the foot approximates the transverse alignment of the tibia (Fig. 2-4), assuming the foot does not present with increased forefoot abduction/adduction. More

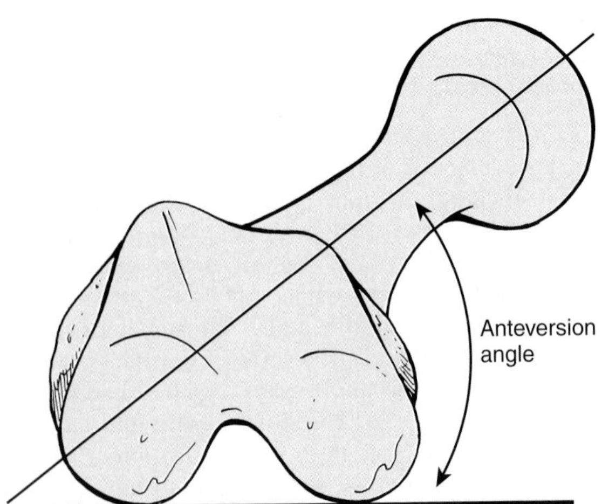

Figure 2-2 The femoral anteversion angle is the angle between the long axis of the femoral neck and a line drawn through the medial and lateral condyles of the femur.

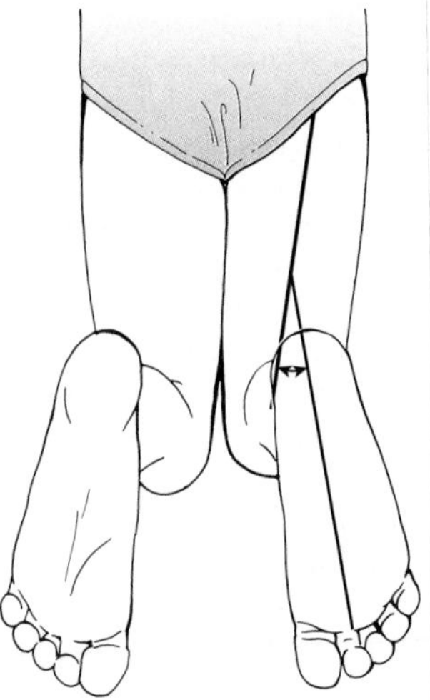

Figure 2-4 The thigh–foot angle is the angle formed between the thigh and the long axis of the foot, which approximates the transverse alignment of the tibia.

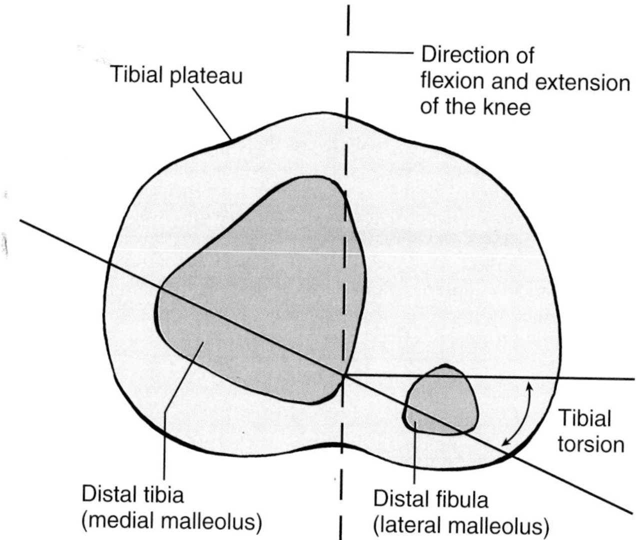

Figure 2-5 Tibial torsion is defined as the angle between the line perpendicular to the axis of knee flexion/extension and the tibial transmalleolar axis.

precisely this alignment is defined by the angle between the line perpendicular to the axis of knee flexion/extension and the tibial transmalleolar axis (Fig. 2-5). Persistence of internal torsion through the tibia is called internal tibial torsion, a common cause of in-toeing in the toddler age group.

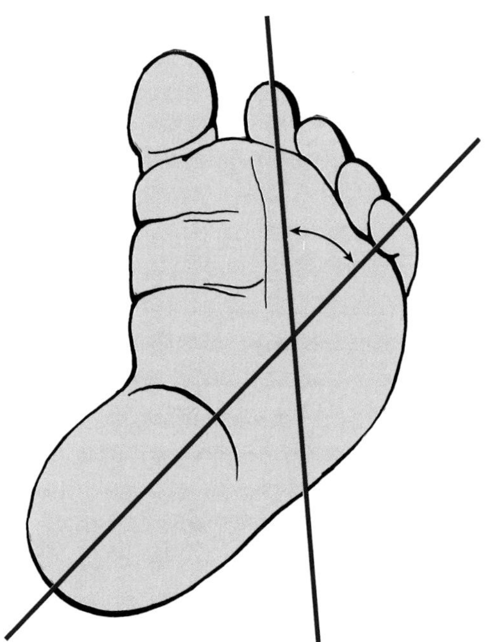

Figure 2-6 Metatarsus adductus.

The *foot morphology* itself is the final component of the rotational profile. Most commonly, metatarsus adductus or other foot deformities can independently cause in-toeing (Fig. 2-6). These tend to present earlier than femoral or tibial deformities, since foot deformities are apparent prior to ambulation. Deformities of the foot are discussed specifically in a different chapter.

Of course, the general physical exam is important in the workup of a child with a rotational abnormality. The possibility of neurologic disorders, skeletal dysplasias, joint or ligamentous laxity, and metabolic disorders should be evaluated. The deformity can occur at more than one level as well, either exaggerating or compensating for another deformity.

Ultimately, rotational deformities are dynamic conditions, and repeat follow-up over time may be necessary to evaluate patients and the progression of the deformity. The following factors raise clinical suspicion and require additional follow-up:

- Unilateral conditions
- History of progression
- Deformities causing functional symptoms
- Pain
- Asymmetry
- Trend not as suspected.

TREATMENT

Rotational deformities very rarely require treatment. Spontaneous resolution is the norm. Only persistent deformity that fails to resolve with growth and produces functional or cosmetic concerns warrants further investigation. Ultimately, when treatment is indicated, the only solution is a surgical correction. There has not been any proven benefit to brace therapy of any kind for tibial or femoral rotational deformities.

In the past, surgical treatment for anterior femoral torsion was thought to protect against early arthrosis of the hip due to abnormal forces across the joint. This has not been substantiated. The indication for surgical treatment of persistent increased anterior femoral torsion is functional or cosmetic deformity in a child older than 8 years. Usually the residual femoral anteversion has to be greater than 50 degrees to create significant functional/cosmetic problems. Intertrochanteric or supracondylar derotational femoral osteotomy is the treatment of choice, with use of K-wires to determine the exact amount of angular correction intraoperatively.

Tibial torsion tends to resolve spontaneously in most children. Disability rarely comes from increased/decreased tibial torsion, since there is such a wide range of normal values. Once indicated by individual functional or cosmetic deformity, surgical correction should be delayed until at least 8 years of age. Most advocate a supramalleolar osteotomy stabilized with pins or a dynamic compression plate and a short- or long-leg cast.

The combination of increased femoral anteversion and increased *external* tibial torsion deserves special notation.

This "malignant malalignment syndrome" tends to induce patellofemoral maltracking and pain, and is more likely to require intervention than single level deformity. Again, no brace or nonoperative treatment has shown any benefit. These patients are surgical candidates from about the time that the patellofemoral symptoms are increasing with their activities, usually around 10 years of age. In most cases, both deformities must be addressed surgically for a successful outcome. This can be best achieved by two-level osteotomy of the distal femur and proximal tibia. Improvement in knee pain, gait patterns, and cosmetic appearance can be expected.

SUGGESTED READING

Delgado ED, Schoenecker PL, Rich MM, et al. Treatment of severe torsional malalignment syndrome. J Pediatr Orthop 1996;16: 484–488.

Herring JA, ed. Tachdjian's pediatric orthopaedics, 3rd ed. Philadelphia: WB Saunders, 2002.

Staheli L. Rotational problems in children: an instructional course lecture, the American Academy of Orthopaedic Surgeons. J Bone Joint Surg 1993;75A:939–949.

Staheli LT, Corbett M, Wyss C, et al. Lower extremity: rotational problems in children. J Bone Joint Surg 1986;67A:39–47.

Svennigsen S, Terjesen T, Auflem M, et al. Hip rotation and in-toeing gait. Clin Orthop Rel Res 1990;251:177.

ANGULAR DEFORMITIES OF THE LOWER EXTREMITIES

JAN S. GRUDZIAK
PATRICK BOSCH

Angular deformities of the lower extremities in children often present very dramatically and lead to a great deal of anxiety for parents and families. Most are physiologically normal variants that will resolve spontaneously. However, pathologic forms of deformity that can result in serious disability and persistent deformity without treatment must be differentiated from a benign condition. This differentiation is not always apparent on the initial examination. Recognizing the different patterns of deformity and how they evolve is the key to understanding and treating angular deformities in children.

CORONAL PLANE DEFORMITY

PATHOGENESIS

Coronal plane deformity of the lower extremities, "bowlegs" or "knock-knees," can present at varying stages of a child's development. The natural development of the coronal leg alignment or femoral–tibial angle must be appreciated. At birth, the child has 10 to 15 degrees of varus at the knee. This bowleg appearance persists in most children until 14 to 18 months, and sometimes up to 24 months of age, when the femoral–tibial angle becomes neutral. The alignment progresses to maximal valgus (knock-kneed) position by 3 or 4 years of age and then gradually resolves into adult physiologic valgus (around 7 degrees) by the age of 8 years (Fig. 3-1).

DIAGNOSIS

Physical examination of children with coronal plane deformity generally relies on measurements of the distance between the child's medial femoral condyles for varus deformity, and between the medial maleoli for valgus deformity position. Although these numbers can be recorded, they are a pseudo-quantification of the child's gross appearance; they can however be used for monitoring pur-

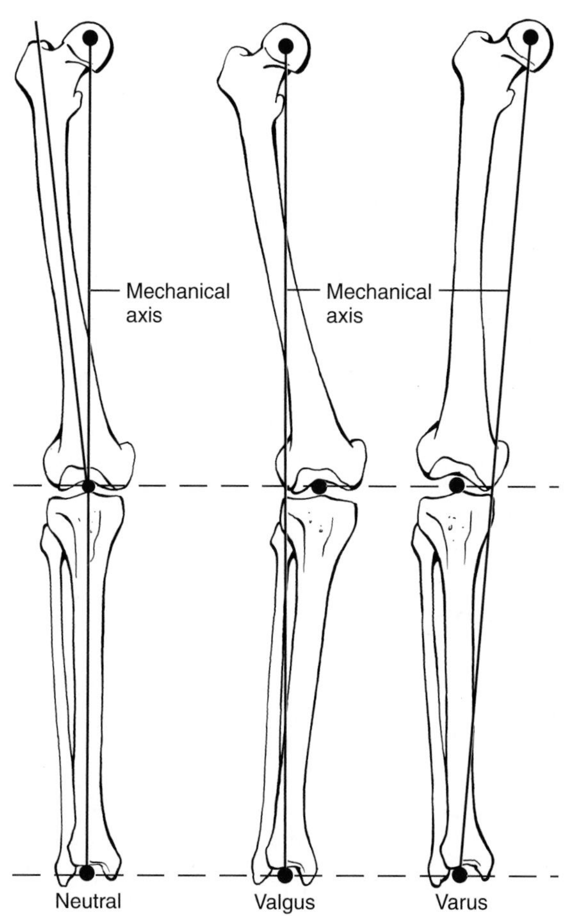

Figure 3-1 Mechanical alignment of the lower extremity: normal (neutral), valgus, varus.

poses. A standing anteroposterior radiograph of both lower extremities is indicated for the following:

- Trend not as expected
- Unilateral involvement
- Asymmetry
- Pain
- Generalized growth abnormality

Various measurements, including a femoral–tibial angle, can be determined from these films. A scanogram may also be indicated in children over 3 years of age to evaluate concomitant leg length discrepancy.

INFANTILE TIBIA VARA (BLOUNT'S DISEASE)

PATHOGENESIS

Parents frequently bring a toddler with bowlegs, or genu varum, for orthopedic evaluation. Differential diagnosis of an ambulating toddler with excessive femoral–tibial varus alignment includes the following:

- Physiologic bowing
- Infantile tibia vara, Blount's disease
- Metabolic disorders, rickets
- Skeletal dysplasias, focal fibrocartilaginous dysplasia, chondrodysplasias

Most of these children have physiologic bowing. This is a benign variant of normal development, which usually resolves by 30 to 48 months of age. In some children, however, the varus alignment does not correct and progresses as the proximal medial tibial physis undergoes pathologic changes, failing to grow properly. This is known as infantile tibia vara, or Blount's disease. Less frequently, genu varum is the result of metabolic disorders or skeletal dysplasias. These last two categories of disorders can usually be screened based on overall child growth (less than fifth percentile growth would suggest a dysplasia), radiographic appearance (changes in physes elsewhere in the body), or lab values (changes in calcium, phosphate, alkaline phosphatase, vitamin D, or 1,25-dihydroxy vitamin D in rickets).

DIAGNOSIS

The differentiation between physiologic and pathologic bowing is often difficult on initial presentation. Some experts consider the two processes to be on a continuum. Blount's disease usually presents with an acute bowing at the proximal tibia whereas smooth, evenly distributed bowing of the tibia is usually indicative of physiologic genu varum. The pathologic genu varum may occur when the compressive forces exerted by the deformity irreversibly injure the medial aspect of the proximal tibial physis and metaphysis. In the case of pathologic genu varum, there might be simultaneous changes in other physes (ankle, femur, spine).

TABLE 3-1 LANGENSKIÖLD'S CLASSIFICATION OF BLOUNT'S DISEASE

Stage	Description
I	Irregular metaphyseal ossification with protrusion of the metaphysis
II–IV	Progressive depression of the medial metaphysis The epiphysis slopes more medially as the disease progresses
V	Definite sloping of the epiphysis with a cleft separating the medial and lateral aspects of the epiphysis
VI	Well-seen bony bridge across medial epiphysis and metaphysis that additionally hampers the development of the proximal tibia, increasing the varus angulation

Radiographic features that are diagnostic of infantile tibia vara rely on identification of the physeal damage. They were classically clarified and categorized by Langenskiöld, who published a six-stage classification system for Blount's disease based both on the radiographic appearance of the proximal tibial physis and on patient age (Table 3-1). Unfortunately, these criteria are not useful for initial diagnosis, since most changes in the proximal tibia are not evident until after 3 years of age. In addition, interobserver

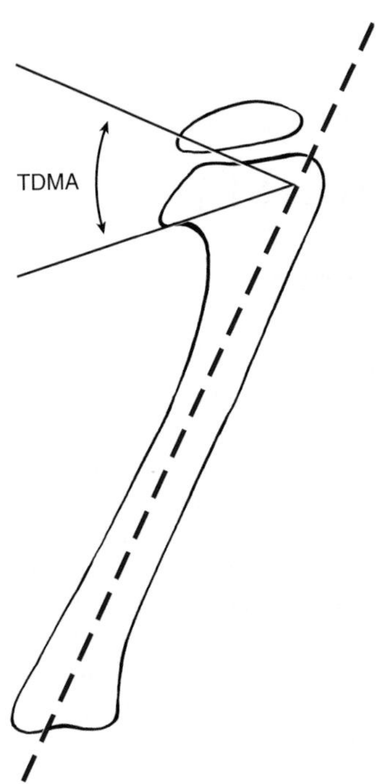

Figure 3-2 Tibial metaphyseal–diaphyseal angle (TDMA) of Levine and Drennan. The angle lies between a line drawn through the most distal point on the medial and lateral breaks of the tibial metaphysic and perpendicular to the long axis of the tibia.

reliability is poor (50%) with this classification system and it is especially difficult to distinguish between stages II and IV, which might affect the ultimate outcome of treatment of Blount's disease.

Various radiographic measurements have been proposed to differentiate physiologic and pathologic tibia vara prior to the development of changes in the physis as described by Langenskiöld. The tibial metaphyseal–diaphyseal angle (TDMA) was originally described with a threshold at 11 degrees, beyond which infantile tibia vara was suspected (Fig. 3-2). More recently investigators, raising the threshold to 16 degrees, have modified the criteria for the TDMA. The "gray zone" of TDMA between 10 and 16 degrees warrants special attention as pathologic genu varum might develop. When in doubt, magnetic resonance imaging is a useful tool to identify pathologic changes in the proximal tibial physis.

TREATMENT

The treatment of infantile tibia vara depends on both patient age and proximal tibial physeal changes. Brace treatment may be recommended for children under 3 years of age with a TDMA measured at least 16 degrees or presenting with Langenskiold stage I or II. It should continue for no longer than 1 year and should be discontinued if deformity persists to age 4 years or progresses to stage III. Bracing may be accomplished with one of a variety of various orthoses that exert valgus movement on the proximal tibia. Traditionally, a knee–ankle–foot orthosis (KAFO) is used. There are conflicting reports on whether nighttime or daytime brace wear is sufficiently effective. The more a brace is worn (as close to 24 hours a day as feasible), the more effective it should be. However, it remains controversial, as its efficacy has not been proved.

Results and Outcome

Operative intervention is most effective when performed early. Practically, the definitive diagnosis of Blount's disease is made around 3 years of age, when Langenskiöld changes become evident. A corrective valgus osteotomy is indicated for children who present at age 4 years or older, with Langenskiöld stage III or higher even at a younger age, or who have not benefited from bracing. There are numerous potential complications with this procedure:

- Recurrence of deformity:
  - Especially when done in older children
  - Inadequate correction: one should overcorrect infantile tibia vara to slight valgus alignment
  - Failure to laterally displace the distal segment
- Compartment syndrome: prophylactic fasciotomy should be done
- Peroneal nerve palsy: fibular osteotomy should be done at a more distal site, in the diaphysis, to avoid injury to common peroneal nerve
- Growth disturbance, which progresses to recurvatum deformity of proximal tibia: reason the osteotomy is performed distal to the tibial tubercle.

More advanced lesions, Langenskiöld stage IV to VI, with medial epiphyseal deformity, and in children approaching maturity require more complex surgical intervention. An osseous bar excision with or without interposition of fat or bony cement and elevation of the medial epiphysis to resolve the contour of the joint surface might be combined with lateral physeal stapling to reverse the pathologic changes of the proximal tibia.

ADOLESCENT TIBIA VARA

PATHOGENESIS

True adolescent Blount's disease usually occurs in morbidly obese boys approaching skeletal maturity without previous history of fracture or infection. A recent onset of deformity without previous bowing should raise suspicions about adolescent Blount's disease. The workup of these children should include a long cassette radiograph with patella centered over the femur to avoid rotational error. The etiology of adolescent Blount's disease is thought to be varus deformity forced by the large thighs of these obese children generating increased force across the medial aspect of the proximal tibial physis. Unlike infantile Blount's disease, however, the more mature physis is stunted but not as profoundly deformed. The physis will show widening on radiographs; however, the epiphysis will not be as collapsed as in the infantile form.

There are special issues concerning patients with adolescent Blount's disease. Since most are far above the ninety-fifth percentile for weight at their age, proper instrumentation must be used and operative beds must be provided for these "large adult"-sized patients being treated in a pediatric hospital. Many experts also recommend sleep studies to evaluate for sleep apnea, which is present to some degree in most of these patients. Furthermore, a slipped capital femoral epiphysis should *always* be considered in this population.

TREATMENT

The treatment of adolescent tibia vara is overwhelmingly operative. There is no role for bracing in this condition. Good results have been reported with a number of approaches:

- Osteotomy and internal fixation: usually closing wedge through proximal medial tibia, with avoiding overcorrection in *adolescent* Blount's.
- Lateral epiphysiodesis: if adequate growth is remaining to slowly correct the varus (may be done by stapling, which is potentially reversible).
- Gradual correction of deformity with external fixator: numerous techniques have been designed to correct the deformity in multiple planes if necessary.

Surgical treatment of the adolescent tibia vara has been proven successful, and an overall good final result should be expected. Complications are not uncommon, however, and careful preoperative planning is necessary with these procedures.

PATHOLOGIC GENU VALGUM

PATHOGENESIS

Most children who present for evaluation of knock-knees are 3 to 5 years of age, when the maximal valgus angulation of the lower extremities occurs. However, if that deformity persists beyond 8 years of age and is outside 2 standard deviations of the norm, it is defined as pathologic. As with other deformities, the level of deformity needs to be evaluated on long cassette standing radiographs. Most commonly, the deformity is in the distal femur, however, proximal tibia and joint laxity should also be considered. Classification of the degree of deformity can be made based on how far laterally the mechanical axis of the extremity falls from the center of the knee.

TREATMENT

Treatment options for pathologic genu valgum should be individualized. As with most deformities the severity of deformity, the functional and cosmetic ramifications, and the unilateral involvement are considered. Possible treatment options include:

- Hemi-epiphysiodesis: staple epiphysiodesis either permanent or transient, depending on remaining growth; less predictable but lower morbidity than osteotomy.
- Osteotomy: in the skeletally mature; most often a closing medial wedge osteotomy of the distal femur is performed.

The goal of valgus correction is to mechanically achieve sound alignment of the lower extremity with a horizontally positioned tibial plateau and ankle joint.

BOWING OF THE TIBIA

Tibial bowing present at birth, often termed *congenital,* falls into three categories—posteromedial, anterolateral, and anterior.

Posteromedial Bowing

Posteromedial bowing of the tibia presents as a severe-looking deformity in a newborn, with a calcaneus positioned foot and dorsiflexion contracture at the ankle. This is a benign condition. The etiology is presumed to be an intrauterine packaging phenomenon, without any associated abnormalities. The abnormal position of the foot resolves with simple parental stretching and plantar foot stimulation. Serial casting is rarely necessary. The tibia deformity resolves by 2 years of age in nearly all cases. Ultimately the affected limb will end up with a smaller calf musculature and leg length discrepancy. Typically, the discrepancy is between 3 and 8 cm. Contralateral epiphysiodesis is the most common treatment. Investigators have reported a correlation between the degree of initial angulation and the eventual growth retardation.

Anterolateral Angulation or Congenital Pseudoarthrosis

Anterolateral angulation of the tibia is a very rare disorder, affecting 1 in 140,000 to 190,000 newborns. Often there is no fracture at the time of birth; however, the abnormal structure of the bone usually leads to inevitable fracture. This deformity is closely associated with neurofibromatosis. Approximately 5% of patients with neurofibromatosis have the deformity, and over half of the children with a congenital pseudoarthrosis are eventually diagnosed with neurofibromatosis. An association with fibrous dysplasia is also reported. Classification schemes for this entity are based on the radiographic appearance of the bone at the pseudoarthrosis. The most commonly cited is the Boyd classification (Table 3-2).

Treatment for anterolateral bowing of the tibia has consistently been difficult. If fracture has not yet occurred, a total contact orthosis is recommended to protect the extremity until maturity. Once fractured, the pseudoarthrosis will generally not heal without surgery. Surgical princi-

TABLE 3-2 BOYD'S CLASSIFICATION OF NEUROFIBROMATOSIS

Type	Description
I	Anterior bow and tibial defect
II	Anterior bow with hourglass constriction of the tibia Tibia ends are tapered and sclerotic Medullary canal is obliterated Fractures occur typically by 2 years of age
III	Bone cyst located between middle and distal third of the tibia; discovered either before or after fracture
IV	Anterior bow with sclerotic fragment of the tibia Sclerotic bone segment with partially or entirely obliterated medullary canal "Insufficiency" fracture of the sclerotic fragment routinely evolves to pseudoarthrosis
V	Anterior bow with associated dysplastic fibula Develops into pseudoarthrosis of the fibula or tibia
VI	With intraosseous neurofibroma or schwannoma

ples for this problem include excision of the fibrous tissue present at the pseudoarthrosis and then obtaining rigid fixation. Surgical approaches include the following:

- Intramedullary fixation, initially crossing ankle and subtalar joint
- Vascularized fibular transfer
- Distraction osteogenesis, Ilizarov techniques.

Despite fairly predictable union at the pseudoarthrosis site, particularly with intramedullary fixation, late complications are common. Refracture, joint stiffness, and leg length discrepancies severely limit the success of any surgical approach to this problem. Trans-pseudoarthrosis, below knee or Syme amputation is not an uncommon salvage procedure.

Anterior or Anteromedial Bowing

Such bowing of the tibia is often associated with varying degrees of fibular hypoplasia. In the more severe forms, complete absence of the fibula might present with an anteromedial bow of a shortened tibia, a ball and socket ankle joint, tarsal coalitions, and absence of one or more lateral rays of the foot. These patients might present with structural anomalies of the upper extremities as well. Proximal focal femoral deficiency (PFFD) frequently coexists with fibular hypoplasia. Treatment depends on the severity of the fibular hypoplasia. Treatment for limbs with absent fibula and more extensive hypoplasia with unstable foot is most commonly treated with a modified Syme amputation. Less involved limbs with fibular hypoplasia and a stable plantigrade foot might benefit from simple treatment of the leg length discrepancy and do fine.

SUGGESTED READING

Anderson DJ, Schoenecker PL, Sheridan JJ, et al. Use of an intramedullary rod for the treatment of congenital pseudoarthrosis of the tibia. J Bone Joint Surg 1992;4A:161–168.

Boyd HB. Pathology and natural history of congenital pseudoarthrosis of the tibia. Clin Orthop Rel Res 1982;166:5–13.

Feldman MD, Schoenecker PL. Use of the metaphyseal–diaphyseal angle in the evaluation of bowed legs. J Bone Joint Surg 1993;75A: 1602–1609.

Herring JA, ed. Tachdjian's pediatric orthopaedics, 3rd ed. Philadelphia: WB Saunders, 2002:840–850.

Hofmann A, Wenger DR. Posteromedial bowing of the tibia. J Bone Joint Surg 1981;63A:384–388.

Langenskiold A. Tibia vara: osteochondrosis deformans tibiae. Clin Orthop Rel Res 1981;158:77–82.

Levine AM, Drennan JC. Physiological bowing and tibia vara: the metaphyseal–diaphyseal angle in the measurement of bowleg deformities. J Bone Joint Surg 1982;64A:1158–1163.

Paley D, Tetsworth K. Mechanical axis deviation of the lower limbs. Clin Orthop Rel Res 1992;280:48–64.

Salenius P, Vanka E. The development of the tibiofemoral angle in children. J Bone Joint Surg 1975;57A:259–261.

Steven PM, Maquire M, Dales MD, et al. Physeal stapling for the idiopathic genu valgum. J Pediatr Orthop 1999;19:645–649.

Stricker SJ, Edwards PM, Tidwell MA. Langenskiold classification of tibia vara: an assessment of interobserver variability. J Pediatr Orthop 1994;14:152–155.

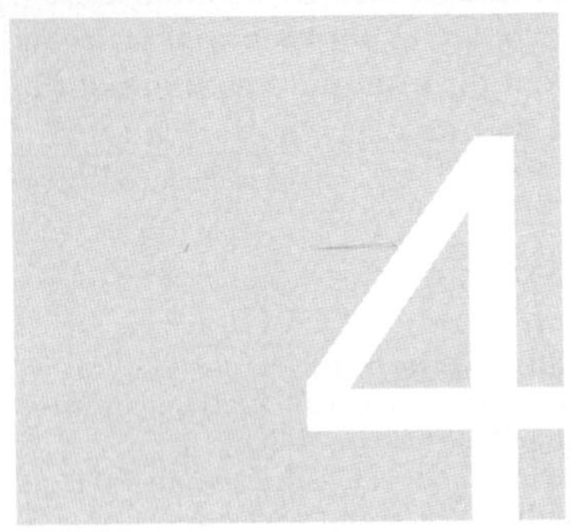

FOOT DISORDERS

4.1 METATARSUS ADDUCTUS

WILLIAM L. HENNRIKUS

Metatarsus adductus refers to a foot with a C- or bean-shaped configuration. The lateral border of the foot is curved rather than straight. The forefoot is deviated inward relative to the hindfoot. The hindfoot is in neutral or slight valgus. The ankle is supple. Metatarsus adductus is usually noted at birth but it may be present at any age. Metatarsus adductus is a common cause of in-toeing in otherwise normal newborns and infants.

PATHOGENESIS

Etiology

Metatarsus adductus is believed to be caused by intrauterine compression or "packaging". This etiology has not been proven. Presumably, the feet are compressed during intrauterine development.

Epidemiology

About 1% of infants will demonstrate metatarsus adductus. The condition may persist longer in premature babies. First-born babies, large babies, and twinning may predispose to metatarsus adductus due to intrauterine crowding. Metatarsus adductus is reportedly seen in association with developmental dysplasia of the hip, although several large series have not borne this out. Theoretically, the packaging problem that leads to metatarsus adductus can also affect the adducted hip. Therefore, the child presenting with metatarsus adductus should have a careful hip examination. Pelvic imaging is necessary only if there is a positive finding on the hip examination.

Pathophysiology

Medial subluxation of the tarsometatarsal joints, adduction of the metaphysis of the second through the fifth metatarsals, and medial deviation of the articular surface of the medial cuneiform have been demonstrated in stillborn infants with metatarsus adductus.

Classification

Metatarsus adductus can be classified based on the flexibility of the deformity. The three classification grades are: actively correctable, passively correctable, or rigid. Actively correctable feet straighten out when the lateral border of the foot is stroked by the examiner's finger and the muscles of the child's foot contract correcting the C-shape to neutral. The passively correctable foot straightens out with gentle manipulation. To manipulate the foot, grasp the heel with one hand and push the inward-turning forefoot outward with your other hand in order to realign the foot in a straight position and reverse the C-shaped outer border of the foot. The rigid metatarsus adductus does not correct with manipulation. The rigid case typically has a medial soft tissue crease at the tarsometatarsal level with a medial soft tissue contracture. As the forefoot is pushed laterally, the great toe will abduct and a tight abductor hallucis can be palpated medially.

The amount of adduction can be quantified grossly by extrapolation of a line bisecting the heel up to the toes (Fig. 4.1-1). This heel bisector should hit between the second and third rays of the foot. If it hits the third ray, the metatarsus adductus is mild; the fourth ray, moderate; and the fifth ray, severe. This measurement can be used to follow the deformity over time.

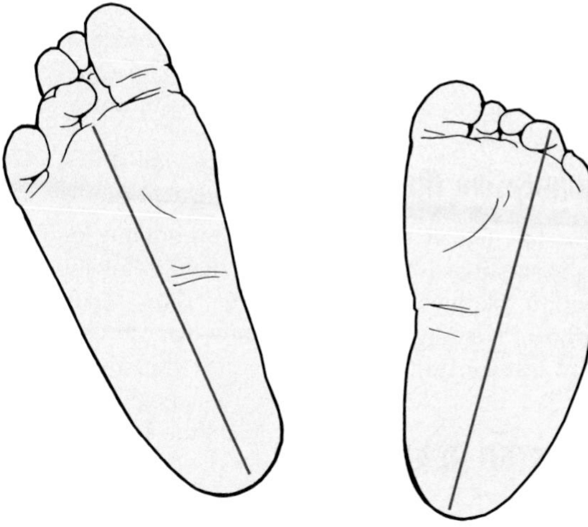

Figure 4.1-1 Severity of metatarsus adductus can be assessed by extrapolating from a line that bisects the heel and extends through the toes. In normal feet (**left**) this line hits between the second and third rays of the foot. With the line hitting the fourth ray, the degree of adduction in the root on the right is moderate.

DIAGNOSIS

Clinical Features

The diagnosis of metatarsus adductus is made clinically (Box 4.1-1). Radiographs are rarely needed. The outer border of the foot is curved or C-shaped. When viewed from the dorsal surface, the entire foot appears to be turned inward. When the foot is viewed from the plantar surface, the sole of the foot has the shape of a bean. The base of the fifth metatarsal may appear prominent. The arch may appear high. The space between the first and second toe may appear wide. The first toe often seems to be reaching medially. The ankle joint and heel alignment are normal or in slight valgus in metatarsus adductus. If the foot demonstrates a fixed valgus hindfoot then the child does not have metatarsus adduction: instead the diagnosis of skewfoot (forefoot adductor, midfoot abduction, and heel valgus) should be considered. The ankle joint is supple in metatarsus adductus. For example, the foot could easily dorsiflex above the neutral position. If the foot demonstrates fixed equinus and cannot dorsiflex, and the hindfoot is in a varus position, then the child does not have metatarsus adductus: instead the diagnosis of clubfoot should be considered.

BOX 4.1-1 CHARACTERISTIC FEATURES OF METATARSUS ADDUCTUS

- Spontaneous active medial deviation of the foot
- High arch
- Concave medial border of the foot
- Separation of the first and second toes
- Fixed adduction of the forefoot when the hindfoot is held in neutral
- Bean-shaped sole of the foot

Radiologic Features

Radiographs of the feet are rarely needed for the diagnosis or treatment of metatarsus adductus. Radiographs are taken in the rare case undergoing surgery or in the patient being evaluated for possible skewfoot. Radiographs should be taken in the weightbearing position. Metatarsus adductus radiographs show medial deviation of the metatarsals at the tarsometatarsal joints and in some cases medial deviation of the metatarsal shafts. Radiographs in adults followed long-term for metatarsus adductus demonstrate obliquity of the medial cuneiform–metatarsal joint.

TREATMENT

Nonsurgical Indications/Contraindications

Flexible actively correctable metatarsus adductus does not require treatment. About 90% of metatarsus adductus is flexible and actively correctable. These cases correct spontaneously during the first 2 years of normal growth and development. Reassurance and education for the parents about the natural history of the deformity is indicated.

Treatment of the passively correctable metatarsus adductus is controversial. Some authors recommend observation of the foot and reassurance and education for the parents because many of these feet will correct without intervention. Other authors recommend that the passively correctable foot with metatarsus adductus can be treated by passive stretching exercises of the foot by the child's parents. The exercises are performed by holding the heel in one hand and pushing the forefoot outward to correct the C-shape of the foot. The foot is stretched in this manner for about 3 seconds and repeated 5 times. The exercises can be easily performed at each diaper change. Reverse last shoes can be used to maintain correction. Although exercises and reverse last shoes are commonly used, their efficacy has not been proven.

Rigid metatarsus adductus or partly correctable metatarsus adductus that has failed an attempt at stretching exercises for 3 months can be treated with serial manipulation and casting. Short-leg or long-leg casts have both been used successfully. Casts are removed and the foot is remanipulated at 1- to 2-week intervals until the convexity of the lateral border of the foot is straightened. Correct molding of the cast is very important. After application of the plaster, molding is performed with the lateral fulcrum at the calcanealcuboid joint. The calcaneus is pushed medially and the forefoot is pushed laterally. Once correction is achieved, reverse last shoes can be used to maintain the correction. Adding a Denis Browne bar to the reverse last shoe is not recommended because of the tendency of the bar to produce correction through the subtalar joint resulting in hindfoot valgus and a flatfoot. Casting is reported to be most effective in children younger than 8 months of age; however, improvement has been reported in children as old as 2 years of age. A Wheaton brace, a removable plastic version of a stretch cast, is also an option.

A simple method of documenting the metatarsus adductus at presentation and documenting the changes in the shape of the foot over time during observation or active treatment involves taking photocopies of the foot in the weightbearing position.

Surgical Indications/Contraindications

Rare cases of rigid metatarsus adductus may benefit from surgical correction. Surgical indications include the rigid foot that has failed serial casting and the older child who presents with fixed adduction deformity and shoe-fitting problems.

Results and Outcomes

Multiple surgical procedures have been reported for treatment of rigid metatarsus adductus. Outcomes are reportedly good in most cases; however a standardized outcome measure does not exist. Surgery can include tendon releases, joint releases, osteotomies or combinations of any of these. In the young child the simplest surgical procedure includes release of the abductor hallucis tendon with or without capsulotomy of the first tarsometatarsal joint followed by casting. Release of the tarsometatarsal joints of all five toes has also been reported. However, reports of the development of degenerative arthritis at the operated joints have tempered enthusiasm for this once-popular operation. In the older child, metatarsal osteotomies can be performed. Complications specific to this procedure include cross-union of the osteotomies and iatrogenic closure of the proximal first metatarsal physis. In the child older than 5 years of age, a lateral closing wedge osteotomy of the cuboid combined with a medial opening wedge osteotomy of the first cuneiform can be performed. The graft from the cuboid can be used to hold the medial osteotomy open.

Postoperative Management

Casting for 4 to 8 weeks followed by bracing or wearing reverse last shoes is commonly practiced following surgical correction of metatarsus adductus. The recommended duration of bracing or special shoe wear varies by author but can last for up to 2 years.

SUGGESTED READING

Asirvatham R, Stevens PM. Idiopathic forefoot-adduction deformity: medial capsulotomy and abductor hallucis lengthening for resistant and severe deformities. J Pediatr Orthop 1997;17:496–500.

Brink DS, Levitsky DR. Cuneiform and cuboid wedge osteotomies for correction of residual metatarsus adductus: a surgical review. J Foot Ankle Surg 1995;34:371–378.

Farsetti P, Weinstein SL, Ponseti IV. The long-term functional and radiographic outcomes of untreated and non-operatively treated metatarsus adductus. J Bone Joint Surg 1994;76A:257–265.

Katz K, David R, Soudry M. Below-knee plaster cast for the treatment of metatarsus adductus. J Pediatr Orthop 1999;19:49–50.

Kite JH. Congenital metatarsus varus. J Bone Joint Surg 1967;49A: 388–397.

Kumar JS, MacEwen GD. The incidence of hip dysplasia and metatarsus adductus. Clin Orthop 1982;164:234–235.

Lichtblau S. Section of the abductor hallucis tendon for correction of metatarsus varus deformity. Clin Orthop 1975;110:227–232.

Ponsetti IV, Becker JR. Congenital metatarsus adductus: the results of treatment. J Bone Joint Surg 1966;48A:702–708.

Rushforth GF. The natural history of hooked forefoot. J Bone Joint Surg 1978;60B:530–532.

Smith JT, Bleck EE, Gamble JG, et al. A simple method of documenting metatarsus adductus. J Pediatr Orthop 1991;11:679–680.

Stark JB, Johanson JE, Winter RB. The Heyman-Herndon tarsometatarsal capsulotomy for metatarsus adductus: results in 48 feet. J Pediatr Orthop 1987;7:305–310.

Wide T, Aaro S, Elmstedt E. Foot deformities in the newborn: incidence and prognosis. Acta Orthop Scand 1998;59:176–179.

4.2 CLUBFOOT

B. DAVID HORN

Clubfoot is a congenital foot deformity characterized by hindfoot equinus, forefoot adduction, subtalar joint varus, and cavus of the foot. It is present at birth and the affected foot may exhibit varying degrees of deformity and rigidity. This condition is also known as congenital talipes equinovarus. Clubfoot has been described since antiquity, and the early literature recommended manipulation and immobilization for treatment. These concepts remain the basis of clubfoot treatment today.

The four types of clubfoot are described in Box 4.2-1.

BOX 4.2-1 THE FOUR TYPES OF CLUBFOOT

Idiopathic: rigid clubfoot; this is an isolated finding
Postural: supple clubfoot from intrauterine molding
Neurogenic: rigid clubfoot associated with neurologic conditions such as myelomeningocele
Syndromic: rigid clubfoot found in association with known syndromes such as arthrogryposis

INCIDENCE

The incidence of clubfoot varies with the population studied:

- 7 per 1,000 in South Pacific Islanders
- 1.2 per 1,000 in Caucasians
- 0.5 per 1,000 in Asians

Despite these differing incidences, there are some consistent features:

- Male:female ratio of 2:1
- 50% bilateral

ETIOLOGY

The cause of clubfoot remains unknown. Multiple etiologies have been proposed as a cause of clubfoot. These include:

- Intrauterine molding
- Myopathic process
- Neuropathic process
- Retracting fibrosis
- Bone dysplasia (germ plasm defect theory)
- Prenatal viral infection
- Primary vascular defect

Current concepts regarding the etiology of clubfoot recognize both environmental and genetic factors. A neuropathic process is supported by histologic studies that demonstrate abnormal muscle fiber type within the clubfoot, with a predominance of type I muscle fiber and a deficiency of type IIb fibers. This fiber type predominance as well as the presence of abnormal fiber grouping and other cytostructural changes are cited as evidence of a neuropathic etiology of clubfeet. An abnormal number of myofibroblasts have also been reported in the deltoid ligament resected in children with clubfeet. These cells are involved in wound and scar contracture and it has been hypothesized that the myofibroblasts may cause a localized soft tissue contracture contributing to the clubfoot.

There is also a strong genetic component to clubfeet. The precise mechanism of transmission has not been elaborated, but it is thought to be either autosomal dominant with variable penetrance or multifactorial.

- If both parents have normal feet and have one affected child with clubfoot, there is a 2% to 5% chance of the next child having clubfoot.
- If one parent has a clubfoot and one child has a clubfoot, there is 10% to 25% risk of subsequent children having clubfeet.
- There is a concordance rate of 32.5% in monozygotic twins, compared to a concordance rate of 2.9% in heterozygotic twins.
- Clubfeet may also occur in conjunction with other neuromuscular and genetic conditions such as arthrogryposis, spina bifida, and myotonic muscular dystrophy.

PATHOLOGIC ANATOMY

Clubfoot represents a dysplasia of the entire affected extremity, with much of the clinically significant pathologic anatomy involving the hindfoot and midfoot. There is controversy about some of the anatomic findings in the clubfoot, but there are also areas of general agreement (Box 4.2-2).

PHYSICAL EXAMINATION

Diagnosis of clubfoot usually is made on the basis of the physical examination. In all cases, a thorough physical exam, including a neurologic examination, should be performed in order to exclude other conditions associated with a clubfoot. In patients with idiopathic clubfoot, positive physical findings include the following (Fig. 4.2-1):

- Shortening of the entire lower extremity
- Calf atrophy
- In unilateral cases the clubfoot will be shorter and wider than the normal foot.

The above three findings are permanent and persist regardless of treatment. This should be discussed with the

BOX 4.2-2 ANATOMIC FINDINGS IN CLUBFOOT

- The neck of the *talus* is medially rotated, shortened, and plantarflexed.
- The *subtalar joint* is held in internal rotation, equinus, and supination by soft tissue contractures.
- The *calcaneus* is rotated medially about the talocalcaneal interosseous ligament and is pulled into equinus.
- The plane of the talocalcaneal joint is oblique. Medial rotation of the calcaneus results in simultaneous *adduction and varus of the calcaneus.*
- This medial rotation of the calcaneus also results in approximation of the posterior tuberosity of the calcaneus to the fibula with *resulting contractures of the calcaneofibular ligament.*
- The *navicular* is medially displaced and there may be a pseudoarticulation present between the navicular and the medial malleolus.
- The *cuboid* may exhibit medial subluxation or dislocation secondary to a medial tilt of the calcaneocuboid joint.
- The *soft tissues* of the clubfoot are also contracted and fibrotic. There are contractures of the spring ligament, the posterior tibial tendon, the Achilles tendon, the flexor digitorum longus tendon, the flexor hallucis longus tendon, the plantar fascia, the short plantar muscles, tendon sheaths, and the talocalcaneal interosseous ligament.
- *Joint capsules,* particularly involving the posterior ankle and subtalar joint have contractures in the rigid clubfoot.
- The amount and direction of tibial torsion and rotation of the body of the talus in the ankle mortise are controversial.

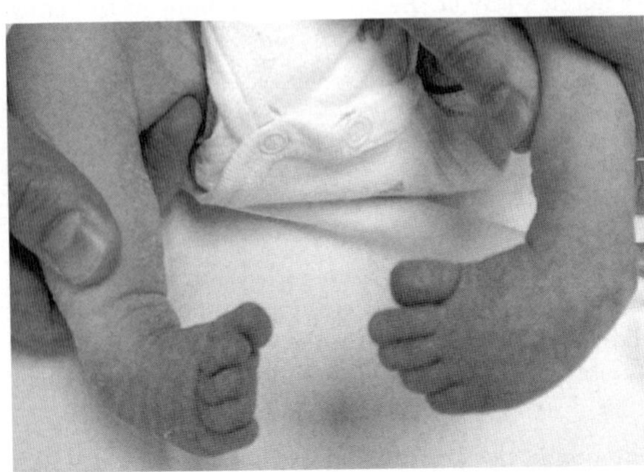

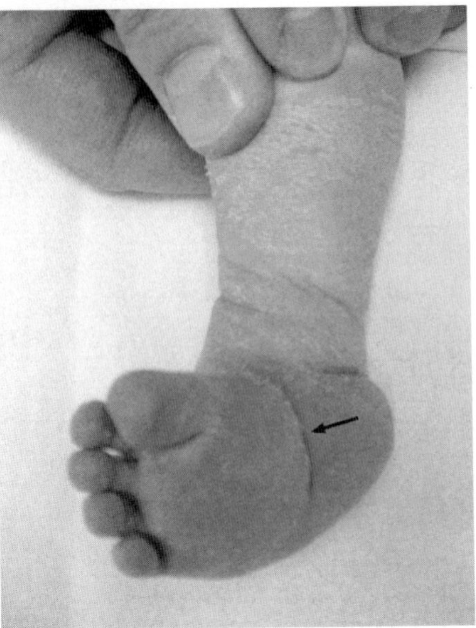

A B

Figure 4.2-1 (A) Six-week-old boy with bilateral clubfoot. Note the cavus, adduction, varus, and equinus position of the foot. (B) The *arrow* indicates a medial crease in the midfoot.

patient's family at the onset of treatment. Other physical findings include:

- Cavus, forefoot *a*dductus, subtalar joint *v*arus, and hindfoot *e*quinus, (mnemonic = *CAVE*)
- Empty calcaneal fat pad due to proximal migration of the calcaneus
- Head of talus palpable on dorsolateral foot
- A medial plantar skin crease, which denotes a more rigid foot

The flexibility of the foot should be documented as well. The presence of rigid hindfoot equinus differentiates a clubfoot from metatarsus adductus. Several classification systems have been proposed but none are universally accepted.

RADIOGRAPHS

Radiographs are of limited value in the initial evaluation and treatment of clubfoot. The bones in an infant's foot are primarily cartilaginous and any ossification centers present are frequently located eccentrically, making radiographic interpretation difficult. Radiographs, however, may have a role intraoperatively or in the older infant or child to confirm correction or to analyze deformity. Anteroposterior (AP) and lateral foot radiographs should be taken in a weightbearing position. In children who are not yet standing, this is enacted through simulated weightbearing radiographs done with maximum ankle dorsiflexion. In severe deformity separate radiographs may be needed of the ankle and foot, since orthogonal radiographs of one area may result in oblique views of the other. The AP and lateral talocalcaneal angles should be measured. On both of these projections this angle will be decreased (normal is 25 to 45 degrees) and there will be increased parallelism between the talus and calcaneus (Fig. 4.2-2).

NATURAL HISTORY

The untreated clubfoot will not correct spontaneously. With ambulation, weightbearing occurs on the dorsolateral aspect of the foot and ankle. Normal shoe wear is not possible and a callus and bursa forms over the dorsolateral foot. This typically becomes painful over time and makes ambulation difficult.

TREATMENT

Initial treatment in children with clubfeet is nonoperative. Techniques using serial manipulation with casting, splinting, taping, physical therapy, and the use of continuous passive range of motion machines have all been described. Serial manipulation and casting is currently the standard for initial treatment in the United States. There are two prevailing schools of thought regarding serial casting. The Kite technique corrects the foot through the use of short leg casts changed every 1 to 2 weeks. The foot is rotated about the calcaneocuboid joint and the clubfoot is corrected in a specific order: adduction is corrected first, followed by varus and equinus. Success rates for this technique have been reported to be between 15% and 50%. The Ponseti technique has recently become popular due to its reported high success rate and low complication rate in the treatment of clubfeet. This currently is the preferred technique. The Ponseti method relies on serial casting, and incorporates several very important differences when compared to the Kite technique. Conceptually, the Ponseti

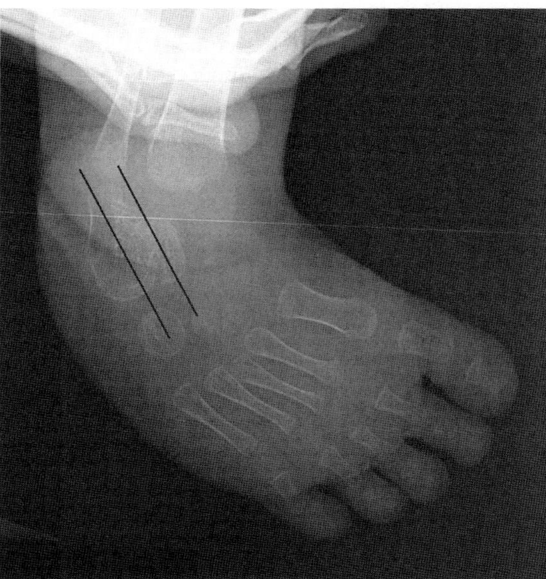
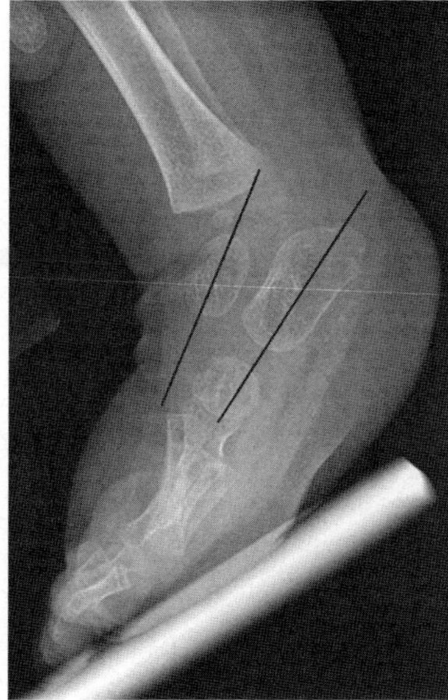

A B

Figure 4.2-2 Anteroposterior (A) and lateral (B) radiographs of clubfoot in a 1-year-old child. Both views show parallelism between the talus and the calcaneus.

technique emphasizes external rotation of the midfoot and forefoot about the talus while initially maintaining the foot in supination. This is achieved by:

- Using weekly manipulations and long leg casts. The foot is corrected in a precise order.
- Dorsiflexing the first ray to stretch the plantar fascia and to unlock the talonavicular joint, which loosens the foot and allows for correction.
- Supinating the foot for the initial casts.
- Abducting the forefoot around the talus using the talar head as the center of rotation. This results in simultaneous correction of supination, adduction, and varus as the calcaneus midfoot and forefoot rotate about the talus.
- Dorsiflexing the hindfoot once the other components have been corrected.

An Achilles tenotomy is needed 90% of the time to fully correct hindfoot equinus. This may be done as an outpatient procedure in the office. Patients are then maintained fulltime in a Denis Browne bar until they start to stand and nighttime bracing is continued for 2 to 3 years. Due to recurrence, 30% of patients require a transfer of the anterior tibialis tendon at 3 to 4 years of age.

Proponents of the Ponseti technique cite its high success rate, with 78% good or excellent results at an average 30-year follow-up. Regardless of the method chosen casting should begin within the first few weeks of life. Complications of casting include:

- Rocker bottom foot formation with dorsiflexion occurring through the midfoot instead of the ankle
- Deformation of the cartilage resulting in joint stiffness
- Physeal injury

Careful attention to the details and technique of serial casting is required to avoid complications and achieve the best results.

Surgical Management

Clubfeet resistant to nonoperative treatment or those with clubfeet secondary to neuromuscular or congenital condition often require operative intervention. Surgery is generally done between 6 to 12 months of age. Multiple surgeries have been described for clubfoot and many surgeons will tailor the procedure to the needs of the individual, creating an "a la carte" approach to clubfoot surgery. Multiple incisions have also been described for the surgery. The two most commonly used incisions are:

- The Cincinnati incision, which is a circumferential incision around the posterior of the foot.
- A two-incision (medial and lateral) technique can also be safely and effectively used.

All procedures can be adequately performed through either approach; in all cases, this phrase applies: "the decision (of which structures to release) is more important than the incision."

A comprehensive clubfoot release includes the following four components:

- Release of the plantar structures including the plantar fascia to correct cavus.
- A medial and posteromedial release with lengthening of the posterior tibial tendon, the flexor hallucis longus tendon, the flexor digitorum longus tendon, and release of their tendon sheaths into the knot of Henry. The abductor hallucis muscle is taken down and released. A

talonavicular joint capsulotomy is performed to allow reduction of the navicular onto the talar head. A medial subtalar joint release is also performed while preserving the talocalcaneal interosseous ligament (although some surgeons release this ligament as well).

- A posterior release including Achilles tendon lengthening, posterior ankle capsulotomy and posterior subtalar join capsulotomy is also performed to correct the equinus.
- Posterolateral and lateral releases are also often performed during surgical correction of a clubfoot. A posterolateral release involves dividing the calcaneofibular ligament and peroneal tendon sheath to allow external rotation of the calcaneus. A calcaneocuboid capsulotomy may also be performed in order to realign the cuboid with the long axis of the calcaneus and produce a straight lateral border of the foot.

Internal fixation may be used to help stabilize the foot after surgery, particularly after more extensive releases. Typically, a smooth 0.062-inch Kirschner wire is used to transfix the talonavicular joint for 4 to 6 weeks. Postoperative casting and care varies. Generally some type of bracing is used after surgery, but the type and duration varies widely from surgeon to surgeon.

Complications of surgery are numerous. They include:

- Neurovascular injury
- Cartilage damage
- Direct bone injury
- Avascular necrosis of the talus and navicular
- Wound healing problems
- Recurrence
- Stiffness
- Dorsal bunion
- Undercorrection
- Overcorrection
- Residual deformity—the most common residual deformity after clubfoot surgery is forefoot adduction.

Treatment of these complications is difficult, and must be individualized. Repeat soft tissue releases, tendon transfers, osteotomies, and fusions may all be used alone or in combination to treat the recurrent, residual, or overcorrected clubfoot.

SUGGESTED READING

Barker S, Chesney D, Miedzbrodzka Z, et al. Genetics and epidemiology of idiopathic congenital talipes equinovarus. J Pediatr Orthop 2003:23:265–272.

Bensahel H, Csukonyi Z, Desgrippes Y, et al. Surgery in residual clubfoot: one-stage medioposterior release "a la carte." J Pediatr Orthop 1987;7:145–148.

Crawford AH, Marxen JL, Osterfeld DL. The Cincinnati incision: a comprehensive approach for surgical procedures of the foot and ankle in childhood. J Bone Joint Surg (Am) 1982;64: 1355–1358.

Irani RN, Sherman MS. The pathological anatomy of idiopathic clubfoot. Clin Orthop 1972;84:14–20.

Kite JH. Nonoperative treatment of congenital clubfoot. Clin Orthop 1972;84:29–38.

Laaveg SJ, Ponseti IV. Long-term results of treatment of congenital clubfoot. J Bone Joint Surg (Am) 1980;62:23–31.

McKay DW. New concept of and approach to clubfoot treatment: II. Correction of the clubfoot. J Pediatr Orthop 1983;3:10–21.

Ponseti IV, ed. Congenital clubfoot: fundamentals of treatment. Oxford, UK: Oxford University Press, 1996:51–52.

Tarraf YN, Carroll NC. Analysis of the components of residual deformity in clubfeet presenting for reoperation. J Pediatr Orthop 1992;12:207–216.

Turco VJ. Resistant congenital clubfoot: one-stage posteromedial release with internal fixation: a follow-up report of a fifteen-year experience. J Bone Joint Surg Am 1979:61:805–814.

4.3 CONGENITAL VERTICAL TALUS

REGGIE C. HAMDY

Congenital vertical talus (CVT) is a rare condition of unknown etiology that was first described by Henken in 1914. Other synonyms for this deformity include rocker bottom foot, rigid flatfoot, and convex pes valgus. About half of all CVT cases occur as an isolated deformity; the remainder have additional pathology. The hallmark of this condition is the fixed vertical position of the talus that does not correct with maximum plantarflexion of the foot.

CORONAL PLANE DEFORMITY

PATHOGENESIS

Etiology

The exact etiology is unknown. In about half the cases, CVT is associated with other abnormalities or is part of genetic or neuromuscular conditions. Box 4.3-1 lists conditions associated with CVT.

Epidemiology

- CVT is a rare condition.
- It is bilateral in approximately 50% of cases.
- There is no definite gender or racial difference.

Pathologic Anatomy

CVT can be described as a *triad* of:

1. Dorsal dislocation of the talonavicular joint where the navicular lies dorsal to the talus
2. Equinus position of the talus
3. Equinus position of the calcaneus

The pathologic changes can best be subdivided into osseous, ligamentous, retinacular, and muscular.

- Osseous changes (Figs. 4.3-1 and 4.3-2)
  - The *talus* is plantarflexed and medially deviated. This deformity is rigid.
  - The *os calcis* is in equinovalgus and is abducted or laterally subluxed underneath the talus. It is in close contact with the lateral malleolus.
  - The *navicular* is dorsally dislocated on the talar neck.
  - As a result of these primary changes, secondary adaptive changes develop. The dislocated navicular adapts to this new position and becomes wedge-shaped with a hypoplastic plantar segment. The sustentaculum becomes hypoplastic and offers no support to the talar head. The calcaneocuboid joint gradually subluxes.
  - The *cuboid* becomes displaced laterally and dorsally.
  - This calcaneocuboid subluxation—together with the talonavicular dislocation—causes a break in the midtarsal joints. Subsequently, this causes the lateral

BOX 4.3-1 CONDITIONS ASSOCIATED WITH CONGENITAL VERTICAL TALUS

Arthrogryposis
Neural tube defects
- Myelomeningocele
- Diastematomyelia
- Hydrocephalus

Sacral agenesis
Neuromuscular disorders
- Cerebral palsy
- Poliomyelitis

Spinal muscular atrophy
Iatrogenic, secondary to clubfoot correction
Genetic conditions
- Trisomies 13, 15, 17, and 18

Turner syndrome
Malformation syndromes
- Freeman-Sheldon disorder
- Nail patella syndrome
- Marfan syndrome

Multiple pterygium syndrome
Visceral anomalies (cardiovascular, gastrointestinal)

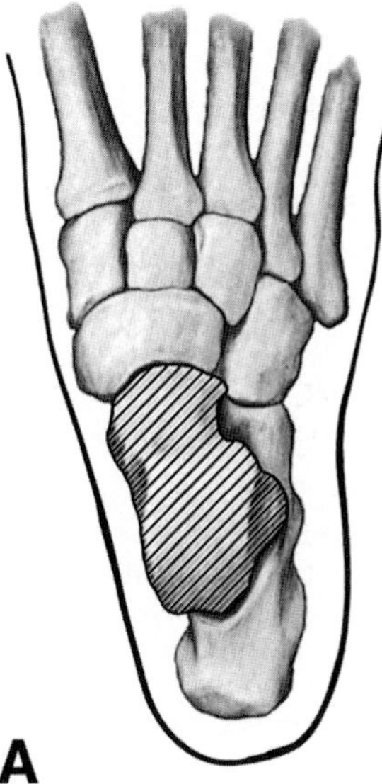

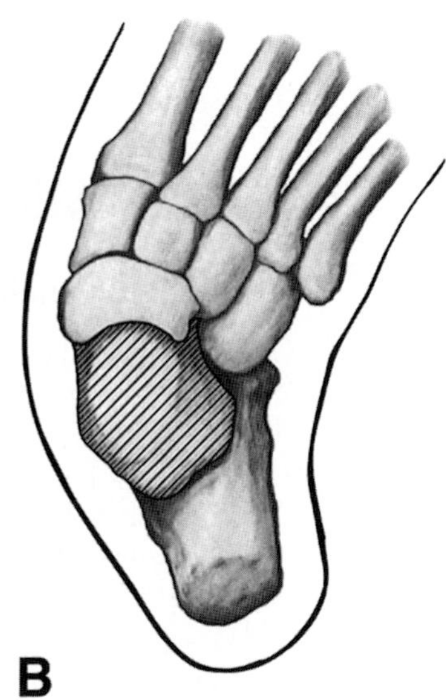

Figure 4.3-1 Osseous changes as viewed from the top. (**A**) Normal foot. (**B**) Foot with vertical talus. (Adapted from Kumar SJ, Cowell HR, Ramsey PL. Foot problems in children. AAOS Instr Course Lect 1982;31:235–251.)

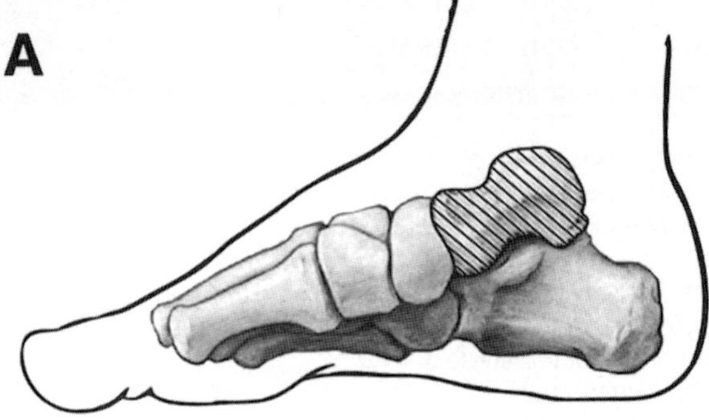

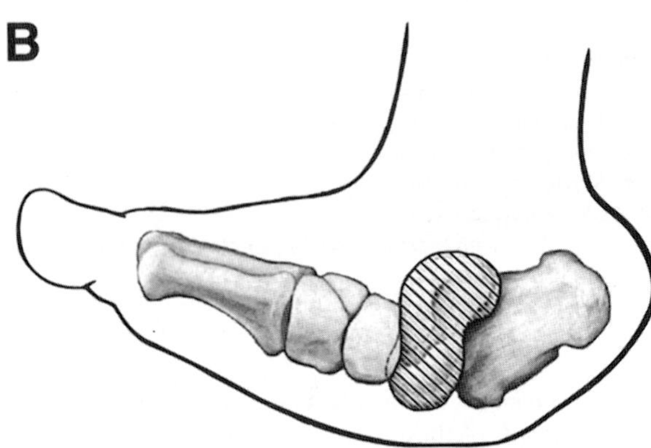

Figure 4.3-2 Osseous anatomy as seen from a medial view. (**A**) Normal foot. (**B**) Elongated talar neck in congenital vertical talus. (Adapted from Kumar SJ, Cowell HR, Ramsey PL. Foot problems in children. AAOS Instr Course Lect 1982;31:235–251.)

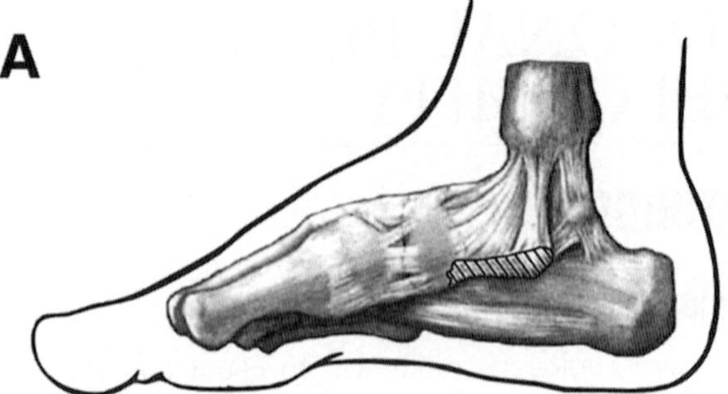

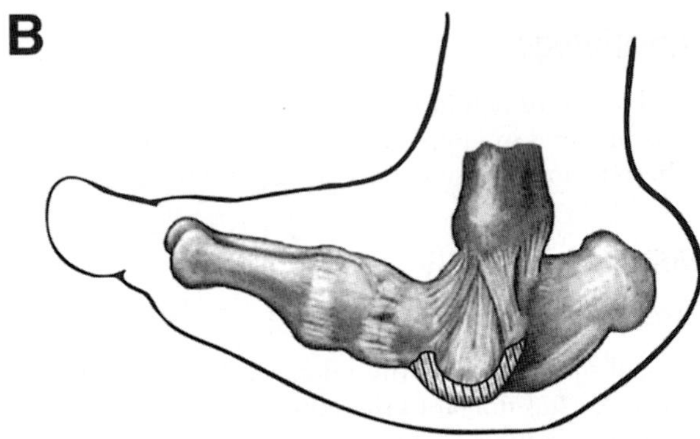

Figure 4.3-3 The plantar calcaneonavicular ligament is stretched and attenuated in a foot with vertical talus. Note the contrast between the normal foot (**A**) and the deformed foot (**B**). This structure is not clearly visualized during surgery. (Adapted from Kumar SJ, Cowell HR, Ramsey PL. Foot problems in children. AAOS Instr Course Lect 1982;31:235–251.)

border of the foot to look shortened and concave and the medial border elongated and convex.

- Ligamentous changes (Fig. 4.3-3):
  - Stretching of the calcaneonavicular or spring ligament.
  - Contractures of the lateral part of the talonavicular capsule, the calcaneofibular, the interosseous talocalcaneal ligament, and the posterior capsule of the ankle and subtalar joints. The dorsolateral part of the calcaneocuboid capsule may also be contracted.
- Muscular and tendinous changes:
  - Contractures of:
    - Tibialis anterior tendon
    - Long extensors of the toes
    - Peroneal tendons
    - Tendo Achilles
  - Anterior subluxation of:
    - Tibialis posterior tendon (Fig. 4.3-4)
    - Peroneal tendons
- Retinacular changes (Fig. 4.3-5):
  - The dorsal extensor retinaculum is thickened and contracted.
  - The superior peroneal retinaculum is stretched.

Classification

Numerous classifications for CVT have been described. Lichtblau described three types according to etiology: teratogenic, neurogenic, and acquired. Pouliquen suggested a radiologic classification based on the talocalcaneal angle and reducibility of the equinus of the os calcis on the lateral x-ray of the foot. The most practical classification, however, is the one described by Ogata and colleagues:

- Primary isolated form
- Associated form without neurologic deficit (e.g., dislocated hip, clubfoot, hand anomalies)
- Associated form, with neurologic deficit

DIAGNOSIS

Clinical Features

The typical appearance of CVT is that of a "Persian slipper foot" and consists of the following triad (Fig. 4.3-6):

1. Equinusvalgus position of the hindfoot
2. Rocker bottom deformity of the midfoot (formed by the dislocated head of the talus which can be palpated on the medial and plantar aspect of the foot)
3. Dorsiflexion and abduction of the forefoot

This deformity is *rigid* and becomes more rigid if untreated.

Pain is usually not a problem in early childhood. However, plantar callosities may develop in adolescence under-

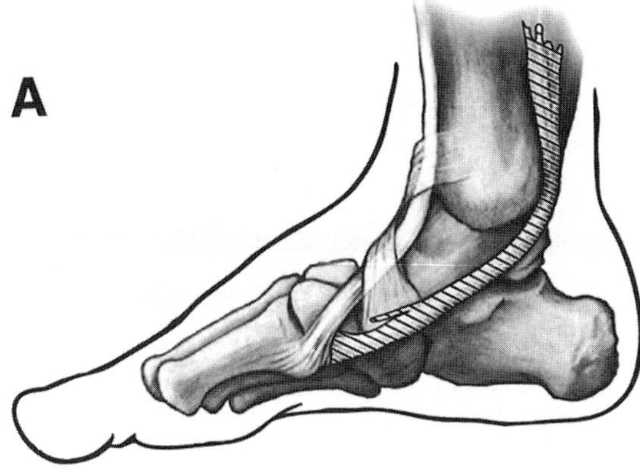

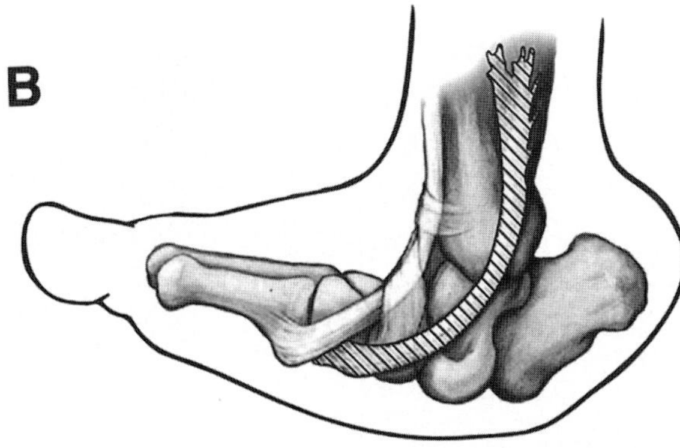

Figure 4.3-4 Orientation of the anterior and posterior tibial tendons. (**A**) Normal foot. (**B**) Foot with vertical talus, showing contracture of the tibialis anterior tendon and subluxation of the tibialis posterior tendon. (Adapted from Kumar SJ, Cowell HR, Ramsey PL. Foot problems in children. AAOS Instr Course Lect 1982;31:235–251.)

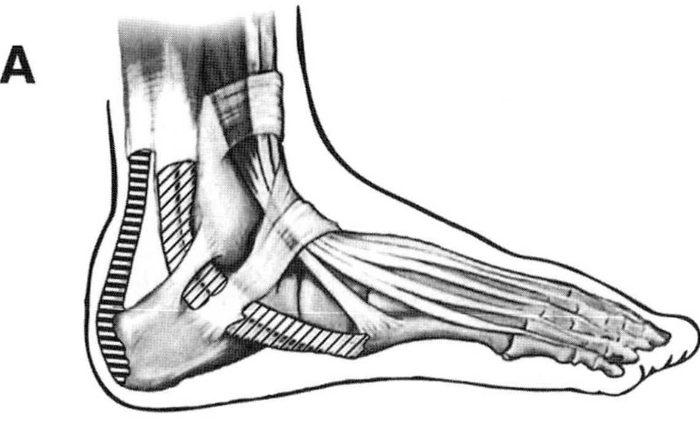

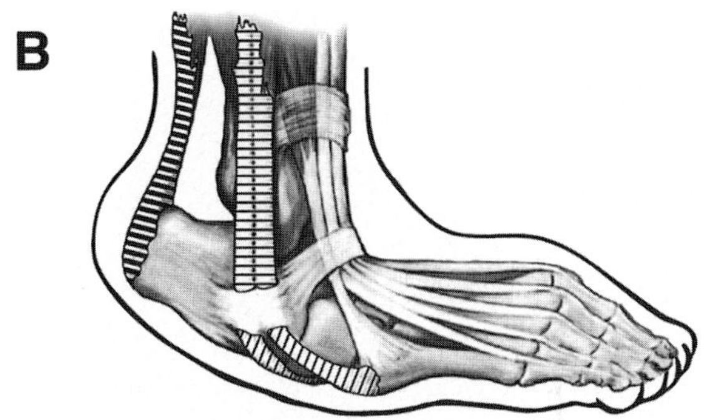

Figure 4.3-5 Tendons on the lateral and posterior aspect of the foot. (**A**) Normal foot. (**B**) A foot with vertical talus has a contracted tendo Achilles, anterior subluxation of the peroneal tendons, contracture of the dorsal extensor retinaculum, and attenuation of the superior peroneal retinaculum. In addition, the course taken by the peroneus tertius is straighter. (Adapted from Kumar SJ, Cowell HR, Ramsey PL. Foot problems in children. AAOS Instr Course Lect 1982;31:235–251.)

neath the dislocated head of the talus and this may cause pain. Most of the weightbearing area of the foot is centered over the dislocated head of the talus.

Walking is not delayed if the condition is not treated. However, the gait may be awkward and clumsy. Wearing of shoes may cause problems.

Associated Features

As previously mentioned, about half of all CVT cases are associated with other abnormalities such as dislocation of the hip or are part of neuromuscular conditions such as arthrogryposis, spinal dysraphism, and cerebral palsy.

As soon as a diagnosis of congenital vertical talus is suspected, a complete physical and neurologic examination of the child should be performed. Magnetic resonance imaging (MRI) of the spine is recommended.

Radiologic Features

At birth, most of the tarsal bones are still cartilaginous. The ossification center of the cuboid appears within the first month of life, while that of the navicular appears

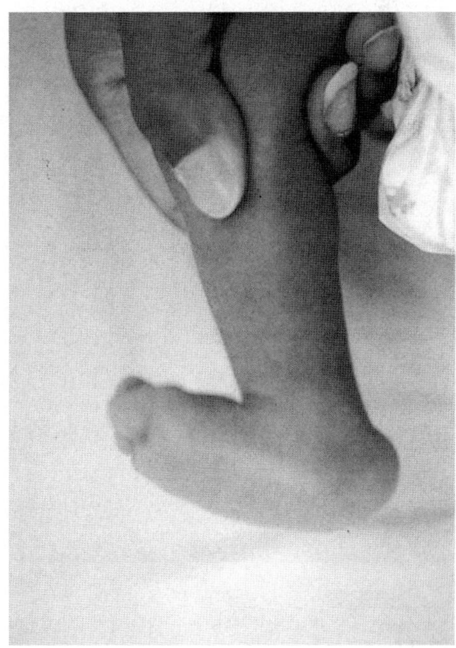

Figure 4.3-6 Clinical appearance of congenital vertical talus.

between 2 and 5 years of age. However, a radiologic diagnosis of CVT can still be made in the neonate by the appearance of the fixed vertical position of the talus.

The lateral view of the foot and ankle is the most important view, both in neutral and maximal plantar flexion as this will differentiate between an oblique and a vertical talus. In the neutral view, both oblique talus and CVT may appear the same. However, in the maximum plantarflexion view, an oblique talus will reduce and there is realignment of the long axis of the talus with that of the first metatarsal, as shown in Figure 4.3-7. This does not occur in cases of CVT, as shown in Figure 4.3-8. Other angles measured in the lateral view include:

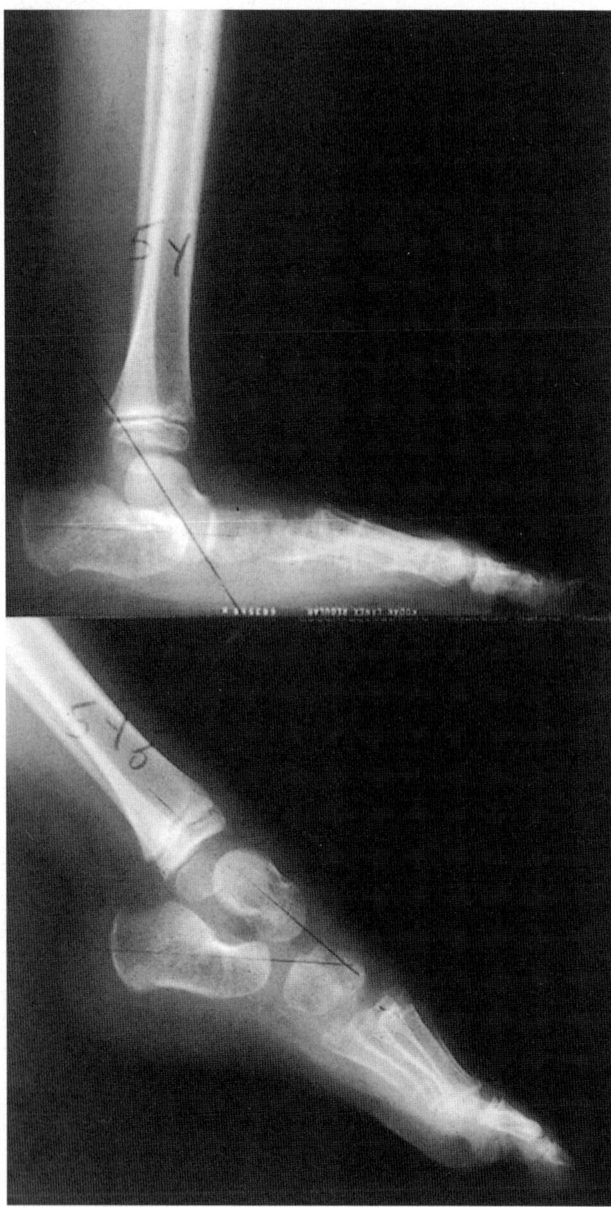

Figure 4.3-7 Radiologic appearance of oblique talus showing restoration of the normal talo-first metatarsal angle in maximal plantarflexion.

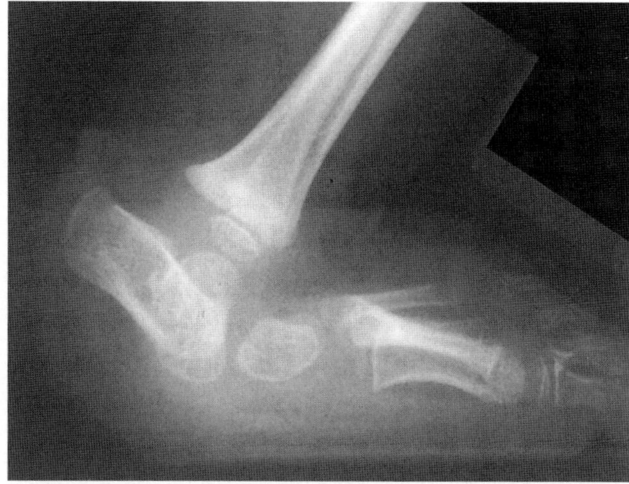

A

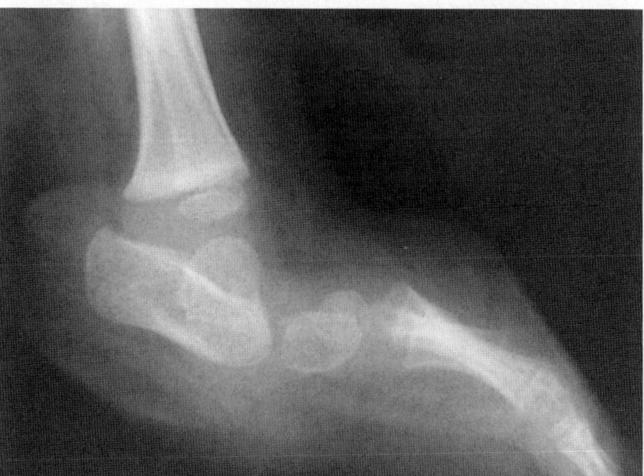

B

Figure 4.3-8 Lateral view of congenital vertical talus (**A**) showing vertical position of the talus that will not correct with maximum plantarflexion (**B**).

- Talocalcaneal angle: either increased or decreased
- Tibiocalcaneal angle: measures the amount of equinus of the os calcis
- Talo-first metatarsal angle: increased (normal 0 to 10 degrees).

In the anteroposterior view of the foot and ankle (Fig. 4.3-9), the following angles are measured:

- Talocalcaneal angle: increased
- Talo-first metatarsal angle: increased
- Calcaneo-fifth metatarsal angle: increased

Differential Diagnosis

Talipes Calcaneovalgus (Fig 4.3-10)

- This is the most common differential diagnosis in the neonatal period.
- There is no equinus of the heel but rather a pure calcaneus deformity.

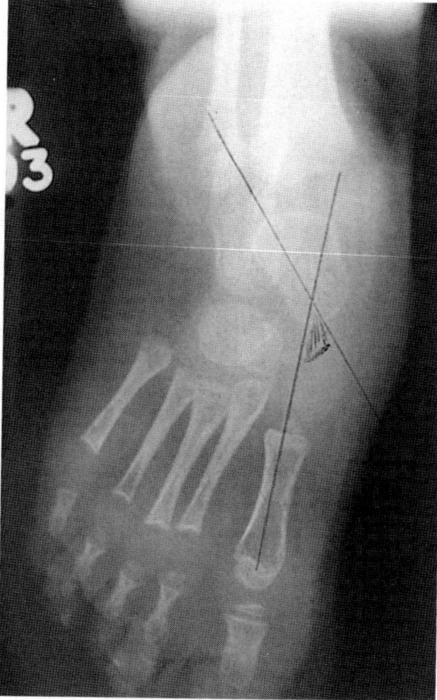

Figure 4.3-9 Anteroposterior view showing increased talo-first metatarsal angle.

- The calcaneovalgus deformity responds very well to passive manipulation and corrects completely after a few weeks or months of stretching.

Oblique Talus

- Oblique talus usually presents as a severe flatfoot deformity, either idiopathic flatfoot or associated with other conditions such as Down syndrome. An oblique talus is flexible in contrast with CVT, which is a rigid deformity.
- Usually there are no associated neurologic abnormalities.

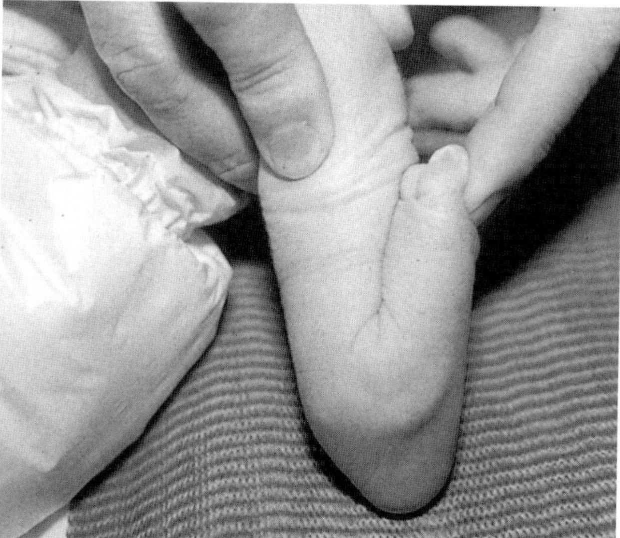

Figure 4.3-10 Clinical appearance of a calcaneovalgus foot.

- The differentiation between an oblique and a vertical talus is made on a lateral view of the foot and ankle in neutral and in maximal plantar flexion as previously mentioned.
- The treatment of oblique talus is completely different than that of vertical talus. If the deformity is flexible, usually no surgical treatment is indicated. In cases where there is contracture of the tendo Achilles, treatment includes stretching of the tendon and repeated casting or lengthening of the tendon. Many surgical procedures have been described for the treatment of oblique talus (the same as for severe flatfoot deformities).

Rigid Flatfoot Secondary to Tarsal Coalition

- In these cases, there is very limited subtalar motion. Radiologic examination reveals the coalition most commonly in the calcaneonavicular or talocalcaneal joints.

Iatrogenic Vertical Talus

- This may develop as a complication of clubfoot surgery.

TREATMENT

The treatment of a congenital vertical talus is almost always surgical. Casting is applied usually for stretching of the anteriorly contracted structures. Surgery is usually indicated before walking age, around 9 to 12 months of age.

Goals

- Reduction of the talonavicular dislocation
- Restoration of normal weightbearing area of the foot
- Obtain a plantigrade and braceable foot in cases where braces are indicated.

Technique

Two-Stage Procedure

The first stage is aimed at correcting the talonavicular subluxation and the second stage (6 weeks later) is directed at correcting the equinus deformity of the heel. The main disadvantage of this technique is the high incidence of avascular necrosis (AVN) of the talus.

One-Stage Procedure

All the deformities are corrected during the same surgery. Details of this procedure are well described by Drennan, Tachdjian, and Kumar (Fig. 4.3-11). A single Cincinnati skin incision or a combination of two or three incisions can be used. Releases are performed posteriorly, laterally, and medially:

- Posterior approach:
  - ☐ Achilles tendon is lengthened.
  - ☐ Ankle and subtalar joints are released.
  - ☐ Talofibular and calcaneofibular ligaments are incised.
- Lateral approach (centered over the sinus tarsi):

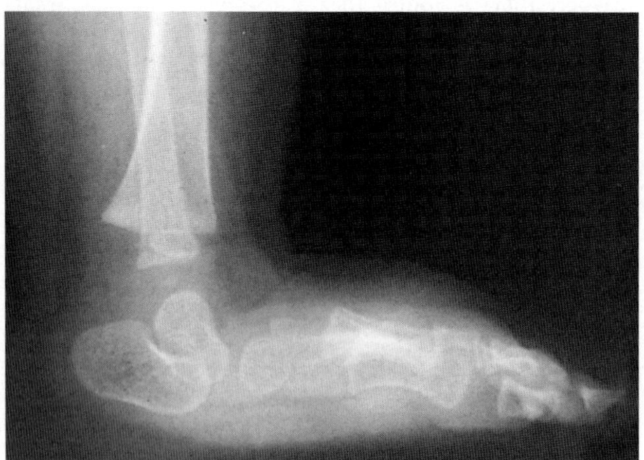
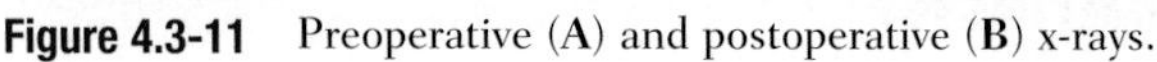
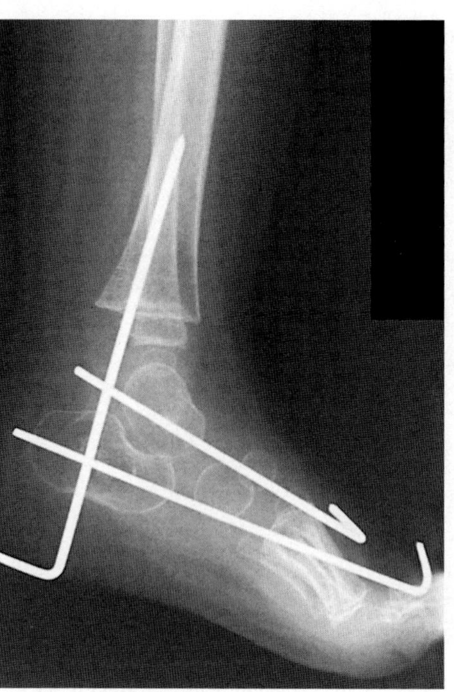

Figure 4.3-11 Preoperative (**A**) and postoperative (**B**) x-rays.

- Extensor digitorum brevis muscle is reflected.
- Sinus tarsi is cleaned.
- Calcaneocuboid joint is opened.
- Interosseous talocalcaneal ligament is incised.
- Peroneal tendons are lengthened.

- Medial approach:
  - Complete capsulotomy of the talonavicular joint is performed.
  - Capsule is incised near the navicular to avoid AVN of the talus.
  - Tibialis posterior tendon is dissected and incised.
- The following tendons are lengthened:
  - Tibialis anterior
  - Extensor hallucis longus
  - Extensor digitorum longus
- Reduction of the talonavicular dislocation:
  - Kirschner wire (K-wire) is inserted in the posterior aspect of the talus and used as a lever to reduce the talonavicular joint.
  - Equinus position of the calcaneus is corrected with a K-wire and the calcaneocuboid joint reduced if necessary and held in place with a K-wire.
  - Capsulorrhaphy of the talonavicular joint is performed.
  - The tibialis posterior tendon is transferred to the plantar aspect of the navicular to support the head of the talus.
  - Transfer of the tibialis anterior to the neck of the talus through a drill hole in the neck of the talus may be performed (Fig. 4.3-12).

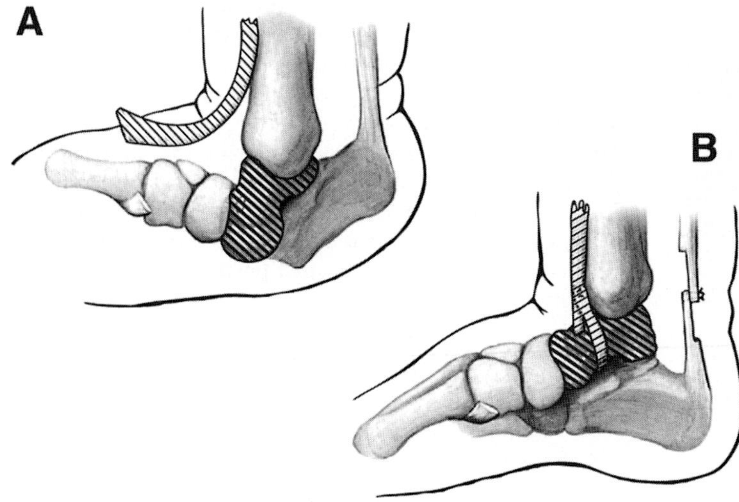

Figure 4.3-12 (**A**) Isolation of the anterior tibial tendon and placement of the drill hole in the talar neck. Depending on the size of the tendon, either the whole tendon or, preferably, only two-thirds of it is detached. (**B**) Tendon threaded through the drill hole and sutured onto itself. (Adapted from Kumar SJ, Cowell HR, Ramsey PL. Foot problems in children. AAOS Instr Course Lect 1982;31:235–251.)

- Other bony procedures described in the treatment of CVT include:
  - ☐ Excision of the navicular
  - ☐ Talectomy
  - ☐ Grice procedure
  - ☐ Triple arthrodesis.

These procedures are usually indicated in severe or recurrent cases in which a standard soft tissue release as previously described fails to correct the deformity.

Postoperative Management

- The pins are removed after 2 months.
- Total period of cast immobilization is 3 to 4 months.

Complications

- Complications are common and include skin necrosis, infection, AVN of the talus, and, most important, recurrence of the talonavicular dislocation.

Results and Outcome

Results of surgery can be evaluated using the scoring system developed by Adelaar, as shown in Box 4.3-2. However, the numerous surgical procedures reported, as well as the wide range of rigidity and severity of the deformity, make it very difficult to compare the results of published series.

There is a high recurrence rate following surgical correction and parents should be made aware of this complication. The prognosis for very rigid feet, especially when associated with neuromuscular or other conditions, should be guarded.

BOX 4.3-2 ADELAAR-WILLIAMS-GOULD SCORING SYSTEM FOR CONGENITAL VERTICAL TALUS (10 POINTS)

Clinical appearance
- Poor cosmetic appearance
- Ankle plus subtalar motion loss
- Prominent talar head
- Loss of medial longitudinal arch
- Hindfoot valgus
- Abnormal shoe wear

Radiographic appearance (weightbearing)
- Abnormal appearance
- Hindfoot equinus
- Talometatarsal axis
- Talonavicular subluxation

Adapted from Adelaar RS, Williams RM, Gould JS. Congenital convex pes valgus: results of an early comprehensive release. Foot Ankle 1980;1:62–73.

PEARLS

- Whenever a diagnosis of CVT is made, other associated conditions should be sought and a complete neurologic examination performed. MRI of the spine is recommended.
- Radiologic examination of the foot and ankle in maximal plantarflexion on the lateral view is part of the diagnosis and should always be performed.
- Congenital vertical talus usually does not respond to casting and surgery is nearly always recommended.
- Recurrence rate is high. This should be explained to the child's parents.

SUGGESTED READING

Adelaar RS, Williams RM, Gould JS. Congenital convex pes valgus: results of an early comprehensive release. Foot Ankle 1980;1:62–73.

Coleman SS, Stelling FH, Jarrett J. Pathomechanics and treatment of congenital vertical talus. Clin Orthop 1970;70:62–72.

Drennan JC. Congenital vertical talus. AAOS Instr Course Lect 1996;45:315–322.

Duncan RD, Fixsen JA. Congenital convex pes valgus. J Bone Joint Surg (Br) 1999;81:250–254.

Harrold AJ. The problem of congenital vertical talus. Clin Orthop 1973;97:133–143.

Jacobsen ST, Crawford AH. Congenital vertical talus. J Pediatr Orthop 1983;3:306–310.

Kodros SA, Dias LS. Single-stage surgical correction of congenital vertical talus. J Pediatr Orthop 1999;19:42–48.

Kumar SJ, Cowell HR, Ramsey PL. Foot problems in children. AAOS Instr Course Lect 1982;31:235–251.

Lichtblau S. Congenital vertical talus. Bull Hosp Joint Dis 1978;39:165–179.

Ogata K, Schoenecker PL, Sheridan J. Congenital vertical talus and its familial occurrence: an analysis of 36 patients. Clin Orthop 1979;139:128–132.

Rigault P. Le pied convexe congenital. SOFCOT. Orthop Pediatr 1990;1:87–107.

Tachdjian M. Congenital vertical talus. In: Pediatric orthopaedics, 2nd ed. Philadelphia: WB Saunders, 1990:2557–2578.

4.4 TARSAL COALITION

ANDREW W. HOWARD ■ ANDREW M. WAINWRIGHT

Tarsal coalition is defined as a fibrous, cartilaginous, or bony connection between bones of the hindfoot or midfoot. It is frequently congenital (but may occasionally be acquired), and is usually between the calcaneus and talus or navicular. Coalitions may cause pain and stiffness and a flatfoot in adolescence, and may be responsible for recurrent ankle sprains. Younger children with coalitions are often asymptomatic. Adults may also have asymptomatic coalitions.

Radiographs often demonstrate the bony coalition, but computed tomography (CT) or magnetic resonance imaging (MRI) may be required. Initial treatment should be nonoperative. However, many will require an operation. Surgery may involve resection of the fusion (with or without interposition of material to stop recurrence) or arthrodesis. Results of these operations are good, at least in the short to medium term.

PATHOGENESIS

Anatomy

The normal anatomy (Fig. 4.4-1) of the hindfoot is complicated. The two bones below the ankle joint lie on top of each other—the talus above and the calcaneus below. They meet at the subtalar joint, which has three facets—posterior, middle, and anterior. Distal to this are two bones that lie side by side: the navicular on the medial side and the cuboid on the lateral side. The anterior calcaneus articulates with the cuboid, and the anterior talus articulates with the navicular.

The most common coalitions are seen between the talus and calcaneus (i.e., bridging the middle facet) and between the calcaneus and the navicular (which do not normally form an articulation).

Etiology

Congenital

- Failure of segmentation of the mesenchymal anlage
- Bone malformation in the hindfoot
- Coalitions frequently associated with congenital deficiencies

Acquired

- Untreated clubfoot
- Inflammatory arthritis
- Intraarticular fractures
- Osteonecrosis

Pathophysiology

- Coalitions alter normal motion that acts as a shock absorber and torque converter:

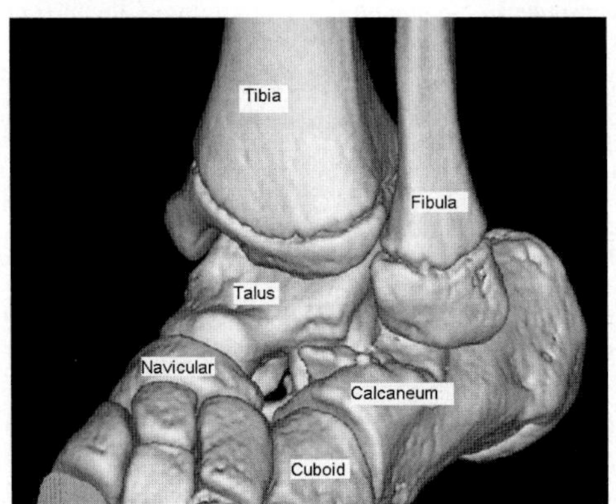

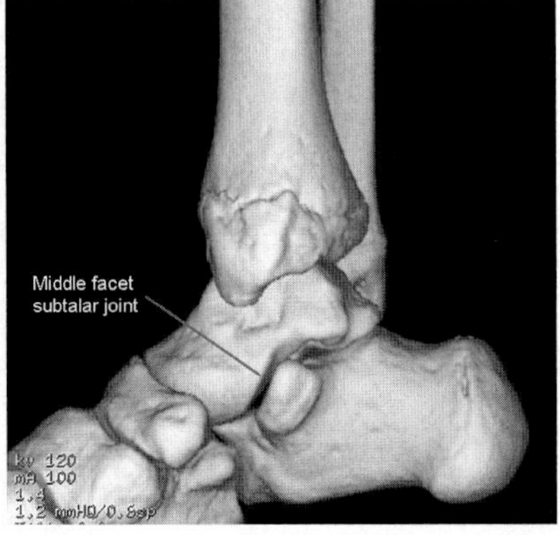

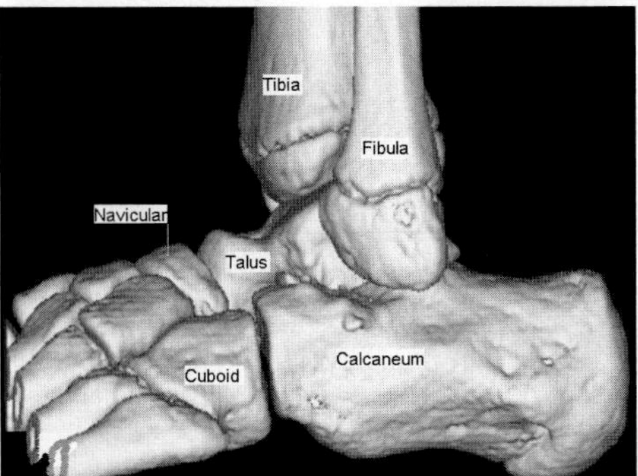

Figure 4.4-1 Normal osseous anatomy of the hindfoot taken from a three-dimensional computed tomography reconstruction as seen from the dorsolateral side of the left foot (**A**), the lateral side of the left foot (**B**), and the medial side of the right foot (**C**).

- Subtalar joint (rotatory, gliding)
- Transverse tarsal joint ("socket" navicular around "ball" of the talar head)
- Ankle joint (talar dome flexing and extending within mortise)

- Coalitions lead to abnormal stresses on adjacent joints resulting in painful symptoms or compensatory adaptations:
  - Ball-and-socket ankle joint (abnormal inversion and eversion)
  - Traction on talonavicular dorsal capsule (talar beaking)
  - Loss of subtalar motion with variable hindfoot valgus

Epidemiology

- Incidence: 0.03% to 2% of general population (not all coalitions are symptomatic)
  - Calcaneonavicular: 53%
  - Talocalcaneal: 37%
- No racial predilection
- 40% to 68% are bilateral
- Multiple coalitions occur in the same foot in up to 20% of cases
- Genetics: 39% of first-degree relatives of an affected individual have a coalition, suggesting unifactorial autosomal dominant trait

Classification

Site

- Calcaneonavicular (CNC)
- Talocalcaneal (TCC):
  - Middle facet—most common
  - Posterior facet
  - Anterior facet
- Other:
  - Talonavicular (TNC)
  - Calcaneocuboid
  - Naviculocuneiform
  - Cubonavicular

Tissue

- Type 1: Osseous
- Type 2: Cartilaginous
- Type 3: Fibrous

DIAGNOSIS (ALGORITHM 4.4-1)

History and Physical Examination

Clinical Features

Symptoms

- Pain initially with activities
- Repetitive sprains
- Onset based on ossification:
  - CNC: 8 to 12 years
  - TNC: 3 to 5 years
  - TCC: 12 to 16 years
- Progress: Becomes during symptomatic during teenage years
- Location:
  - Anterolateral or lateral: sinus tarsi
  - Peroneal muscles (spasm)

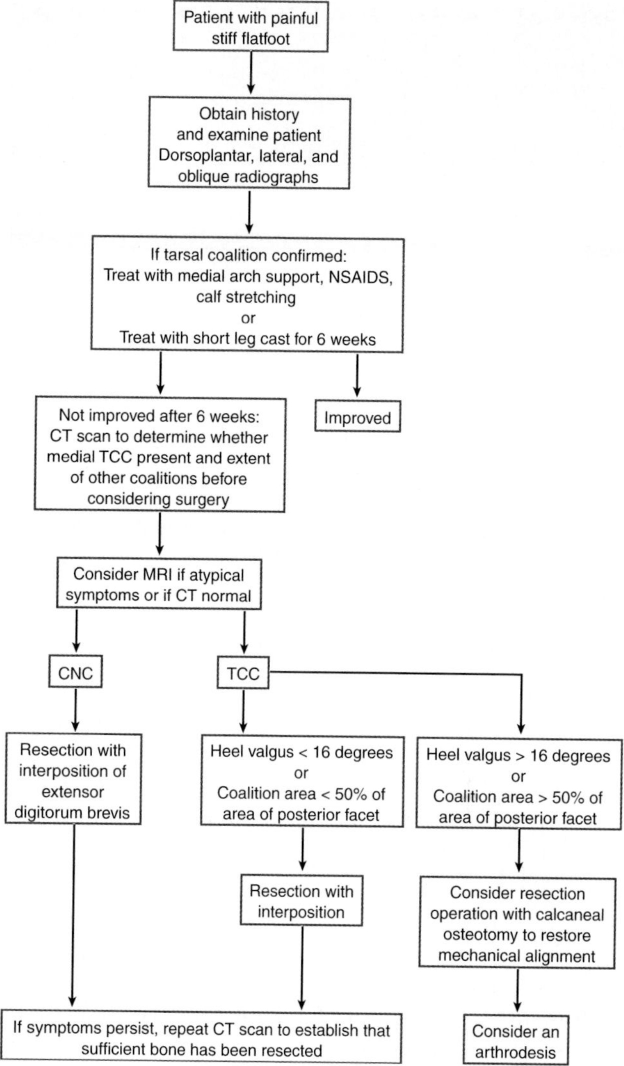

Algorithm 4.4-1 Algorithm for the diagnostic workup of tarsal coalitions.

Signs

- Limited or no subtalar motion (easier to identify if coalition is unilateral)
- No correction of heel valgus or reformation of longitudinal arch on tiptoe
- Pes planus
- Hindfoot valgus
- Flat medial longitudinal arch
- Midfoot pronation
- Antalgic gait
- Peroneal muscle spasm (spastic flatfoot)

Differential Diagnosis

- Rheumatoid arthritis
- Osteoid osteoma
- Injury

Radiologic Features

Radiographs

- Anteroposterior (dorsoplantar) weightbearing:
  - Coalition seen between talus and navicular (TNC)
  - Ball-and-socket ankle

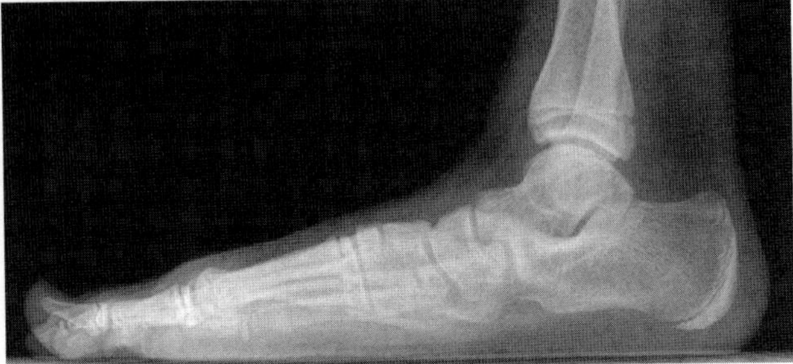

Figure 4.4-2 Lateral weightbearing view of the hindfoot in a patient with a stiff flatfoot caused by a calcaneonavicular coalition.

- Lateral weightbearing (Fig. 4.4-2):
  - ☐ Anteater nose (CNC)
  - ☐ Talar beaking (not degenerative sign) (TCC)
  - ☐ C sign (of Lateur): Initially thought to be a reliable indicator for middle facet TCC but is actually specific for *flatfoot*, not coalition)
  - ☐ Rounding/flattening talar lateral process
  - ☐ Concave plantar surface: talar neck
  - ☐ Narrowing of the posterior subtalar facet (TCC)
  - ☐ Failure to visualize middle subtalar facet (TCC)
- Internal oblique (45-degree angle, Sloman view) (Fig. 4.4-3):
  - ☐ No gap between calcaneum and navicular (CNC)
  - ☐ Asymmetry of the anterior subtalar joints (TCC)
- Axial (Harris-Beath view):
  - ☐ Middle facet TCC

Computed Tomography

- To identify associated unseen coalitions (useful for cases preoperatively)
- If there is clinical suspicion despite normal x-rays
- If secondary radiologic signs are present
- If there is middle facet TCC (Fig. 4.4-4)
- To differentiate between fibrous, cartilaginous, and osseous.

Magnetic Resonance Imaging

- If clinical suggestion is apparent, but CT is normal
- To differentiate between fibrous and cartilaginous
- To help detect differential pathology.

Technetium-99 Bone Scan

- A screening procedure
- Useful for localization of pathology

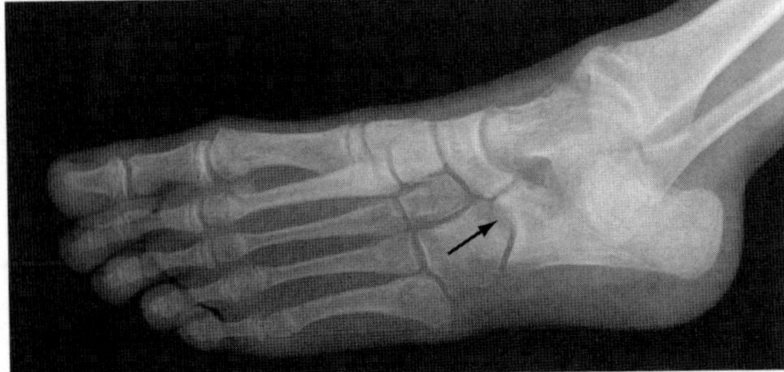

Figure 4.4-3 Internal oblique view (45-degree angle, Sloman view) of a stiff flatfoot showing signs of a fibrous calcaneonavicular coalition.

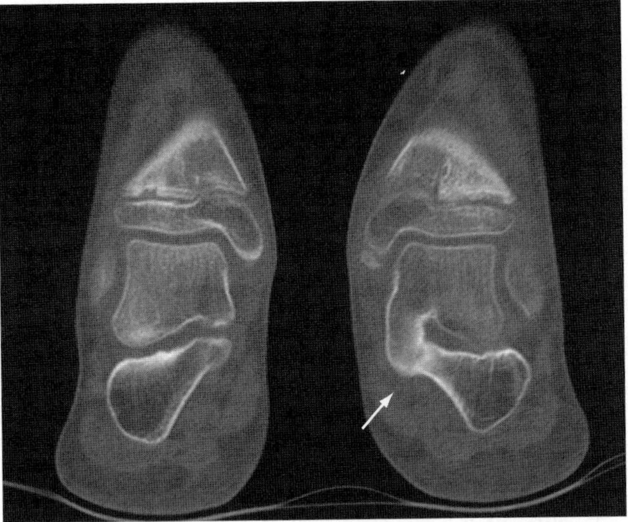

Figure 4.4-4 Coronal computed tomography through both hindfeet showing a middle facet talocalcaneal osseous coalition compared with a normal middle facet on the contralateral foot.

TREATMENT

Nonoperative

- Initial management for all symptomatic coalitions
- Success rate:
  - ☐ Less than 33% sustained long-term relief
  - ☐ Less success for weightbearing coalitions

Aims

- Decrease stress
- Support/correct valgus hindfoot, pronated midfoot
- Reduce inflammation in mobile joints
- Decrease peroneal spasm

Methods

- Short leg non-weightbearing/weightbearing casts
- Shoe inserts (UCBL)
- Calf muscle stretching

Operative

Surgical Indications/Contraindications

- Failed nonoperative treatment prior to degenerative changes
- CN coalitions
- Joint degenerative

Aims

- Relieve symptoms
- Improve range of motion
- Realign foot

Methods

- Excision of coalition with or without interposition

Calcaneonavicular

- Make Ollier incision (oblique over sinus tarsi). Be careful not to injure superficial peroneal nerve.
- Mobilize extensor digitorum brevis (proximolateral to distomedial).

- Define bone to avoid injury to talonavicular joint.
- Perform bone resection parallel in all planes. Beware of tendency to converge toward sole.
- Interpose extensor digitorum brevis into resection using pull-through suture.
- Confirm complete resection with intraoperative radiograph.
- Examine range of motion to confirm increase.

Talocalcaneal

- Make medial curved incision (part of Cincinnati incision)
- Identify medial (posterior tibial) neurovascular bundle
- Find the subtalar joint:
  - ☐ Open sheaths of tibialis posterior and flexor digitorum longus
  - ☐ Find posterior subtalar joint through flexor hallucis longus sheath
  - ☐ Find anterior subtalar joint by following sustentaculum tali anteriorly then laterally around the corner to anterior process of calcaneum
  - ☐ Excise bar with burr and rongeurs
  - ☐ Interpose sheath of flexor hallucis longus, fat, or Gelfoam material
  - ☐ If heel in valgus, use calcaneal osteotomy

Subtalar Arthrodesis: Dennyson-Fulford Technique

- Make curved incision on lateral foot over subtalar joint
- Place calcaneum in neutral position (i.e., below talus)
- Insert cancellous bone graft in sinus tarsi
- Place cannulated screw through talar neck, across sinus tarsi, into posterolateral calcaneum

Triple Arthrodesis

- Surgical fusion:
  - ☐ Talocalcaneal joint
  - ☐ Calcaneocuboid joint
  - ☐ Talonavicular joint
- For severe planovalgus foot or degeneration:
  - ☐ Make curved incision over sinus tarsi
  - ☐ Expose and resect the three joints with removal of enough bone to fuse joints in corrected position
- Fix with staples or screws
- Add cancellous bone graft as necessary

Postoperative Management

- Following resection operations: 1–2 weeks partial weightbearing in below-knee cast
- Following arthrodesis: 12 weeks in a non-weightbearing cast

Results and Outcome

- Natural history of untreated peroneal spastic foot at 21 years after diagnosis:
  - ☐ Only 10% have severe disability
  - ☐ Average duration of symptoms with bars is 18 months
  - ☐ Severe tarsal arthritis is unusual
- Results of a survey of 3,600 Canadian male army recruits:
  - ☐ 74 (2%) had peroneal spastic flatfoot; caused disability
  - ☐ 217 (6%) had flexible flatfeet; no symptoms or disability
- Results of surgery reported to be good (Table 4.4-1)

TABLE 4.4-1 RESULTS OF SURGERY

Author	Coalition	Treatment	Follow-up	No. of Feet	Results				Comments
					Excellent	Good	Fair	Poor	
Asher/Olney	TCC	Excision, fat graft	42 mo	10	5	3	1	1	
Wilde	TCC	Excision, fat graft	12–21 mo	20	8	2	4	6	Area coalition/ valgus
Gonzalez	CNC	Excision, interpose EDB	2–23 yr	75	20	38	12	5	
Chambers	CNC	Excision, interpose EDB[a]	3–14 yr	31	—	—	—	—	Function/gait assessed
Swiontkowski	TCC	Excision or arthrodesis	3.1 yr	13	11	2	—	1	
	CNC	Excision or arthrodesis	4.6 yr	44	29	7	—	4	
Kitakoa (1997)	TCC	Excision ± fat interposition	6 yr	14	5	4	3	2	Gait abnormal
Takaura	TCC	Excision	—	—	24	7	2	—	
Kumar (1992)	TCC	Excision ± interpose fat/FHL	4 yr	18	8	8	1	1	
Scranton	TCC	Excision	>2 yr	14	—	13	1	0	
Raikin	TCC	Excision, interpose split FHL	51 mo	14	11	1	1	1	
McCormack	TCC	Excision and fat graft	11.2 yr	9	—	—	—	1	

[a]Two arthrodeses.
CNC, calcaneonavicular coalition; EDB, extensor digitorum brevis; FHL, flexor hallucis longus; TCC, talocalcaneal coalition.

- Of those who had surgery, failures were attributed to:
  - ☐ Preexisting talonavicular or subtalar arthritis
  - ☐ Incomplete excision
  - ☐ Recurrence of coalition
- Gait analysis 2 to 16 years after TCC resection showed gait abnormality (despite good clinical results)

SUGGESTED READING

Harris RI, Beath T. Etiology of peroneal spastic flat foot. J Bone Joint Surg 1948;30B:624–634.

Jayakumar S, Cowell HR. Rigid flatfoot. Clin Orthop Rel Res 1976; 122:77–84.

Tachdjian MO. Paediatric orthopaedics, 3rd ed. Philadelphia: WB Saunders, 2001.

Wenger DR, Rang M. The art and practice of children's orthopaedics. New York: Raven Press, 1992.

4.5 PES PLANUS

MICHAEL SCHRECK ■ ELIANA DELGADO

When presented with a child whose parents are concerned that their child's feet appear to be too flat (Fig. 4.5-1), keep in mind that this condition is very common and is usually asymptomatic. Approximately 20% of adults have flatfeet, and in 65% of these adults the condition causes no disability.

PATHOGENESIS

Flatfeet may be described as flexible or rigid. A flexible flatfoot forms an arch when the patient stands on the tip of his or her toes. There are two forms of flexible flatfeet: those with and those without a tight or short Achilles tendon. Though a plain flatfoot is a benign condition, the flexible flatfoot with a short Achilles tendon is somewhat more likely to cause pain and disability. In the patient with a short Achilles tendon, the subtalar and midtarsal joints pronate to bypass the tight heel cord and get the heel down to the ground.

Rigid flatfeet do not form an arch in the tiptoe position. They generally present during adolescence. Rigid flatfeet are more likely to be painful. They are usually caused by tarsal coalitions but may also be the result of the following vertical talus, talipes calcaneovalgus, compensated metatarsus adductus or skewfoot deformity, trauma, infections, arthritides, polio, cerebral palsy, myelodysplasias, or neoplasms.

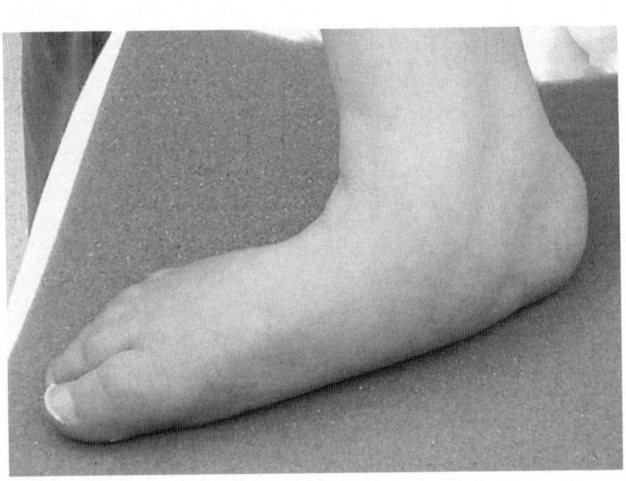

Figure 4.5-1 A normally presenting low arch without pain or biomechanical problems: pes planus.

DIAGNOSIS

History and Physical Examination

The overall exam should begin with appropriate history, noting any problems at birth and the age at which the onset of ambulation began. Clinically, one should evaluate rotation of the hips, tibial/malleolar torsion, foot deformities (i.e., metatarsus adductus), joint laxity, limb lengths (a flat, pronated foot may indicate a compensatory mechanism to lower or shorten a longer limb), tightness of Achilles tendon, Hubscher maneuver (discussed later), foot callosities, shoe wear patterns, patellar position, and forefoot to hindfoot relationships.

Clinical Features

The clinical examination of the child should be performed in two ways. The first is the bench exam while the child is sitting. The other includes a dynamic exam with the child standing and walking. First, determine whether the flatfoot is flexible or rigid. The foot may appear to have an arch when non-weightbearing (Fig. 4.5-2A) and present with a lowering or collapsing of the arch when weightbearing (see Fig. 4.5-2B) indicating flexible flatfoot. This is easily differentiated from the rigid flatfoot, which will have no arch in both non-weightbearing and weightbearing circumstances.

The Hubscher maneuver can also be performed to determine flatfoot flexibility. This test is performed with the patient in a weightbearing position and involves dorsiflexion of the hallux. If a flexible deformity exists, you should see the first ray plantarflex, the plantar fascia shorten and tighten, the medial arch rise, the calcaneus invert, and the leg externally rotate. This movement is a

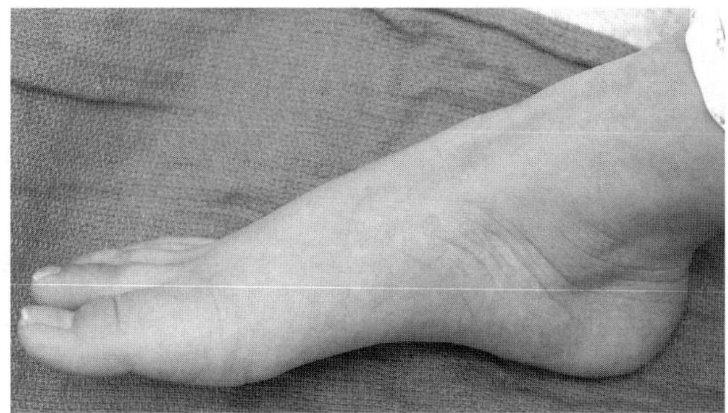

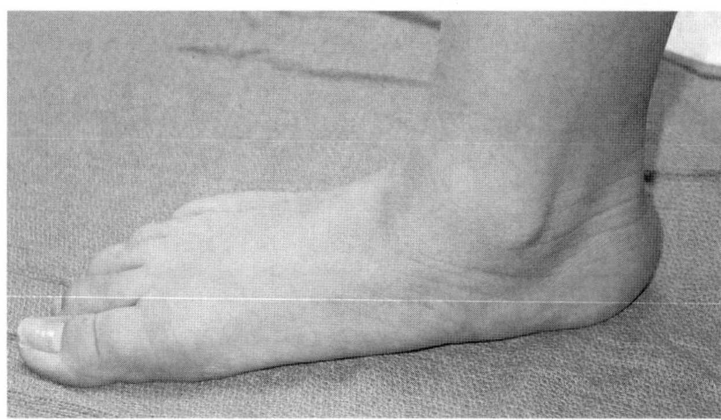

Figure 4.5-2 (A) Normal arch appearing when non-weightbearing takes place. (B) Arch collapses with weightbearing, indicating a flexible flatfoot.

good sign that the flatfoot is flexible and the patient should respond well to orthotics.

Next, the heel dorsiflexion should be assessed with the Silverskiöld test. This test is used to determine a gastrocnemius equinus versus a soleus equinus. With the leg extended (Fig 4.5-3) the foot is dorsiflexed. If the examiner is unable to acquire 10 to 15 degrees of dorsiflexion with the subtalar joint (STJ) in neutral position, the knee is then flexed to eliminate the activity of the gastrocnemius. The foot is again dorsiflexed. If 10 to 15 degrees of dorsiflexion is still unattainable, a gastrosoleus equinus exists. If dorsiflexion is available, a gastrocnemius equinus exists.

During the gait exam, observe for level shoulders, any twisting or bent position of the back (compensating for any scoliosis), patellar position in the frontal plane, rotation of the leg, heel strike, toe walking, and foot position. A limp may indicate a leg length discrepancy with a pronating foot as a compensatory mechanism. Pronating the foot helps to shorten the longer leg. The normal heel position at heel strike should be central-lateral. Overpronation results in a more medial heel strike which results in excessive wear of shoes. Some hindfoot and midfoot pronation during gait is normal and allows adaptation to uneven terrain.

Radiologic Features

Painless flatfeet do not require radiologic exam; however, a painful or rigid flatfoot may benefit from imaging, particularly in order to look for tarsal coalitions. The flatfoot on x-ray can be evaluated by using many different angles and measurements. Note that in growing children, bones may not be fully ossified; therefore, certain angles and measurements may not be able to be determined.

Standard radiographic views include an anteroposterior (AP), lateral, oblique, and calcaneal axial (Harris-Beath view), in a weightbearing position if possible. This gives the truest representation of the structural relationships of the foot. The AP view shows transverse plane deformities, particularly the talocalcaneal angle (Fig 4.5-4) formed by the bisection of the calcaneus and talus. As the calcaneus everts and the talus plantarflexes and adducts with pronation, this angle increases. Normal pediatric values range from 35 to 50 degrees at birth to 5 years of age and decrease to 15 to 35 degrees in children more than 5 years of age. Normal adult values are around 18 degrees. The relationship between the talus and navicular can also be evaluated. The navicular normally overlaps the talus approximately 75%. In the abducted, pronated flatfoot, as the talus begins to plantarflex and

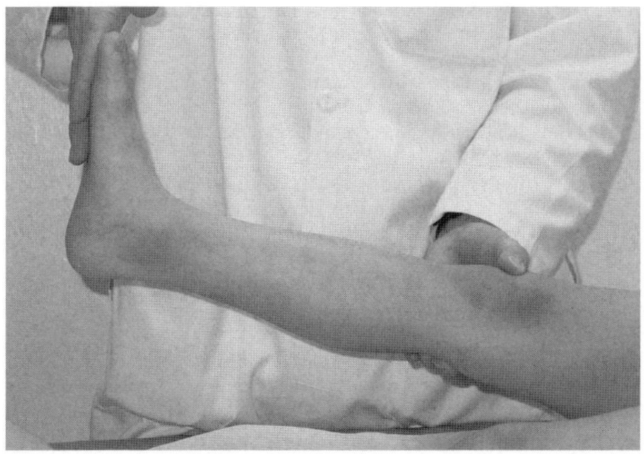

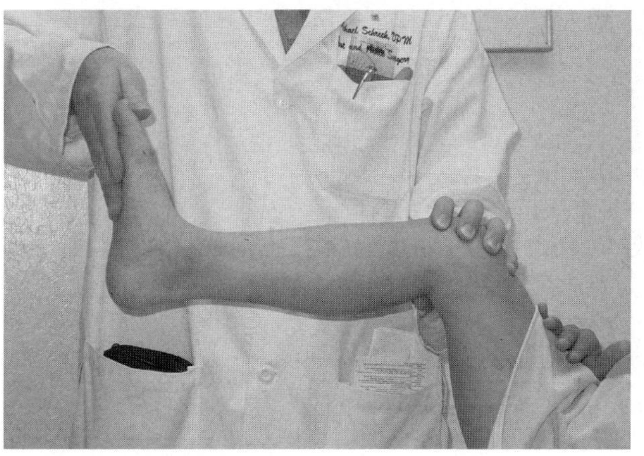

Figure 4.5-3 (A) Silverskiöld test. Leg is straight and foot is dorsiflexed. Foot acquires less than neutral dorsiflexion. (B) Gastrocnemius is eliminated by flexing the knee. Foot dorsiflexes to approximately neutral. Gastrocsoleus equinus exists.

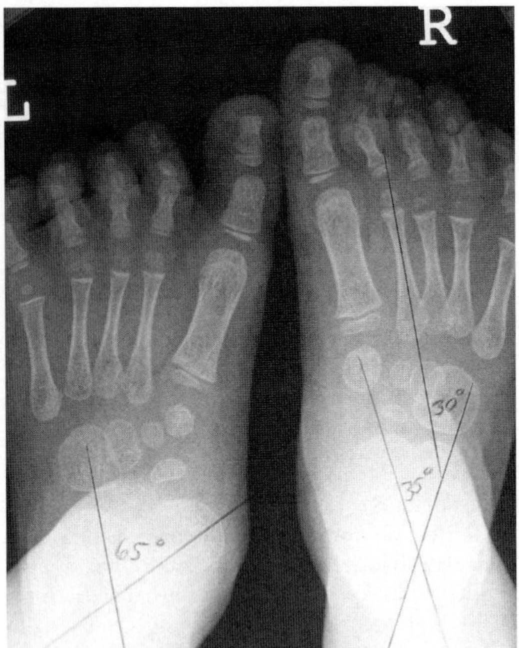

Figure 4.5-4 Sixty-five-degree talocalcaneal angle on left foot. This angle increases with pronation.

adduct, the navicular covers it less, depending on the severity of the deformity.

On the lateral view, the calcaneal inclination angle can be measured (Fig 4.5-5). This is formed by a line drawn tangential from the medial tubercle of the calcaneus along the anterior process bisecting a line drawn along the weightbearing portion of the foot along the fifth metatarsal head and calcaneus. While this angle can decrease in severe forms of flatfoot, it is a structural angle, meaning that it could be large in cases of a cavus foot that has a

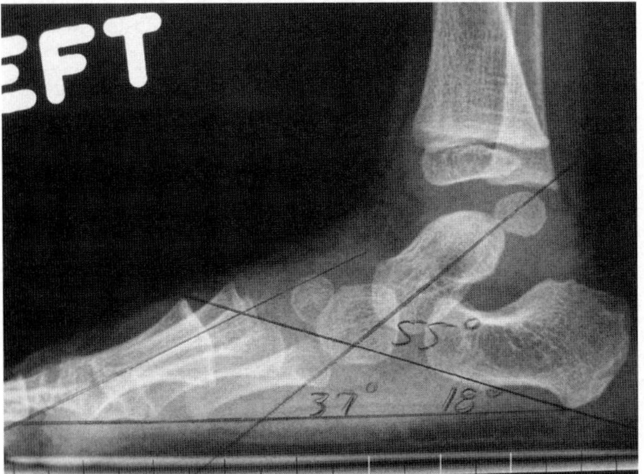

Figure 4.5-5 Calcaneal inclination angle: 18 degrees. Talar-declination angle: 37 degrees. Talocalcaneal angle: 55 degrees.

pronated STJ and midtarsal joint. Normal values are around 21 degrees.

The talar declination angle is formed from the intersecting of a line bisecting the talus and a line drawn along the weightbearing plane in reference to the fifth metatarsal as previously described. This angle usually increases with pronation and normally runs about 21 degrees. If you combine this angle with that of the calcaneal inclination angle, you get the lateral talocalcaneal angle formed by bisecting the talus and intersecting it with a line tangential to the medial tubercle and anterior process of the calcaneus. This angle also increases with pronation and is about 45 degrees. Calcaneonavicular coalitions may be seen on the 45-degree oblique view and talocalcaneal coalitions are sometimes seen on the Harris-Beath view.

TREATMENT

Surgical Indications/Contraindications

Painless, flexible flatfeet require no treatment. Flexible flatfeet that ache may be managed with orthoses. Orthoses are contraindicated in flexible flatfeet with a tight Achilles tendon, as raising the arch exacerbates the underlying problem. Treatment in this case is stretching the Achilles tendon through physical therapy or casting. Rigid flatfeet may respond temporarily to orthoses but are more likely to require surgical treatment to correct the underlying defect or deformity. Various osteotomies of the hindfoot and midfoot have been described to correct bony deformity. Arthrodesis is rarely indicated in children and is used primarily as a salvage procedure in cases of severe subtalar joint arthrosis.

SUGGESTED READING

Banks AS, Downey MS, Martin DE, et al, eds. McGlamry's comprehensive textbook of foot and ankle surgery, 3rd ed. Philadelphia: Lippincott Williams & Wilkins, 2001.

Crim J, Cracchiolo A, Hall R. Imaging of the foot and ankle. Philadelphia: JB Lippincott Co, 1996.

DeRosa GP, Ahlfeld SK. Congenital vertical talus. The Riley experience. Foot Ankle 1984; 5:118–124.

Jay RM. Pediatric foot and ankle surgery. Philadelphia: WB Saunders, 1999.

Page JC. Symptomatic flatfoot: etiology and diagnosis. J Am Podiatr Med Assoc 1983;73:393–399.

Powell HDW, Cantab MA. Pes planovalgus in children. Clin Orthop 1983;177:133–139.

Root ML. A discussion of biomechanical considerations for treatment of the infant foot. Arch Podiatr Foot Surg 1973;1:41–46.

Rose GK, Welton EA, Marshall T. The diagnosis of flatfoot in the child. J Bone Joint Surg 1985;67B:71–78.

Staheli LT. Evaluation of planovalgus foot deformities with special reference to the natural history. J Am Podiatr Med Assoc 1987;77: 2–6.

Valmassy RL. Biomechanical evaluation of the child. Clin Podiatr 1984;1:563–579.

Valmassey RL. Clinical biomechanics of the lower extremities. St. Louis: Mosby, 1996.

4.6. CONGENITAL ANOMALIES OF THE TOE

JUAN A. REALYVASQUEZ

Congenital anomalies of the toes are common and are usually familial disorders. They are often associated with other anomalies or syndromes.

ANOMALIES OF THE GREAT TOE

Congenital Hallux Varus

Congenital hallux varus is a rare deformity and is bilateral in one-third of cases. It is classified as either primary or secondary. *Primary congenital hallux varus* is a supernumerary cartilaginous toe anlage presenting on the medial aspect of the foot (Fig. 4.6-1). It is not associated with any other anomalies.

Secondary congenital hallux varus is associated with other anomalies especially polydactyly, true metatarsus varus, and dysplasia of bone such as dystrophic dwarfism and Apert syndrome. In secondary congenital hallux, the first metatarsal is broad and shortened. It is often associated with bracket epiphysis.

Surgery for this condition must be tailored to meet the needs of the individual deformity. In both types, it is important that sufficient skin be maintained medially to ensure complete correction. Sometimes it is necessary to develop a flap to lengthen the shortened medial side. All the structures medially, including a metatarsal phalangeal joint capsule and the abductor halluces must be released to obtain complete correction. If associated with bony deformities of the distal phalanx (Fig. 4.6-2), an osteotomy is required to prevent recurrence of the deformity.

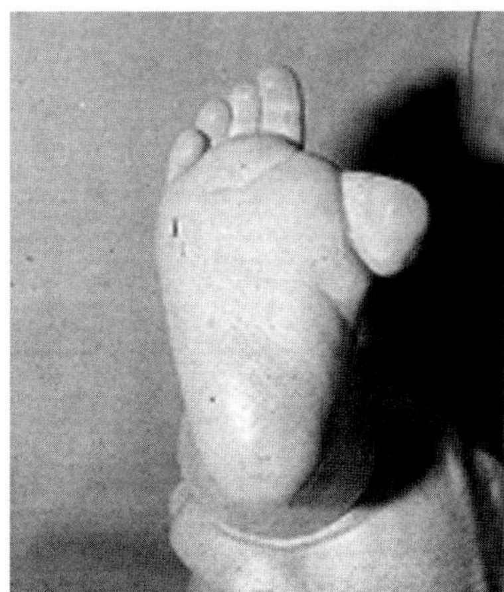

Figure 4.6-1 Primary congenital hallux varus.

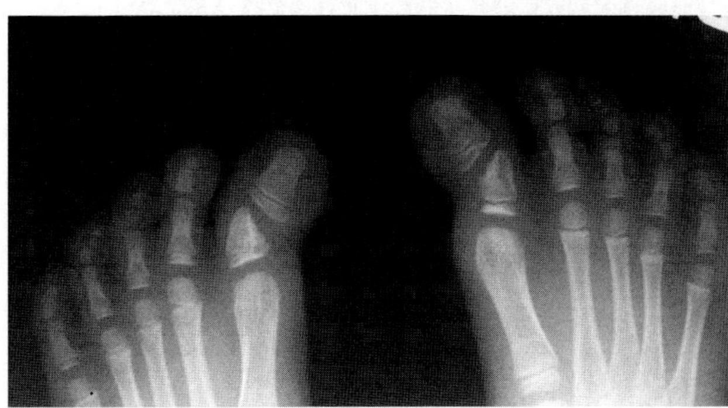

Figure 4.6-2 Joint deformity in residual secondary congenital hallux varus.

Congenital Hallux Valgus

Congenital hallux valgus, the result of deformity of the distal phalanx of the great toe, is deviated laterally toward the second toe at the interphalangeal joint (Fig. 4.6-3). It is

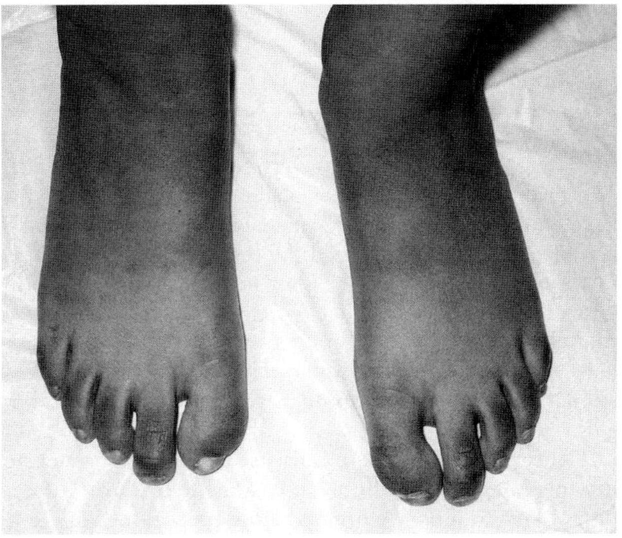

Figure 4.6-3 Congenital hallux valgus—deformity at interphalangeal joint.

associated with syndromes and is also seen in neurologic conditions such as cerebral palsy. Treatment is indicated with severe deformities that result in callus and nail problems. In the younger individual, a wedge resection of the proximal phalanx is done to realign the toe. In the older child, an interphalangeal joint fusion is required because of the adaptive changes that occur at the interphalangeal joint.

PROBLEMS OF THE LESSER TOES

Mallet Toe

Mallet toe is a result of a flexion deformity of the distal interphalangeal joint and usually involves a single toe. It is usually asymptomatic in young children, but can become painful in adolescence with shoe wear leading to corns as the toe strikes the sole of the shoe. In infancy treatment consists of stretching and adhesive strapping to the adjacent toes. Sectioning of the long flexor can treat more severe deformities, especially on the second or third toe if the deformity is still flexible. A fusion of the distal interphalangeal joint is required in the mature foot with a rigid deformity.

Congenital Hammertoe

Congenital hammertoe is a flexion deformity of the proximal interphalangeal joint. Hammertoe deformity is congenital in origin and often familial. It will often become symptomatic by causing pressure on the dorsum of the toe by the shoe. Treatment in the infant consists of stretching exercises in conjunction with adhesive strapping in corrected position. Flexor tendon transfer can be done in a flexible deformity in the preadolescent and adolescent. Any fixed deformity requires fusion of the interphalangeal joint. A flexor tenotomy is also required in the rigid deformity.

Claw Toe Deformities

Claw toe deformities are the result of muscle imbalance. The distal and proximal interphalangeal joints are hyperflexed and the metatarsophalangeal joint is hyperextended and often dorsally subluxated. All toes are usually involved in contrast to a mallet toe. Claw toes are associated with cavus feet seen in neurologic conditions such as Charcot-Marie-Tooth disease, cerebral palsy, and polio; or as residuals of compartment syndrome. The condition is listed as idiopathic only after a thorough search for known etiologies.

Conservative treatment consists of orthotics to elevate the metatarsal heads. Surgical treatment requires correction of any hindfoot deformity before proceeding with correction of the forefoot. Flexor tendon transfer to the dorsum of the toe (Girdlestone-Taylor procedure) along with extensor tenotomies and metatarsophalangeal joint capsulotomy are used in flexible deformities. In fixed deformities, a resection of the distal proximal phalanx with extensive dorsal capsulotomies is preferred. The proximal interphalangeal joint is fixed with a Kirschner wire for 6 weeks to maintain alignment while soft tissue healing occurs and stabilizes the digit. In the great toe, the Jones procedure and arthrodesis of the interphalangeal joint and a transfer of the extensor hallucis longus to the first metatarsal is used to align the toe.

Macrodactyly or Gigantism

This is often a manifestation of a generalized disease such as neurofibromatosis, hemangiomatosis, lipomatosis, and arteriovenous fistula. It can be part of the Proteus syndrome and Klippel-Trenaunay-Weber syndrome. Localized gigantism most frequently involves the second and third toes and the accompanying metatarsal. The soft tissue is enlarged with tissue of the primary disease. Magnetic resonance imaging can be used to distinguish localized macrodystrophia lipomatosis from other conditions causing local gigantism. In lipomatosis there is an increase in fibrofatty tissue, bony hypertrophy, and fatty infiltration of muscle. In neurofibromatosis there is fibrofatty infiltration of neural fascicles.

Surgical treatment requires evaluation of toe deformity as well as the systemic disease associated with it. The major objective of surgery is to reduce the size of the foot to improve function and cosmesis. For a single toe, early epiphysiodesis can be used to control some of the growth. Epiphysiodesis is unpredictable and resection of middle or distal phalanx is often indicated to shorten the digit. Amputation or ray resection is indicated for severe enlargement, multiple previous failed procedures, and in the insensate toe. Amputation of a toe should be exercised with care in localized gigantism as secondary deformities have been described. Amputation of the second toe may lead to development of hallux valgus. In some cases, partial toe amputation can help with shoe wear. Complications such as skin necrosis, infection, and recurrence are common.

Congenital Curly Toe

Congenital curly toe is the most common congenital deformity of the lesser toes (Fig. 4.6-4). It is usually bilateral and has a high familial incidence. It commonly involves the lateral three toes. The toe is deviated medially under the adjacent medial toe. It is considered to be secondary to a hypoplasia of the intrinsic muscles. Curly toe is usually asymptomatic. In the infant, strapping has been found ineffective. Severe deformities can be treated either by a tenotomy of the flexion digitorum longus and flexus digitorum brevis or a Girdlestone-Taylor tendon transfer. Contracted deformity will often require an osteotomy of the phalanx. In contrast to congenital overlapping toe, surgery is less frequent, but still requires special attention to the available skin.

Congenital Overlapping of the Fifth Toe

Congenital overlapping (digitus minimus varus) is commonly seen with the fifth toe overlapping the fourth toe.

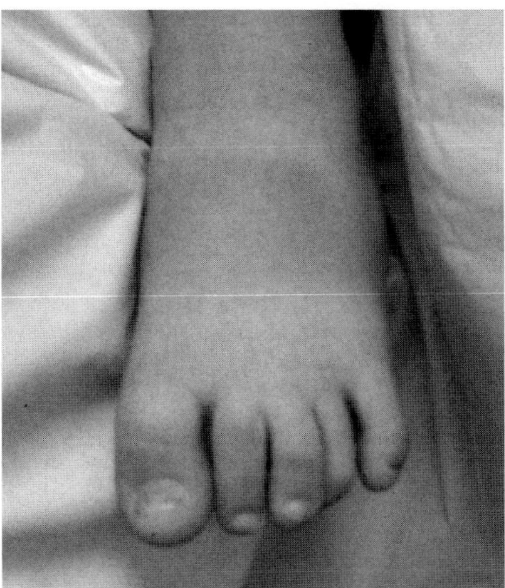

Figure 4.6-4 Congenital curly toe (fourth toe).

There is dorsiflexion of the metatarsus phalangeal joint with abduction external rotation of the digit (Fig. 4.6-5). The condition is usually bilateral and is also familial. In contrast to congenital curly toe, this condition is symptomatic and can cause problems with shoe wear. Early treatment requires stretching of the medial ligaments and structures and the dorsal medial capsule. Taping is done in the correct position. Surgery, however, is the definitive treatment. Lengthening of the extensor tendons and dorsal and plantar capsulotomies are often required. The skin incision must be carefully planned as it is also contracted. Amputation is not recommended because it results in pain and pressure on the metatarsal head.

Polydactyly

Polydactyly refers to supernumerary digits of the foot. Postaxial (fibular) polydactyly is transmitted as an autosomal dominant trait and may be associated with polydactyly of the hand. It is more common in African Americans, occurring at a rate as high as 1 in 100. Preaxial polydactyly occurs on the tibial side and is more common among Caucasians. Morphologically, polydactyly may present as:

- A redundant soft tissue mass that is devoid of bone and cartilage
- A duplication of the digit or part of the digit that articulates with a hypotrophic metatarsal or bifid metatarsal
- A complete duplication of the digit with its own metatarsal

Surgical treatment is indicated for difficulty in fitting and wearing shoes. The optimum age for surgery is 9 to 12 months, when the child is beginning to walk. Two principles are important in performing any surgery on a multidigited foot:

- Maintenance of the normal contour of the foot
- Restoration of normal muscle ligament and tendon insertions. The most lateral and medial digit is usually ablated

The duplicated phalanx is usually excised and its accompanying metatarsal can be narrowed if the head is too large or duplicated.

On the medial side, adequate soft tissue and bone must be removed. Polydactyly of the first ray is often accompanied by congenital hallux varus and a bracket epiphysis. Excision of the medial ray, lengthening of the abductor, and plication of the adductor into the metatarsophalangeal capsule of the first ray is recommended. If there is significant accompanying varus of the first ray, syndactylization of the first and second toes may be necessary.

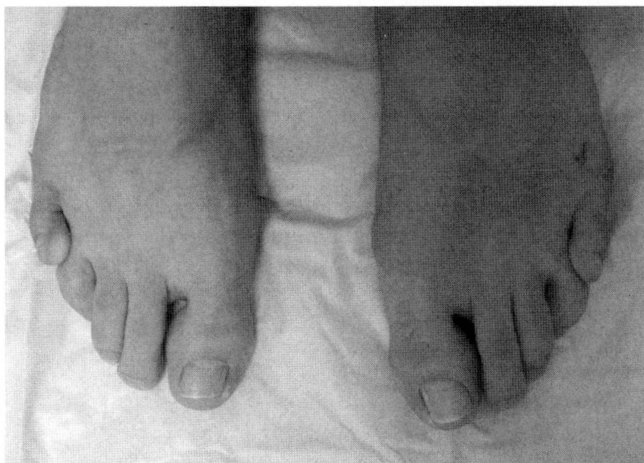

Figure 4.6-5 Congenital overlapping fifth toe.

Syndactyly

Congenital webbing of the toes does not usually lead to a functional problem. It is most common between the second and third toes. It is ten times more common in whites than blacks and may be associated with polydactyly, brachydactyly, phalangeal fusion, and annular bands. It can be seen as an isolated anomaly or as part of a syndrome. Surgery is rarely indicated, but when it is necessary, the same principles and techniques for surgical separation of syndactyly of the hand apply.

Temtamy and McKusick classified isolated syndactyly into five types. These three are seen in the feet:

- Zygodactyly—complete or partial webbing to the nail base
- Synpolydactyly—syndactyly of latter two toes and polydactyly of the fifth within the syndactyly
- Syndactyly with metatarsal fusion

Syndactyly may be a predominant feature in Poland syndrome, Apert syndrome, and other forms of acrocephalosyndactyly. It is an occasional feature in chromosomal abnormalities such as Down syndrome, trisomy 18, and Cri-du-Chat syndrome. Syndactyly is also seen in Möbius, Silver, Cornelia de Lange, and Prader-Willi syndromes.

Treatment is indicated because shoe fitting is often a problem and peers often ridicule children with webbed feet. In the foot, treatment is indicated in syndactyly associated with polydactyly and fusion of the metatarsals. Treatment is aimed at reconstruction of the commissure and reconstruction of the digits. The incision is never linear and consists of a series of flaps with use of skin graft where necessary.

Toenail Problems

Ingrown toenail problems in children are rare and are due to hypertrophy of the nail folds, hypertrophy of the nail bed, and hypertrophy of the distal pulp. Hypertrophy of the lateral nail folds results in tissue overgrowth over the nail and occludes the nail groove. In resistant cases, a resection of 50% of the nail and resection of lateral nail wall usually solves the problem. In severe cases wedge resections of the lateral nail fold can open up the nail groove. In the infant, the nail can be so sharp that it can grow directly into a hypertrophied distal pulp. Massaging the bulbous tip underneath the nail is sometimes useful and its recurrence can be prevented by the use of appropriate size shoes and socks. Some genetic disorders with nail changes are the *nail–patella syndrome* characterized by lunula, and atrophy of the nail. A dislocating hypoplastic patella, iliac horns, hypermobility, and dislocated radial heads also characterize this autosomal dominant condition. *Darier disease* is an autosomal dominant condition with distal subungual wedge-shaped keratosis, red and white longitudinal striations, and thinning of the nail bed. *Pachyonychia congenita* is characterized by massive hypertrophy of the nail plates with a brown and yellowish discoloration. It is also an autosomal dominant condition. *Dyskeratosis congenita* is an X-linked recessive or autosomal dominant condition with atrophy of the nail plate and ridges and fusion of the proximal nail fold. *Deafness, onycho-osteodystrophy, mental retardation (DOOR) syndrome* is an autosomal recessive disorder with anonychia or atrophied nails.

ASSOCIATED ANOMALIES

Congenital toe anomalies are seen with other syndromes and other conditions. *Congenital short metatarsal* or *brachymetatarsia, Streeter syndrome* or *multiple congenital bands*, and a *congenital split* or *cleft foot (lobster claw)* deserve special mention. *Congenital short metatarsal* is not uncommon. It is usually bilateral and more common in females. When more than one metatarsal is involved, it is known as brachymetapodia. The etiology is thought to be a premature close of the physis. It has been found in association with Down syndrome, Albright disease, pseudohypoparathyroidism, and multiple epiphyseal dysplasias. The fourth metatarsal is most commonly involved. When affecting the first metatarsal, the condition is known as metatarsus primus atavicus, and is often associated with congenital hallux varus. Congenital shortening of the third and fourth metatarsal usually requires no treatment. Metatarsal lengthening is difficult, has many complications, and is not recommended for cosmesis. Lengthening of the first metatarsal should not exceed 36% of the original length.

Congenital lobster claw or *cleft foot* is a deformity in which the central three rays are dysplastic or absent and the phalanges of the remaining toes are deviated to the center of the foot. The hindfoot is normal. This rare condition is usually bilateral and inherited as an autosomal dominant trait. The gene has been mapped to the long arm of chromosome 7. It can occur as an isolated deformity, but more typically is associated with other anomalies such as cleft hand, cleft lip, syndactyly, and triphalangeal thumb. Surgery to realign the divergent toes and metatarsals and narrow the foot is indicated to facilitate shoe wear. Abraham's classification is simple and his results in 32 feet in 16 patients were satisfactory. Treatment is as follows:

- Type 1, central partial forefoot is treated by syndactylism and partial hallux valgus correction, if needed.
- Type 2, a complete forefoot cleft to the tarsus requires syndactylism, and first ray osteotomy is performed before age 5. If after age 5, first ray amputation is advised.
- Type 3, complete absence of the first through fourth ray, does not need forefoot surgery.

CONGENITAL CONSTRICTION BAND SYNDROME

Streeter Dysplasia

Streeter dysplasia is a spectrum of deformities thought to be secondary to a rupture of the amnion and results in bands of tissue that wrap around the fetus' extremities *in utero*. Four types of constriction band deformities are described:

- A simple ring around the limb or digit
- A deeper ring often associated with abnormalities of the distal limb and lymphedema
- Fenestrated syndactyly or acrosyndactyly
- Intrauterine amputations

Distal rings are more common, as is involvement of the central digits.

Treatment is indicated in the deep rings that cause interference with circulation. If the ring is circumferential, a staged procedure relaxing half the band at a time is preferred. The ring is excised down to normal tissue and multiple Z-plasties are performed to ensure adequate skin coverage. Acrosyndactyly should be treated early because all the digits are fused at the tip and can result in deformities if left untreated.

SUGGESTED READING

Abraham E, Waxman B, Shirali S, et al. Congenital cleft-foot deformity treatment. J Pediatr Orthop 1999;19:404–410.

Bamvorth JS. Amniotic band sequence: Streeter's hypothesis reexamined. Am J Med Genet 1992;44:280–287.

Caldwell BD. Genetics of split hand and split foot: a case study. J Am Podiatr Med Assoc 1996;86:244–248.

Coughlin MJ, Mann RA. Lesser toe deformities. AAOS Instruct Course Lect 1987;36:137–160.

Honig PJ, Spitzer A, Bernstein R, et al. Congenital ingrown toenails: clinical significance. Clin Pediatr 1982;21:424–426.

Jay RM. Pediatric foot and ankle surgery. Philadelphia: WB Saunders, 1999.

Ruby L, Goldberg MJ. Syndactyly and polydactyly. Orthop Clin North Am 1976;7:361–374.

Steedman JT, Peterson HA. Brachymetatarsia of the first metatarsal treated by surgical lengthening. J Pediatr Orthop 1992;12: 780–785.

Sweetman R. Congenital curley toe: an investigation into the value of treatment. Lancet 1968;2:398.

Temtamy SA, McKusick VT. The Genetics of Hand Malformations; Birth Defects: Original Article Series. 14(3):I-xviii. 1–619,1978.

Topoleski TA, Ganel A, Grogan DP. Effect of proximal phalangeal epiphysiodesis in the treatment of macrodactyly. Foot Ankle Int 1997;18;500–503.

Turra S, Santini S, Cagnoni G, et al. Gigantism of the foot: our experience in seven cases. J Pediatr Orthop 1998;18;337–345.

Urano Y, Kobayashi A. Bone lengthening for shortness of the fourth toe. J. Bone Joint Surg 1978;60A:91–93.

Venn-Watson E. Problems in polydactyly of the foot. Orthop Clin North Am 1976;7:909–927.

DEVELOPMENTAL DYSPLASIA OF THE HIP

RUSSELL J. CRIDER

Developmental dysplasia of the hip (DDH) refers to an abnormal configuration of, or relationship between, the femoral head and the acetabulum. It is a continuum of disorders that ranges from shallowness of the acetabulum, to instability and subluxation of the femoral head, to frank dislocation. The term *development dysplasia of the hip* has replaced the former term "congenital dislocation of the hip" (CDH) to acknowledge that the disorder may not be present at birth, and can change or progress with growth and development.

PATHOGENESIS

The classification of DDH is listed in Table 5-1.

Teratologic Type

The teratologic type of DDH is rare, often includes malformation of the components of the hip joint, and is usually associated with a syndrome such as arthrogryposis or Larsen's syndrome. It is thought to be secondary to an underlying "germ plasm" defect.

Typical Type

Perinatal positioning contributes to the etiology of the typical form of DDH. A strong hereditary component is also known; first-degree relatives of a person with DDH have a much higher incidence than the general population. The persistence of maternal relaxin hormone in the infant's bloodstream at the time of birth has been implicated in DDH, but recent studies have not supported this theory.

EPIDEMIOLOGY

The rate of DDH in the general population in North America and Europe is approximately 0.15% (i.e., 1.5 per 1,000). A positive family history increases the incidence of DDH approximately 35 times. Girls are more frequently affected than boys by a ratio of approximately 4 to 1. The left hip is more frequently involved. Breech presentation increases the incidence of DDH to approximately 20%. Some cultures, including certain Native Americans and Laplanders, have a markedly high rate of DDH, but this increased incidence is probably due to positioning in traditional infant swaddling, rather than to a genetic predisposition.

TABLE 5-1 CLASSIFICATION OF DEVELOPMENTAL DYSPLASIA OF THE HIP

Classification	Description
Teratologic	Dysplasia due to primary malformation of the femoral head or acetabulum
Typical	Dysplasia caused by factors allowing the dislocation or subluxation of a hip with relatively normal formed components
Subluxed	The femoral head is not dislocated from the acetabulum but is not concentrically reduced (i.e., there is some contact between the cartilage of the acetabulum and the femoral head)
Dislocatable	The hip is reduced, but can be dislocated by certain maneuvers
Dislocated	There is no contact between the cartilage of the femoral head and the acetabulum; the femoral head is completely out of the acetabulum

PATHOPHYSIOLOGY

Teratologic Type

The acetabulum is frequently plate-like in nature, the femoral head broad, and the femoral neck quite anteverted.

Typical Type

The early manifestations of hip dislocation include:

- Increased fat in the depths of the acetabulum
- A tight iliopsoas muscle
- Capsular constriction at the mouth of the acetabulum
- Anteversion of the femoral neck
- Decreased depth of the acetabulum
- Hypertrophy of the transverse ligament
- Hypertrophy of the ligamentum teres
- The development of a neolimbus.

The longer the hip is left unreduced, the more pronounced the aforementioned changes become.

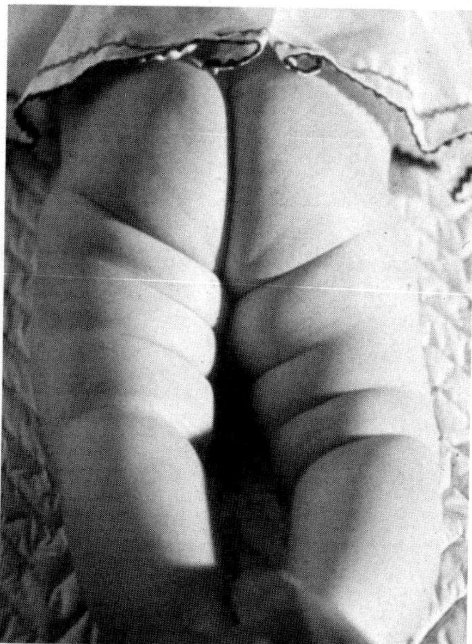

Figure 5-1 Asymmetry of the thigh folds due to a dislocated left hip.

DIAGNOSIS

Breech or footling position at the time of delivery indicates increased risk for DDH. Also, a history of other family members with DDH is significant.

PHYSICAL EXAMINATION

Clinical Features (Box 5-1)

During the physical exam, the infant should be comfortable and relaxed (feeding can be helpful). Initially, inspection of the child is carried out so that any asymmetry in the number of thigh folds anteriorly and posteriorly (Fig. 5-1), flexion deformities, or spinal deformities can be noted. The height of the knees with the knees and hips flexed at 90 degrees is observed (Galeazzi sign; Fig. 5-2). In a child with a posteriorly subluxed or dislocated hip, the femur is functionally shortened, thus the knee on the affected side will appear lower. This is also the reason for the increased thigh folds: the normal length musculature of the thigh bunches up around the "short" femur.

The two tests, the Ortolani and Barlow, are then performed. These should be done with the baby fully undressed, on a relatively firm surface to provide the necessary resistance.

BOX 5-1 CLINICAL FEATURES OF DEVELOPMENTAL DYSPLASIA OF THE HIP

Suggestive Signs
- Decreased abduction (less than 60 degrees)
- Asymmetry of thigh folds (anteriorly and posteriorly)
- Positive Galeazzi sign (Fig. 5-2)

Diagnostic Signs
- Positive Ortolani sign[a]
- Positive Barlow sign[a]

[a]Since the signs depend upon the relocation of the dislocated or dislocatable hip they gradually become negative; by the age of 6 months they can rarely be elicited. They may also be negative in irreducibly dislocated hips.

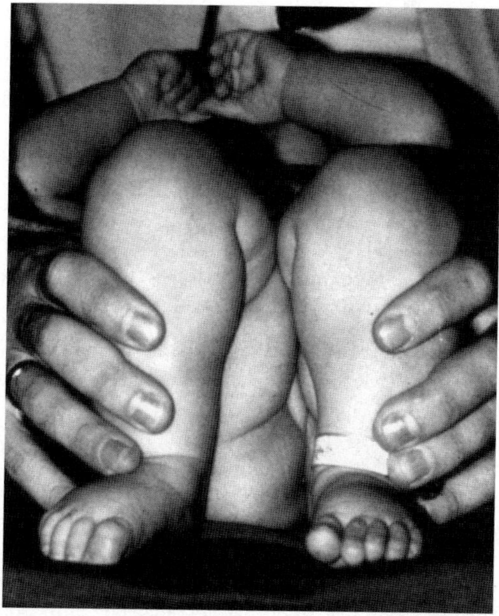

Figure 5-2 A positive Galeazzi sign indicating apparent shortening of the left femur due to a dislocated hip.

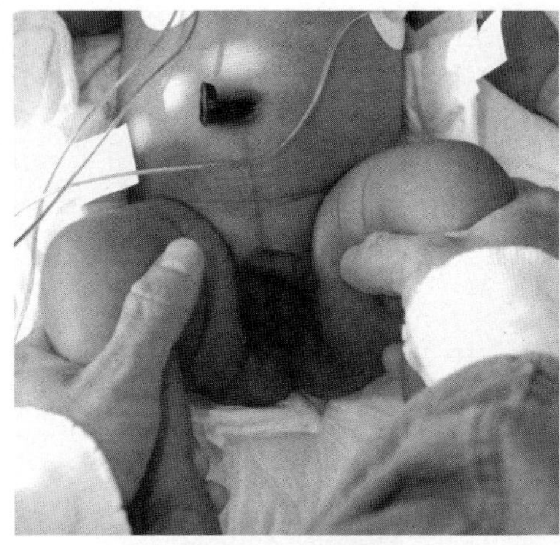
A

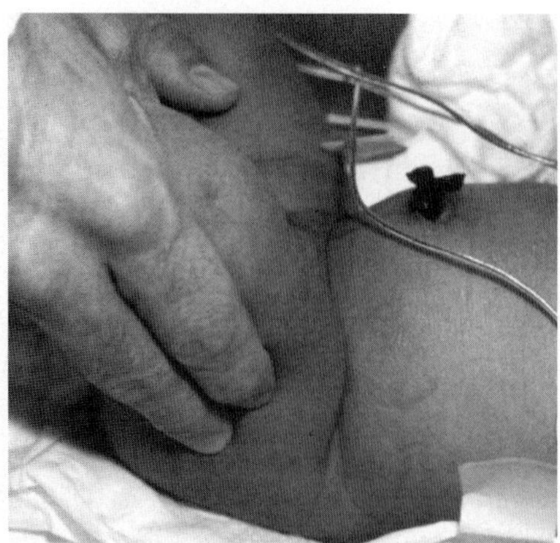
B

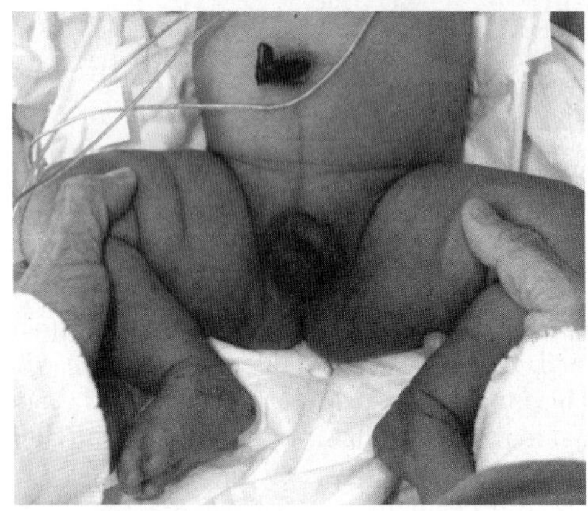
C

Figure 5-3 Appropriate way of examining a newborn's hip. One hand is holding the hip and pelvis stable (**A**) and the other hand is performing the maneuvers (**B**). (**C**) The middle finger is placed on the greater trochanter to detect a shift in position as seen in an Ortolani or Barlow sign.

Ortolani Test

- The examiner holds the patient's flexed lower extremity so that the thumb is on the internal aspect of the thigh, the patient's knee is in the thenar web space, and the examiner's index or middle finger is placed over the greater trochanter (Fig. 5-3).
- The hips are then gently abducted, one at a time, with anterior pressure on the greater trochanter.
- A positive Ortolani sign is a palpable shift in position (clunk) of the hip with the initial abduction of the hip.

Barlow Test

- The hip is brought into adduction with gentle posterior pressure, and the Ortolani maneuver is repeated.

A positive Ortolani test indicates a dislocated hip, whereas a negative Ortolani test and a positive Barlow test indicate a dislocatable hip.

One should also note the amount of full abduction of the hip and the amount of adduction at which the hip re-dislocates (this approximates the "safe zone"; Fig. 5-4). Some signs are more specific for DDH than others (i.e., suggestive signs) as indicated in Box 5-1.

In the child older than 6 months to 1 year, the Ortolani and Barlow signs are likely to be negative, but the functional leg length discrepancy in a unilateral dislocation will manifest as a limp or toe-walking on the affected side. If both hips are dislocated, the older child will tend to walk with a waddle, have decreased abduction bilaterally, and have an increased lumbar lordosis. In the child over 6 months of age, decreased abduction bilaterally (less than 60 degrees) might be the only sign of bilateral dislocations of the hips and should be investigated with x-ray studies. Another indicator of bilateral abnormality is the Klisic line. This is a line extrapolated through the greater trochanter and anterior superior iliac spine. It should fall

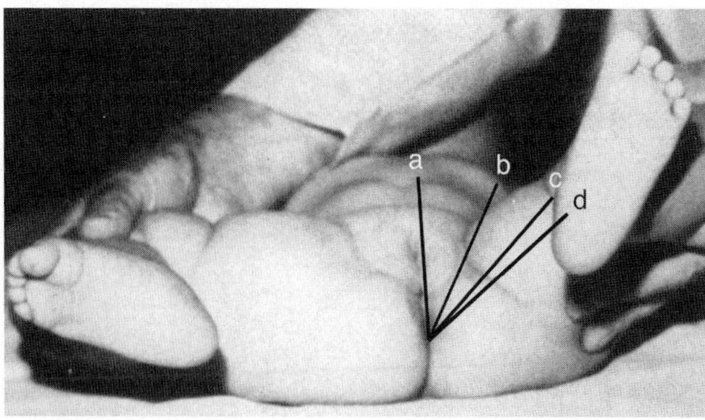

Figure 5-4 The angle a–d represents full abduction of the hip, angle a–c is 10 degrees less than full abduction, and angle a–b is the abduction at which the hip re-dislocates. The angle b–c is the "safe zone."

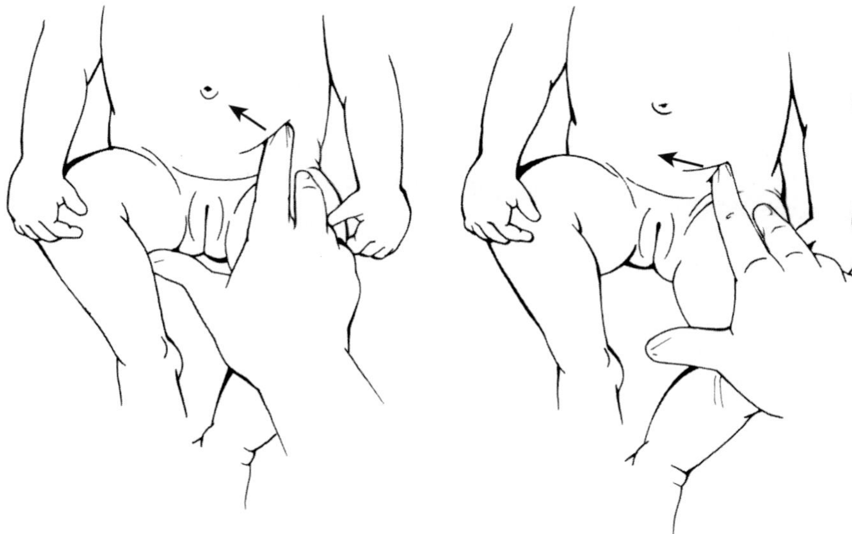

Figure 5-5 Klisic line test.

through or superior to the umbilicus and is independent of the contralateral side. If the Klisic line falls inferior to the umbilicus, this indicates a possible posterior subluxation/dislocation (Fig. 5-5).

RADIOGRAPHIC FEATURES

Ultrasound

The ultrasound examination of the hips is most valuable prior to the appearance of the ossific nucleus of the femoral head at the age of 4 to 6 months. There are frequent false-positives in newborns younger than 2 weeks of age, and because of this many ultrasonographers prefer to obtain the initial study at 4 to 6 weeks of age. Though routine ultrasound screening of all newborns is the norm in some parts of Europe, it is not currently the standard in the United States. In the United States ultrasonography (US) is generally used to evaluate cases in which there is a high-risk history or abnormal or equivocal physical exam. It can also be used to evaluate the results of treatment with a Pavlic harness, and to help determine when it is safe to terminate the Pavlic treatment.

Two methods of hip US evaluation are used, and it is important to know which one your ultrasonographer uses in order to interpret the results. The Graf method is a static exam of the hip in the coronal plane, and uses the relationship of the bony and cartilaginous components of the hip joint to describe a variety of angles, which can be followed over time (Fig. 5-6). The Harcke method is a dynamic exam which evaluates instability of the hip joint.

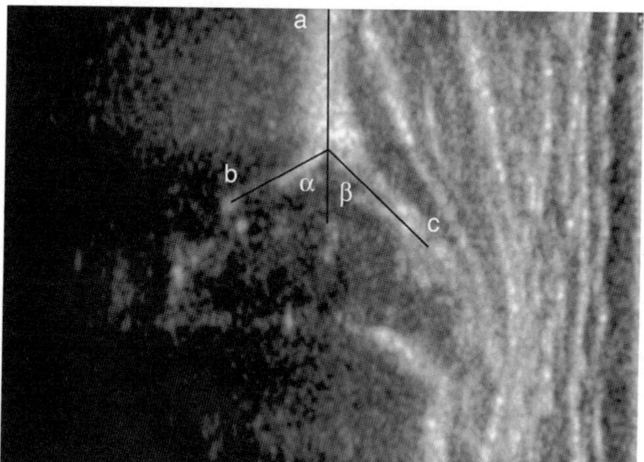

Figure 5-6 A normal static ultrasound picture is present with the α-angle (*a–b*) showing acetabular bony coverage more than 60 degrees and the β-angle (*a–c*) indicating the cartilaginous coverage of more than 55 degrees. Line *a* indicates the iliac ring.

Plain Radiography

The anteroposterior (AP) pelvic x-ray is useful after the formation of the secondary ossific nucleus of the proximal femur (Box 5-2).

- Acetabular angle (AI): Normal is less than 30 degrees. Newborns typically have an AI of about 40 degrees. In

BOX 5-2 X-RAY SIGNS OF DEVELOPMENTAL DYSPLASIA OF THE HIP

- Acetabular angle (acetabular index) less than 30 degrees
- Break in Shenton's line
- Ossific nucleus not in lower inner quadrant
- Decrease of center-edge angle of Wiberg (in children older than 6 years)
- Distortion of the acetabular teardrop
- Increased femoral metaphyseal–acetabular teardrop distance
- Change in normal sourcil

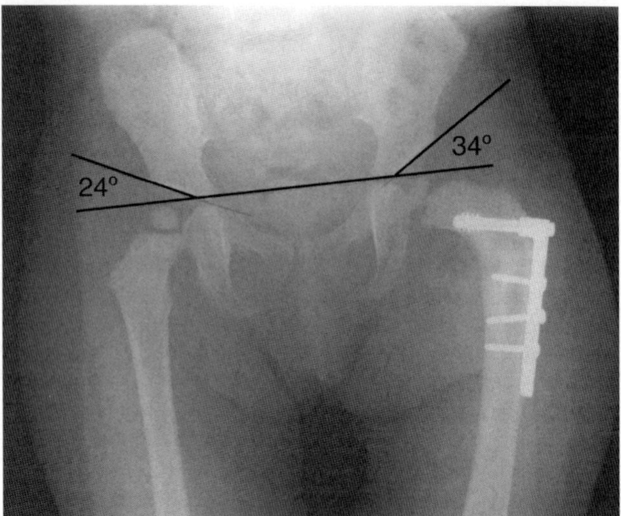

Figure 5-7 The hip is concentrically reduced after a femoral osteotomy and the acetabular angle is improved, but not below 30 degrees. The patient will probably require a pelvic osteotomy.

concentrically reduced hips, the AI should decrease about 1.5 degrees per month (Fig. 5-7).

- Shenton's line: The curved line drawn from the inferior femoral neck to the superior aspect of the obturator foramen in the normal hip. This sign indicates no subluxation is present if the arc is unbroken (Fig. 5-8).
- Quadrants: Four quadrants are formed by the conjunction of the horizontal line of Hilgenreiner and the perpendicular line of Perkins. The reduced femoral head resides in the lower inner quadrant (see Fig. 5-8).

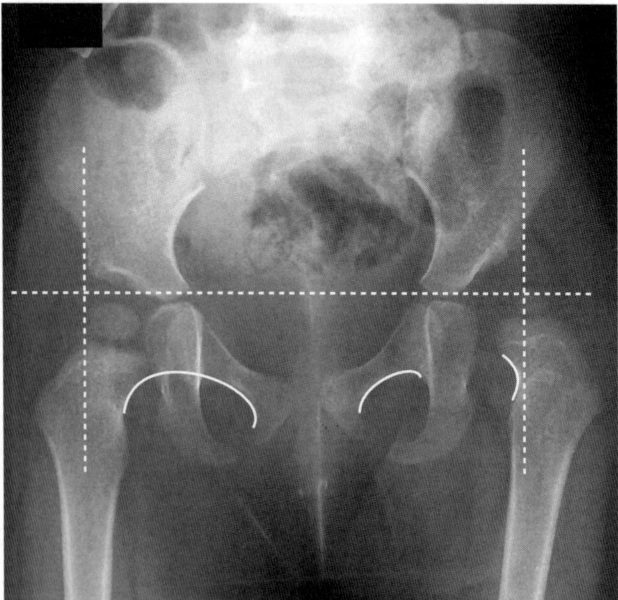

Figure 5-8 Dislocation of the left hip is present. The dashed lines reveal that the femoral head is outside and lower in the quadrant. The curved lines at right reveal a break in the Shenton's line.

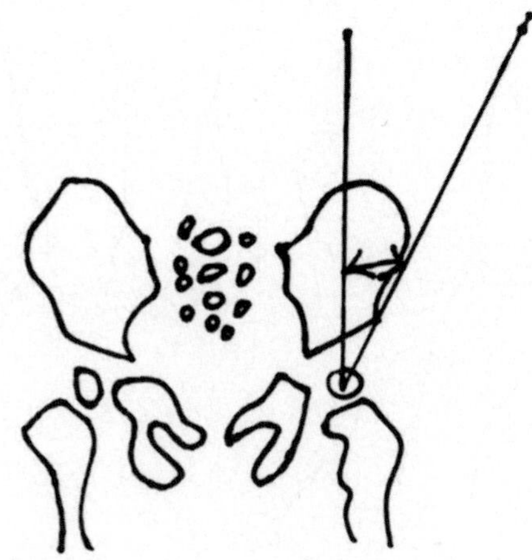

Figure 5-9 The center-edge angle of Wiberg.

- Center-edge angle of Wiberg: In children older than 6 years, the center of the femoral head is located on an AP x-ray and a line is drawn vertically from this point. Another line is drawn to the superior edge of the bony acetabulum and the angle formed by these lines is recorded (Fig. 5-9).

TREATMENT

Since the acetabulum and femoral head grow and develop in response to each other when in the reduced position, the principles of treatment of DDH can be summarized as follows: The goal of the treatment of DDH is to obtain and maintain, as early as possible, a concentric reduction of the hip without force and by avoiding extremes of position. The modes of treatment discussed in the subsequent paragraphs are simply means to achieve this goal depending on the patient's age.

Birth to 6 Months

The hip can frequently be reduced gently and held in a stable abducted position with the use of the Pavlic harness. There is a 90% to 95% success rate using this device. It must be applied properly and the parents must be instructed in its care. The body strap is positioned immediately below the nipple line, the anterior flexion strap lies in front of the knee, and the posterior abduction strap is loose to allow the baby some active motion while limiting adduction to maintain the reduction while the soft tissues contract and stabilize the hip. The hips are flexed to about 100 degrees (Fig. 5-10). The Pavlic harness has been shown to stabilize reduction in 85% of hips within 2 to 3 weeks. If, after 3 weeks of use, the hip is not reduced on ultrasound, the use of the harness should be discontinued to prevent complications and plans should be made for a closed reduction arthrogram and spica casting under general anesthesia. Complications of the use of the harness are enumerated in Box 5-3.

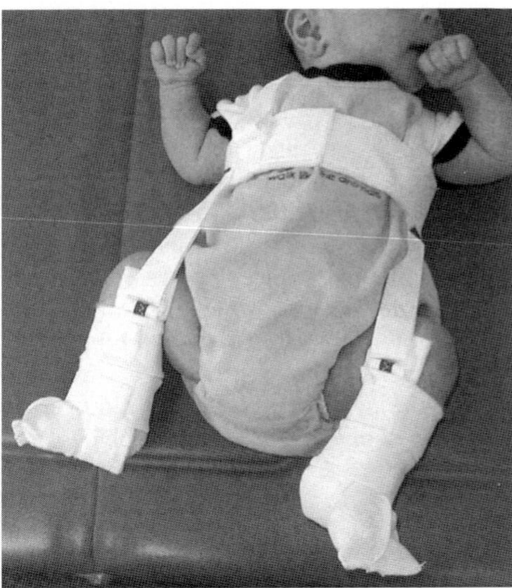

Figure 5-10 The proper positioning of the straps of the Pavlic harness with the anterior straps against the medial aspect of the thigh producing sustained flexion of about 100 degrees, but no more. The posterior straps remain somewhat loose.

BOX 5-3 COMPLICATIONS OF USE OF THE PAVLIC HARNESS IN DEVELOPMENTAL DYSPLASIA OF THE HIP

- Inferior subluxation caused by too much flexion
- Femoral nerve palsy caused by too much flexion
- Skin breakdown caused by lack of skin care
- Cartilage damage or AVN caused by excessively tight straps or continued use after 3 weeks of nonreduction of the hip

If, after 3 weeks, the hip is reduced, use of the harness is continued until the physical examination and ultrasound examination of the hips are within normal limits. A very rough rule of the thumb is that the harness needs to be used for the total time of the sum of the patient's age at the beginning of treatment plus 6 weeks (i.e., if an infant is 3 weeks old at the onset of treatment, the harness should be used for about 3 weeks plus 6 weeks, for a total of 9 weeks).

The safe zone is defined as the arc of hip motion from a few degrees less than full abduction to the point of dislocation on adduction. Immobilization in full abduction can cause avascular necrosis and should be avoided, whereas dislocation results from too little abduction. Thus, the safe zone is between these extremes (see Fig. 5-4). The smaller the safe zone in an individual patient, the more difficult the hip is to treat successfully nonoperatively.

Age 6 to 18 Months

Children are generally too big for treatment with a Pavlic harness in this age group. Traditionally, skin traction has been used to gradually and gently pull the femoral head distally so that it descends past the superior edge of the acetabulum allowing a closed reduction to be performed without excessive force, thus resulting in a lower incidence of avascular necrosis (AVN). Traction can be performed at home, if the facilities exist, but must be checked frequently since skin complications and compartment syndromes are not unusual. A percutaneous adductor tenotomy is usually employed to assist in this treatment by improving the safe zone.

Many pediatric orthopedists have found that the routine skin traction is not necessary to safely reduce the hip in this group, and elect to perform a percutaneous adductor tenotomy, a hip arthrogram (Fig. 5-11), and gentle closed reduction under general anesthesia, followed by the maintenance of this reduction in a double hip spica cast in the

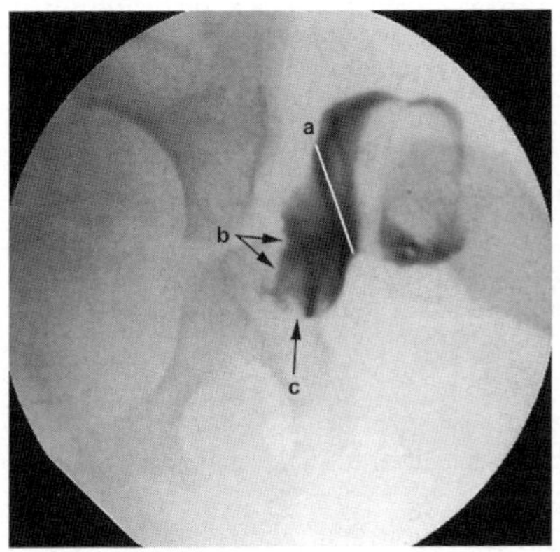

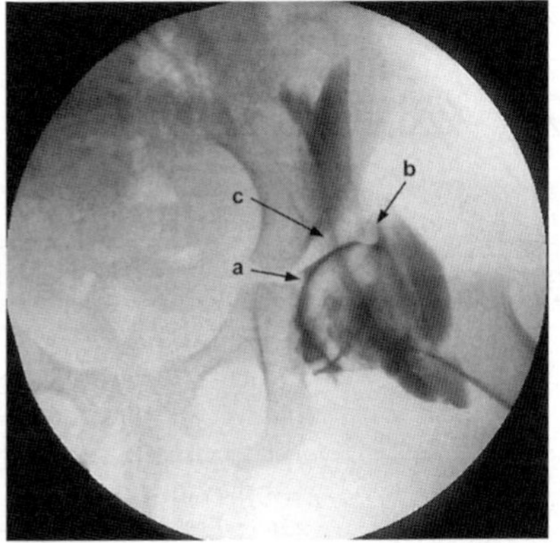

Figure 5-11 (A) Arthrogram revealing narrowing of the capsule at the entrance of the acetabulum (a), medial soft tissue filling the acetabulum (b), and transverse acetabular ligament, which could possibly inhibit concentric reduction (c). (B) With abduction and internal rotation, there is a slight bit of medial dye-pooling (a), good coverage although the labrum is somewhat blunted (b). Dye is extravasated into the iliopsoas tendon sheath (c).

BOX 5-4 CRITERIA INDICATING FAVORABLE PROGNOSIS FOR FUTURE HIP DEVELOPMENT AFTER CLOSED REDUCTION OF DEVELOPMENTAL DYSPLASIA OF THE HIP[a]

- Shenton line essentially intact
- Acetabular angle less than 30 degrees
- Less than 2-mm difference between the teardrop distances
- Femoral head in lower inner quadrant

[a]When these criteria are met, closed treatment may be discontinued but continued follow-up is essential.

"human position" (abduction of about 45 degrees and flexion of about 100 degrees). A postoperative computed tomography scan is usually necessary to confirm concentric reduction in the hip spica cast. Spica casting is continued for 6 weeks to 6 months, with periodic changes, and a plastic abduction brace is used at least until the child is walking, and usually until the standing AP x-ray of the hips is within normal limits. Treatment is discontinued if the criteria in Box 5-4 are met.

If closed reduction fails, adductor tenotomy, arthrogram, and open reduction must be performed. Although European studies have suggested that an open reduction has a lower incidence of AVN after the appearance of the ossific nucleus (at about 6 months of age) this observation has not been borne out in other literature, and the timing of surgery remains somewhat controversial. If open reduction is required in a child under the age of 12 months, a medial approach (Ludloff, Staheli) or anterior-medial approach (Ponseti-Weinstein) can be performed. I prefer the traditional anterior approach (Smith-Petersen), since it affords visualization of the entire femoral head and acetabulum and plication of the capsule can be done to ensure stability of the hip. A "bikini" incision is used, since this incision is cosmetically pleasing. In children over the age of 1 year, the medial approach has a higher complication rate and is not recommended.

If the reduction in a walking position is not maintained in children between 12 and 18 months of age, a femoral osteotomy or pelvic osteotomy can be performed. A variety of pelvic osteotomies may be employed. Femoral and pelvic osteotomies can also be used together (Box 5-5). In the child older than 2 to 3 years of age, a femoral shortening should be performed in addition to the open reduction and femoral or pelvic osteotomies, in order to minimize the risk of AVN. In the child older than age 6 years, a unilateral dislocation will require an open reduction, femoral shortening (with varus de-rotation as needed), adductor release, iliopsoas release, and acetabular procedure such as a Salter osteotomy (less than 8 years). In the child over 8 years, a triple (Steele) or double (Southerland) pelvic osteotomy, or a shelf procedure (e.g., Staheli) should be used. If the growth plates are closed, a Chiari, Wagner, Dial (Eppright), triple, or double pelvic osteotomy can be performed in addition to the soft tissue releases, femoral shortening, and varus derotation osteotomy. The use of native cartilage is theoretically preferable to cover the femoral head (e.g., Salter, triple osteotomy) rather than relying on the development of fibrocartilage (e.g., Chiari).

In bilaterally dislocated hips in an older child (8 to 10 years of age), the option of no treatment should be considered. These patients frequently have a relatively pain-free existence up to the age of about 50 years of age and the risks of surgical treatment are considerable.

The surgical treatment of the teratologic hip dislocation carries a complication rate of about 50% including re-dislocation and AVN. Therefore, one should consider not treating these hips, depending upon the patient's overall health and functional status. The signs and symptoms of untreated DDH are outlined in Box 5-6.

The development of avascular necrosis is often an iatrogenic complication and produces poor results. AVN can be usually prevented by avoiding extremes of position and excessive force during casting. Signs of AVN are listed in Box 5-7.

Postoperative Regimen

After open reduction, the patient remains in a double hip spica cast for 2 to 3 months, and an abduction brace until

BOX 5-5 SURGICAL OPTIONS TO MAINTAIN (STABILIZE) A PREVIOUSLY CONCENTRICALLY REDUCED HIP IN A WALKING POSITION

1 Year of Age
- Varus derotation osteotomy of the femur, Pemberton

18 Months to 8 Years
- Salter osteotomy
- Dega osteotomy
- Pemberton osteotomy
- Staheli shelf
- ± Femoral osteotomy with shortening

8 Years to Adulthood
- Triple osteotomy (Steele)
- Double pelvic osteotomy (Southerland)
- Staheli shelf
- ± Femoral shortening and osteotomy

Adult (Growth Plates Closed)
- Dial acetabular osteotomy (Eppright)
- Wagner/Ganz
- Chiari osteotomy
- Femoral shortening osteotomy

BOX 5-6 SYMPTOMS OF UNTREATED DEVELOPMENTAL DYSPLASIA OF THE HIPS

Unilateral
- Apparent leg length discrepancy
- Scoliosis
- Ipsilateral knee pain
- Ipsilateral valgus knee deformity with degenerative arthritis
- Gait disturbance
- Pain (with false acetabulum)
- Lumbar spine degeneration and pain

Bilateral
- Waddling gait (bilateral positive Trendelenburg gait)
- Hyperlordosis
- Back pain and early arthritis
- Fatigue (early)
- Pain (if false acetabulum present)

Subluxation
- Positive Trendelenburg and antalgic gait
- Early degenerative arthritis with severe pain (by 15–25 years of age); very early total hip replacement

the hip is stable in a walking position and a standing AP of the hips appears normal.

RESULTS

Obtaining and maintaining a concentric reduction of the hips without excessive force or extremes of position before the age of 4 usually results in hips that are very close to normal. Long-term follow-up should consist of yearly office visits until the patient attains skeletal maturity. It should be remembered that the contralateral hip demonstrates abnormality in 50% of the cases of DDH and should also be watched. Unrecognized subluxed hips or dislocated hips can result in early degenerative changes, causing pain and disability by the age of 15 to 25. This situation can necessitate early total hip replacement, arthrodesis, or pelvic osteotomy.

BOX 5-7 SIGNS OF AVASCULAR NECROSIS OF THE FEMORAL HEAD AFTER TREATMENT FOR DEVELOPMENTAL DYSPLASIA OF THE HIP[a]

- Failure of appearance of ossific nucleus within 1 year after reduction
- No increase in size of the existing ossific nucleus for 1 year after reduction
- Widening of femoral neck within 1 year after reduction
- Fragmentation or increased density of ossific nucleus
- Deformation of ossified femoral head or neck

[a]It must be remembered that avascular necrosis in DDH has an iatrogenic cause.

SUGGESTED READING

Barlow TG. Early diagnosis and treatment of CDH. J Bone Joint Surg (Br) 1962;44:292.

Dahr S, Taylor JF, et al. Early open reduction for congenital dislocation of the hip. J Bone Joint Surg (Br) 1990;72:175–180.

Doudoulakis JK, Cavadias A. Open reduction of CDH before one year of age. 69 hips followed for thirteen years. ACTA Orthop Scand 1993;64:188–192.

Forlin E, Choi IH, Gille JT, et al. Prognostic factors in congenital dislocation of the hip treated with closed reduction. The importance of arthrographic evaluation. J Bone Joint Surg (Am) 1992;74:1140–1152.

Graf R. Hip ultrasonography in infancy: procedure and clinical significance. Fort Med 1985;103:62.

Harcke HT. The role of ultrasound in the diagnosis and management of congenital dislocation and dysplasia of the hip. J Bone Joint Surg (Am) 1991;73:622.

Herring JA. Conservative treatment of congenital dislocation of the hip in the newborn and infant. Clin Orthop 1992;281:41–47.

Ing HO, Chen Kuo KN, Lubicky JP. Prognosticating factors in acetabular development following reduction of development dysplasia of the hip. J Pediatr Orthop 1994;14:3–8.

Klisic P, Jankovic L. Combined procedure of open reduction and shortening of the femur in the treatment of congenital dislocation of the hips in older children. Clin Orthop 1976;119:60.

Pavlika. The functional method of treatment using a harness with stirrups as a primary method of conservative therapy for infants with congenital dislocation of the hip. Clin Orthop 1992;281:4–10.

Smith JT, Matan A, Coleman SS, et al. The predictive value of the development of the acetabular teardrop figure and developmental dysplasia of the hip. J Pediatr Orthop 1997;17:165–169.

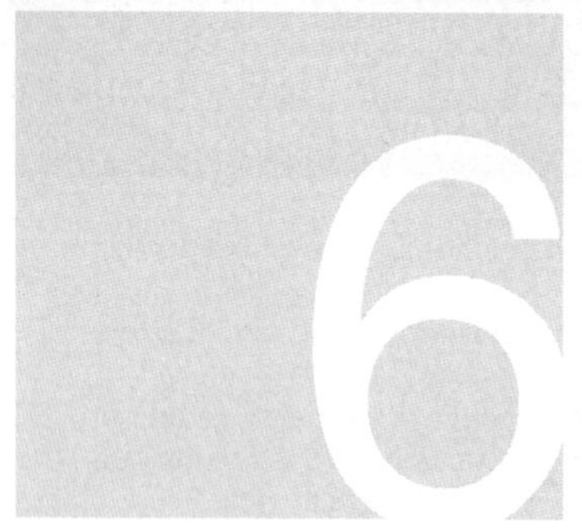

LEGG-CALVÉ-PERTHES DISEASE

ROBERT J. BIELSKI

Legg-Calvé-Perthes disease is a disorder of the hip of young children that causes collapse of the femoral head. It closely resembles avascular necrosis in its radiographic appearance. It is a very common cause of hip, knee, and thigh pain in children ages 3 to 10 years, and is a frequent cause of limp in this age group. Although it has been recognized as a distinct entity for almost 100 years, its exact etiology is not known, and the proper methods of treatment remain controversial.

PATHOGENESIS

Etiology

The etiology of this disease remains unclear, although most current theories center on disruption of blood flow to the femoral head. In the age group that is affected by Perthes disease, the blood flow to the femoral head comes from a ring of vessels formed by the medial and lateral circumflex arteries. The medial circumflex artery is the primary source of blood flow to the posterior ring, and the branches that come from the posterior ring give the majority of the blood flow to the femoral head. The lateral ascending cervical vessel, a termination of the medial femoral circumflex artery, is the most important contributor of flow to the femoral head.

Many authors believe that Perthes disease is not a result of a single vascular occlusion, but multiple infarctions over time. Single vascular insults in animal models have failed to produce typical Perthes changes, but repeat vascular insults can produce the changes. This has led investigators to question if patients with this disorder are thrombophilic (i.e., experiencing thrombosis in the vessels of the blood supply to the femoral head). The results have been mixed. Studies by Eldridge and Glueck found a high percentage of children with Perthes disease who had abnormal coagulation profiles. Similar studies by other authors have found little tendency toward thrombophilia in their patients with Perthes disease. Recent studies have also implicated secondhand smoking as a risk factor for Perthes disease.

Epidemiology

Perthes disease is primarily a disease of boys, by a ratio of 4 or 5 to 1. The peak incidence of the disease is between the ages 4 to 8 years, although it presents as early as age 2 and may present in children older than 10. Bilaterality is about 10%, but the heads are usually in different stages of collapse. The overall incidence in the United States is about 1 in 1,200 children.

Children with this disorder tend to be smaller than their peers and some reports have found them to have a delay in their bone age. There is a higher incidence of Perthes disease in children who have a positive family history, but there is no current evidence that it is an inherited condition.

Pathology

Very few histologic sections have been done on humans with Perthes disease. The epiphysis shows areas of bone with avascular necrosis, but there are also strands of cartilage that form clefts that connect the articular surface to the physeal plate. This supports the idea that this entity is different from avascular necrosis seen in the adult population.

Classification

The course of Perthes disease can be classified in four radiographic stages (Box 6-1). It is the shape of the femoral head and the acetabulum at the *healed* stage that appears to determine the risk of degenerative joint disease.

The Stulberg classification (Table 6-1) is a system that correlates radiographic appearance of the femoral head and acetabulum in the healed stage to the long-term risk for degenerative joint disease. It is based on the sphericity of the femoral head and acetabulum. Higher Stulberg classes carry the worst long-term results, with very early degeneration of class 5 hips. Stulberg 1 and 2 hips generally have a good long-term prognosis.

The Herring lateral pillar classification is the most widely used radiographic classification system for helping to determine treatment and prognosis during the *active*

BOX 6-1 CLASSIFICATION OF PERTHES DISEASE ACCORDING TO ITS COURSE

Initial: Marked by joint space widening, increased density of the femoral epiphysis, and the appearance of a subchondral fracture (the crescent sign).
Fragmentation: Collapse of the epiphysis with fragmentation of the bone.
Reossification: Appearance of new bone with normal density. The epiphysis begins to take on a more normal appearance.
Healed: At the conclusion of the reossification phase, the femoral head and neck are left with residual deformity, such as flattening of the femoral head or coxa magna.

stage of the disease. It has replaced the Catterall method because it is easier to apply, has better inter- and intraobserver reliability, and has been shown to be a strong predictor of final clinical and radiographic outcome.

The lateral pillar is defined by Herring as the lateral 15% to 30% of the femoral head width on an anteroposterior radiograph of the hip. Classification is based on several radiographs taken during the early fragmentation stage. The radiograph with the greatest involvement of the lateral pillar is used for classification (Fig. 6-1 and Table 6-2).

Patients with a greater degree of lateral pillar involvement have slower reossification, which leads to more femoral head flattening. Patients in group A typically have a uniformly good outcome with mainly Stulberg 1 and 2 results. Patients in group B have a good outcome when

TABLE 6-1 STULBERG CLASSIFICATION OF RADIOGRAPHIC FINDINGS IN PERTHES DISEASE

Class	Radiographic Findings	Congruency
1	Normal hip	Spherical
2	Spherical femoral head with some abnormalities such as coxa magna, abnormally steep acetabulum	Spherical
3	Ovoid but not flat femoral head, with abnormally steep acetabulum	Aspherical
4	Flat femoral head with abnormalities of the head, neck, and acetabulum	Aspherical
5	Flat femoral head, normal neck and acetabulum	Aspherical incongruency

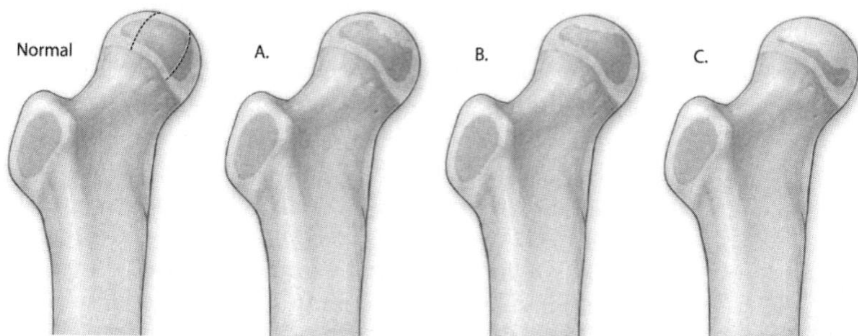

Figure 6-1 The Herring lateral pillar classification of Perthes disease. Normal: In the diagram of the normal hip, the femoral head is divided into three pillars. The lateral pillar occupies the lateral 15% to 30% of the femoral head. The central pillar represents about 50% of the head width, and the medial pillar occupies 20% to 35% of the head width. (A) In group A, the lateral pillar is radiographically normal, even though there is collapse in the central or medial pillars. (B) In group B, there is some collapse of the lateral pillar, but it maintains 50% to 100% of the height of the normal lateral pillar. (C) In group C, there is more collapse of the lateral pillar, and the height is less than 50% of the height of the normal lateral pillar.

TABLE 6-2 LATERAL PILLAR CLASSIFICATION

Group	Lateral Pillar
A	No involvement
B	>50% of lateral pillar height maintained
C	<50% of lateral pillar height maintained

they are less than 9 years of age at onset of disease, and patients in group C have a poor prognosis regardless of the age at onset.

Because of the poor prognosis seen in group C hips, surgical intervention is more common in children with group C hips.

DIAGNOSIS

Symptoms

- Thigh pain
- Knee pain
- Limp, with Trendelenburg gait
- Rare complaints of "hip pain"

Physical Examination

- Decreased hip abduction
- Decreased hip internal rotation
- Slight limb length discrepancy
- Positive Trendelenburg test

Radiographic Findings

Early

- Joint space widening
- Increased density of femoral epiphysis
- Subchondral fracture, or "crescent sign," seen on lateral radiograph

Midstage

- Fragmentation and flattening of head (Fig. 6-2)
- Widening of the physis
- Femoral neck cysts
- Extrusion of the femoral head

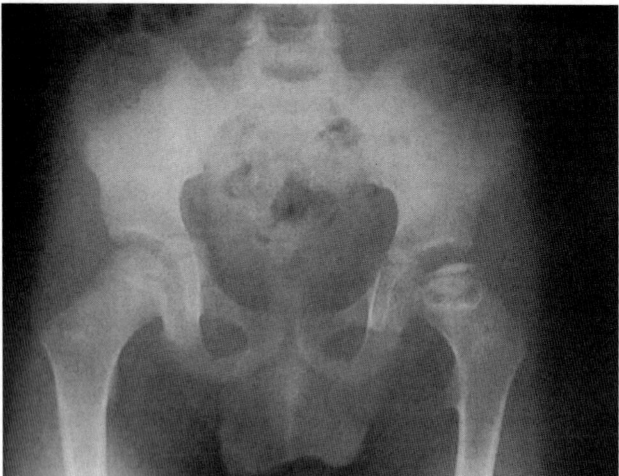

Figure 6-2 Flattening and sclerosis of the femoral head in Perthes disease.

BOX 6-2 DIFFERENTIAL DIAGNOSIS OF LEGG-CALVÉ-PERTHES DISEASE

- Toxic synovitis
- Multiple epiphyseal dysplasia
- Spondyloepiphyseal dysplasia
- Hypothyroidism
- Gaucher disease
- Sickle cell disease
- Meyer dysplasia
- Traumatic avascular necrosis

Long Term

- Coxa magna
- High-riding trochanter
- Flattened femoral head
- Irregular articular surface

Bone scan and magnetic resonance imaging are rarely needed to make the diagnosis of Perthes disease. Although some authors have proposed classification systems based on these studies, plain radiographs remain the most important imaging studies for Perthes disease at this time.

Differential Diagnosis

In most cases of unilateral Perthes disease, the clinical presentation and radiographic appearance are typical, and the diagnosis is not difficult. In the very early stages of disease, before femoral head collapse, the disease may be mistaken for toxic synovitis (Box 6-2).

Although Perthes is occasionally bilateral, it is rare that both hips are in the exact same stages of collapse. Symmetric Perthes changes should always raise the suspicion of a skeletal dysplasia, or diffuse metabolic process. Multiple epiphyseal dysplasia is a common cause of bilateral Perthes-like changes in the femoral head. Meyer dysplasia is a poorly understood process that causes collapse of the femoral head similar to Perthes disease, but the disease runs its course quickly, and usually has a benign outcome.

TREATMENT

Not all patients with Perthes disease need active treatment. Patients with lateral pillar group A disease tend to do well without any formal treatment. Patients with group B disease who maintain a good range of motion and do not show femoral head extrusion may also need minimal intervention.

Almost all patients with group C disease do better with treatment, and patients in group B who present above the age of 8 years or have significant pain and stiffness tend to benefit from active treatment.

The proper treatment methods for Perthes disease remain controversial. The generally accepted basic principles are:

1. Restoration of range of motion.
2. "Containment" of the femoral head: The concept of containment is to keep the femoral head within the limits of the acetabulum as it reossifies. By keeping the head contained, it is believed that the head will remodel with a more spherical contour. Abduction braces such as the Scottish Rite brace have been used in the past as a means of nonsurgical containment, but long-term studies have failed to support their efficacy. Support can be found in the literature for surgical containment by femoral, pelvic, or combined osteotomies, with the use of the shelf for selected cases.

Range of Motion Restoration

- Nonsteroidal antiinflammatory drugs—to decrease synovitis in the hip
- Physical therapy
- Traction
- Nighttime abduction splints
- Petrie casts (long leg casts separated with an abduction bar and internally rotated)
- Adductor tenotomy (often in conjunction with Petrie casts)

Containment of the Femoral Head

- Varus (femoral) osteotomy
  - Reproducible results
  - Causes limb shortening
  - Residual abductor weakness
  - Second surgery required for hardware removal
- Pelvic osteotomy
  - Usually a Salter osteotomy
  - Reproducible results
  - Lengthens limb
  - Technically more demanding
  - Requires good range of motion preoperatively
  - May cause loss of motion
- Combined varus and pelvic osteotomy
  - Good for hips that need maximum containment
  - No significant shortening or lengthening
  - Increases operative time and blood loss
- Shelf arthroplasty
  - Fewer clinical studies
  - Usually used in older patients (more than 8 years of age)
  - Good for hips that have large extrusion or hinge abduction that are not candidates for varus or pelvic osteotomy

SUGGESTED READING

Atsumi T, Yamano K, Muraki M, et al. The blood supply of the lateral epiphyseal arteries in Perthes disease. J Bone Joint Surg (Br) 2000;82:392.

Coates CJ, Paterson JM, Woods KR, et al. Femoral osteotomy in Perthes' disease. Results at maturity. J Bone Joint Surg (Br) 1990; 72:581.

Eldridge J, Dilley A, Austin H, et al. The role of protein C, protein S, and resistance to activated protein C in Legg-Perthes disease. Pediatrics 2001;107:1329.

Glueck CJ, Crawford A, Roy D, et al. Association of antithrombotic factor deficiencies and hypofibrinolysis with Legg-Perthes disease. J Bone Joint Surg (Am) 1996;78:3.

Hayek S, Kenet G, Lubetsky A, et al. Does thrombophilia play an aetiological role in Legg-Calve-Perthes disease? J Bone Joint Surg (Br) 1999;81:686.

Herring JA. The treatment of Legg-Calve-Perthes disease. A critical review of the literature. J Bone Joint Surg (Am) 1994;76:448.

Herring JA, Neustadt JB, Williams JJ, et al. The lateral pillar classification of Legg-Calve-Perthes disease. J Pediatr Orthop 1992;12:143.

Kruse RW, Guille JT, Bowen JR. Shelf arthroplasty in patients who have Legg-Calve-Perthes disease. A study of long-term results. J Bone Joint Surg (Am) 1991;73:1338.

Mata SG, Aicua EA, Ovejero AH, et al. Legg-Calve-Perthes disease and passive smoking. J Pediatr Orthop 2000;20:326.

McAndrew MP, Weinstein SL. A long term follow-up of Legg-Calve-Perthes disease. J Bone Joint Surg (Am) 1984;66:860.

Meehan PL, Angel D, Nelson JM. The Scottish Rite abduction orthosis for the treatment of Legg-Perthes disease. A radiographic analysis. J Bone Joint Surg (Am) 1992;74:2

Ogden JA. Changing patterns of proximal femoral vascularity. J Bone Joint Surg (Am) 1974;56:941.

Olney BW, Asher MA. Combined innominate and femoral osteotomy for the treatment of severe Legg-Calve-Perthes disease. J Pediatr Orthop 1985;5:645.

Sponseller PD, Desai SS, Millis MB. Comparison of femoral and innominate osteotomies for the treatment of Legg-Calve-Perthes disease. J Bone Joint Surg (Am) 1988;70:1131.

Stulberg SD, Cooperman DR, Wallensten R. The natural history of Legg-Calve-Perthes disease. J Bone Joint Surg (Am) 1981;63:1095.

Weinstein SL. Legg-Calve-Perthes syndrome. In Morrissy RT, Weinstein SL, eds. 4th ed. Philadelphia: Lippincott-Raven, 1996:951–991.

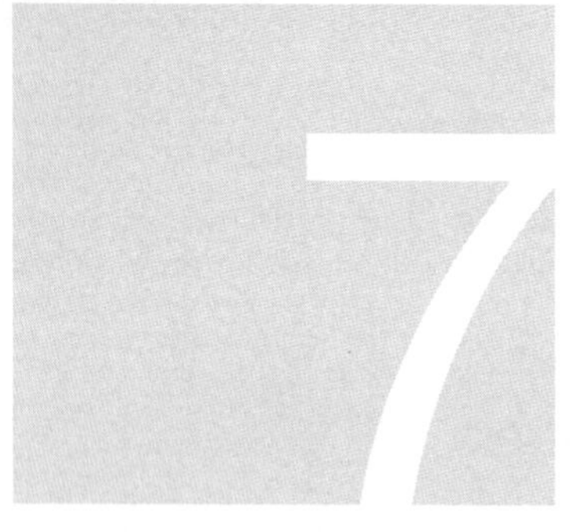

SPINE

STEPHEN KARL STORER
MICHAEL VITALE
DAVID L. SKAGGS

7.1 IDIOPATHIC SCOLIOSIS

Scoliosis is a curvature of the spine in the coronal plane greater than 10 degrees associated with a variable degree of rotational deformity. A measurable curve less than 10 degrees is referred to as a *spinal asymmetry* and is of little consequence. Idiopathic scoliosis refers to scoliosis without a known etiology. It is a diagnosis of exclusion.

Three categories of idiopathic scoliosis have been described based on the patient's age at onset: infantile (0 to 3 years), juvenile (4 to 10 years), and adolescent (older than 10 years). Prognosis and treatment for each type differ.

ADOLESCENT IDIOPATHIC SCOLIOSIS

PATHOGENESIS

Adolescent idiopathic scoliosis (AIS) is the most common form of idiopathic scoliosis with a prevalence of approximately 3%. Though various potential etiologies have been examined, to date available evidence does not support any single causative factor. The role of genetic factors is widely documented but a specific mode of inheritance remains undetermined. Boys and girls are affected equally by AIS, but the risk of curve progression is seven times greater in girls than in boys.

DIAGNOSIS

Curves are usually discovered during routine examination or school screening programs. Occasionally parents notice that their child's clothing does not hang correctly or that the child's posture is awkward. Pain is not characteristic of AIS. The history should always include questioning for pain and neurologic complaints. A painful scoliosis should prompt further evaluation for other conditions including neoplasm and infection.

Physical Examination

Minor curves may not be readily apparent when the patient is standing erect. Physical exam should document uneven shoulder elevation and waistline asymmetry, even though these findings may be present in the absence of scoliosis. The Adams forward bending test is the most sensitive clinical exam to screen for scoliosis (Fig. 7.1-1). The examiner should observe the patient from the back as he or she bends forward with feet together, knees straight, and arms hanging free. This test accentuates the rotational component of scoliosis and allows the examiner to appreciate rib or lumbar paravertebral prominences. Inability to flex forward in a supple manner should alert the examiner and prompt further workup. Assessment of leg lengths, trunk shift, sagittal plane balance, and complete neurologic examination including abdominal reflexes are mandatory. Positive neurologic findings should prompt further workup for intraspinal pathology including syringomyelia and neoplasm. Left-sided thoracic curves have a significant association with spinal cord pathology and again should prompt further diagnostic workup, including screening magnetic resonance imaging (MRI) of the spinal cord.

Radiographic Features

Radiographic analysis should include standing full-length posteroanterior and lateral views of the spine. A determination of skeletal maturity should be based on the *Risser sign* (Fig. 7.1-2). The *Cobb technique* is the standard method used to quantify the degree of curvature in scolio-

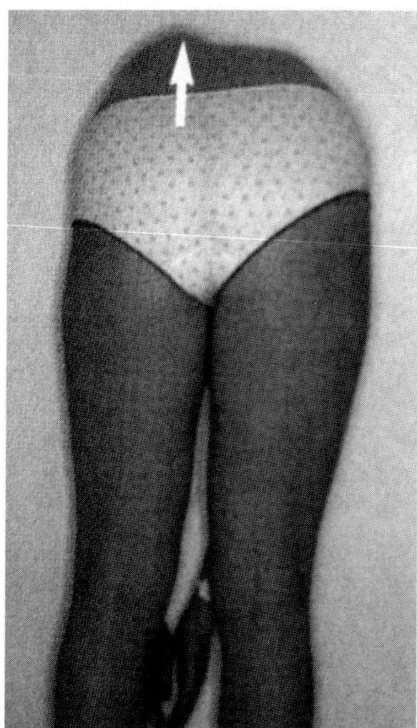

Figure 7.1-1 The Adams forward bending test gives the best visualization of truncal asymmetries.

sis. The Cobb angle for a particular curve is the angle formed by the intersection of a line parallel to the superior end plate of the most cephalad vertebra of the curve to a line parallel to the inferior end plate of the most caudad

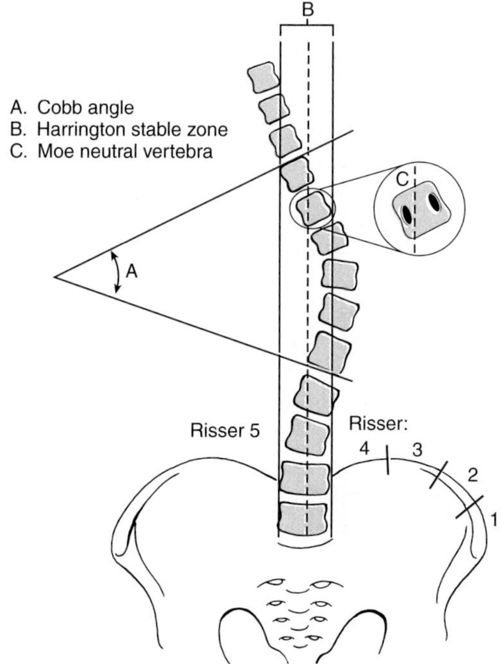

Figure 7.1-2 Measurements for scoliosis. (From Stephens RM, Fridian MA. Pediatric orthopaedics. In: Miller X, ed. Review of orthopaedics, 3rd ed. Philadelphia, WB Saunders, 2000:165.)

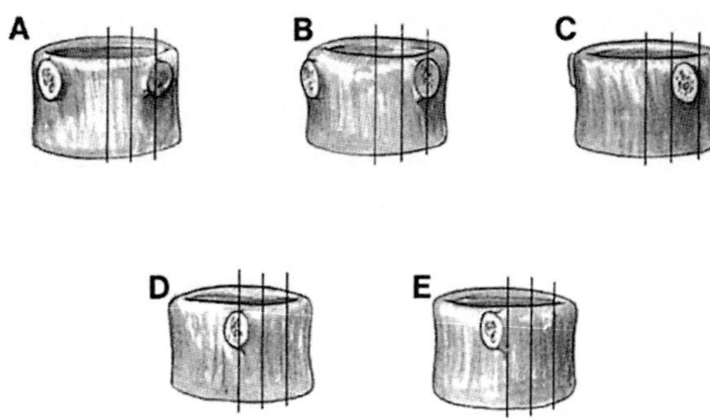

Figure 7.1-3 Nash-Moe method of determining vertebral body rotation. Grade of rotation is determined by the location of the convex pedicle. As more rotation occurs, the concave pedicle disappears, and the convex pedicle moves into the apparent midpoint of the vertebral body. (From Bridwell KH. Adolescent idiopathic scoliosis: surgery. In: Weinstein SL. The pediatric spine: principles and practice, 2nd ed. Philadelphia: Lippincott Williams & Wilkins, 2001:386.)

vertebra of the curve. Vertebral rotation should also be noted (Fig. 7.1-3). Curves are described by the location and direction of their apical convexity (Table 7.1-1). The most common curve types in AIS, in order of frequency, are isolated right thoracic, right thoracic/left lumbar, left lumbar, and right lumbar.

Most patients with AIS live normal lives without pain or functional limitations. Approximately 10% of patients require treatment other than observation. Risk factors for curve progression include female sex, younger age at presentation (less than 12 years), relative skeletal immaturity (Risser less than 2), premenarchal status, and curve magnitude at presentation (more than 20 degrees) (Tables 7.1-2 and 7.1-3). Progression of curves after skeletal maturity is possible. Curves less than 50 degrees at skeletal maturity usually remain static while curves greater than 60 degrees have a significant risk of progression with subsequent cardiopulmonary compromise and early death. Cardiopulmonary function is not usually impaired in otherwise healthy patients until the curve measures 90 degrees. The risk of disabling back pain in adulthood in patients with modest curves (40 to 50 degrees) is similar to that of the general population.

TABLE 7.1-1 CURVE DESCRIPTION BY APICAL VERTEBRA

Vertebrae	Curve
C1-C6	Cervical
C6-T1	Cervicothoracic
T2-T11	Thoracic
T12-L1	Thoracolumbar
L2-L4	Lumbar
L5-S1	Lumbosacral

TABLE 7.1-2 INCIDENCE OF PROGRESSION BY RISSER SIGN AND CURVE MAGNITUDE AT PRESENTATION

Risser Sign	5–19 Degrees	20–29 Degrees
0, 1	22%	68%
2, 3, 4	1.6%	23%

Adapted from Lonstein JE, Carlson JM. The prediction of curve progression in untreated idiopathic scoliosis during growth. J Bone Joint Surg (Am) 1984;66:1061–1071.

TABLE 7.1-3 PROBABILITY OF PROGRESSION BY CURVE MAGNITUDE AND AGE AT PRESENTATION

Curve Magnitude	10–12 Yr (%)	13–15 Yr (%)	16 Yr (%)
<19 degrees	25	10	0
20–29 degrees	60	40	10
30–59 degrees	90	70	30
>60 degrees	100	90	70

Adapted from Nachemenson A, Lonstein J, Weinstein S. Report of the SRS Prevalence and Natural History Committee 1982. Presented at SRS Meeting, Denver, 1982.

TREATMENT

Treatment of AIS depends on the magnitude of the curve, its progression, and the skeletal maturity of the patient (Table 7.1-4). Options include observation, bracing, and surgery. Curves less than 20 degrees in skeletally immature patients should be followed regularly by clinical and radiographic examination. Documented progression of greater than 5 degrees warrants consideration of bracing in the skeletally immature. Children presenting with curves greater then 30 degrees at first visit should also be considered for bracing. Bracing is not considered efficacious in curves more than 40 degrees. Surgery may be considered for curves over 45 to 50 degrees, as curves over 50 degrees at maturity have a risk of significant progression over the patient's lifetime.

The efficacy of bracing is quite controversial, though most surgeons who treat scoliosis believe that bracing has a role in the prevention of curve progression in the immature patient. The ultimate goal of bracing is to halt curve progression until the patient reaches skeletal maturity, at which time the risk of progression of curves less than 50 degrees is low. Bracing does not permanently reduce the magnitude of an established curve. Its effectiveness at halting progression seems to be "dose-related" (i.e., related to the extent of brace use), although there are reports showing comparable results between full-time use (23 hours per day) and part-time use (16 hours per day).

The underarm TLSO is generally well-accepted and is useful for curves with the apex at T8 or below. Curves with the apex cephalad to T8 are uncommon, and require the Milwaukee type brace, which has a chin extension and is less well accepted by children. The Charleston nighttime brace holds the patient bent in a position opposite to the major curve. Its efficacy has been reported to be greatest in single curves less than 35 degrees. To evaluate a brace, in-brace radiographs are taken. An in-brace x-ray showing more than 50% reduction of curve magnitude correlates with successful outcomes. Brace treatment should continue until a girl is 2 years' postmenarcheal and is Risser 4 and a boy is Risser 5. Whenever bracing is discontinued, a "rebound" phenomenon of an increase in curve magnitude may be expected.

The indications for surgery for AIS are curves greater than 45 to 50 degrees in skeletally immature patients. There are multiple spinal instrumentation systems available that provide excellent segmental fixation of the vertebral column. Whatever system is used, the goal of surgery is to halt progression and partially correct the curve while maintaining acceptable sagittal and coronal balance. The basic options for the surgical treatment of AIS are anterior spinal fusion with instrumentation, posterior spinal fusion with instrumentation, or both anterior and posterior approaches. The type of curve determines the approach used. King and Moe identified five patterns of scoliosis and proposed a method for the selection of fusion levels in thoracic idiopathic curves using first and second generation segmental spinal fixation systems (Fig. 7.1-4). The choice of fusion levels shows some variability and is generally based on the *stable* and *neutral* vertebrae. Stable vertebrae are defined as those vertebrae bisected by the central sacral line. Bending films identify the neutral disc as that disc which opens both to the right and left on supine bending films. Historically, Harrington

TABLE 7.1-4 TREATMENT RECOMMENDATIONS

Curve Magnitude	Curve Progression	Skeletal Maturity	Treatment Recommendation
0–20 degrees		Immature	Observation
20–30 degrees	5–10 degrees	Immature	Bracing
30–40 degrees		Immature	Bracing
>45–50 degrees		Immature	Surgery
>50 degrees		Mature	Surgery

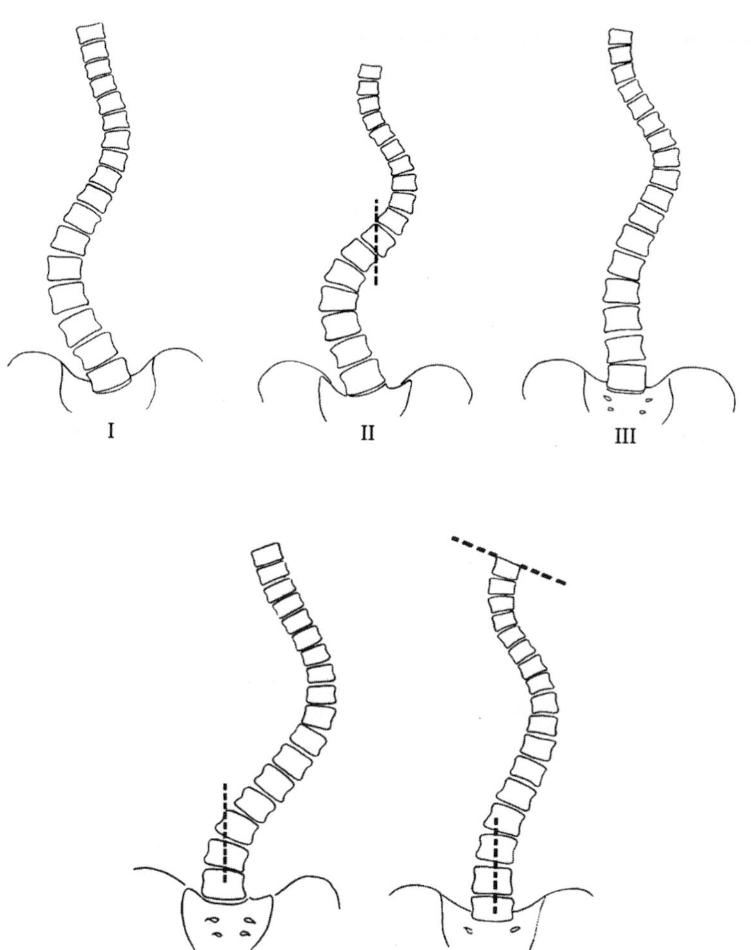

Figure 7.1-4 King classification of scoliotic curves. (From King HA, Moe JH, Bradford DS, et al. The selection of fusion levels in thoracic idiopathic scoliosis. J Bone Joint Surg (Am) 1983;65:1302–1313.)

instrumentation involved fusion from stable vertebra to stable vertebra. With newer, more powerful instrumentation including the use of pedicle screws, it may be possible to successfully end the fusion on the vertebrae above the neutral disc. Anterior instrumentation also provides more powerful correction than Harrington instrumentation and allows for potentially shorter fusions. Long-term follow-up has revealed an increased incidence of late, low back pain with fusion to L5, though this is controversial. Some believe that low back pain in spinal fusions to the lower lumbar regions is more related to loss of lordosis with earlier systems than to the level of fusion. A new classification has been proposed to attempt to better guide treatment options given the development of newer, more powerful segmental instrumentation systems (Fig. 7.1-5).

Bone grafting in spinal fusions is necessary for a spinal fusion. The traditional iliac crest bone grafting is associated with high rates of long-term pain, and has become less popular. Allograft bone grafting has been shown to be safe and efficacious in multiple series. A rib resection of the most prominent concave ribs may provide autograft, with significant cosmetic improvements as well.

The most common complications of surgery include infection, hardware failure, and pseudoarthrosis, and the overall reoperation rate has been described by numerous authors as between 5% to 15%. The most devastating complication of surgery is irreversible neurologic impairment, with an incidence of about 1 per 1,000 patients. The widespread use of intraoperative somatosensory and motor evoked potential monitoring minimizes this complication and has largely replaced the use of the Stagnara wake-up test. Excessive blood loss and the need for homologous transfusion are minimized by the use of preoperative recombinant erythropoietin, intraoperative cell saver, hypotensive anesthesia, and autologous blood donation. The *crankshaft phenomenon* occurs in skeletally immature patients after posterior spinal fusion, as anterior spinal growth progresses without restraint. The result is rotational and sagittal deformity over the fused levels. Anterior fusion should be considered with or without posterior fusion and instrumentation for children with more than 3 years of remaining growth. Late complications such as the crankshaft phenomenon and decompensation below fused levels are best avoided by careful preoperative planning.

CURVE TYPE				
Type	Proximal Thoracic	Main Thoracic	Thoracolumbar/ Lumbar	Curve Type
1	Nonstructural	Structural (major)	Nonstructural	Main thoracic (MT)
2	Structural	Structural (major)	Nonstructural	Double thoracic (DT)
3	Nonstructural	Structural (major)	Structural	Double major (DM)
4	Structural	Structural (major)	Structural	Triple major (TM)
5	Nonstructural	Nonstructural	Structural (major)	Thoracolumbar/lumbar (TL/L)
6	Nonstructural	Structural	Structural (major)	Thoracolumbar/lumbar–main thoracic (TL/L-MT)

Major = Largest Cobb measurement, always structural; minor = all other curves with structural criteria applied.

STRUCTURAL CRITERIA
(Minor Curves)

Proximal thoracic:	Side-bending Cobb ≥25°
	T2–T5 kyphosis ≥20°
Main thoracic:	Side-bending Cobb ≥25°
	T10–L2 kyphosis ≥20°
Thoracolumbar/lumbar:	Side-bending Cobb ≥25°
	T10–L2 kyphosis ≥20°

LOCATION OF APEX
(SRS Definition)

Curve	Apex
Thoracic	T2–T11-12 disc
Thoracolumbar	T12–L1
Lumbar	L1-2 disc–L4

MODIFIERS			
Lumbar Spine Modifier	CSVL to Lumbar Apex	Thoracic Sagittal Modifier (T5-T12)	Degrees
A	CSVL between pedicles	**–** (hypo)	<10
B	CSVL touches apical body(ies)	**N** (normal)	10–40
C	CSVL completely medial	**+** (hyper)	>40

CLASSIFICATION

Curve type (**1–6**) + lumbar spine modifier (**A, B, C**) + thoracic sagittal modifier (**–, N, +**) = classification, such as **1B+**

Figure 7.1-5 Synopsis of all necessary criteria for curve classification. *SRS*, Scoliosis Research Society; *CSVL*, center sacral vertical line. (From Lenke LG, Betz RR, Harms J, et al. Adolescent idiopathic scoliosis, a new classification to determine extent of spinal arthrodesis. J Bone Joint Surg [Am] 2001;83A:1169–1181.)

INFANTILE IDIOPATHIC SCOLIOSIS

PATHOGENESIS

Infantile idiopathic scoliosis is much less common than AIS. It accounts for less than 1% of all cases of idiopathic scoliosis in the United States. It occurs in children younger than 3 years, but deformity is usually noticed during the first 6 months of life.

The etiology of infantile idiopathic scoliosis is unknown. Significant geographic variability in its incidence has led some to suggest pressure molding from postnatal positioning as a possible etiology. In Europe, where the incidence of infantile idiopathic scoliosis has been higher, children are customarily placed in the supine or lateral decubitus position. In the United States the earlier trends had been to place children in the prone position. This difference may account for the geographic variation in prevalence and play a role in the etiology of the disease. If this theory is correct, as more children in the U.S. are placed supine because of the fear of sudden infant death syndrome, an increased incidence may be seen.

DIAGNOSIS

Unlike AIS, the majority of infantile idiopathic curves are left-sided. In addition, there is a strong male predominance. The curves are generally located in the thoracic and thoracolumbar regions. Associated anomalies include plagiocephaly, congenital muscular torticollis, and developmental hip dysplasia. It is imperative to rule out other causes of scoliosis in this age group, including congenital scoliosis, neuromuscular scoliosis, and scoliosis secondary to intraspinal pathology.

Supine anteroposterior and lateral radiographs of the entire spine and pelvis, including both hips, should be examined carefully for the presence of congenital abnormalities. Cobb angle measurements and the apical rib–vertebra angle difference (RVAD) should be recorded at each evaluation (Fig. 7.1-6). Risk of curve progression depends on the patient's age at time of presentation, curve magnitude at presentation, and the RVAD. Older children (more than 1 year of age) with larger curves have a greater risk of progression. Most curves less than 25 degrees with an RVAD less than 20 degrees will tend to resolve spontaneously.

TREATMENT

All children with curves greater than 25 degrees, RVAD greater than 20 degrees, or documented progressive curves require screening MRI of the brainstem and spinal cord. Serial casting or bracing is traditionally considered the first line of treatment for these patients. If the correction is maintained, the patient may be gradually weaned from the brace with close observation to maturity. Surgery should be considered in children who progress despite bracing. Surgery is problematic in such young children, as significant growth retardation is possible. Traditional surgical options include instrumentation without fusion (growing rod) and limited short segment circumferential fusion. Instrumentation without fusion involves exposing the cephalad and caudad ends of the curve, achieving fixation at these sites and distracting through these sites with a subcutaneous rod. The rod is lengthened or replaced every 6 months, as additional length is needed to accommodate growth. This theoretically allows continued growth of the spine with delay of formal fusion until the patient is closer to skeletal maturity, though actual growth reported in many series is disappointing.

A thoracotomy with implantation of a vertical titanium rib prosthesis, with subsequent lengthening two to three times each year, is a new and promising technique. Initial reports demonstrate significant improvement of scoliosis, acceleration of spinal growth on the concave side, and chest expansion, which encourages lung growth in the collapsed hemithorax during the critical period of alveolar development.

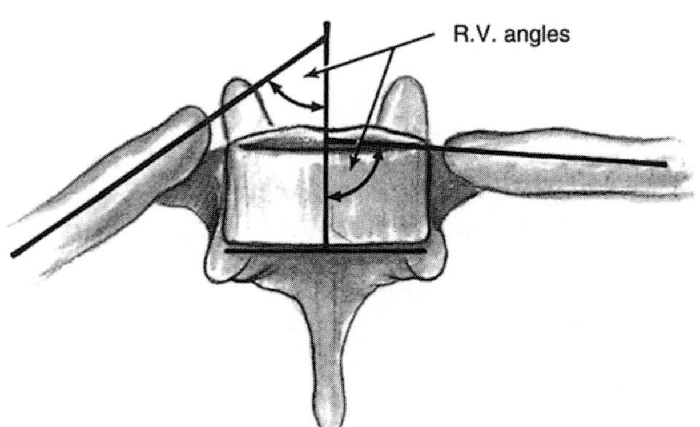

Figure 7.1-6 Measurement of rib–vertebra angle difference. (From Warner WC Jr. Juvenile idiopathic scoliosis. In: Weinstein SL. The pediatric spine: principles and practice, 2nd ed. Philadelphia: Lippincott Williams & Wilkins, 2001:333.)

JUVENILE IDIOPATHIC SCOLIOSIS

PATHOGENESIS

Juvenile idiopathic scoliosis is defined as idiopathic scoliosis detected between the ages of 3 to 10 years. It accounts for 12% to 21% of patients with idiopathic scoliosis. Its etiology is unknown and may differ depending on the age of presentation. Patients classified as having juvenile idiopathic scoliosis may actually have late-onset infantile idiopathic scoliosis or early onset AIS but fall into the juvenile category based on age. In children between 3 and 6 years, the female-to-male ratio is 1:1. In children between 6 and 10 years, girls are more frequently affected and often present with larger curves.

The curve patterns of juvenile idiopathic scoliosis resemble AIS with a right thoracic and right thoracic/left lumbar double major predominance. The left thoracic curves common in infantile idiopathic scoliosis are not typical in this age range and, as in AIS, should prompt further workup to rule out intraspinal pathology.

Unlike AIS, the natural history of juvenile scoliosis is more aggressive. Approximately 70% of juvenile curves progress and require some form of treatment. A thorough history and physical including neurologic examination is important to rule out any underlying cause of the curvature. The loss of abdominal reflexes is sometimes the only clinical finding in a patient with scoliosis with an underlying dysraphism. Factors associated with curve progression include curves greater than 45 degrees at presentation and thoracic kyphosis of less than 20 degrees. The RVAD is less useful in determining prognosis in juvenile idiopathic scoliosis than in infantile idiopathic scoliosis.

TREATMENT

Clinical and radiographic follow-up is appropriate for curves less than 20 degrees at initial presentation. Curves larger than 20 degrees or smaller curves with documented progression of 5 degrees or more should be braced because of a high risk of progression. Children younger than 6 years should be treated in the same manner as infantile curves discussed previously. When curves continue to progress despite bracing, bracing may still be continued to allow for further spine growth prior to fusion. Once a curve reaches 50 degrees, surgery should be considered.

The type of surgery performed depends on the age of the child and the amount of spinal growth available. Options are similar to those discussed with infantile idiopathic scoliosis. Spinal stabilization without fusion may be considered in children younger than 8 years. This may involve a growing rod, a Luque trolley construct, or a titanium rib implant. Combined anterior/posterior fusion should be considered in children over 8 years of age who have a Risser 0 sign with open triradiates cartilages. The following shortening formula provides a quick and easy way to predict spinal shortening after spinal fusion, though height may be gained with a decrease in the spinal curvature after surgery:

$$0.07 \times \text{spinal segments fused} \times \text{years of remaining growth} = \text{expected amount of shortening (in cm)}$$

SUGGESTED READING

Burwell RG, Cole AA, Cook TA, et al. Pathogenesis of idiopathic scoliosis: the Nottonhham concept. Acta Orthop Belg 1992;58 [Suppl]:33.

Figueiredo UM, James JIP. Juvenile idiopathic scoliosis. J Bone Joint Surg (Br) 1981;63:61–66.

James JIP, Lloyd-Roberts GC, Pilcher ME. Patterns in idiopathic structural scoliosis. J Bone Joint Surg (Br) 1959;41:719.

King HA, Moe JH, Bradford DS, et al. The selection of fusion levels in thoracic idiopathic scoliosis. J Bone Joint Surg (Am) 1983;65: 1302–1313.

Lloyd-Roberts GC, Pilcher MF. Structural idiopathic scoliosis in infancy: a study of the natural history of 100 patients. J Bone Joint Surg (Br) 1965;47:520–523.

Lonstein JE, Carison JM. The prediction of curve progression in untreated idiopathic scoliosis during growth. J Bone Joint Surg (Am) 1984;66:1067.

Ponseti IV, Friedman B. Prognosis in idiopathic scoliosis. J Bone Joint Surg (Am) 1950;32:381–395.

Sanders JO, Herring JA, Browne RH. Posterior arthrodesis and instrumentation in the immature spine in idiopathic scoliosis. J Bone Joint Surg (Am) 1995;77:39.

Weinstein SL, Zavala DC, Ponseti IV. Idiopathic scoliosis: long-term follow-up and prognosis in untreated patients. J Bone Joint Surg (Am) 1981;63:702–712.

Wynne-Davies R. Familial (idiopathic) scoliosis. J Bone Joint Surg (Br) 1968;50:24–30.

7.2 NEUROMUSCULAR SCOLIOSIS

Neuromuscular scoliosis is a scoliosis in patients with disorders of the neuromuscular system. The diseases associated with neuromuscular scoliosis are quite diverse but share many common features. They can be classified into either neuropathic, myopathic, or mixed disease states (Box 7.2-1). Although the specific disorder dictates the type of curve encountered and its risk of progression, the classification simplifies patterns of natural history, evaluation, and management.

DIAGNOSIS

Clinical Features

Neuromuscular scoliosis is characterized by an early onset with rapid progression during growth and continued progression after skeletal maturity. The curves are generally long, extend into the sacrum, and are associated with pelvic obliquity. Kyphosis is an important part of the neuromuscular deformity pattern and must be carefully considered in the evaluation of these deformities. Severe deformities commonly compromise sitting ability and pulmonary function in patients with baseline dysfunction. Characteristically, these patients have poor head control, lack of neck and trunk balance, and poor coordination. Disuse osteopenia and medication-associated osteomalacia frequently present treatment challenges in this patient population.

BOX 7.2-1 CONDITIONS ASSOCIATED WITH NEUROMUSCULAR SCOLIOSIS

1. Neuropathic

Upper Motor Neuron

- Cerebral palsy
- Syringomyelia
- Spinal cord tumor
- Spinal cord trauma
- Spinocerebellar degeneration

Lower Motor Neuron

- Poliomyelitis
- Spinal muscular atrophy
- Dysautonomia

2. Myopathic

- Muscular dystrophy
- Arthrogryposis
- Congenital hypotonia
- Myotonia dystrophica

3. Mixed

TREATMENT

The goal for nonoperative management of patients with neuromuscular scoliosis is to maintain the spine in a balanced position in both the coronal and sagittal planes over a level pelvis. Bracing is sometimes effective at controlling structural curves prior to the adolescent growth spurt, delaying the need for surgical stabilization. With the onset of puberty, control is often lost necessitating operative intervention. Prior to that, wheelchair seating adaptations allow for upright trunk positioning and provide some control of pathologic reflexes. Additionally, they have the advantage of not being as restrictive as spinal orthoses. In general however, bracing in the patient with neuromuscular scoliosis should be viewed as slowing the inevitable progression of the curve until the child can safely undergo definitive spinal surgery.

Operative treatment of patients with neuromuscular scoliosis is associated with much higher rates of complication than those encountered with the surgical treatment of AIS. The general state of the patient's health, poor bone quality, poor nutritional status, impaired respiratory function, and susceptibility to infection all may adversely affect outcome. Prior to embarking on surgical stabilization patients with neuromuscular scoliosis should have a thorough evaluation of respiratory and cardiac function, nutritional status, and risk for seizure. Patients with preoperative vital capacity less than 30% of the predicted normal value may require prolonged postoperative respiratory support. An albumin of less than 3.5 mg/dL is associated with a higher rate of infection, prolonged intubation, and longer hospitalization. Evaluation and treatment of low-grade urosepsis and metabolic bone disease is equally important.

The goal of surgical treatment of patients with neuromuscular scoliosis is to produce a stable, balanced spine over a stable, balanced pelvis. This maximizes pulmonary function, sitting ability, functional independence, and ease of handling. Usually this involves fusion from the thoracic spine to the pelvis with segmental spinal instrumentation.

Cerebral Palsy

Scoliosis is common in children with cerebral palsy. It is most prevalent in patients with quadriplegia and total body involvement. In general, the severity of the scoliosis parallels the severity of the neurologic involvement. Functional decline in these patients parallels progression of the spinal deformity. Progressive functional impairment may limit walking tolerance in ambulatory patients and sitting tolerance in nonambulatory patients. Patients may even entirely lose the ability to sit or stand.

The functional gains in treating scoliosis in patients are sometimes difficult to gauge. In general, if progression compromises function, causes pain, or increases nursing care demands, the deformity should be treated. Benefits from adaptive seating devices, frequent positional changes by caregivers, and the judicious use of braces should be maximized prior to surgical intervention. Surgery should be considered in patients with severe (more than 50 degrees) progressive curves that cause problems with seating. Medical comorbidities, including poor nutritional status, must be addressed prior to surgery. This may involve a nutritional improvement schedule or placement of a gastrostomy or gastrojejunostomy feeding tube prior to spinal surgery.

Lonstein and Akbarnia have identified two curve patterns in patients with cerebral palsy (Fig.7.2-1). Group I curves are single or double curves without pelvic obliquity. They usually occur in ambulatory patients and resemble curve patterns seen in idiopathic scoliosis. Group II curves are long thoracolumbar or lumbar curves with pelvic obliquity. They occur most often in nonambulatory patients. While fusion to the pelvis should be avoided in group I patients, it is advocated in patients with group II curves. In both types of patients fusion should extend proximally above the thoracic kyphosis, to reduce the tendency toward thoracic hyperkyphosis. Preoperative bending or traction radiographs help determine the flexibility of the curve and the necessity of anterior fusion. When traction radiographs fail to balance the thorax over the pelvis, an anterior/posterior fusion is usually indicated. Combined anterior/posterior fusion should also be considered in patients with large lumbar curves, rigid pelvic obliquity, and significant

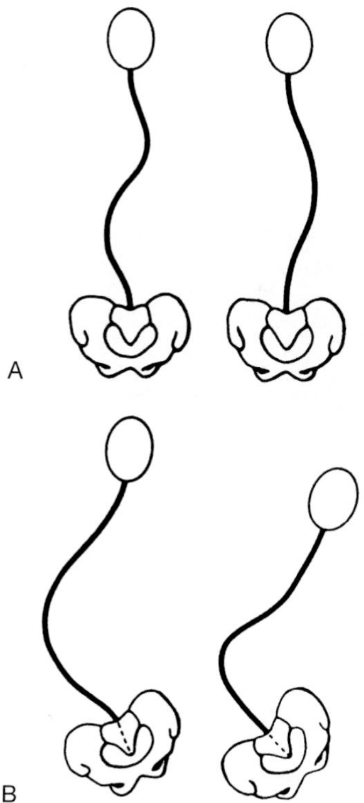

Figure 7.2-1 Curve patterns of cerebral palsy scoliosis. Group I curves (**A**) are double curves with thoracic and lumbar components. There is little pelvic obliquity. Group II curves (**B**) are large lumbar or thoracolumbar curves with marked pelvic obliquity. (Lonstein JE. Spine deformities due to cerebral palsy. In: Weinstein SL. The pediatric spine: principles and practice, 2nd ed. Philadelphia: Lippincott Williams & Wilkins, 2001:800.)

anterior growth potential. Data suggest that combined anterior/posterior procedures facilitate spinal correction and a higher fusion rate in the neuromuscular population. Whether to perform combined anterior/posterior surgery in one sitting or as a staged procedure is subject to debate.

Postoperative care requires intensive care monitoring by multidiscipline intensive care specialists. Short-term goals include stabilization of pulmonary function, reinstitution of nutritional supplementation, and achieving upright posture.

Muscular Dystrophy

Muscular dystrophy refers to a group of hereditary progressive diseases with unique phenotypic and genetic features. Duchenne muscular dystrophy is most common, with an incidence of 30 per 100,000 liveborn males. It is inherited as a sex-linked recessive trait characterized by a mutation of the gene coding for the structural protein dystrophin. The pathogenesis involves rapid deterioration and regeneration of muscle fibers until the repair capacity is overrun. Eventually irreversible degradation occurs and fat and connective tissue replace muscle cells. The disorder is present at birth, but only becomes apparent between ages 3 and 5. By age 12, most patients are confined to a wheelchair. It is universally fatal by early adulthood.

The majority of children with Duchenne muscular dystrophy develop a progressive scoliosis. Treatment objectives include maintaining the patient in an upright, ambulatory status for as long as possible. This involves judicious use of lower extremity surgery and bracing. Scoliosis progresses rapidly once the child is wheelchair-bound and spinal orthoses are ineffective in preventing progression. The spinal deformity and the myopathy itself result in a progressive restrictive lung disease. By 14 years of age, the functional vital capacity is usually less than 50% of predicted normal values. With decreasing pulmonary function, respiratory complications rise. Surgery is indicated for curves 25 degrees or greater in patients with a functional vital capacity of at least 20% to 30% of the normal predicted value. The goals of surgery are to maintain the patient's sitting ability, relieve pain, and improve quality of life. Standard surgical procedure involves posterior spinal fusion with instrumentation from T2 to L5 or the pelvis if there is significant pelvic obliquity. Postoperative goals include aggressive weaning of ventilatory support and rapid mobilization to an upright posture.

SUGGESTED READING

Bonnett C, Brown J, Grow T. Thoracolumbar scoliosis in cerebral palsy. J Bone Joint Surg (Am) 1976;58:328.

Lonstein J, Akbarnia B. Operative treatment of spinal deformities in patients with cerebral palsy or mental retardation. J Bone Joint Surg (Am) 1983;65:43.

Lonstein JE, Winter RB, Moe JH, et al. Neurological deficits secondary to spinal deformity: a review of the literature and report of 43 cases. Spine 1980;5:331.

McDonald C, Abresch R, Carter G, et al. Profiles of neuromuscular diseases. Am J Phys Med Rehabil 1995;74[Suppl]:S70.

Siegel I. Scoliosis in muscular dystrophy: some comments about diagnosis, observations on prognosis, and suggestions for therapy. Clin Orthop 1973;93:235.

7.3 CONGENITAL SPINE DEFORMITY

The development of the vertebral bodies and posterior elements begins with the migration of ectodermal cells between the endoderm and ectoderm to form the mesoderm at the end of the second week of development. The mesoderm forms pairs of somites that line both sides of the notochord and develop into the dermatomes, myotomes, and sclerotomes. Sclerotomal cells further differentiate to ultimately surround the notochord to form the vertebral bodies and posterior elements. Each sclerotome contributes the intervertebral disc and the caudal half of the vertebra above and the cephalad half of the vertebra below. Congenital spinal disorders result from a developmental defect in the formation and differentiation of the sclerotome during the fourth to sixth weeks of development. The resulting defects are classified as errors of segmentation, errors of formation, or mixed types (Fig. 7.3-1).

Patients with congenital spine anomalies frequently have congenital anomalies involving other organ systems. The genitourinary tract is most commonly affected with an incidence between 20% and 33%. Many of the genitourinary anomalies do not demand treatment because they are anatomic variants with normal renal function, but obstructive uropathy is not uncommon. Thus, all patients with congenital spine anomalies should have an evaluation of the genitourinary system by ultrasound or MRI. Cardiac anomalies are present in 10% to 15% of patients and may go undiagnosed until the spine anomalies are discovered.

A high frequency of spinal dysraphism in patients with congenital spine anomalies has been observed. Careful neurologic examination, including abdominal reflexes, may uncover subtle deficits resulting from tethered cord, diastematomyelia, or syringomyelia. Examination of the skin overlying the vertebral column is important. Hair patches, dimples, and subtle pigmentation often herald underlying spinal dysraphism. Radiographs should be examined for interpedicular widening and midline bony

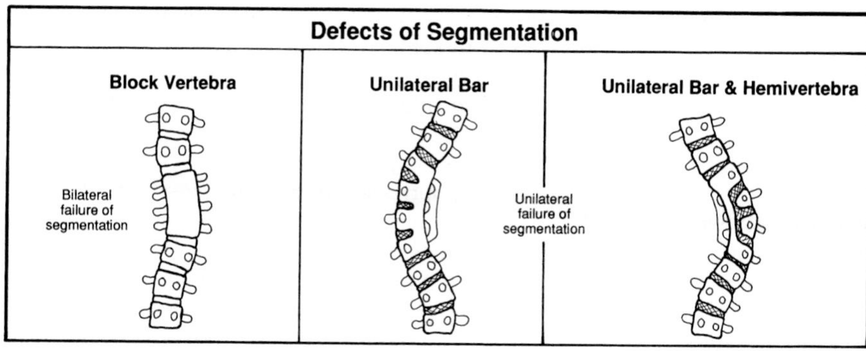

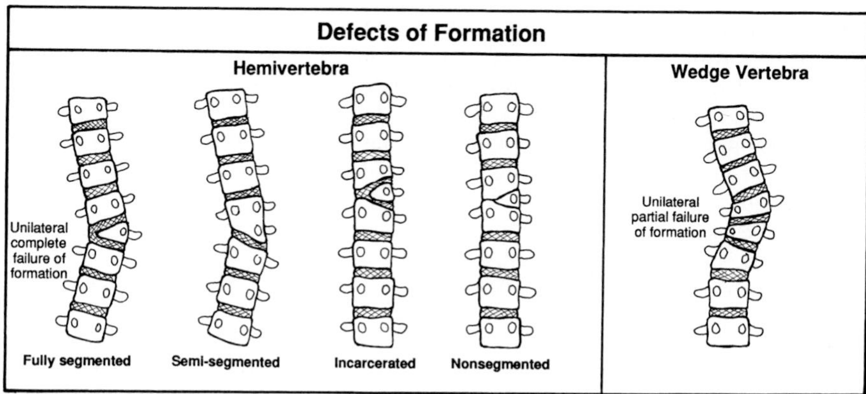

Figure 7.3-1 Congenital scoliosis. (From McMaster MJ. Congenital scoliosis. In: Weinstein SL. The pediatric spine. New York: Raven Press, 1994:229.)

speckles. Screening MRI should be obtained in all patients being treated for congenital spinal anomalies.

CONGENITAL SCOLIOSIS

PATHOGENESIS

Congenital scoliosis is scoliosis caused by abnormal vertebral development. It is classified into errors of formation, errors of segmentation, or mixed deformities (Fig. 7.3-1). Errors of formation include hemivertebra and wedge vertebra. Errors of segmentation include unilateral bars and block vertebrae. Associated sagittal plane deformity is common.

Careful characterization of the deformity is important. One must accurately document the type of anomaly and its magnitude from the initial radiographs. All congenital curves must be examined periodically to determine whether they are progressive or not. Some curves never progress while others that have been stable for many years suddenly progress with the adolescent growth spurt. The majority of congenital curves, however, are progressive.

Knowledge of the natural history of some specific anomalies is essential as it guides prognosis and treatment. The rate of progression depends on the area of spine involved and the type of anomaly. Thoracic curves have a poor prognosis. Unilateral thoracic unsegmented bars with contralateral, fully segmented vertebrae carry the worst prognosis and have the greatest likelihood of progression. Other anomalies with high rates of progression include unilateral unsegmented bar, double ipsilateral hemivertebrae, and single fully segmented hemivertebra. Block vertebrae have the best prognosis. The most common anomaly is a single hemivertebra. Its risk of progression is unpredictable. Hemivertebra at the lumbosacral junction should be of particular concern because there is no room for natural compensation to occur below the anomaly. These patients often have a progressive list to one side. Similarly, unbalanced hemivertebrae at the cervicothoracic junction often result in a progressive head tilt.

TREATMENT

Patients with anomalies whose natural history is reliably progressive should have early fusion before the deformity becomes rigid and more difficult to treat successfully with surgery. Such anomalies include the unilateral unsegmented bar with or without contralateral hemivertebra. Close observation is essential in care of patients with anomalies whose natural history is less reliable, such as hemivertebrae and mixed deformities. Such patients must be examined both clinically and radiographically every 4 to 6 months, especially during the first 4 years of life and the adolescent growth spurt. Close comparisons of films at successive visits is essential.

Orthotic treatment has a limited role in the treatment of congenital scoliosis. Braces should not be used with short rigid curves, unsegmented bars, and congenital kyphosis. Their role should be limited to mixed flexible anomalies with progressive secondary curves. They will always fail if used to treat curves whose natural history dictates surgical intervention.

Surgery is frequently the treatment of choice in congenital scoliosis. Any intraspinal pathology must be addressed prior to instrumentation and fusion. There is no single algorithm to determine what procedure to perform or at what age it should be done. Patients with unilateral unsegmented bars with or without contralateral hemivertebrae and those with two ipsilateral hemivertebrae have reliably progressive curves and should undergo early operative intervention. Documented progressive curves should also be treated surgically. Options include hemivertebra excision, convex growth arrest (hemiarthrodesis/hemiepiphysiodesis), posterior fusion *in situ*, instrumentation without fusion, and combined anterior and posterior fusion. In immature patients circumferential fusion should be considered to avoid the crankshaft phenomenon. If fusion without instrumentation is performed, postoperative casting may favorably affect correction. Instrumentation generally is used to stabilize the spine rather than to impart corrective forces. In general, treatment should be directed at early intervention to avoid severe rigid curves that are technically more difficult to treat.

CONGENITAL KYPHOSIS

PATHOGENESIS

Congenital kyphosis is deformity in the sagittal plane caused by errors of formation or errors of segmentation of the vertebral elements. Pure anterior failure of formation results in pure kyphosis while anterolateral errors of formation result in kyphoscoliosis. Complex errors of formation may even result in sagittal translation of the vertebral column or narrowing of the spinal canal. Such deformities are known as congenital spondylolisthesis and segmental spinal dysgenesis, respectively.

Although kyphotic deformities are less common than scoliosis, they are complicated more often by neurologic compromise including paraplegia. This is of particular concern with errors of formation in the upper thoracic area where the blood supply to the cord is tenuous. The paraplegia may occur early in life but is more common during the adolescent growth spurt with rapid progression of the kyphosis. Errors of segmentation causing kyphosis may involve single or multiple levels resulting in a rounded kyphosis with little risk of neurologic compromise. The rate of progression in deformity due to errors of segmentation is usually less than that due to errors of formation because the bars form late in the juvenile years, and the growth discrepancy is not as great.

TREATMENT

The natural history for congenital kyphosis is universally poor, especially for errors of formation. There is usually no role for nonoperative treatment, including bracing. Surgical options include posterior fusion and combined anterior and posterior fusion. Patients with neurologic findings also often require anterior decompression.

SUGGESTED READING

Kuhns JE, Hormell RS. Management of congenital scoliosis. Arch Surg 1952;65:250.

MacEwen GD, Winter RB, Hardy JH. Evaluation of kidney anomalies in congenital scoliosis. J Bone Joint Surg (Am) 1972;54:1451.

McMaster MJ, Ohtsuka K. The natural history of congenital scoliosis: a study of two hundred and fifty-one patients. J Bone Joint Surg (Am) 1982;64:1128.

Winter RB, Moe JH, MacEwen GD, et al. The Milwaukee brace in the nonoperative treatment of congenital scoliosis. Spine 1986;1:85.

7.4 CERVICAL SPINE DISORDERS

The care of cervical spine disorders in children requires an understanding of distinctive anatomic and biologic characteristics that differ significantly from adults. While cervical spine disorders in adults usually present with pain, infants and children usually present with deformity as the primary symptom. The pediatric cervical spine approaches the adult configuration at 8 years of age. Hypermobility, incomplete ossification, and hyperlaxity of ligamentous and capsular structures are all characteristics of the normal immature cervical spine. The relative laxity and horizontal orientation of the facet joints allow for increased mobility in children. Congenital abnormalities and developmental alterations further complicate evaluation and treatment. Connective tissue disorders and syndromes associated with ligamentous laxity may accentuate the baseline hypermobility and cause progres-

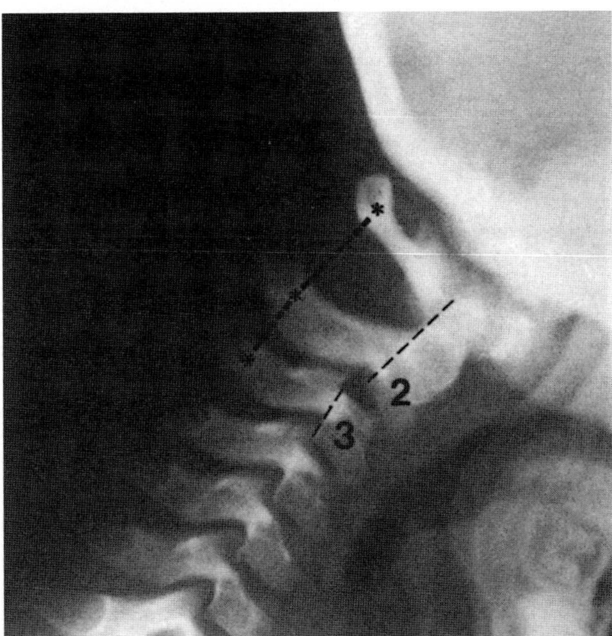

Figure 7.4-1 Lateral cervical radiograph of a child with pseudosubluxation at C2-C3. The step-off at C2-C3 is present, but the posterior cervical line of Swischuk is normal. (From Loder RT, Hensinger RN. Developmental abnormalities of the cervical spine. In: Weinstein SL. The pediatric spine: principles and practice, 2nd ed. Philadelphia: Lippincott Williams & Wilkins, 2001:317.)

sive instability and serous neurologic injury or sudden death.

Radiographic evaluation of the cervical spine in children should include anteroposterior, lateral, and open-mouth views. Misinterpretation of normal findings as pathologic is not uncommon. *Pseudosubluxation* is commonly misdiagnosed as pathologic instability (Fig.7.4-1). Persistence of the basilar synchondrosis of C2, loss of normal cervical lordosis, and variations in prevertebral soft tissue appearance may be normal findings in some children. Instability is best evaluated by flexion–extension lateral views.

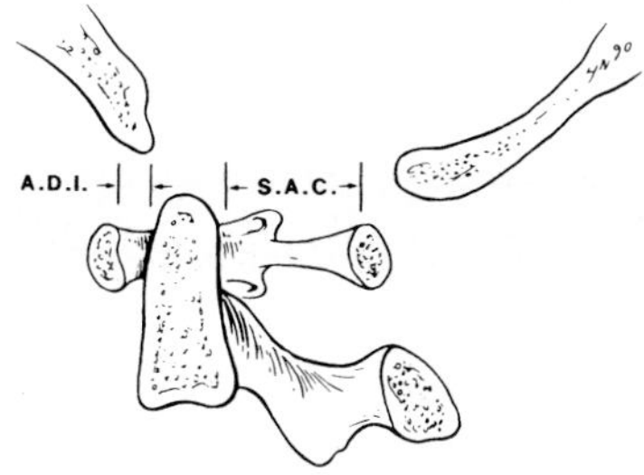

Figure 7.4-2 Atlantoaxial joint demonstrating the normal atlas-dens interval (ADI) and the normal space available for the spinal cord (SAC). (From Moskovitch R. Cervical instability [rheumatoid, dwarfism, degenerative, others]. In: Bridwell KH, DeWald RL, eds. The textbook of spinal surgery, 2nd ed. Vol 1. Philadelphia: Lippincott-Raven, 1997:970.)

Two commonly used measurements include the *atlanto-dens interval* (ADI) and the *space available for the cord* (SAC) (Fig. 7.4-2). The ADI is used to measure the stability of the atlantoaxial articulation and is measured on a flexion-lateral view of the C-spine. Normal is 4.5 mm or less in a child, and 3.5 mm or less in an adult. An increased ADI indicates potential C1-C2 instability. In this setting, a decreased SAC signals possible catastrophic encroachment of the cord. Computed tomography (CT) scanning is indicated to more clearly define complex anomalous bony anatomy. MRI is useful for evaluating paracervical soft tissues and spinal cord pathology.

DIFFERENTIAL DIAGNOSIS

Down Syndrome

Down syndrome is a common genetic disorder that occurs in 1 in 700 live births. It is the result of a nonsegregation of chromosome 21 during meiosis, causing trisomy 21. Phenotypic features of affected individuals include characteristic facies, mental retardation, congenital heart disease, and ligamentous laxity. Cervical instability is common in those with Down syndrome. Progressive instability with neurologic deficits is seen more commonly in boys than in girls. Patients with instability may present with gait abnormalities. Careful regular neurologic examination is mandatory. Surveillance cervical spine flexion–extension views should be obtained at least every 3 years. Recommendations for asymptomatic patients with an ADI greater than 5 mm include avoidance of activities that stress the cervical spine including contact sports and diving. Symptomatic patients and patients with an ADI greater than 10 mm regardless of symptomatology should undergo C1-C2 fusion. Surgical complications, including pseudoarthrosis and high mortality occur more frequently in patients with Down syndrome.

Klippel-Feil Syndrome

Klippel-Feil syndrome refers to a complex of osseous and visceral anomalies with a variable phenotypic presentation. The classic triad of fusion of cervical vertebra, shortening of the neck, and a low hairline is only present in 50% of patients. The term *Klippel-Feil syndrome* is used for any patient with fusion of the cervical vertebrae. Associated findings include a 70% incidence of scoliosis, deafness, Sprengel deformity, synkinesis, cervical ribs, and congenital heart and renal disease. Children with Klippel-Feil usually present with concerns relating to the appearance and motion of the neck or complaints of neck pain. Physical examination is usually notable for decreased neck range of motion, especially lateral bending and rotation. A thorough neurologic examination is mandatory. Positive findings may include cranial nerve abnormalities, cervical radiculopathy, or even myelopathy. Radiographic analysis should include standing full-length posteroanterior and lateral views of the entire spine as well as flexion–extension lateral views of the cervical spine. It is believed that children with multiple fused segments are at greater risk for instability through the unfused segments, and should be kept out of contact sports to prevent catastrophic injury. Patients with radiographic evidence of progressive instability clearly are at risk for early neurologic injury. Treatment recommendations include regular flexion–extension radiographic examination in asymptomatic children. The treatment of symptomatic patients includes activity limitations, use of cervical orthoses, and traction. Posterior cervical fusion is recommended for progressive symptomatic segmental instability or neurologic compromise.

Osteochondrodysplasias

The osteochondrodysplasias are a group of heritable disorders of bone and cartilage growth with variable phenotypic presentations of dwarfism. Angular deformities of the extremities, premature degenerative joint disease, and spinal disorders including cervical instability are common clinical features of these disorders. The diagnosis is often made during early growth when disproportion of the trunk and limbs becomes apparent. Any child below the fifth percentile in growth should be evaluated for a skeletal dysplasia or metabolic disorder. Identification of the exact skeletal dysplasia is often difficult and should be made in consultation with a geneticist.

Spondyloepiphyseal dysplasia (SED) refers to a subgroup of osteochondrodysplasias that are characterized by primary epiphyseal and vertebral involvement. Despite some clinical heterogeneity, they all result in short-trunk dwarfism. Associated anomalies include pectus carinatum, scoliosis, genu valgum, and hip flexion contractures. Radiographic features include delayed vertebral body and epiphyseal ossification, platyspondyly, and coxa vara. Up to 40% of children with SED develop atlantoaxial instability. Odontoid hypoplasia and os odontoideum are common features that predispose to this instability. Persistent hypotonia and delay in motor milestones are early manifestations of neurologic compromise caused by the instability. Lateral cervical spine flexion–extension radiographic examination is mandatory for all patients with SED. Surveillance radiographs should be obtained at least every 3 years. Surgical stabilization is recommended for children with instability with neurologic compromise. Prophylactic stabilization should be considered for asymptomatic children with instability greater than 5 mm.

The *mucopolysaccharidoses* are another subgroup of osteochondrodysplasias with a high incidence of significant cervical spine involvement. Although they share many features, specific clinical features and the natural history of these disorders vary depending on the specific enzyme deficiency. These disorders produce a proportionate dwarfism caused by the accumulation of mucopolysaccharides due to an inherited hydrolase enzyme deficiency. The diagnosis is made by urine screening for mucopolysaccharides and confirmed by serum testing for the specific sugar abnormality. Morquio syndrome is the most common form and is characterized by the inability to metabolize keratin sulfate. Clinical manifestations include coarse facial features, abnormal dentition, kyphosis, corneal clouding, ligamentous laxity, and joint stiffness. Radiographic features include oval-shaped vertebral bodies with anterior beaking, coxa vara with unossified femoral heads, bullet-shaped metacarpals, and wide, flat ilia. Odontoid hypoplasia is common in children with Morquio syndrome. Atlantoaxial instability with progressive myelopathy is one of the most disabling features. Lateral cervical spine flexion–extension radiographic examination is mandatory for all patients with mucopolysaccharidoses. Surveillance radiographs should be obtained at least every 3 years. Surgical stabilization is recommended for children with instability with neurologic compromise. Prophylactic stabilization should be considered for asymptomatic children with instability greater than 5 mm.

Achondroplasia is the most common osteochondrodysplasias. It results in disproportionate short-limb dwarfism. It is an autosomal dominant condition caused by abnormal endochondral bone formation. Clinical features include frontal bossing, flattened nasal bridge with midface hypoplasia, trident hands, kyphosis, and lumbar stenosis. Atlantoaxial instability is uncommon but stenosis of the foramen magnum may present with sleep apnea or sudden death. Foramen magnum decompression should be performed for repeated apneic episodes or evidence of neurologic compromise. Prophylactic decompression is not recommended.

Torticollis

Torticollis is a combined head tilt and rotation deformity of the cervical spine. Its presence is usually indicative of an atlantoaxial problem, as 50% of cervical spine rotation occurs through this joint. A number of conditions are associated with torticollis (Box 7.4-1) but *congenital muscular torticollis* and *atlantoaxial rotary subluxation* are the most common causes in children.

Congenital muscular torticollis is the most common type of torticollis in the infant and young child. The deformity is usually discovered within the first 2 months of life and is caused by a contracture of the sternocleidomastoid muscle. The exact etiology is unknown but current theory suggests that it is the result of a compartment syndrome of that muscle. The head tilts toward the side with a tight sternocleidomastoid and the chin rotates toward the opposite shoulder. The right sternocleidomastoid muscle is involved 75% of the time. Occasionally an "olive-like" mass is palpable within the muscle belly. Cervical spine radiographs should be obtained to rule out congenital vertebral

BOX 7.4-1 CAUSES OF TORTICOLLIS

Congenital muscular torticollis
Atlantoaxial rotatory subluxation
Sandifer syndrome
Basilar impression
Arnold-Chiari malformation
Familial cervical dysplasia
Central nervous system neoplasm
Grisel's syndrome

anomalies. Careful examination of the hips, including a screening ultrasound, is mandatory since 20% of children with congenital muscular torticollis also have developmental dysplasia of the hip. Initial treatment is nonoperative and includes a home stretching program supervised by a physical therapist. This is effective in 90% of cases. Surgical release is indicated if the deformity persists after 1 year of age, since stretching is usually ineffective in older children. If untreated, skull and facial flattening (plagiocephaly) may result during the first year of the child's life.

Atlantoaxial rotatory subluxation is the most common cause of acquired childhood torticollis. The patient generally presents with discomfort and a torticollis that has developed following trauma, an upper respiratory infection, or following head and neck surgery. Even routine events, like vomiting, may cause subluxation. *Grisel syndrome* is spontaneous atlantoaxial subluxation that follows an upper respiratory infection. It is caused by an inflammatory ligamentous laxity following the infectious process.

On physical examination, it is important to differentiate which sternocleidomastoid muscle is tight. In torticollis associated with atlantoaxial rotatory subluxation the sternocleidomastoid muscle opposite to the head tilt is stretched causing the muscle to go into spasm. In congenital muscular torticollis the head tilts toward the shoulder on the same side as the involved contracted muscle. Plain radiographs are often difficult to obtain because the child cannot be positioned properly. The open-mouth odontoid view may show a medial and lateral offset of the lateral masses. A dynamic CT scan of C1-C2 in which the head is rotated maximally to both sides should be obtained in all suspected cases. A fixed relationship of C1 to C2 is diagnostic.

Treatment of atlantoaxial rotatory subluxation is based on the duration and severity of symptoms. Patients who have had the symptoms for less than 1 month should be hospitalized and treated with cervical traction. This usually reduces the subluxation and corrects the torticollis. After confirmation of reduction by CT scan, the patient should be immobilized in a soft collar for 4 to 6 weeks. For subluxations that have been present for more than 1 month, posterior spinal fusion of C1 and C2 is usually required because the deformity is either irreducible or persistently recurs when the patient is removed from traction.

SUGGESTED READING

Hensinger R, Lang JE, MacEwen GD. Klippel-Feil syndrome: a constellation of associated anomalies. J Bone Joint Surg (Am) 1974; 56:1246–1253.

7.5 BACK PAIN

The exact prevalence of back pain in children and adolescents is unknown. The literature suggests that significantly more children have back pain than the number who actually seek medical attention. The differential diagnosis of back pain in children, unlike adults, more often includes neoplastic, developmental, and inflammatory conditions (Box 7.5-1). Overuse and lumbar strain should be diagnoses of inclusion after all other causes for back pain have been excluded. The evaluation of a child with back pain must include a detailed history, physical examination, radiographic evaluation, and appropriate laboratory and diagnostic imaging studies when indicated.

BOX 7.5-1 DIFFERENTIAL DIAGNOSIS OF BACK PAIN IN CHILDREN AND ADOLESCENTS

Mechanical
- Overuse syndrome
- Herniated disc

Developmental
- Spondylolysis/spondylolisthesis
- Scheuermann disease

Neoplastic
- Benign
- Malignant

Inflammatory
- Discitis
- Osteomyelitis
- Rheumatologic disorders

Adapted from Bunnell WA. Back pain in children. Orthop Clin North Am 1982;13:587–604.

DIAGNOSIS

History and Physical Examination

The history should begin with general questions regarding the onset, location, frequency, severity, and duration of symptoms. Alleviating and aggravating factors must be addressed specifically. Pain that is promptly relieved by nonsteroidal antiinflammatory drugs (NSAIDs) may be related to an osteoid osteoma. Back pain associated with pain in other joints relieved by NSAIDs is usually related to an underlying rheumatologic disorder.

It is important to assess the child's baseline activity level and degree of sport participation. Competitive gymnasts, for example, have a relatively high incidence of spondylolisthesis. Traumatic events and changes in activity or athletic participation require careful exploration. The exam-

iner must learn from both the patient and the parent how the pain is affecting the child's normal activities and routines. A child who self-limits enjoyable activities because of pain requires a thorough evaluation.

Night pain is a significant symptom to identify. A child who wakes in the middle of the night with pain and is unable to return to sleep must be considered to have a neoplastic or inflammatory condition until proven otherwise. Other common causes of back pain in children including overuse syndromes, spondylolysis, and Scheuermann's disease typically improve at night with rest.

Neurologic complaints including pain radiating to the legs and changes in bowel and bladder habits must be carefully documented. Similarly, it is important to note symptoms of weight loss, fever, chills, lethargy, rashes, and infections.

Physical examination should begin with a general orthopedic screening examination including assessment of both upper and lower extremities and the patient's gait. Subtle changes in gait may reflect an underlying neurologic problem. The evaluation of the spine should include the Adams forward bending test. Inability to flex forward in a supple manner should alert the examiner as such patients may have a spondylolysis or spinal cord neoplasm. Similarly, lumbosacral pain that worsens with hyperextension seems to correlate well with spondylolysis and spondylolisthesis. Assessment of leg lengths, trunk shift, sagittal plane balance, and complete neurologic examination including abdominal reflexes are mandatory.

Radiographic evaluation should begin with anteroposterior and lateral views of the spine in all children presenting with pain. Thereafter, the working differential diagnosis should guide additional radiographic and laboratory tests. Oblique views are useful in children with suspected spondylolysis. Children with normal radiographs and significant pain should have a technetium bone scan. Single-photon emission computed tomography (SPECT) bone scans have shown an increased sensitivity and specificity in finding fractures in the lumbar spine as compared to traditional bone scans. SPECT may provide further insight in patients with suspected spondylolysis and negative plain bone scans. CT scans are useful to more clearly define bone pathology detected by bone scan. MRI is useful for patients with neurologic signs or symptoms. It is invaluable in diagnosing spinal cord tumors, syringomyelia, tethered cord, and disc herniations.

DIFFERENTIAL DIAGNOSIS

Disc Herniation

Intervertebral disc herniation, while common in adults, is relatively uncommon in children and adolescents. Children with disc herniations may present with back pain with or without leg pain. Symptoms are often related to traumatic events. On physical examination patients usually demonstrate a positive straight leg raise test but neurologic deficits are uncommon. Most disc herniations occur at the L4-L5 and L5-S1 levels. MRI is the best test to demonstrate a herniated disc. Treatment is the same as in adults.

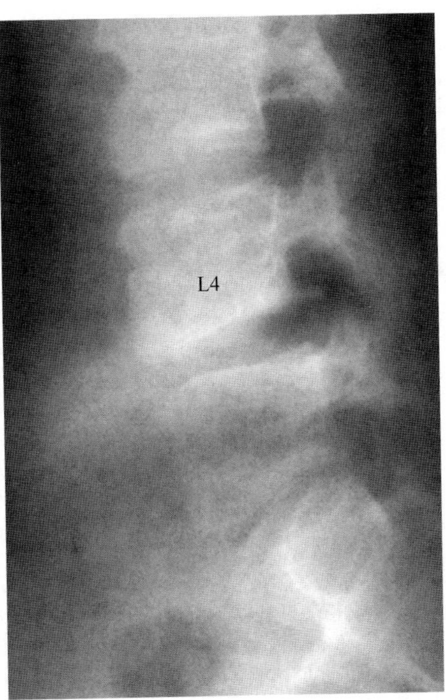

Figure 7.5-1 A 15-year-old patient complained for several months of severe right sciatica after having lifted a heavy weight. The spot lateral lumbar spine shows a localized kyphosis at L4-L5 and an avulsed piece from the inferior border of L4. (From Arlet V, Fassier F. Herniated nucleus pulposis and slipped vertebral apophysis. In: Weinstein SL. The pediatric spine: principles and practice, 2nd ed. Philadelphia: Lippincott Williams & Wilkins, 2001:461.)

Rest, NSAIDs, and physical therapy comprise the initial line of treatment. Patients who fail nonoperative treatment usually improve with disc excision without fusion.

The diagnosis of a *slipped vertebral apophysis* must be excluded prior to initiating treatment for an intervertebral disc herniation (Fig. 7.5-1). It most often occurs in adolescents following trauma and presents similar to a disc herniation. It can be visualized as a bony fleck within the spinal canal but is best visualized by CT. Treatment is surgical excision.

Spondylolysis/Spondylolisthesis

Spondylolysis is a defect of the *pars interarticularis*, the area between the superior and inferior articular facets of the posterior vertebral arch. The defect may be unilateral or bilateral. Spondylolisthesis occurs in the setting of a spondylolysis when one vertebral body slips forward in relation to the vertebral body below. It is graded by the percentage of uncovered length of the superior border of the vertebral body below the slip measured on standing lateral radiographs (Fig. 7.5-2). The *slip angle* is used to quantify the resulting lumbosacral kyphosis in high-grade slips (Fig.7.5-3). Spondylolysis and spondylolisthesis are common causes of back pain in children and adolescents older than 10 years.

In children, spondylolysis may be either *dysplastic* or *isthmic*. Dysplastic spondylolysis is characterized by con-

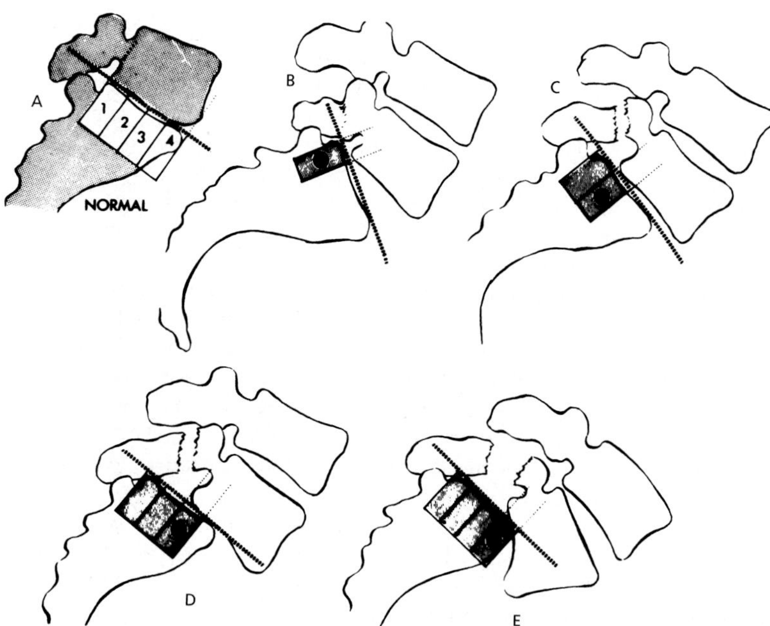

Figure 7.5-2 Meyerding classification of spondylolisthesis. (**A**) Normal or grade 0. (**B**) 1% to 25% slippage is grade I. (**C**) Up to 50% is grade II. (**D**) Up to 75% is grade III. (**E**) 76% to 100% slippage is grade IV. (From Hu SS, Bradford DS. Spondylolysis and spondylolisthesis. In: Weinstein SL. The pediatric spine: principles and practice, 2nd ed. Philadelphia: Lippincott Williams & Wilkins, 2001:436.)

genital dysplasia of the L5-S1 facet joint that allows forward slippage of L5 on the sacrum. Isthmic spondylolysis is characterized by a developmental defect of the pars interarticularis. The defect is usually in L5 or the sacrum. The etiology is believed to be a stress fracture of the pars interarticularis caused by repetitive lumbar hyperextension. It is common in young gymnasts, wrestlers, and football linemen. The defect generally develops between the ages of 5 and 8. Its incidence is 6% in the general population.

Many individuals with spondylolysis and spondylolisthesis are asymptomatic. Patients with symptomatic spondylolysis present with complaints of activity-related back pain. Symptoms can be acute and associated with trauma but usually are insidious in onset. They may be mild or quite severe, causing the child to limit sporting activities. The severity of the slip may not correlate with the severity of symptoms. Patients may present with hamstring tightness and a knee-flexed, hip-flexed gait (*Phalen-Dickson sign*). Neurologic signs and symptoms are rare, but can occur with severe slips.

The diagnosis can usually be made with plain radiographs including oblique views (Fig. 7.5-4). Bone scan with SPECT imaging may reveal the diagnosis in children with suspected

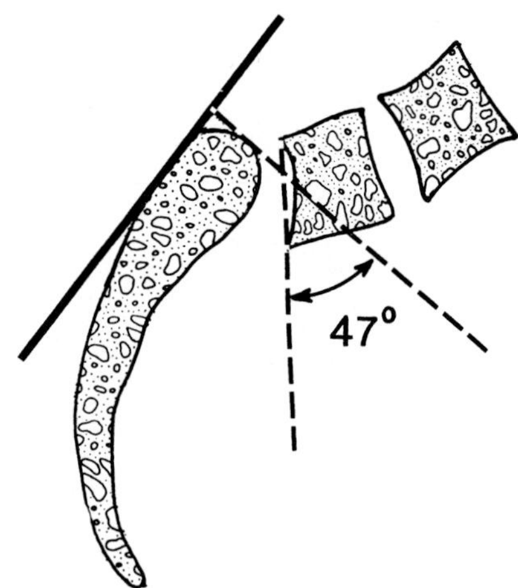

Figure 7.5-3 The slip angle (47 degrees shown) is determined by drawing a line along the posterior cortex of the sacrum and measuring the angle between its perpendicular and a line drawn along the inferior border of L5. (From Hu SS, Bradford DS. Spondylolysis and spondylolisthesis. In: Weinstein SL. The pediatric spine: principles and practice, 2nd ed. Philadelphia: Lippincott Williams & Wilkins, 2001:436.)

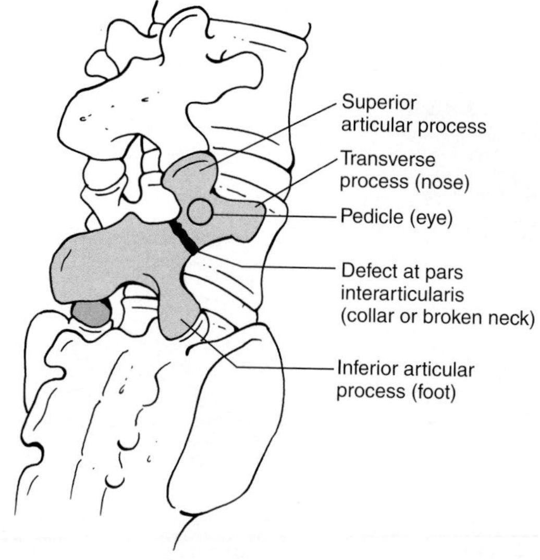

Figure 7.5-4 "Scotty dog" seen on oblique views of the lumbar spine. (From Smith JA, Hu SS, et al. Management of spondylolysis and spondylolisthesis in the pediatric and adolescent population. Orthop Clin North Am 1999;30:488.)

spondylolysis and negative plain radiographs. It is also useful in determining the acuity of the fracture. CT imaging can differentiate a pars defect from other entities that may result in a positive bone scan, including neoplasms.

Activity modification, rest, NSAIDs, and physical therapy comprise the initial line of treatment for patients with a symptomatic spondylolysis or low-grade spondylolisthesis. Brace immobilization with a modified TLSO to reduce lumbar lordosis is also useful in alleviating symptoms, and may even heal early defects. The risk of progression of a spondylolisthesis is related to the patient's age and the grade of slip at presentation.

Surgery is reserved for patients who do not respond to nonoperative treatment and patients who present with high-grade slips. Young patients with a spondylolysis but no spondylolisthesis may undergo direct repair of the pars defect. This involves debridement of the defect, autogenous bone grafting, and internal fixation with either screws or wires. Alternatively, such patients may be treated with lateral *in situ* fusion with or without instrumentation. The addition of pedicle screw fixation enables rapid patient mobilization and obviates the need for prolonged postoperative bracing. Skeletally immature patients with slips greater than 50% or with slip angles greater than 45 degrees have a high rate of progression and should undergo surgery regardless of their symptomatology. Patients with nerve root or thecal sac compression require decompression in addition. There is considerable debate regarding the role of reduction of high-grade slips. Spondyloptosis is usually treated with fusion *in situ* with a fibula strut graft or vertebral column shortening with a L5 vertebrectomy. Complications include slip progression, pseudoarthrosis, and neurologic compromise.

Scheuermann's Disease

Scheuermann's disease refers to a rigid kyphosis of the thoracic or thoracolumbar spine. It is the most common cause of structural kyphosis in adolescence. Its prevalence is reported to be between 4% and 8%, affecting boys and girls equally. Its etiology is unknown although there appears to be underlying genetic factors.

The onset of Scheuermann's disease occurs near puberty. Cosmetic concerns usually cause the patient's parents to seek medical attention. Occasionally, the deformity is attributed to poor posture delaying the diagnosis and treatment. Pain and fatigue are common complaints but are usually mild and related to exercise or prolonged sitting. When present, the pain is usually localized to the apex of the deformity and disappears with skeletal maturity. Severe, activity-limiting pain is uncommon with Scheuermann's disease. Persistent or severe low back pain in patients with Scheuermann's disease may be related to spondylolisthesis, which is noted with an increased incidence in these patients.

The kyphotic deformity of the patient with Scheuermann's disease is readily apparent on physical examination. Observation from the side with the patient standing erect reveals a thoracic or thoracolumbar kyphosis (Fig. 7.5-5). It is sharply angulated and fixed, even with hyperextension of the spine. The kyphosis becomes more prominent in the position of the Adams forward bending test and is likened to an "A-frame" deformity. Typically, the cervical spine and the lumbar spine display increased flexible lordosis, while the overall sagittal balance is well maintained. This lumbar hyperlordosis and subsequent degenerative disc and facet arthropathy predispose adults to low back pain. The shoulder girdles are often rotated anteriorly, which in combination with the kyphosis can produce an awkward stooped appearance. The arms and legs will appear relatively long compared with the shortened truck. Concomitant scoliosis occurs in about one-third of patients. Hamstring tightness is a common finding. Neurologic dysfunction has been reported but is rare and, if present, requires a thorough evaluation including MRI of the spinal cord. Cardiopulmonary complaints are extremely rare on initial presenta-

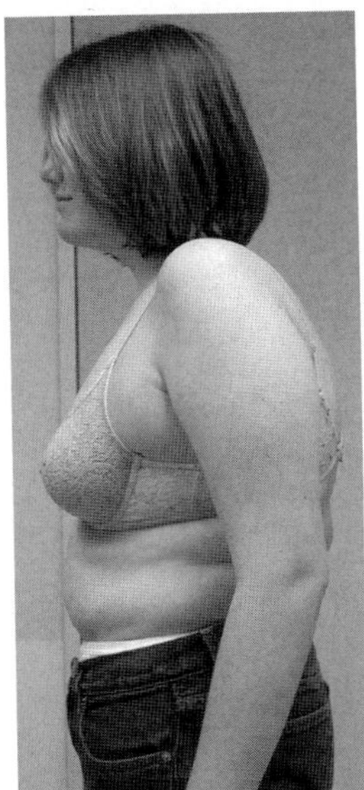

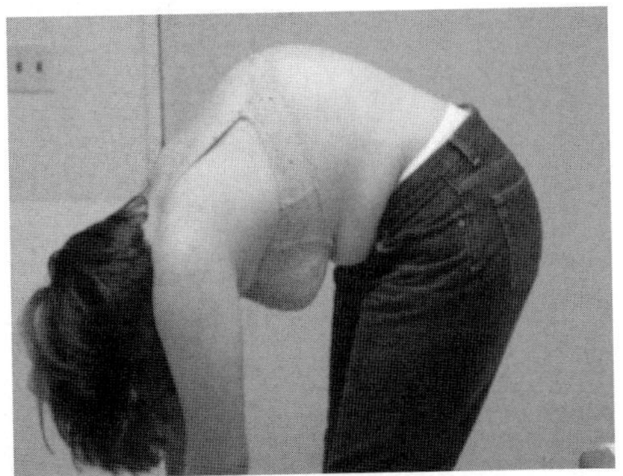

Figure 7.5-5 (A) A 14-year-old patient with Scheuermann kyphosis. (B) Note the "A-frame" deformity on forward bending.

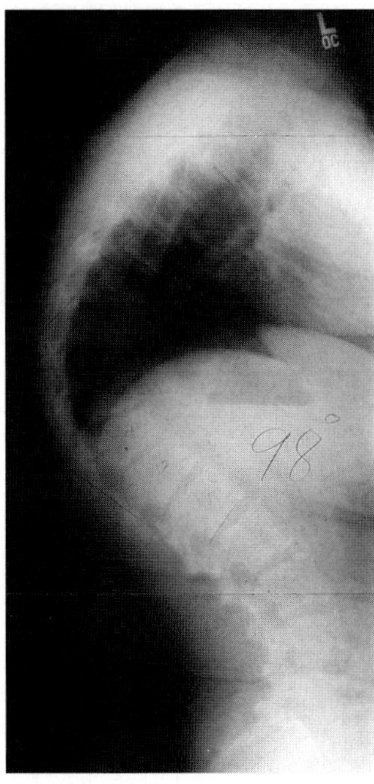

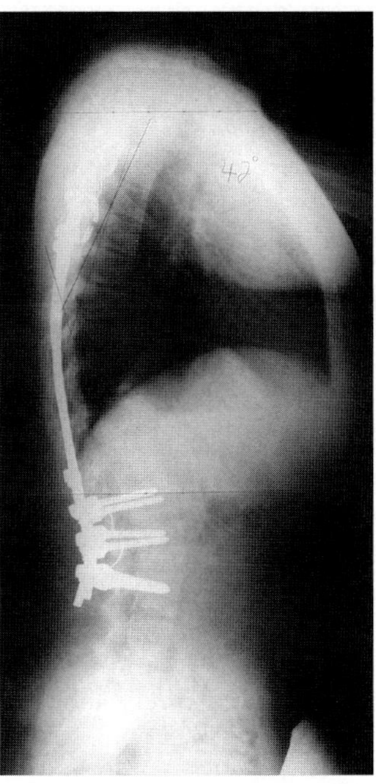

A,B

Figure 7.5-6 (A) Standing lateral radiograph of a patient with Scheuermann's disease. (B) After anterior releases and posterior spinal fusion with instrumentation.

tion, although restrictive pulmonary disease can be seen in patients with kyphosis measuring greater than 100 degrees.

Routine radiographic evaluation should include standing long cassette posteroanterior and lateral views as well as a supine hyperextension lateral view over a bolster. Normal thoracic kyphosis in adolescents is 20 to 45 degrees, although it varies with age and is slightly greater in women than in men. The radiographic criteria for Scheuermann's disease, include increased thoracic kyphosis with anterior wedging of 5 degrees or more of at least three adjacent vertebral bodies. Both the vertebral wedging and the kyphosis should be measured by the Cobb technique. When evaluating serial radiographs, care should be taken to ensure that the same levels are being measured. Associated radiographic findings include Schmorl nodes, irregularity and flattening of the vertebral end plates, narrowing of the intervertebral disc spaces, and anteroposterior elongation of the apical vertebral bodies. Radiographic examination with forced extension films is the most helpful tool in differentiating Scheuermann's disease from postural kyphosis (Fig. 7.5-6).

Treatment of Scheuermann's disease is primarily nonoperative and based on the magnitude of the deformity, the presence of pain, and the age of the patient. Adolescents with a thoracic kyphosis of less than 60 degrees should be treated with NSAIDs and a thoracic extension exercise program. Skeletally immature patients with kyphosis measuring greater than 60 degrees should also undergo brace treatment. The brace should be a Milwaukee type with a neck ring. It can be weaned with the onset of skeletal maturity. Surgical treatment is reserved for patients with severe deformity (more than 75 degrees) and those with neurologic compromise. Surgical options include posterior spinal fusion with instrumentation and combined anterior release with posterior fusion with instrumentation. The posterior-only approach is generally reserved for skeletally immature patients or skeletally mature patients with a kyphosis that corrects to at least 50 degrees on hyperextension lateral views. The anterior approach may be performed either open or thoracoscopically. Overcorrection should be avoided. Complications include the development of a junctional deformity either above or below the fusion and neurologic compromise.

SUGGESTED READING

Aufdermaur M. Juvenile kyphosis (Scheuermann's disease): Radiography, histology, and pathogenesis. Clin Orthop 1981;154:166–174.

Bailey DK. The normal cervical spine in infants and children. Radiology 1952;59:712–719.

Bodner RJ, Heyman S, Drummond DS, et al. The use of single photon emission computed tomography (SPECT) in the diagnosis of low-back pain in young patients. Spine 1988;13:1155–1160.

Bunnell WA. Back pain in children. Orthop Clin North Am 1982;13: 587–604.

Epstein JA, Epstein NE, Marc J, et al. Lumbar intervertebral disc herniation in teenage children: recognition and management of associated anomalies. Spine 1984;9:427.

King HA. Back pain in children. Pediatr Clin North Am 1984;31: 1083–1095.

Koptis SE. Orthopaedic complications of dwarfism. Clin Orthop 1976;114:153–179.

Lowe TG. Current concepts review: Scheuermann's disease. J Bone Joint Surg (Am) 1990;72:940–945.

Olsen TL, Anderson RL, Dearwater SR, et al. The epidemiology of low back pain in adolescent population. Am J Public Health 1992;82: 606–609.

Skaggs DL, Samuelson MA, Hale JM, et al. Complications of posterior iliac crest bone grafting in spine surgery in children. Spine 2000;25:2400–2402.

Turner PG, Hancock PG, Green JH, et al. Back pain in childhood. Spine 1989;14:812–814.

Vitale MG, Stazzone EJ, Gelijns AC, et al. The effectiveness of preoperative erythropoietin in avoiding allogeneic blood transfusion among children undergoing scoliosis surgery. J Pediatr Orthop (Br) 1998;7: 203–209.

Wiltse L. Spondylolisthesis: classification and etiology. Symposium on the spine. American Academy of Orthopedic Surgeons. St. Louis: Mosby, 1969:143–166.

LEG LENGTH INEQUALITY

KENNETH GUIDERA

Leg length inequality is a relatively common orthopaedic problem encountered in children. The treatment is complicated by the need to consider the growth of the limb and estimate discrepancies at skeletal maturity.

PATHOGENESIS

Leg length discrepancies may be congenital, developmental, or acquired. There are numerous etiologies within each category (Table 8-1).

Congenital or developmental etiologies include shortening or absence of the femur, fibula or tibia, hemihypertrophy, hemiatrophy, and skeletal dysplasias. The congenital causes may have associated anomalies that complicate management (i.e., foot abnormalities with fibular hemimelia; knee anomalies with tibial dysplasias). Other etiologies include Ollier disease, multiple hereditary exostoses, developmental dysplasia of the hip, clubfoot, Blount's disease, Legg-Calvé-Perthes disease (LCP), and slipped capital femoral epiphysis (SCFE).

Acquired causes include trauma, infection, inflammation, irradiation, tumors, and mechanical causes. Trauma may cause direct shortening, overgrowth, or growth-plate injuries. Infections and tumors may retard or stimulate growth.

It is important to understand the etiologies so that appropriate interventions may be planned. In addition, hemihypertrophy and hemiatrophy are associated with Wilms tumor and hepatic neoplasms, necessitating screening ultrasounds of the abdomen and pelvis throughout childhood.

DIAGNOSIS

Clinical Features

The management of limb length inequalities requires careful clinical and radiographic evaluation over extended periods of time. Clinical assessment requires gross inspection of the discrepancy, as well as evaluation for other anomalies includ-

TABLE 8-1 ETIOLOGY OF LEG LENGTH INEQUALITY

	Decreased Growth	Increased Growth
Congenital/ developmental	Femoral deficiency (proximal femoral focal deficiency, short femur) Fibular deficiency Tibial deficiency Hemiatrophy Developmental dysplasia of the hip Clubfoot Ollier disease	Hemihypertrophy Klippel-Trenaunay-Weber syndrome
Acquired	Infection Tumor Trauma Burns Radiation Legg-Calvé-Perthes disease Slipped capital femoral epiphysis	Infection Tumor Trauma

TABLE 8-2 RADIOGRAPHIC METHODS OF ASSESSMENT OF LEG LENGTH INEQUALITY

Method	Advantages	Disadvantages
Teleoradiograph	Simple, one exposure, can see limb deformities	Magnification error
Orthoroentograph	Simple, less magnification error	Patient must remain still
Scanogram	Less magnification error, smaller films	Patient must remain still, limb deformities not visualized
Computed tomography scan	Accurate, low radiation, can visualize entire limb	Not available in offices, expensive

ing angular deformities, joint contractures, joint instability, spine deformities, and vascular malformations. Gait must be assessed and compensatory mechanisms considered. Children are quite adept at compensating for leg length discrepancies. Compensation mechanisms include toe-walking on the shorter limb, flexing the hip or thigh of the longer limb, and circumducting or vaulting over the longer limb.

Measurements to be obtained include real leg length (measured from anterosuperior iliac spine to the tip of the medial malleolus) and apparent leg length (measured from umbilicus to the tip of the medial malleolus). Blocks are used to measure leg length discrepancy by placing incrementally larger blocks under the shorter limb until the pelvis is level.

Radiographic Features

Several means of radiographic evaluation of leg length discrepancy are available (Table 8-2). The teleoradiograph (Fig. 8-1A) is a single exposure of both legs on a long film with a ruler. Its advantages include visualization of angular deformities and the requirement of only a single exposure

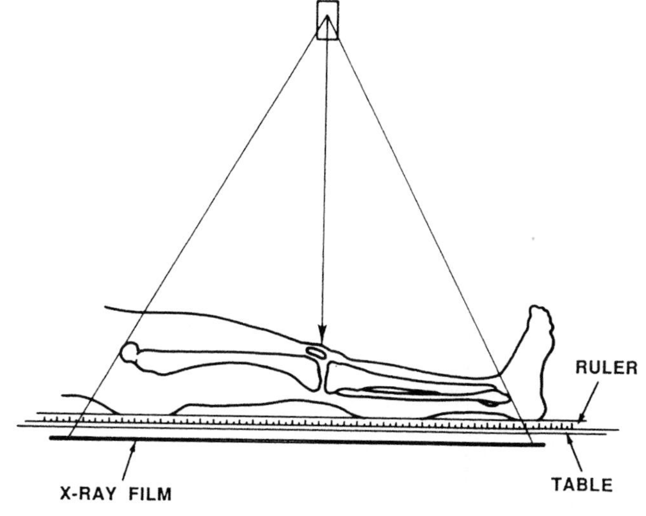

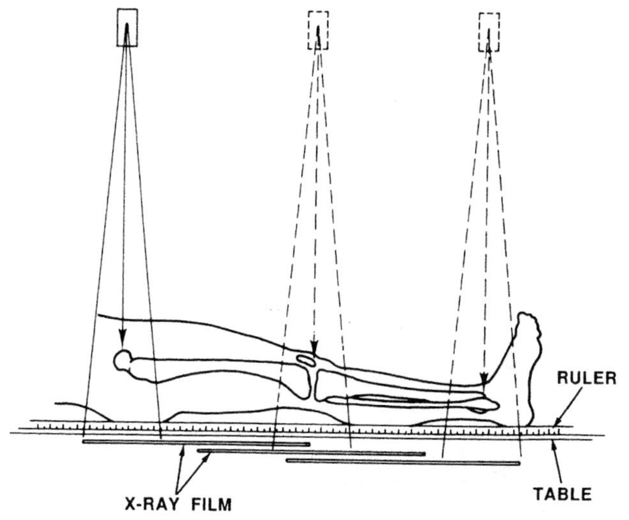

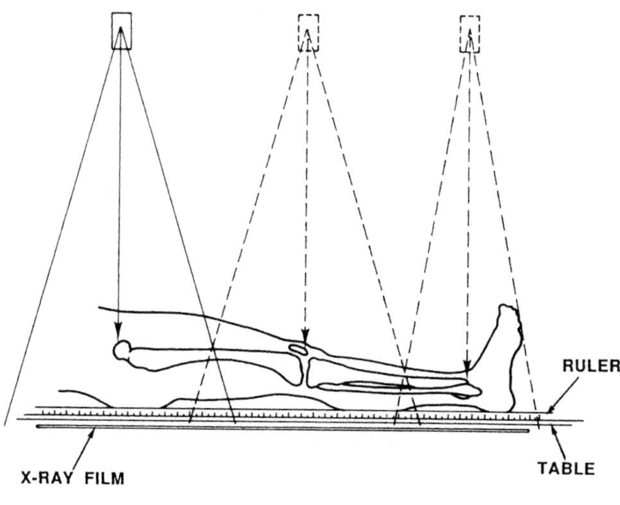

Figure 8-1 (**A**) Diagram of teleroentgenogram technique. This technique shows angular deformity but is subject to errors of magnification. It is probably the best technique for children who cannot reliably comply with instructions to remain still for multiple exposures. (**B**) Diagram of orthoroentgenograph technique. This technique exposes each joint individually, ensuring that the beam through each joint is perpendicular to the x-ray film, thereby avoiding errors of magnification. (**C**) Diagram of scanogram technique. This technique avoids magnification error in the same manner as does the orthoroentgenograph and is the preferred technique for children who cannot remain still for three exposures. (From Mosley CF. Leg length discrepancy. In: Morrissey RT, Weinsten SL, eds. Lovell and Winter's pediatric orthopaedics, 5th ed. Philadelphia: Lippincott Williams & Wilkins, 2001:1106–1150.)

(making it easier to obtain in small children who have difficulty remaining still during the procedure). However, the single exposure introduces a magnification error that decreases the accuracy.

The orthoroentgenograph (Fig. 8-1B) is similar to the teleoradiograph but it uses three separate exposures over the hips, knees, and ankles on one long film with a ruler. This results in less magnification error, but requires a cooperative patient.

The scanogram (Fig. 8-1C) is acquired by moving the radiographic tube and the film for the three exposures. This again diminishes magnification error and results in smaller, more manageable films, but does require the patient to be cooperative and still. It also does not allow for assessment of overall limb alignment. A flexion contracture may diminish its accuracy.

Computed tomography scans are highly accurate for measuring leg length discrepancy. They use decreased radiation and are less sensitive to errors secondary to positioning or contractures and measurements in the lateral plane can be obtained. They also visualize the entire limb, allowing for assessment of other deformities.

Ultrasound also has a role in the assessment of leg length discrepancy. It is more popular in Europe, and a primary reason for its popularity is that it does not use ionizing radiation.

Growth Calculation

To effectively plan treatment, methods to assess growth and predict outcomes have been devised.

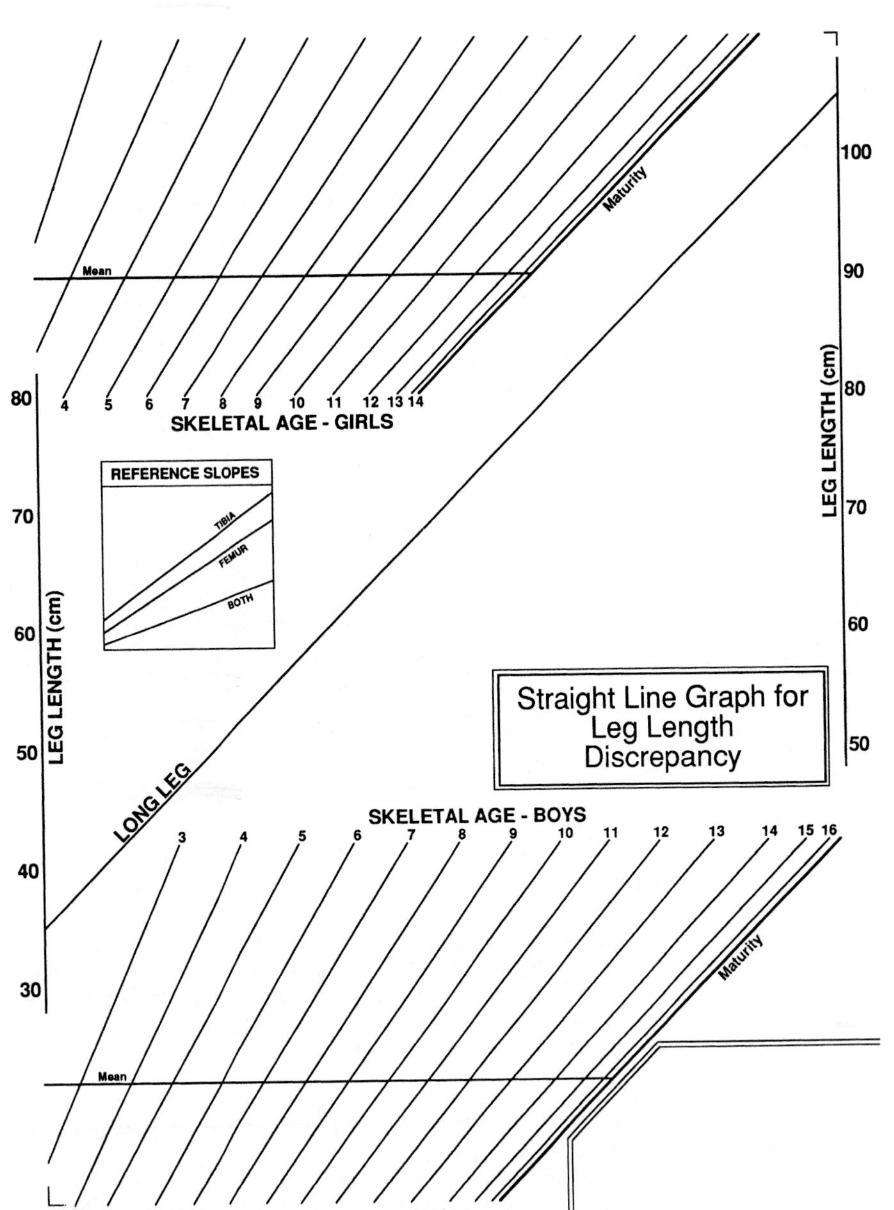

Figure 8-2 The straight-line graph consists of three parts: the leg-length area with the predefined line for the growth of the long leg, areas of sloping lines for the plotting of skeletal ages, and reference slopes to predict growth after epiphysiodesis. (From Mosley CF. Leg length discrepancy. In: Morrissey RT, Weinstein SL, eds. Lovell and Winter's pediatric orthopaedics, 5th ed. Philadelphia: Lippincott Williams & Wilkins, 2001:1106–1150.)

The arithmetic method or Menelaus method is based on several assumptions. The first is that boys grow until age 16 and girls until age 14. The second is that the distal femur contributes ⅜-inch per year to growth and the proximal tibia contributes ¼-inch per year. The third is that the discrepancy increases by ⅛-inch year. These assumptions allow for mathematical calculations of growth and estimation of timing for epiphysiodesis (surgical closure of the growth plates).

The Anderson-Green-Messner growth remaining method predicts future growth based on skeletal age rather than chronologic age. Graphs are used to determine growth percentile of the child, future growth of the long leg, and the effects of epiphysiodesis. Information required for these calculations includes the length of the limbs, skeletal age, chronologic age, and percent of growth inhibition.

Moseley expanded on this method and created straight-line graphs that are used to record, analyze, and predict growth (Fig. 8-2). The Moseley graph relies on the assumptions that the growth of legs can be represented graphically by straight lines and that the leg length discrepancy is the vertical difference between the two lines. The percentage of inhibition of growth is the difference between the slopes of the two lines, with the slope of the normal leg equal to 100%. A leg that is lengthened is represented by a straight line of the same slope displaced upward by the amount lengthened. After epiphysiodesis, the straight line will have a decrease in slope equal to the percent contribution that the growth plate would have made, with the proximal tibia contributing 28% and the distal femur contributing 37% (Fig. 8-3). This method enables better prediction of the effects of surgery, enabling timing to be planned. It is the most commonly used method, and there are now computer programs available to perform the calculations.

With a thorough understanding of the evaluation of leg length discrepancy, it is possible to formulate a treatment plan.

TREATMENT

Operative Treatment of Limb Length Discrepancy

Observation/Lift

The treatment of limb length inequality should be highly individualized (Table 8-3). Observation is the best treatment for small discrepancies under 2 cm. Most of these patients do well with a lift, although some adolescents and teenagers will reject this. The parents should be reassured that, in general, small discrepancies do not cause significant spine or hip problems. A lift up to ½-inch can be fit inside the shoe, making it more cosmetically pleasing for the patient.

Shortening Procedures

For moderate discrepancies (i.e., 2 to 4 cm), the treatment may consist of epiphysiodesis or shortening of the long side. With an epiphysiodesis, the growth charts must be consulted and the patient evaluated at least 3 times at 6-month intervals. The growth charts can assist in the determination of where and when the procedure is to be done. For example, a larger discrepancy may require a distal femoral and proximal tibial epiphysiodesis at 1 to 2 years before the end of growth, while a smaller discrepancy may need only a proximal tibial ablation in the last year of growth. The surgery itself is not overly challenging but the timing is crucial. Poor timing may result in a persistent limb length inequality. Because the procedure is irreversible, the surgical decision must be made carefully. Overall growth and stature of the patient and the patient's parents must be given consideration. For example, a child with small stature may not want a shortening procedure, whereas a tall child may be more accepting of this. A short child with tall parents may have more growth potential than realized. Again, one is faced with shortening the overall stature and operating on the normal, longer, lower extremity.

An epiphysiodesis may be done with either the open or closed method on the long side. The open method involves cutting a piece of bone out from each side of the growth plate, turning it, and reinserting in a manner to produce a bony bridge (Fig. 8-4). A postoperative cast is required for about 6 weeks. The closed or percutaneous method is done under the C-arm using a small incision with a drill or burr being inserted to ablate the growth plate. Both medial and lateral sides must be ablated or an angular deformity may result. The epiphyseal plate is undulating rather than horizontal in contour so care must be taken to burr its entirety. A knee immobilizer is used postoperatively for about 4 weeks and partial weightbearing is allowed. Serial outpatient radiographs are taken to follow the closure of the growth plate.

For larger discrepancies, or those not amenable to epiphysiodesis due to age and cessation of growth, a femoral or tibial shortening may be performed. This may also be done in either a closed or open method. In the open technique, a midshaft approach is made to either the femur or tibia, the desired amount of bone is removed, and the ends are brought together and held with a plate and screws. The closed technique is more technically demanding, requiring intramedullary reaming, cutting, and rodding for stability. However, the patient has less morbidity and a smaller scar. Surgical shortening of greater than 2 inches may result in clumping of the soft tissues, giving a bulky appearance and possibly weakness of the underlying muscles due to the shortening.

Limb Lengthening

The decision to perform or undergo a limb lengthening procedure should not be made lightly. The patient and family must be carefully evaluated as to whether this is the best procedure for them and are they prepared, physically and psychologically, to deal with the long and involved procedure. The general principle consists of making an osteotomy in the bone to be lengthened, stabilizing it with an external frame, and then gradually distracting the two ends of ends of the bone to allow the bone to lengthen as it heals (Fig. 8-5). Each lengthening takes about 1 year to complete, with 6 months in the frame, and 6 months consolidating in an orthosis. The patient and family must be

Determining Leg Length Discrepancy: The Straight Line Graph Method

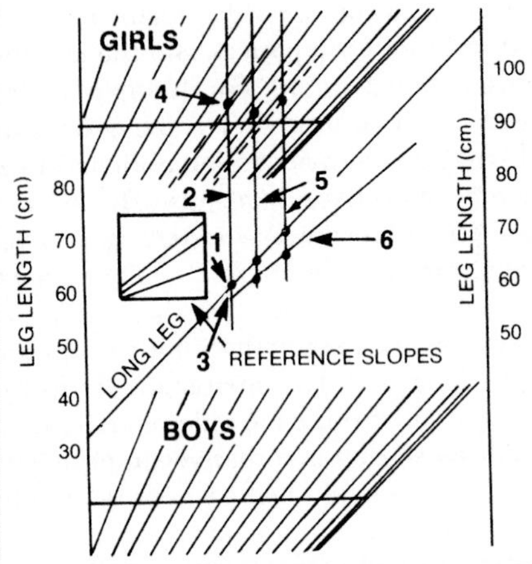

A Assessment of past growth

1. Plot the point for the long leg on the sloping line labeled "LONG LEG" at the appropriate length.
2. Draw a vertical line through that point representing the current assessment.
3. Plot the point for the short leg on the vertical line.
4. Plot the point for skeletal age with reference to the sloping lines in the nomogram.
5. Plot successive visits in the same fashion.
6. Draw a straight line through the short leg points to represent the growth of the short leg.

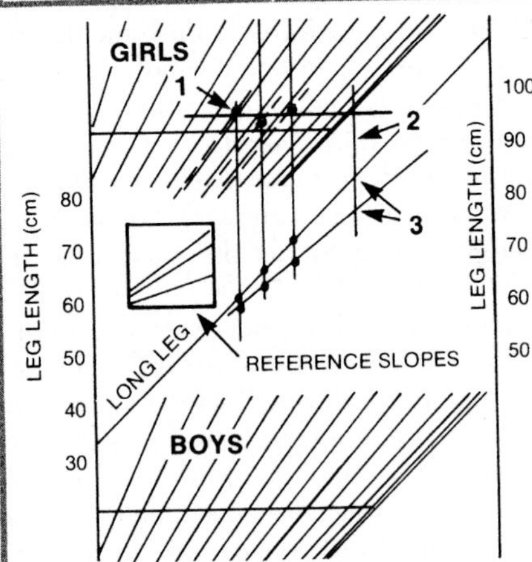

B Prediction of future growth

1. Draw the horizontal straight line that best fits the points previously plotted for skeletal age. The fit to later points is more important than to earlier points. This is the growth percentile line.
2. From the intersection of the growth percentile line with the maturity skeletal age line, draw a vertical line to intersect the growth lines of the two legs. This line represents the end of growth.
3. The points of intersection of the vertical line with the two growth lines indicate the predicted lengths of the legs at maturity.

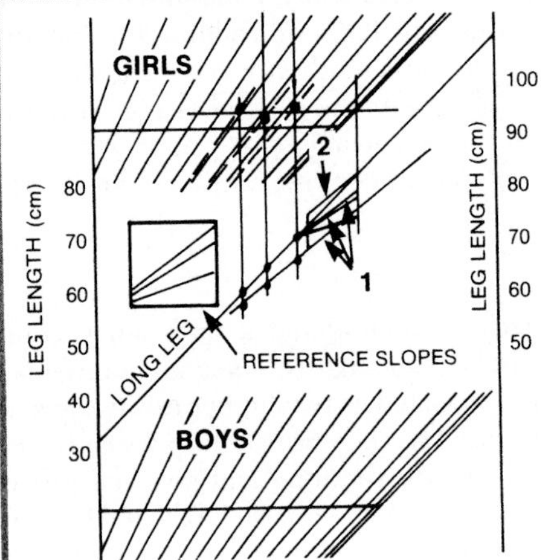

C Prediction of effect of surgery

1. To predict the outcome after epiphysiodesis, draw three lines to the right from the last point for the long leg parallel to the three reference slopes. The intersections of these lines with the vertical line representing the end of growth indicates the predicted lengths of the long leg after the three possible types of epiphysiodesis.
2. To predict the outcome after leg lengthening, draw a line parallel to the growth line of the short leg but elevated above it by the amount of length gained.

Figure 8-3 Step-by-step instructions for using the straight-line graph in determining remaining growth. Data used are an example. (From Mosley CF. Leg length discrepancy. In: Morrissey RT, Weinsten SL, eds. Lovell and Winter's pediatric orthopaedics, 5th ed. Philadelphia: Lippincott Williams & Wilkins, 2001:1106–1150.)

TABLE 8-3 TREATMENT OF LEG LENGTH INEQUALITY

Discrepancy	Treatment
0–2 cm	Observation, shoe lift
2–5 cm	Epihphysiodesis, contralateral shortening, shoe lift
5–17 cm	Limb lengthening (possibly staged)
>17 cm	Staged lengthenings, amputation, prosthetic fitting

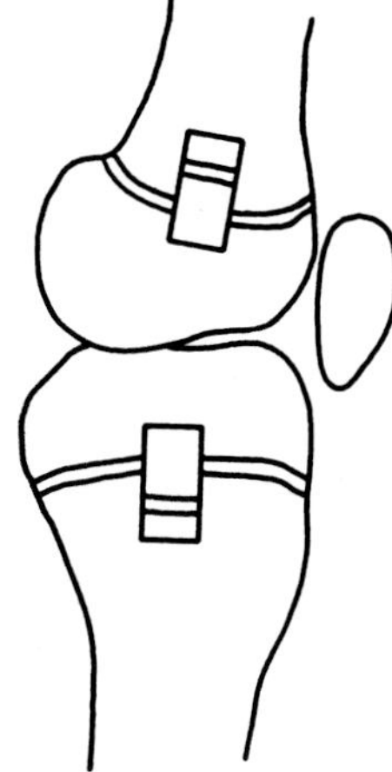

Figure 8-4 Epiphysiodesis by the Phemister method. A rectangular bone block is replaced in reversed position to produce a bar across the growth plate. (From Mosley CF. Leg length discrepancy. In: Morrissey RT, Weinsten SL, eds. Lovell and Winter's pediatric orthopaedics, 5th ed. Philadelphia: Lippincott Williams & Wilkins, 2001:1106–1150.)

able to perform the distractions, pin care, and therapy. Complication almost always arise and include pin site infections, broken wires, loss of range of motion, fractures, angulation, lack of consolidation, and pain. A careful clinical, psychological, and social evaluation of the patient and family prior to planning and scheduling this type of procedure is performed. Potential complications and treatment are outlined to the family.

It is beyond the scope of this chapter to present limb lengthening surgical techniques in detail. However, the basic principles are outlined in Box 8-1. Once the decision has been made to lengthen the extremity, there are several techniques available. One may use either a circumferential frame such as an Ilizarov device or a unilateral lengthener. Each one will yield the same type of results. The circumferential frame provides more stability and allows angular correction concurrently with the lengthening. The unilateral device may also provide angular correction, although in many cases not as much. It may be easier to apply to the femur since one does not have to deal with pins and rings extending medially. An advantage of the circular frame is that it can be constructed in a manner to provide both

BOX 8-1 LENGTHENING PRINCIPLES

- Evaluate length discrepancy
- Patient/family evaluation and education
- Proper pin placement; frame stability
- Maintain joint mobility
- Corticotomy vs. osteotomy
- Latency period (for edema), then distract
- Four-times-a-day distractions
- Compress—for pseudarthrosis, poor regenerate bone
- Physical therapy, pin care, pain control

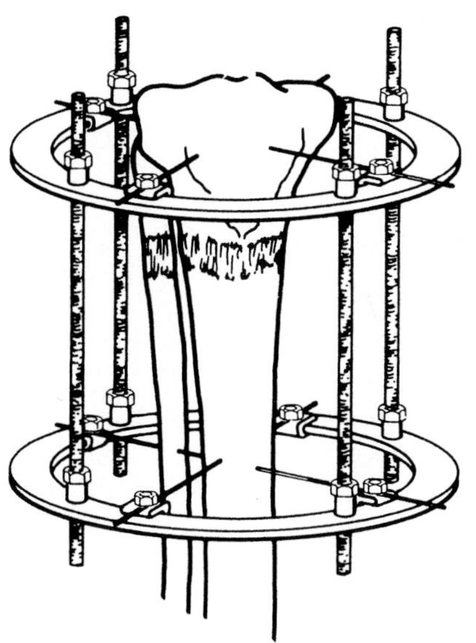

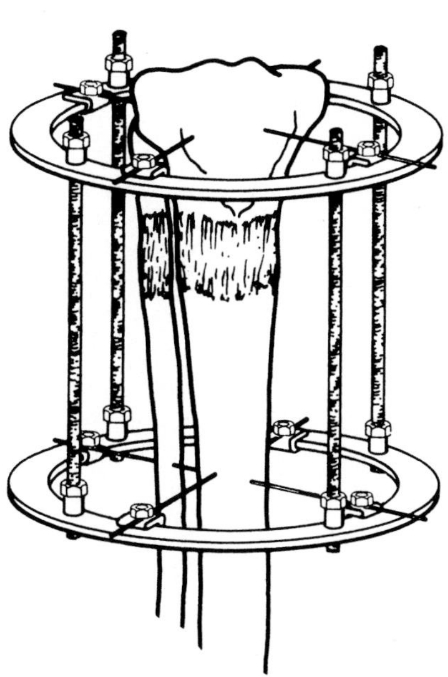

Figure 8-5 Metaphyseal lengthening. Elongation through the metaphysis promotes osteogenesis in the lengthening gap because metaphyseal bone is so active, and it promotes strength by the large cross-sectional area. (From Mosley CF. Leg length discrepancy. In: Morrissey RT, Weinsten SL, eds. Lovell and Winter's pediatric orthopaedics, 5th ed. Philadelphia: Lippincott Williams & Wilkins, 2001:1106–1150.)

compression and distraction if needed (i.e., in a short limb with a pseudarthrosis).

The distraction rate should be 1 mm per day in four equal distractions, which will result in an inch of growth per month. This can be slowed if there is poor callous/regenerate bone formation. In cases of persistent poor regeneration, one can alternately compress and lengthen to stimulate the new bone formation. Distractions should be held for the first 5 to 7 days postoperatively to allow the edema to decrease. At that point, the periosteal new bone formation commences. The osteotomy should be atraumatic to preserve the periosteum and its function. A corticotomy has been recommended by various authors to help preserve the osseous intramedullary circulation. Others have recommended cutting with a Gigli saw.

During the lengthening, physical therapy, pin care and pain management are important adjuncts to treatment. Range of motion of the joints above and below the lengthening are crucial and lengthening may have to be slowed or stopped temporarily if range is significantly lost. Orthotics attached to the frame enhance joint position and prevent loss of motion. Pin care is taught to the patient and family to avoid pin tract infections. Many pins develop drainage which is not a true infection; however, with significant drainage or purulence I prescribe oral antibiotics. Pin care is done with simple soap and water cleansing and saline-soaked sponges. Pain control is dealt with on a team approach at our hospital. Various techniques are used including oral medications, transdermal analgesic patches, and diversion techniques. A combination of these techniques generally results in adequate pain control.

Removal of the device is performed after the consolidation period. This is generally 2 to 3 months after the cessation of lengthening. The patient is placed in an orthosis after removal for about 6 months, until the regenerate bone appears mature. During this period the patient works on range of motion and strengthening. Full weightbearing is allowed and encouraged. This whole process may be repeated after a few years for larger discrepancies, when there is adequate osseous healing.

Many potential complications can arise when lengthening a limb. These range from pin tract infections to fracture (Box 8-2). These should be anticipated and treated promptly and aggressively, while continuing the distractions.

BOX 8-2 COMPLICATIONS OF LENGTHENING

- Infection—pin tract
- Neurovascular injury
- Joint subluxation/dislocation
- Joint contracture—loss of range of motion
- Fracture
- Delayed union/nonunion
- Pain
- Skin compression from fixator
- Psychosocial issues
- Inability to obtain desired length

SUMMARY

Leg length inequality presents a challenge to the pediatric orthopaedist. An understanding of the condition and the ability to predict ultimate discrepancy enables one to formulate a treatment plan. The treatment must be suited to the patient and the family. Treatment may include shoe lift, epiphysiodesis, shortening, or lengthening. A team approach and well-informed and involved family result in the best outcome.

SUGGESTED READING

Andersen M, Green W, Messner M. Growth and predictions of growth in the lower extremities, J Bone Joint Surg (Am) 1963;45:1–14.

Guidera KJ, Helal AA, Zuern KA. Management of pediatric limb length inequality. Adv Pediatr 1996;42:501–543.

Moseley CF. A straight-line graph for leg-length discrepancies. J Bone Joint Surg (Am) 1977;59:174–179.

Mosley CF. Leg length discrepancy. In: Morrissey RT, Weinsten SL, eds. Lovell and Winter's pediatric orthopaedics, 5th ed. Philadelphia: Lippincott Williams & Wilkins, 2001:1106–1150.

Stanitski DF. Limb-length inequality. OKU: Pediatrics 2, AAOS, Chapter 19; 183–190.

TOE-WALKING

BRIAN L. HOTCHKISS

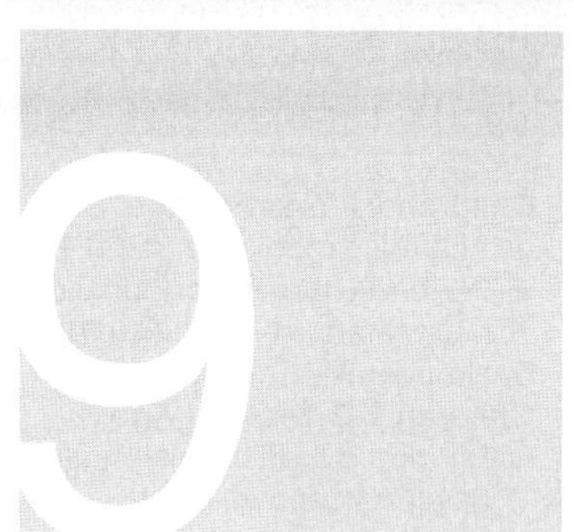

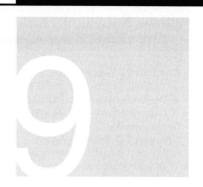

Toe-walking is commonly seen in children, and it is often undertreated. Characteristically the child walks with the foot in an equinus posture, bearing weight mostly or entirely on the forefoot. The child may be able to get the heel down volitionally when standing or walking. This has led to the misleading terms of "habitual" or "volitional" toe-walking. Toe-walking may be a transient developmental variant, associated with neuromuscular conditions, or it may be idiopathic. If persistent into the third year of life, toe-walking deserves medical attention and will likely require treatment.

PATHOGENESIS

Classification

Toe-walking may be developmental, associated with another condition, or idiopathic. Developmental toe-walking is common in normal children during the first year of ambulation. It is bipedal and self-limited. If it is unilateral, other conditions such as developmental hip dislocation, congenitally short femur, or hemiplegia need to be considered.

An associated condition such as cerebral palsy, spinal cord anomaly, muscular dystrophy, or other neurologic conditions needs to be ruled out by history, examination, and diagnostic testing.

Idiopathic toe-walking begins like the developmental type but does not resolve. The diagnosis is established by exclusion if careful exam does not reveal spasticity or other sign of a more generalized neuromuscular disorder.

The child who rises on toes during stance but makes consistently good heel contact is probably developing normally and is not included in this discussion.

Etiology

The cause of toe-walking in otherwise normal children is unknown. There may by a family history of a similar condition.

Pathophysiology

Children with idiopathic toe-walking have been shown to have abnormal electromyographic gait analysis findings. The muscle synergy pattern is abnormal during the toe–toe gait as well as during the heel–toe gait. These changes are reversible with cast treatment. The forefoot adjusts to its weightbearing role by hypertrophy. The heel adjusts to its non-weightbearing role by atrophic growth.

Natural History

It is generally agreed upon that toe-walking in the first year or two of life has a benign prognosis. There is poor agreement in the literature regarding the prognosis in older children. Although some children are said to improve spontaneously, others do not. Persistence leads to enduring gait abnormality, structural foot deformity, and difficulty with shoe wear. Treatment appears to be most effective in children under 5 years of age. The effect of excessive weightbearing by the forefoot in aging adults is not well documented.

DIAGNOSIS

History and Physical Examination

The typical child presents with a history of normal motor development. The toe-walking pattern has usually been present since walking began. It may be static or dynamic. If ankle dorsiflexion can be brought to neutral or beyond, the child can stand flat-footed or walk with the heel down during the initial stance phase of gait. In the static form, the shorter heel cords make it necessary for the child to compensate by knee hyperextension in order to get the heel down. In the less common dynamic form, the range of motion of the ankle is normal. In either form, as soon as the child stops concentrating on walking correctly, the toe–toe gait pattern returns.

If the toe-walking is unilateral, and the bone and joint structure of the extremity is normal, the cause is most likely hemiplegic cerebral palsy. Sustained ankle clonus, abnormal accessory movements of upper extremities dur-

BOX 9-1 DIAGNOSTIC WORKUP OF TOE-WALKING

Children <2 Years of Age
- Acquire a medical and developmental history
- Perform a general orthopaedic examination to rule out neuromuscular condition, bone or joint deformity
- No treatment needed

Children 2–3 Years of Age
- Perform a medical history and physical examination as described above
- Institute treatment if heel cord is short or if plantar skin shows typical pattern of thickening at forefoot

Children >3 Years of Age
- Institute treatment after associated causes of toe--toe gait have been clinically ruled out

Children Not Responding or with Recurrence after Cast Treatment
- Consider electrodiagnostic studies to help detection of subtle forms of cerebral palsy
- Surgical treatment is usually necessary

ing gait, clumsiness with hopping (especially in older children), muscle hypertrophy or atrophy, autism, learning difficulties, bladder problems, cavus feet, or other signs of neurologic impairment need to be considered before settling on a diagnosis of idiopathic toe-walking.

Aside from the characteristic gait abnormality, there are three other characteristic physical findings seen in children who walk on their toes:

- Shortened Achilles tendon is the most obvious.
- Difference in the appearance of the plantar skin.
  - The forefoot skin is thickened and may be calloused.
  - Heel skin is smooth and thinner.
- Underdevelopment of the calcaneus and overdevelopment of the forefoot, leading to wedge-shaped foot with a narrow undeveloped heel and a wide overdeveloped forefoot

Careful examination of the foot can be more important than the observation of walking in the atypical environment of the outpatient clinic. The diagnostic workup is outlined in Box 9-1.

TREATMENT

The role of physical therapy and coaching (instructing the child to volitionally stop walking on toes) for management of idiopathic toe-walking are poorly documented but do not seem to be effective in clinical experience.

Serial casting for a period of 6 to 8 weeks is commonly used, especially in younger children. After casting it may be advisable to splint the ankle in dorsiflexion at night for 6 months and to encourage the parents to perform daily passive stretching techniques during the same time.

Percutaneous heel cord lengthening may be employed as a primary option or as a fallback option for unsuccessful cast treatment.

Botox injection into the triceps surae may be an alternative to consider in children who have failed cast treatment if they don't have significant heel cord shortening.

Results and Outcome

Despite various observations and opinions found in recent articles in the medical literature, I have found consistent success with casting and night splinting:

- Two sets of short leg walking casts are worn for periods of 3 weeks each.
- The casts are applied with the child's forefoot resting on a metal support.
- The foot is kept in maximum dorsiflexion (the child is instructed to drop the heel toward the floor while the parent holds gentle pressure down on the knee).
- Care must be taken not to dorsiflex the foot after the cast material is wrapped to avoid a pressure sore over the anterior ankle.
- If the heel cords are quite short or the child is in the older age group, 3 sets of casts are worn for 2 weeks each.
- All children are kept in dorsiflexion night splints for 6 months.
- Parents are instructed on daily calf muscle stretching.

Recurrences are not common and heel cord lengthening is only infrequently needed. If the condition has been allowed to persist beyond 4 or 5 years of age, treatment is more difficult. Primary care physicians should be encouraged to refer patients between 2 and 3 years of age to orthopaedists.

SUGGESTED READING

Brouwer B, Davidson LK, Olney SJ. Serial casting in idiopathic toe-walkers and children with spastic cerebral palsy. J Pediatr Orthop 2000;20:221–225.

Eastwood DM, Menelaus MB, Dickens DRV, et al. Idiopathic toe-walking: does treatment alter the natural history? J Pediatr Orthop (Part B) 2000;9:47–49.

Griffin PP, Wheelhouse WW, Shiavi R, et al. Habitual toe-walkers: a clinical and electromyographic gait analysis. J Bone Joint Surg (Am) 1977;59:97–101.

Kogan M, Smith J. Simplified approach to idiopathic toe-walking. J Pediatr Orthop 2001;21:790–791.

Policy JF, Torburn L, Rinsky LA, et al. Electromyographic test to differentiate mild diplegic cerebral palsy and idiopathic toe-walking. J Pediatr Orthop 2001;21:784–789.

Stricker SJ, Angulo JC. Idiopathic toe walking: a comparison of treatment methods. J Pediatr Orthop 1998;18:289–293.

LIMPING

RICHARD M. SCHWEND
JON SHERECK

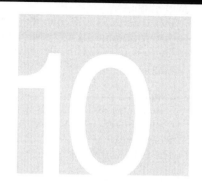

Limping is a common complaint in children of all ages. The child often presents to the primary care physician or to the emergency room with either a limp or has completely stopped walking. It is important to understand normal walking development and mechanics when evaluating the child with a limp.

Although young children fall frequently, they have normal protective reflexes, and being already close to the ground, injuries are rare. The very young child learning to walk relies on a variety of compensations, typically involving proximal body segments, to keep from falling. These include:

- Hands held high
- A wide-based gait
- Hip, knee, and ankle flexion
- Increased time in double stance

Walking maturity follows very predictable developmental milestones (Table 10-1).

PATHOGENESIS

Etiology

Limping is a compensation for a disorder of normal walking mechanics. Limping can be caused by a large variety of conditions from high in the central nervous system such as a brain or spinal cord tumor, or by very distal problems, such as a foreign body in the foot.

TABLE 10-1 DEVELOPMENTAL MILESTONES OF WALKING MATURITY

Age	Milestone
13 mo	Independent walking
18 mo	Reciprocal arm swing, heel-strike
24 mo	Normal knee flexion in stance
36 mo	Mature angular rotations
7 yr	Adult pattern, single-limb stance, velocity, cadence, step length

Pathomechanics

The following disturbances of normal walking mechanics may cause a child to limp. By determining the mechanism for the limp, the physician can more specifically use the physical examination to determine cause.

Pain

Antalgic Gait

- Less time is spent in single-leg-stance. Stride length is shortened. The child walks slowly and cautiously. When severe, the child will refuse to walk.
- Most common reason a child will acutely limp.
- Common conditions include acute fractures, such as a toddler fracture of the tibia or calcaneus, stress fracture, infection (especially in the hip), and foreign body in the foot.

Weakness

Trendelenburg or Waddling Gait

- The hip muscles are stabilizers for single limb stance. The child uses the proximal segments to compensate for distal weakness.
- A trunk shift toward the affected side (Trendelenburg gait) is used to compensate for weak hip abductors.
- Increased lumbar lordosis compensates for anterior pelvic tilt from weak hip extensors.
- The child hikes the hip and flexes the knee excessively during swing phase to clear a dropped foot due to a weak tibialis anterior muscle.
- The Gower sign, in which the child uses the hands to climb up the thighs, is a classic example of using proximal compensation for distal weakness, as seen in Duchenne muscular dystrophy.

Short Limb

- In contrast to adults, children with a very short limb typically compensate by walking on the toes on the involved side.
- Hemiplegia and developmental dysplasia of the hip are frequent causes of a short limb, although other mechanisms also affect the gait in these conditions.

Joint Stiffness

- This is commonly seen in the early stages of Perthes disease with synovitis and restricted hip motion.
- There is typically an adduction contracture and loss of internal rotation and extension.

Spasticity

- Common in children with spastic cerebral palsy.
- Children with spastic diplegia typically have a history of prematurity.
- The child with mild spastic hemiplegia may have a delay in walking (after age 18 months) and a very subtle limp. Asking the child to run accentuates the limp and the upper extremity posturing. The orthopaedic surgeon will frequently be the first physician to recognize this condition.

Poor Balance

- Seen in children with cerebral palsy, Friedrich ataxia, and Charcot-Marie-Tooth disease. Patients with Charcot-Marie-Tooth disease have been described as having a stiff "marionette gait."

BOX 10-1 CLASSIFICATION OF LIMPING BY AGE

All Ages
- Septic hip arthritis
- Trauma and abuse
- Leukemia
- Discitis
- Developmental dysplasia of the hip
- Neoplasia
- Neuromuscular conditions
- Juvenile rheumatoid arthritis
- Epidural abscess
- Discoid lateral meniscus
- Sacroiliac joint infection
- Cellulitis
- Stress fracture
- Foreign body

Toddlers (1–3 Yr)
- Septic hip arthritis
- Tibia fracture
- Calcaneal fracture
- Spastic hemiplegia
- Developmental dysplasia of the hip

Children (4–10 Yr)
- Transient hip synovitis
- Perthes disease
- Juvenile rheumatoid arthritis

Adolesents (>10 Yr)
- Slipped capital femoral epiphysis
- Spondylolisthesis
- Overuse injuries
- Tarsal coalition
- Gonococcal septic arthritis
- Osteonecrosis of the femoral head
- Chondrolysis of the hip

Classifications

Classification can be made based on several factors:

- Age (Box 10-1).
- Limping disasters, both acute and chronic. This is the most important classification (Box 10-2).
- Location (Box 10-3).
- System (Table 10-2).

BOX 10-2 CLASSIFICATION OF LIMPING BY DISASTERS

Acute
- Septic hip arthritis
- Septic arthritis and osteomyelitis
- Unstable slipped capital femoral epiphysis
- Soft tissue infections, necrotizing fasciitis
- Leukemia
- Intraarticular fractures
- Displaced or open fractures
- Child abuse
- Leukemia
- Epidural abscess

Chronic
- Slipped capital femoral epiphysis
- Solid malignant neoplasm
- Spinal cord tumor
- Child abuse
- Treatable neuromuscular conditions
- Leukemia

BOX 10-3 CLASSIFICATION OF LIMPING BY LOCATION

General
- Fractures
- Overuse
- Child abuse
- Leukemia
- Arthritis
- Osteomyelitis
- Soft tissue infection
- Neuromuscular conditions
- Benign bone lesions
- Malignant bone lesions

Abdominal and Pelvic
- Appendicitis
- Kidney infection
- Psoas abscess
- Pelvic abscess
- Pelvic mass

Central Nervous System and Spine
- Cerebral palsy
- Spina bifida
- Spinal cord tumor
- Epidural abscess
  Discitis
- Spondylolysis
- Herniated disc
- Vertebral end-plate fracture
- Hereditary sensory motor neuropathy

Hip
- Septic arthritis
- Transient synovitis
- Perthes disease
- Slipped capital femoral epiphysis
- Pelvic infection

Lower Extremity
- Limb length discrepancy
- Tibia fractures
- Calcaneal fractures
- Foreign body

TABLE 10-2 CLASSIFICATION OF LIMPING BY SYSTEM AND SIGNS AND SYMPTOMS[a]

Condition	Signs, Symptoms, Pearls
Congenital and Developmental	
Developmental hip dysplasia	Unstable hip newborn, limited abduction in older infant
Limb length discrepancy	May walk on toes; measure limb lengths
Torsional deformities	Best detected on prone examination
Idiopathic toe walking	Exclude cerebral palsy or muscle dystrophy
Mild clubfoot	Equinus, heel varus, forefoot adductus
Coxa vara	Trendelenburg limp, radiographic changes
Short femur	Galeazzi sign, confirm on radiograph
Discoid lateral meniscus	Clicking in knee, lack of full knee extension
Intraarticular ganglion	Pain, restricted knee extension
Tarsal coalition	Pain, subtalar stiffness, valgus foot, or varus
Infection-Related	
Septic hip arthritis	Ill, fever, hip pain at rest
Septic arthritis	Fever, pain, stiff swollen joint
Osteomyelitis	Pain, swelling if superficial, fever
Epidural abscess	Pain, fever, won't walk, loss of function
SI joint infection	Pain, fever, pain with FABER
Discitis	Back pain, abdominal pain, won't walk
Lyme disease	Erythema migrans, arthritis
Appendicitis	Pain, loss of apetitite, abdominal tenderness
Pylonephritis	Back pain, fever
Poliomyelitis	Muscle pain, weakness
Tuberculosis of bone	Swelling, radiograph changes, positive PPD
Guillain-Barré syndrome	Ascending generalized weakness
Traumatic and Stress-Related	
Child abuse	Multiple lesions or fractures
Acute fractures	Pain, swelling, deformity
Stress fractures	Pain with activity
Slipped capital femoral epiphysis	Hip pain with activity, loss of internal rotation in flexion
Tibia, calcaneus, and cuboid toddler fractures	Swelling, tender to palpation, often not diagnosed for several weeks
Vertebral end-plate fracture	Trauma, back pain, radiculopathy
Sprains and contusions	Very common
Foreign body	Often missed
Osteochondroses	Pain, swelling, or mechanical symptoms
Neuromuscular	
Cerebral palsy, hemiplegia	Mild delay walking, subtle limp
Spina bifida	Worsening gait may be from tethered cord or shunt malfunction
Duchenne muscular dystrophy	Boys; toe walking or loss of walking ability
Spinal cord tumor	Pain and night pain, loss of function
Hereditary sensory motor neuropathies	Cavus feet, "marionette gait," subtle hip weakness
Friedrich ataxia	Balance problems, may present as scoliosis
Tethered spinal cord	Pain, spasticity, loss of function
Inflammation	
Transient hip synovitis	After viral illness, less ill than septic hip
Juvenile rheumatoid arthritis	Chronic joint pain and effusion
Ankylosing spondylitis	Back and sacroiliac joint pain, stiffness
Henoch-Schönlein purpura	Periarticular findings may precede purpuric rash, abdominal pain and hemorrage, renal
Benign Neoplasia	
Osteoid osteoma	Night pain relieved by aspirin
Osteoblastoma	Pain, lesion larger than 2 cm
Unicameral bone cyst proximal femur	No findings, or pain, or pathologic fracture
Langerhan histiocytosis	Pain, skeletal lesions, diabetes insipidus
Intramuscular hemangioma	Pain, swelling of superficial lesions
Chondroblastoma	Pain and swelling, epiphyseal location
Malignant Neoplasia	
Spinal cord tumors	Pain, night pain, loss of function
Osteogenic sarcoma	Pain, swelling, or mass
Ewing sarcoma	Pain, swelling, or mass
Leukemia	Malaise, fever, joint swelling, pain
Rhabdomyosarcoma	Soft tissue mass, pain

(continued)

TABLE 10-2 (continued)

Condition	Signs, Symptoms, Pearls
General and Metabolic, Genetic	
Sickle cell disease	Pain crisis, osteonecrosis
Hemophilia	Joint pain, swelling, muscle bleeds
Rickets	Pain, swelling, irritable, deformity
Hyperparathyroidism	Skeletal and abdominal pain, irritability, mental status changes
Scurvy	Pain and swelling, bleeding gums, skin rash
Other Causes	
Legg-Calvé-Perthes disease	Hip pain, stiffness, and limp
Conversion reaction	Symptoms do not fit the physical findings

[a]Although by no means complete, this classification is an extensive list of common and uncommon conditions. Use it as a checklist and supplement to the other classifications if the diagnosis is still uncertain.
FABER, flexion, abduction, external rotation; PPD, positive protein derivative; SI, sacral iliac.

DIAGNOSIS

History and Examination

A thorough history and physical examination with thoughtful consideration of pathophysiology and classification should usually determine the most likely location and cause of the limp. During the evaluation, the physician should be particularly suspicious of the limping disasters listed in Box 10-2.

History

- Child's age.
- Acute or chronic onset.
- History of trauma or infection.
- Is pain present? Be very specific about onset, location, quality, intensity, and radiation.
- Constant pain or night pain is always worrisome and suggests infection or tumor.
- Morning pain suggests childhood arthritis.
- Bilateral or unilateral symptoms? Bilateral suggests generalized conditions.
- Is child systemically ill? Limp with lower extremity pain, fever, and malaise lasting for several weeks suggests a serious general condition such as leukemia

Physical Examination

- Undress the child sufficiently to visually observe. Goal is to precisely localize the area of pathology.
- Does the child appear ill or well?
- Is the child protecting or splinting a particular body part, such as the hip? If the child has significant hip pain at *rest*, suspect septic arthritis. Due to the frequency of important pathology found at the hip, a careful examination of this area is essential.
- Gait: If the child seems well, first examine while walking. Observe the feet, knees, hips, and spine during stance and swing phase. Observe with both of normal and abnormal walking mechanics in mind.
- Standing examination: Observe spine for symmetry, lesions, and range of motion.
- Trendelenburg sign.
- Have patient get up off the floor (Gower maneuver).
- Tabletop examination: Observe the patient's most comfortable position. Patients with transient synovitis are typically comfortable at rest, whereas those with septic hip arthritis are not.
- Look for swelling and rash. Lightly touch skin to check for warmth. Have child do active range of motion *before* passive motion is checked. Gently roll the child's foot internally and externally to check hip rotation.

Radiologic Findings

- Children who appear well, but have a limp, have a 96% chance of having a normal radiograph.
- Radiographs should be used to *confirm* the suspected diagnosis, not to *make* the diagnosis.
- Fractures and Legg-Calvé-Perthes disease are the two most common conditions diagnosed on plain radiographs.
- Some fractures such as spiral tibia or calcaneal fractures in the toddler are not apparent on radiographs until 2 or 3 weeks later when new bone is formed.
- Image the entire pelvis—anteroposterior and lateral—when obtaining a hip radiograph. Do *not* use a pelvic shield as it will obscure important findings and often requires the film to be repeated, thus increasing the radiation dose.

Other Imaging Studies

- Ultrasound
  - ☐ Highly sensitive for detecting hip effusion, but less specific to distinguish transient synovitis from septic hip arthritis.
  - ☐ The presence of fluid in hip joint must be explained, especially if the ESR and CRP are elevated.
  - ☐ Ultrasound is useful for examining other joints and soft tissues.
- Bone scan
  - ☐ Sensitive but not very specific.
  - ☐ Rarely is needed urgently to decide treatment.
  - ☐ Useful for screening the entire skeleton in child abuse, suspected discitis, pelvic osteomyelitis, and osteoid osteoma.

- Useful for detecting overuse injuries and stress fractures.
- Test tends to be overused.
- Magnetic resonance imaging
  - Helpful to image suspected spinal cord tumors, epidural abscess, discitis, pelvic abscess and soft tissue lesions.
  - Consult with radiologist *before* test is performed.
  - Always look at the images yourself and preferably *with* the radiologist.

Other Studies

- Complete blood count
  - Use to screen for elevated leukocytes and anemia.
  - With an elevated erythrocyte sedimentation rate (ESR), the combination of thrombocytopenia, anemia, neutropenia, lymphocytosis, and blasts cells present on the peripheral smear is very suggestive of childhood leukemia.
- ESR
  - Sensitive indicator of inflammation and should always be obtained if infection, arthritis, or malignancy is suspected.
  - Slow to rise and fall: It is increased after 24 to 48 hours and may remain elevated for several weeks after appropriate treatment of infection.
  - An ESR over 50 mm per hour is associated with an important diagnosis in three-fourths of limping children.
- C-reactive protein
  - Acute phase protein made in the liver, responds to inflammation.
  - Rises within 6 hours and becomes normal within 6 to 10 days.
  - More sensitive than ESR in following resolution of infection.
- Joint aspiration
  - Aspirate joint if septic arthritis is a possibility.
  - A dry tap in the hip joint may still be an infection. Use arthrography or ultrasound to confirm that needle is *truly* in the joint.
  - Normal fluid less than 200 leukocytes with 25% polymorphonuclear (PMN).
  - 75% of patients with septic arthritis have more than 80,000 PMN.

Putting It All Together

An ill-appearing child who is not walking is always of concern and suggests a serious diagnosis (Box 10-2). The physical examination should locate the area of involvement. Fever, severe or night pain, non-weightbearing and tenderness on palpation, combined with an elevated ESR, suggest a deep inflammatory process such as septic hip arthritis.

TREATMENT

Nonoperative Options

- Treatment depends on an accurate diagnosis.
- Most causes of limping can be treated conservatively.
- Transient synovitis is a frequent cause of limping or refusal to walk. With bed rest and antiinflammatory medication, the child may be markedly improved by the next morning. Hip aspiration is not necessary if the diagnosis is clear and the patient improves.

Surgical Indications/Contraindications

- Septic hip arthritis, epidural abscess, and unstable slipped capital femoral epiphysis require urgent surgical management.
- A patient who has lost the ability to walk should never be sent home from the emergency department without making a clear diagnosis.

Complications

- Septic hip arthritis: Femoral head osteonecrosis, physeal arrest, and arthritis
- Epidural abscess: Permanent loss of neurologic function
- Unstable slipped capital femoral epiphysis: Femoral head osteonecrosis, chondrolysis, and late degenerative arthritis

PEARLS

- Remember the limping disasters (Box 10-2). Missed septic hip arthritis, spinal cord tumor, child abuse, and leukemia are particular disasters to avoid.
- The hip is a common site of limping. Disorders about the hip are commonly misdiagnosed.
- Developmental hip dysplasia and mild hemiplegia in the toddler are common causes of a delay in walking or a persistent limp.
- Always be concerned about the child who loses ability to walk.
- Always consider child abuse in the infant, young child, or the patient with multiple bone and soft tissue injuries.
- Constant pain and night pain are always worrisome.
- If the diagnosis is unclear, reexamine the patient later or consult with a trusted colleague.
- If a case is not following a predicted course for the presumed diagnosis, there may be a different or unexpected diagnosis. Leukemia is classic for prolonged limping with many systemic complaints. Other rare conditions such as vitamin D deficiency and scurvy can show up.
- Be aware of the "cold" or "normal" bone scan of the hip. Instead, this may represent vascular compromise to the femoral head.
- When aspirating a suspected septic hip arthritis and no fluid is obtained, the needle might not be in the hip joint; or, the purulent fluid may be too thick to flow through the narrow gauge needle.
- An adolescent with hip or thigh pain, especially one who cannot walk, should always be suspected for slipped capital femoral epiphysis.

SUGGESTED READING

Barkin RM, Barkin SZ, Barkin AZ. The limping child. J Emerg Med 2000;18:331–339.

Choban S, Killian JT. Evaluation of acute gait abnormalities in preschool children. J Pediatr Orthop 1990;10:74–78.

Flynn JM, Widmann RF. The limping child: evaluation and diagnosis. J Am Acad Orthopaed Surg 2001;989–98.

Kocher MS, Zurakowski D, Kasser JR. Differentiating between septic arthritis and transient synovitis of the hip in children: an evidence-based clinical prediction algorithm. J Bone Joint Surg (Am) 1999; 81:12.

Leet AI, Skaggs DL. Evaluation of the acutely limping child. Am Fam Physician 2000;61:1011–1018.

Richards BS. The limping child. In: Sponseller PD, ed. Orthopaedic knowledge update. Pediatrics 2. Rosemont, IL: Pediatric Society of North America and American Academy of Orthopaedic Surgeons 2002: 3–10.

Sutherland DH, Olshen R, Cooper L, et al. The development of mature gait. J Bone Joint Surg (Am) 1980;62:336–353.

Taylor GR, Clarke NM. Management of the irritable hip: a review of hospital admission policy. Arch Dis Child 1994;71:59–63.

Tuten HR, Gabos PG, Kumar SJ, et al. The limping child: a manifestation of acute leukemia. J Pediatr Orthop 1998;18:625–629.

SLIPPED CAPITAL FEMORAL EPIPHYSIS

DAVID W. MANNING
CHRISTOPHER M. SULLIVAN
SUSAN A. SCHERL

Slipped capital femoral epiphysis (SCFE) is the most common adolescent hip disorder and is defined as displacement between the proximal femoral epiphysis and metaphysis. The displacement occurs through the hypertrophic zone of the proximal femoral physis. Although we often conceptualize the epiphysis "slipping" off the femoral neck, it is the metaphysis that is displaced anterior and proximal with respect to the epiphysis, resulting in a varus deformity of the hip because the acetabulum provides a mechanical constraint to prevent displacement of the epiphysis. Treatment is primarily focused on preventing further displacement and minimizing the risk of sequelae such as avascular necrosis of the epiphysis and hip arthrosis.

PATHOGENESIS

Etiology

The etiology of SCFE is unclear. Several hypotheses (mechanical and endocrine) have been proposed but it is likely that the true etiology is a combination of factors. Evidence supporting a mechanical etiology includes the incidence of obesity, increased physeal obliquity, and femoral retroversion seen in children with SCFE. The result is increased shear stress across the physis. The role of the endocrine system in the development of SCFE is linked to the male predominance as well as the increased incidence in children with hypothyroidism and those with hypogonadism receiving growth hormone supplementation. Clinically, SCFE is a disease of obese adolescents who have increased force transmission across an already widened and possibly weakened physis associated with hormonal changes such as the adolescent growth spurt.

Epidemiology

SCFE has a male predominance reported from 60% to 90% and may occur any time from age 6 to the time of physeal closure. The average age at diagnosis is 13.5 years for boys and slightly younger, at 12 years, for girls. The majority of children are clinically obese. There is a reported ethnic and geographic variation in prevalence. The lowest reported incidence has been reported in Japan (0.2 per 100,000), while one of the highest has been reported in the northeastern United States (10 per 100,000). It has also been reported that SCFE occurs more commonly in the summer in seasonal climates north of 40°N latitude.

Bilaterality has been reported in as many as 60% of cases, nearly half of which may be present at the time of initial presentation. Involvement is usually not symmetric and a high degree of clinical suspicion should be maintained, not only at the initial presentation, but throughout the follow-up period. Independent risk factors for bilateral SCFE include African American heritage and younger age at diagnosis.

Natural History

Failure of the proximal femoral physis and resultant metaphyseal displacement may occur gradually over the course of several months or as an acute event. The course may also be variable with acute events superimposed on a gradual slippage. Progressive slipping through the physis is halted by skeletal maturity or treatment. Despite deformity, patients with uncomplicated SCFE have a normal acetabulum and intact articular cartilage, and clinically perform very well for many years. However, more severe displacement is associated with early onset degenerative arthritis and may also result in injury to the posterosuperior epiphyseal vessels causing avascular necrosis of the femoral head (epiphysis).

Classification

The classification of SCFE is traditionally divided into four categories based on history, physical, and radiographic findings (Table 11-1). The stability classification separates patients based on their ability to ambulate (Table 11-2). The stability classification has proved more useful in predicting prognosis and establishing a treatment plan.

TABLE 11-1 TRADITIONAL CLASSIFICATION OF SLIPPED CAPITAL FEMORAL EPIPHYSIS

Classification	Duration of Symptoms	History	Physical Findings	Radiographic Findings
Preslip	Variable, usually <3 wk	Limp, weakness, pain worse with exertion	Antalgic gait ↓ Internal rotation	Osteopenia of hemipelvis Wide/irregular physis
Acute	<3 wk	Unable to bear weight, severe pain	Unable to ambulate External rotation deformity LLD ↓ Motion secondary to pain	Loss of Klein's line Positive blanch sign Slip angle on frogleg view
Chronic	>3 wk, up to months or years	Groin, thigh, knee pain; limp	Antalgic gait ↓Internal rotation ↓ Abduction LLD External rotation with flexion	Metaphyseal remodeling: Posterior/inferior sclerosis Superior/anterior resorption Pistol grip deformity
Acute-on-chronic	Acute increase in baseline symptoms	Acute increase in baseline symptoms	↓ Motion secondary to pain Antalgic gait ↓ Internal rotation ↓ Abduction LLD External rotation with flexion	Combination of acute and chronic radiographic changes

LLD, limb length discrepancy.

DIAGNOSIS

Clinical Presentation

Patients with SCFE usually present with complaints of groin or thigh pain and a limp. The duration of symptoms is corollary to the different categories in the traditional classification of SCFE (see Table 11-1). Infrequently the patient will complain only of medial knee pain (the referral pattern for the obturator nerve) and a high index of suspicion is needed to make the diagnosis. All pediatric patients with knee or thigh pain should undergo hip evaluation.

Physical Examination Findings

Orthopaedic physical findings are corollary to the different categories in the traditional classification (see Table 11-1) and severity of disease. The physical findings may include:

- Externally rotated and slightly flexed hip positioning with patient supine
- Pain with manipulation of the hip (log roll, flexion, rotation)
- Pain with straight leg raise
- External rotation of the thigh with passive hip flexion (asymmetric)
- Decreased hip flexion
- Decreased hip internal rotation
- Decreased hip abduction
- Limb length discrepancy
- Antalgic gait (shortened stance phase)
- Abductor lurch

Typical Radiographic Features

The gold standard diagnostic test for SCFE is anteroposterior (AP) and frog-leg lateral pelvis radiographs. The frog-

TABLE 11-2 STABILITY CLASSIFICATION OF SLIPPED CAPITAL FEMORAL EPIPHYSIS

	Ambulation	Symptoms	Physical Findings	Treatment	Outcome
Stable	Able to ambulate with or without crutches	Moderate pain, worse with activity	Antalgic gait ↓ internal rotation ↓ abduction	*In situ* pinning	Good to excellent
Unstable	Unable to ambulate with or without crutches	Severe pain groin, thigh, knee	Unable to bear weight Flexed and externally rotated posture ↓ ROM secondary to pain	Gentle (spontaneous) reduction with general anesthetic and pinning	↑ Risk of AVN, chondrolysis, early DJD

AVN, avascular necrosis; DJD, degenerative joint disease; ROM, range of motion.

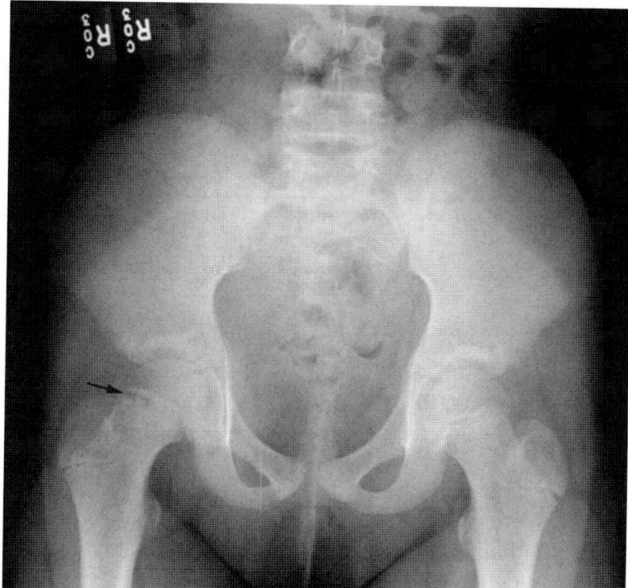

Figure 11-1 Anteroposterior pelvis radiograph showing widening of the right proximal femoral physis.

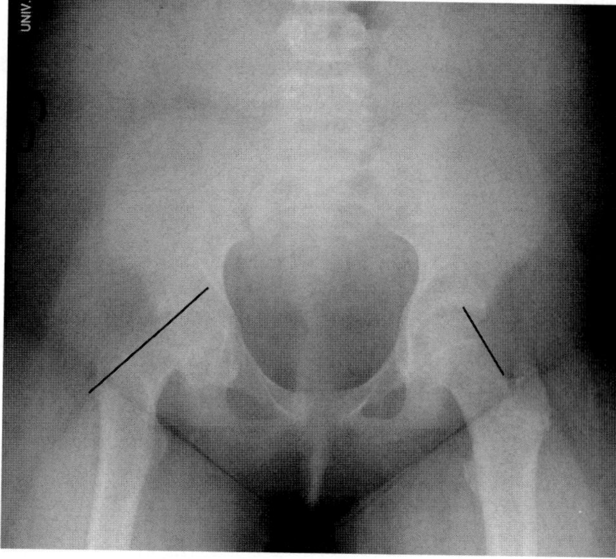

Figure 11-3 Anteroposterior radiograph of a mild slip of the right femoral epiphysis and correspondingasymmetry of Klein's line.

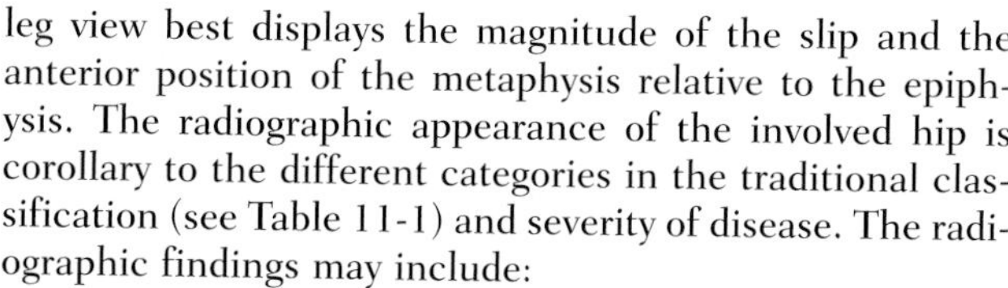

leg view best displays the magnitude of the slip and the anterior position of the metaphysis relative to the epiphysis. The radiographic appearance of the involved hip is corollary to the different categories in the traditional classification (see Table 11-1) and severity of disease. The radiographic findings may include:

- Osteopenia of the hemipelvis and proximal femur
- Widening of the physis (Fig. 11-1)
- Irregularity of the physis
- Subtle displacement of the metaphyseal/epiphyseal relationship (Fig. 11-2)
- Asymmetry of Klein's line, most pronounced on AP projection (Fig. 11-3)
- Metaphyseal blanch sign (overlap of metaphysis on epiphysis)
- Wide displacement of the metaphyseal/epiphyseal relationship
- Metaphyseal remodeling (Fig. 11-4)
- Resorption of superior and anterior proximal metaphysis (see Fig. 11-4)
- Sclerosis of posterior and inferior proximal metaphysis (see Fig. 11-4)
- Varus deformity (see Fig. 11-4)

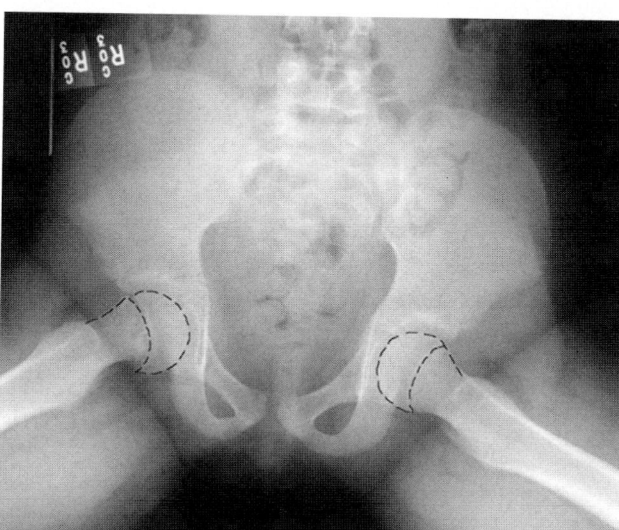

Figure 11-2 Frog-leg radiograph showing mild epiphyseal displacement on the right side.

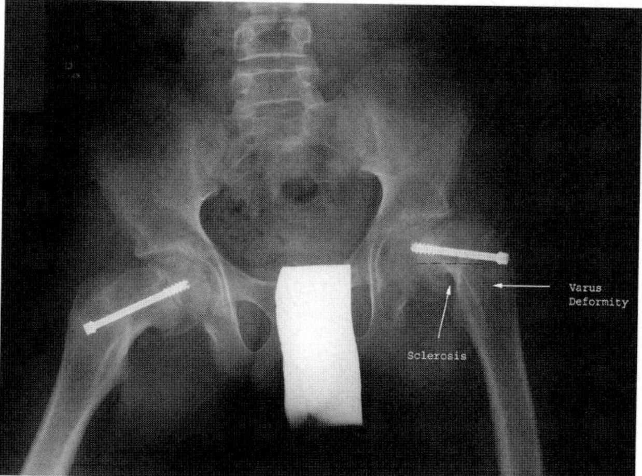

Figure 11-4 Frog-leg radiograph of bilateral chronic slips, after pinning, demonstrating varus deformity and metaphyseal remodeling and sclerosis.

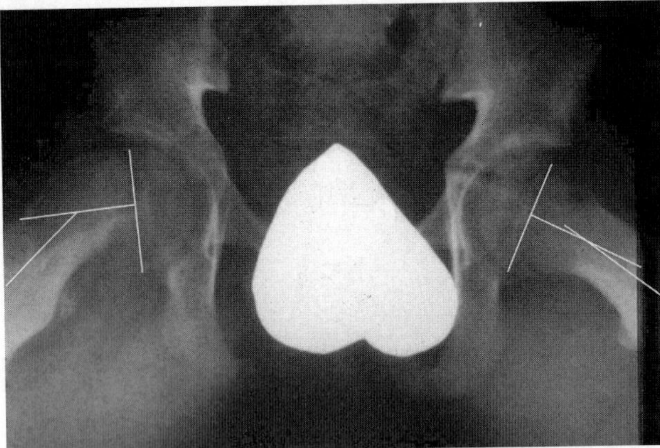

Figure 11-5 Frog-leg projection showing moderate slip of the right femoral epiphysis with corresponding increased Southwick angle.

The severity of SCFE is determined radiographically using two methods:

- AP view displacement of the epiphysis on the metaphysis
  - mild: less than one third
  - moderate: one third to one half
  - severe: greater than one half the width of the femoral neck
- Frog-leg view Southwick angle (epiphyseal shaft angle) (Fig. 11-5)
  - mild: less than 30 degrees
  - moderate: 30 to 50 degrees
  - severe: greater than 50 degrees.

Other Imaging Studies

A pin-hole lateral bone scan can show uptake in early preslip SCFE and may aid in early diagnosis when radiographs are normal. Ultrasound may detect hip joint effusion and metaphyseal remodeling but is usually not needed for diagnosis. The presence of an effusion is thought to correlate with an acute event. Magnetic resonance imaging may be useful in the early detection of avascular necrosis but is not useful in the diagnosis of SCFE.

Differential Diagnosis (Table 11-3)

- Idiopathic (most common)
- Endocrinopathy
  - Hypothyroidism (most common)
  - Hypopituitarism
  - Growth hormone deficiency
  - Hypogonadism
  - Craniopharyngiomas
- Osteodystrophy
- Radiation

Patients between the ages of 10 to 16 years and greater than the fiftieth percentile for weight (negative age/weight test) can routinely be considered to have idiopathic SCFE (Table 11-4). Children who fall outside these boundaries (positive age/weight test) and children less than the tenth percentile for height on a standard Tanner growth chart are significantly more likely to have an underlying endocrine disorder. Preliminary endocrine screening should include thyroid-stimulating hormone and free thyroxine serum levels.

TREATMENT

The ideal management of SCFE should prevent progression of disease, provide pain relief, have few complications, be easy for the patient and family to tolerate, and be technically simple. The gold standard of treatment is immediate bed rest and *in situ* stabilization with single or multiple pins or screws. Postoperatively, the patient is allowed flatfoot weightbearing with crutches. The following section is divided into treatment options for stable and unstable SCFE.

Stable SCFE

Hip Spica Cast

Casting for 3 months was thought to be effective at preventing further progression and also treating or preventing bilateral SCFE. However, progression of slip occurs in up to 10% of cases and spica casting has also been shown to have an unacceptable rate of chondrolysis. Articular cartilage nutrition occurs primarily through diffusion from the synovial fluid and this mechanism is severely hampered by

TABLE 11-3 DIFFERENTIAL DIAGNOSIS OF SLIPPED CAPITAL FEMORAL EPIPHYSIS

Differential Diagnosis	Age (Yr)	Weight	Bilaterality (%)	Mild/Moderate/ Severe (%)
Idiopathic	12.8 ± 1.6	94% ≥ 50th percentile	35	55/26/19
Endocrine	15.3 ± 5.3	No trend	61	60/25/15
Osteodystrophy	11.4 ± 4.4	No trend	90	53/7/43
Radiation	10.5 ± 3.3	No trend	28	81/11/8

Adapted from Reynolds R. Diagnosis and treatment of slipped capital femoral epiphysis. Curr Opin Pediatr 1999;11:1:80–87.

TABLE 11-4 ATYPICAL RESULTS IN SCREENING FOR SLIPPED CAPITAL FEMORAL EPIPHYSIS

Cause	Age/Weight Test (AWT)	Height	Significance
Idiopathic	10–16 yr and ≥50th percentile (negative test)	≥10th percentile	Negative AWT: 93% negative predictive value No need for endocrine evaluation
Endocrine	≥16 yr or ≤10 yr and ≤ percentile (positive test)	≤10th percentile	Positive AWT: 52% positive predictive value Height: 90% sensitivity, 98% negative predictive value necessitate endocrine evaluation
Other	Variable	Variable	History of radiation or renal disease

Adapted from Loder RT, Greenfield MVH. Clinical characteristics of children with atypical and idiopathic slipped capital femoral epiphysis: description of the age-weight test and implications for further diagnostic investigation. J Pediatr Orthoped 2001;21:4:481–487.
Reynolds R. Diagnosis and treatment of slipped capital femoral epiphysis. Curr Opin Pediatr 1999;11: 1:80–87.

immobilization. Treatment in a hip spica cast is not recommended and is of historical value only.

In Situ Pinning

Open or percutaneous pinning of the slip without reduction can be accomplished with a single cannulated screw or pin and is considered the gold standard. The screw or pin should enter the anterior aspect of the proximal femur, cross the physis at 90 degrees, and enter the center of the epiphysis with the tip below subchondral bone. A screw placed in this orientation accommodates the deformity, and has maximal stability with minimal risk of complications (Fig. 11-6). Postoperatively, partial weightbearing with crutches is advanced as tolerated. In stable slips, an additional second screw creates only a minimal increase in stability and theoretically can negatively impact femoral epiphyseal circulation.

Cervical Osteotomy

Open reduction and osteotomy of the femoral neck with multiple pin fixation is associated with an unacceptable rate of avascular necrosis (AVN) and is not recommended.

A
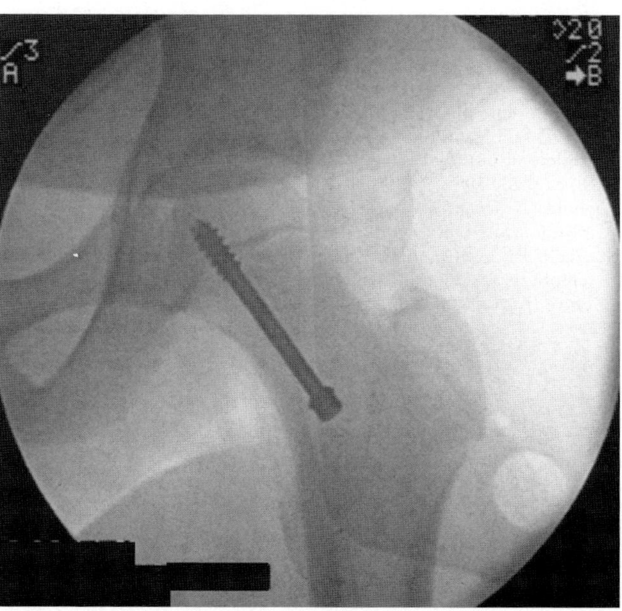

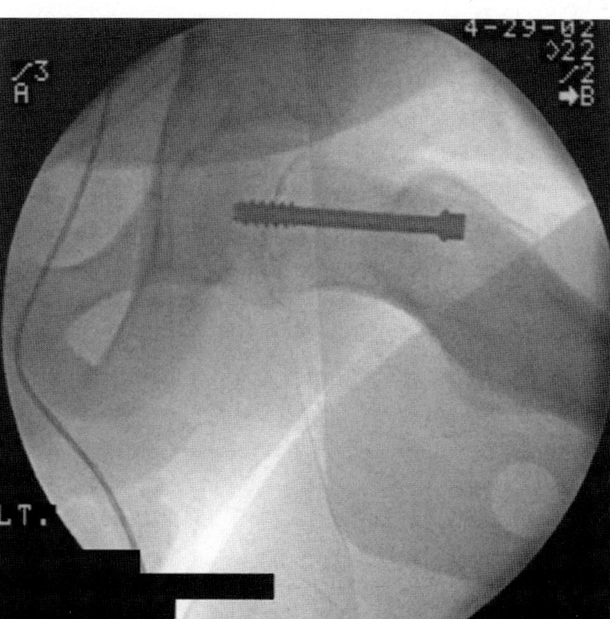

B

Figure 11-6 Operative anteroposterior (**A**) and frog-leg (**B**) radiographs showing single screw fixation.

Intertrochanteric Osteotomy

Anterolateral closing wedge osteotomy at the level of the lesser trochanter and fixation with a compression hip screw can stabilize SCFE and reduce deformity. The result is an improved range of motion at the expense of a more involved procedure that may exacerbate any leg length discrepancy. Osteotomy may be indicated in stable chronic SCFE with a Southwick angle greater than 60 degrees or as a later reconstructive option.

Subtrochanteric Osteotomy

The correction of deformity is inferior to that obtained with an intertrochanteric osteotomy. The procedure is not routinely performed.

Unstable SCFE

The management of unstable SCFE is difficult and the outcome may be poor. Unstable SCFE may be associated with AVN despite adequate treatment because unstable slips tend to be severe and potentially involve injury to the posterosuperior epiphyseal vessels. It has been argued, but not clearly proven, that early decompression of the hip joint (aspiration or open capsulotomy), gentle reduction of deformity, and internal fixation may decrease the incidence of AVN. Frequently, when the patient is anesthetized, a spontaneous partial reduction will occur. In patients with a severe slip angle there is little epiphyseal–metaphyseal overlap and multiple screw fixation may be impossible. Partial reduction often allows two-screw fixation and improved rotational stability in these difficult cases.

At a minimum, the patient with an unstable SCFE should be placed on bed rest until open or percutaneous pinning performed. Flatfoot weightbearing may begin on the first postoperative day and progress to weightbearing as tolerated once radiographic evidence of early callus is seen.

COMPLICATIONS

AVN

AVN is a devastating complication involving necrosis and collapse of the femoral head with resultant pain, stiffness, limp, and degenerative changes. Radiographs confirm the diagnosis. Risk factors include:

- Unstable slip
- Severe slip angle
- Acute slip
- Reduction attempt of chronic slip deformity
- Screw placement in superolateral quadrant of the epiphysis
- Femoral neck osteotomy

Chondrolysis

Chondrolysis is a breakdown of proximal femoral articular cartilage of unknown etiology. Patients present with pain, stiffness, limp, and contracture. Joint space may be narrowed on radiographs and arthrogram. Risk factors include:

- Severe slip
- Prolonged symptoms without treatment
- Cast immobilization
- Unrecognized pin/screw penetration into joint

The complications of AVN and chondrolysis are frequently disabling. Reliable treatment options do not exist.

SUGGESTED READING

Burrow SR, Alman B, Wright JG. short stature as a screening test for endocrinopathy in slipped capital femoral epiphysis. J Bone Joint Surg (Br) 2001;83B:263–268.

Dobbs MB, Weinstein SL. natural history and long-term outcomes of slipped capital femoral epiphysis. Instr Course Lect 2001;50: 571–575.

Loder RT. Unstable slipped capital femoral epiphysis. J Pediatr Orthop 2001;21:5:694–699.

Loder RT, Aronsson DD, Dobbs MB, et al. Slipped capital femoral epiphysis. Instr Course Lect 2001;50:555–570.

Loder RT, Greenfield MVH. Clinical characteristics of children with atypical and idiopathic slipped capital femoral epiphysis: description of the age-weight test and implications for further diagnostic investigation. J Pediatr Orthoped 2001;21:4:481–487.

Loder RT, et al. The demographics of slipped capital femoral epiphysis: an international multicenter study. CORR 1996;322:8–28.

Loder RT, et al. A worldwide study on the seasonal variation of slipped capital femoral epiphysis. CORR 1996;322:28–36.

Maeda S, Kita A, Funayama K, et al. Vascular supply to slipped capital femoral epiphysis. J Pediatr Orthoped 2001;21:5:664–667.

Rattey T, Piehl F, Wright JG. Acute slipped capital femoral epiphysis: review of outcomes and rates of avascular necrosis. J Bone Joint Surg (Am) 1996;78:398–402.

Reynolds R. Diagnosis and treatment of slipped capital femoral epiphysis. Curr Opin Pediatr 1999;11:1:80–87.

Stasikelis PJ, Sullivan CM, Phillips WA, et al. Slipped capital femoral epiphysis: prediction of contralateral involvement. J Bone Joint Surg (Am) 1996;78:1149–1155.

FRACTURES AND DISLOCATIONS

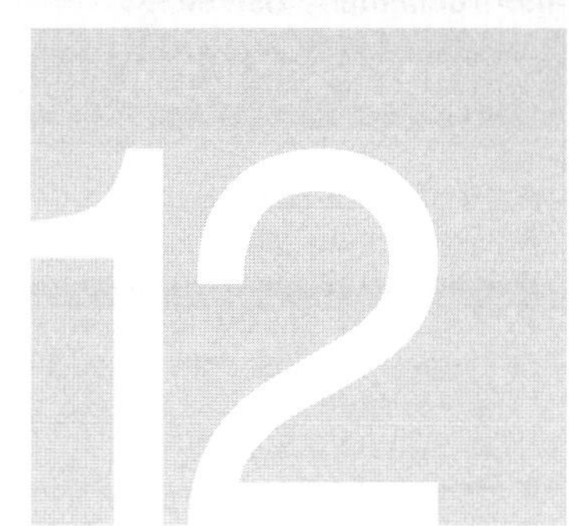

12.1 SPINE

BRUCE L. GILLINGHAM ■ ELOY OCHOA

Pediatric spine fractures are relatively rare. Only 5% of all spinal cord and vertebral column injuries affect those 16 years and under. Although uncommon, spine fractures in children can lead to chronic instability, deformity, neurologic sequelae, and posttraumatic stenosis. Injuries to the spinal column can often be subtle and absent on initial radiographs. Successful treatment is based on knowledge of the radiographic, anatomic, and developmental differences between the pediatric and adult spine.

PATHOGENESIS

Etiology

The location, pattern, and etiology of a child's spine fracture are primarily dependent on the age at the time of injury. Birth trauma is the major cause of spinal trauma in children under age 2. In patients between the ages of 3 and 8 the most frequent mechanisms of injury are falls from height, motor vehicle accidents, and child abuse. Children older than 8 years of age are more commonly injured in motor vehicle accidents, by gunshot wounds, or from sporting activities such as swimming, diving, and surfing.

The views expressed in this chapter are those of the authors and do not reflect the official policy or position of the Department of the Navy, Department of Defense, or the United States Government.

Epidemiology

Less than 5% of all spinal injuries involve children. The majority of spinal column fractures in childhood occur in the thoracolumbar spine. Cervical spine fractures in patients 8 years old or younger involve the upper cervical spine above C4. These most often include the occiput, C1, C2 complex and carry an increased risk of fatality. Patients older than 8 more typically sustain injures below C4 with a much lower fatality rate. Up to 30% of traumatic spine injuries in children present as a traumatic myelopathy known as spinal cord injury without radiographic abnormality (SCIWORA).

Pathophysiology

The patterns and types of spine injuries seen in children reflect features unique to the developing spine (Box 12.1-1).

An appreciation of radiographic features unique to the immature spine is necessary to accurately diagnose spinal trauma. Several developmental features can be misconstrued as evidence of injury to the spine (Table 12.1-1).

After age 8 the spine begins to mature. The ligaments and facet capsules strengthen, the facets become more vertically oriented and the vertebral bodies become more rectangular-shaped. By late childhood the patterns of spinal injuries and healing become similar to the adult.

In addition to knowledge of normal developmental anatomy, it is important to be aware of congenital and genetic conditions manifested in the spine (Table 12.1-2).

BOX 12.1-1 UNIQUE ANATOMIC FEATURES OF CHILDREN AGE 8 AND YOUNGER

- Large head-to-body ratio
- Ligamentous laxity
- Relative muscle weakness
- Horizontal, shallow facet joints
- Increased spinal column elasticity
  - Forces dissipated over several adjacent segments
  - SCIWORA possible
- Presence of the ring apophysis
  - Fractures traverse vertebral body growth plate

TABLE 12.1-1 DEVELOPMENTAL FEATURES THAT CAN BE MISINTERPRETED AS INJURY

Radiographic Finding	Misinterpretation	Explanation
Absent cervical lordosis	Muscle spasm from C-spine injury	Seen in up to 14% of patients less than 8 yr of age
Dentocentral synchondrosis	Odontoid fracture	Usually not fused by age 6; lucency below level of body dens interface
Wedge-shaped vertebrae	Compression fracture	Usually present up to age 8; adjacent bodies similar
Incomplete ossification of ring apophysis (secondary ossification)	Avulsion fracture	Appear at age 5, fuse between age 18 and 25
Notching of anterior and posterior vertebral body in infancy	Vertebral body fracture	Vascular channels. Anterior disappears at age 1. Posterior remains throughout life

TABLE 12.1-2 SELECTED CONGENITAL VERTEBRAL ANOMALIES

Anomaly	Characteristic	Radiographic Significance
Os odontoideum	Rounded hypoplasitic apical segment of dens Remnant of axis at base	Can be confused with dens fracture May represent nonunion May require fusion
Klippel-Feil syndrome	Congenital fusion of two or more vertebrae	Longer lever arm may lead to higher incidence of fractures
Down syndrome	Ligamentous laxity leads to decreased SAC/ADI	Atlanto-axial instability, myelopathy

ADI, atlanto-dens interval; SAC, space available for the cord.

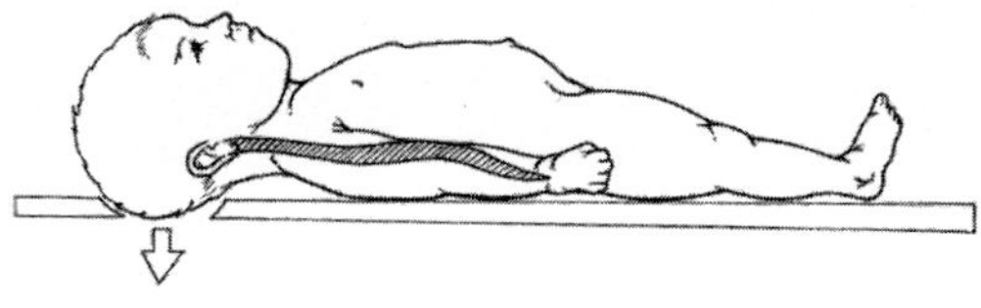

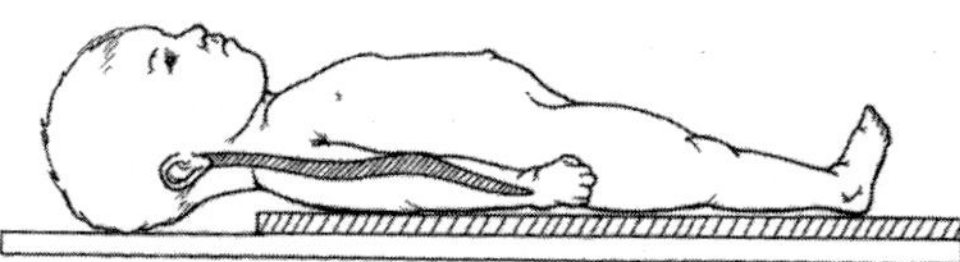

Figure 12.1-1 Diagrams of young children on modified spine boards with either an occipital recess (**top figure**) or a mattress pad (**bottom figure**) to raise the chest. (©1998 American Academy of Orthopaedic Surgeons. Adapted from the Journal of the American Academy of Orthopaedic Surgeons, 1988;6[4]:204–214, with permission.)

DIAGNOSIS

Trauma Evaluation

As with all patients evaluated following a traumatic event, potentially life-threatening conditions must be identified and treated. Once airway, breathing, and circulation are secure, a brief secondary survey can be accomplished. Early proper immobilization in all patients with suspected C-spine injury is essential in order to avoid creating or propagating further spinal cord injury, by increased neck flexion. In a young child with a proportionally large head, this can be done using a spine board with an occipital recess or by placing a mattress or blankets beneath the shoulders and trunk of the child (Fig. 12.1-1). A screening cross-table lateral x-ray of the spine, in addition to anteroposterior (AP) pelvis and chest x-rays, should be standard in the evaluation of all trauma patients.

In addition to proper spine board immobilization, a rigid cervical orthosis, properly designed for infants or children, should be applied. Sandbags on each side of the head will prevent motion. Until the cervical spine is cleared (Box 12.1-2), movement of the patient should only be performed with in-line traction using a log-roll technique.

BOX 12.1-2 SUSPECTED CERVICAL SPINE INJURY

- Loss of consciousness or GCS <13
- Neurologic symptoms or complaints
- Altered mental status
- Mechanism of injury
  - Motor vehicle vs. pedestrian or cyclist
  - Fall from considerable height
  - Motor vehicle accident as unrestrained passenger
  - Neck pain or guarding
  - Head or facial trauma
  - Ecchymosis from seat belt

GCS, Glasgow Coma Scale score (see Table 13-2)

History and Physical Examination

A brief history in the awake, cooperative child is helpful. A spinal cord injury should be suspected in a patient with a history of numbness, tingling, or brief paralysis. Physical examination should begin with inspection of skin for any visible evidence of spinal trauma to include abrasions, edema, or ecchymosis. Pain or step-off along the spinous processes should also raise suspicion. Range of motion should only be attempted when the child is conscious and cooperative and an unstable injury is not suspected.

RADIOLOGIC EVALUATION

Cervical Spine

As in adult victims of trauma, an essential part of the trauma evaluation is clearance of the cervical spine (Algorithm 12.1-1 and Box 12.1-3). The cervical orthosis and spine board precautions should be removed only if the patient has no neck pain or tenderness to palpation and a full painless range of motion.

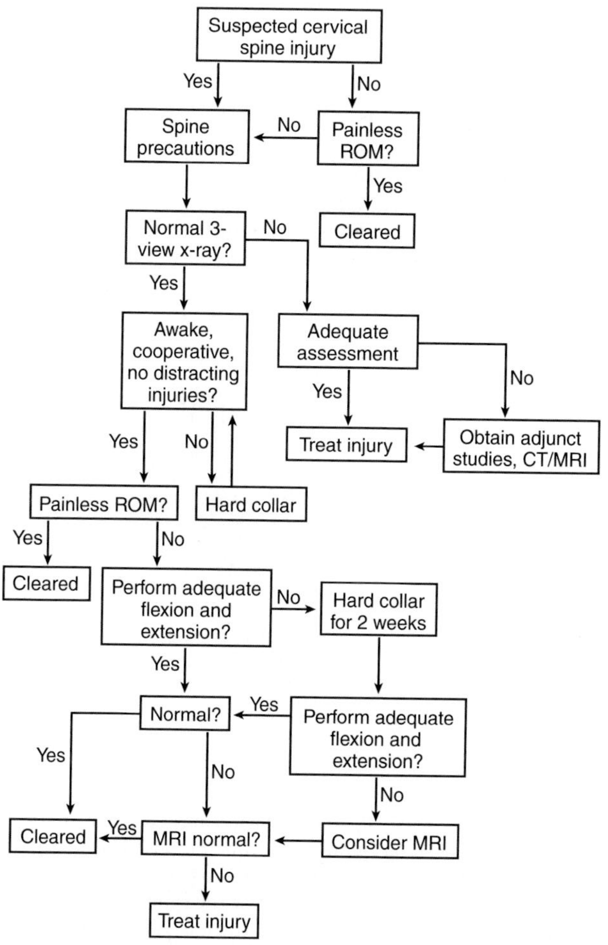

Algorithm 12.1-1 Clearing the cervical spine.

BOX 12.1-3 FACTORS PRECLUDING CLINICAL CLEARANCE OF THE CERVICAL SPINE

- Diverting pain from other injuries
- Altered sensorium
  - Head injury
  - Narcotic pain medication
  - Alcohol use
- Recreational drug use

The cervical spine is evaluated as follows:

- Lateral C-spine radiograph
  - Must see top of T1
- Assess alignment (Fig. 12.1-2)
  - Anterior vertebral line
  - Posterior vertebral line
  - Spinolaminar line
  - Spinous process line
- Check radiographic relationships (Table 12.1-3)
  - Atlanto-dens interval
  - Retropharyngeal and retrotracheal spaces
  - Space available for the cord
- AP and open mouth odontoid views
  - Alignment of lateral masses
  - Odontoid fracture
  - Interpedicular distance
- Flexion–extension views
  - Assess ligamentous stability
  - Active range of motion only
  - Physician-supervised
  - Fully cooperative patient
  - May need to wait until first follow-up visit

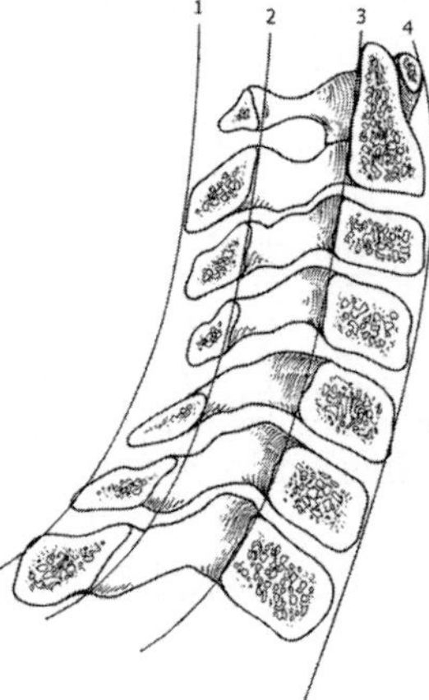

Figure 12.1-2 Normal alignment of the lateral cervical spine. *1,* spinous process line; *2,* spinolaminar line; *3,* posterior vertebral bodyline; *4,* anterior vertebral bodyline. Space available for the cord is the distance between 2 and 3 at the level of C1. (©1998 American Academy of Orthopaedic Surgeons. Adapted from the Journal of the American Academy of Orthopaedic Surgeons, 1998;6:204–214, with permission.)

TABLE 12.1-3 NORMAL PARAMETERS OF THE PEDIATRIC CERVICAL SPINE

Parameter	Normal Value
C-1 facet-occipital condyle distance	≤5 mm
Atlanto-dens interval	≤4 mm
Pseudosubluxation of C2 on C3	≤4 mm
Pseudosubluxation of C3 on C4	≤3 mm
Retropharyngeal space	≤8 mm (at C-2)
Retrotracheal space	≤14 mm (at C-6, under age 15 yr)
Torg ratio (canal to vertebral body)	≥0.8
Space available for cord	≥14 mm

Adapted from Black BE. Spine trauma. In: Sponseller PD, ed. Orthopaedic knowledge update pediatrics 2. Rosemont, IL: American Academy of Orthopaedic Surgery; 2002:134.

There are specific differences in the pediatric patient that one must be aware of when reviewing the cervical spine radiograph (Box 12.1-4).

Thoracic and Lumbar Spine

Mechanisms of injury in thoracolumbar spine fractures include:

- Compression
- Lumbar apophyseal injury

BOX 12.1-4 DIFFERENCES IN THE CERVICAL SPINE SEEN IN PEDIATRIC PATIENTS

Pseudosubluxation
- C2 on C3 or C3 on C4
- Seen in up to 40% of children between 1 and 7 years of age
- Up to 4 mm of stepoff in flexion on AP is acceptable
- Spinolaminar line within 1.5 mm of posterior arch of C1 (Fig. 12.1-2)
- Should reduce in extension
- No treatment necessary

Localized Kyphosis
- Seen in midcervical area
- Seen in up to 14% of children younger than 16 years of age
- Should reduce in extension

Overriding C1 over Tip of Odontoid (C2)
- Seen in extension
- 20% of those between 1 and 7 years of age
- Result of nonossified atlas and tip of odontoid
- Also anterior angulation of odontoid process in as many as 4%

Persistence of Basilar Odontoid Synchondrosis
- Can mimic odontoid fracture
- Sometimes present until 11 years of age
- Appears sclerotic unlike true fracture
- Located well caudad to the base of the odontoid process

- Flexion with compression
- Distraction
- Shear

The region is evaluated as follows:

- Center plain films over injured area.
- Obtain "cone down" views of suspicious findings.
- Always obtain two views 90 degrees apart.
- Oblique views helpful for spondylolysis in lumbosacral spine.

Indications for Special Studies

- Computed tomography (CT) scan best for evaluating bone "architecture"
  - Especially lumbar apophyseal fractures
- Three-dimensional CT often useful in preoperative planning
- Bone scan useful to detect occult tumors/spondylolysis
- Magnetic resonance imaging (MRI) very useful in SCIWORA
- MRI useful in neurocompression by fracture fragments and disc

Clinical and radiographic findings in spine fractures and other conditions are listed in Tables 12.1-4 through 12.1-6

TREATMENT

Atlanto-Occipital Dislocation

- Very unstable
- Require halo immobilization if neurologically intact (Box. 12.1-5)
- Fusion if instability remains or neurologic deficit
- Occiput-C1 fusion if neurologically intact
- Occiput-C2 fusion if neurologically impaired

Atlas Fractures

- Halo immobilization or Minerva brace
- Up to 6 months of immobilization may be necessary
- Surgical intervention rarely indicated

Atlantoaxial (C1-C2) Disruptions

- Rotatory subluxation can be treated with temporary immobilization
- Rarely will require traction for reduction (older than 1 week)
- Dislocation or ligamentous instability less predictable
- Initial treatment with Halo immobilization for 8 to 12 weeks
- C1-C2 fusion if instability persistent

Dens Injuries

- Most heal with closed reduction
- Halo vest or Minerva cast for 4 months
- Posterior C1-C2 fusion if persistent motion or suspected os odontoideum

Hangman Fracture (Pedicle Fracture C2)

- Most respond to closed reduction and halo vest for 8 weeks
- Posterior C1-C3 fusion indicated for non-union or significant disc disruption

C2-C3 Subluxation and Dislocation

- Younger than 8 years, closed reduction and halo vest immobilization
- Older than 8 years, usually require posterior fusion

Middle to Lower Cervical Injuries

- Younger than 8 years, closed reduction and halo vest immobilization
- Initial trial of Halo immobilization for 3 months for ligamentous instability
- Posterior fusion if instability persists beyond 3 months
- Early surgical stabilization for unstable fractures or spinal cord injury

Child Abuse

- Contact child protective services
- Obtain skeletal survey
- Rule out associated injuries
  - Retinal hemorrhages
  - Intracranial or intraocular hemorrhages
  - Visceral injury
- Treat spine injury as indicated

Spinal Cord Injury

- Efficacy of steroids in enhancing recovery not established in children
- Rarely, decompression of spinal cord impingement required
  - Retropulsed disc, bone fragments
- Monitor for late spinal deformity
  - Nearly universal if children are 10 years of age or younger at time of injury
- Recognize late neurologic deterioration
  - Ascending spinal level
  - Assess for posttraumatic syrinx with MRI
    - Drainage usually required

SCIWORA

- Immobilization in a rigid cervical collar or Thoracolumbar spinal orthosis (TLSO)
- Physical activity restriction for 3 months
- Decompression for progressive deficit, discrete lesion
- Prognosis for neurologic recovery
  - Good in mild cases
  - Poor in severe cases
  - Usually affects children less than 8 years

TABLE 12.1-4 CLINICAL AND RADIOLOGIC FEATURES OF SPECIFIC SPINE CONDITIONS OR FRACTURES

Injury	Clinical Features	Radiologic Features
Atlanto-occipital dislocation	Rare, often results in death Survivors often ventilator-dependent Multiple trauma	Massive retropharyngeal/prevertebral swelling Frank atlanto-occipital dislocation
Atlas fractures	Not common Neurologic compromise uncommon Usually results from direct axial load	Open mouth odontoid view is appropriate May be difficult to evaluate or r/o on plain radiograph CT offer most precise imaging
Atlantoaxial (C1-C2) disruptions	Include ligamentous instability, rotatory subluxation and odontoid epiphyseal separation Atlanto-dens interval ≥4 mm Torticollis or cervical muscle spasm	Lateral view space available for cord (SAC) ≤14 mm in flexion Continued pain with motion despite normal static films Open mouth odontoid shows asymmetry of lateral masses Dynamic and axial CT imaging helpful with evaluation of rotatory subluxation or dislocation
Dens injuries	Usually significant trauma Most common pediatric C-spine injuries Patients complain of instability Often hold their head with two hands to prevent motion	Most can be diagnosed with plain three-view trauma series Typically at the base but not extending into body Fractured odontoid moves with C1 on flexion/extension views Can be confused with os odontoideum CT if warranted Flexion–extension MRI/CT may be helpful to evaluate os odonoideum
Hangman fracture (pedicle fracture C2)	Usually results from flexion or extension injuries Isolated	Can be confused with primary spondylolysis Can be confused with synchondrosis of posterior arch CT helpful
C2-C3 subluxation and dislocation	Must be differentiated from pseudosubluxation Typically have associated trauma to head, face, and chest Typically complain of pain	Spinolaminar line (Swischuk line) not disrupted in pseudosubluxation (Fig. 12.1-2) Pseudosubluxation reduces in extension MRI helpful to rule out ligamentous injury/instability
Middle to lower cervical injuries	Typical in children older than 8 yr Average age 13 yr Typically flexion or extension injuries	Widened interspinous spaces on lateral Loss of parallelism of articular facets Kyphosis of the disc space Calcification in the interspinous ligament seen late
Child abuse	Infants and toddlers May see SCIWORA in shaken baby syndrome ▪ Relatively weak cervical musculature ▪ Disproportionately large head Often not recognized Thoracolumbar and lumbar spine injuries most common	Multiple compression fractures Fracture–dislocations with or without spinal cord injury Fractures at different stages of healing
Spinal cord injury	Serial examinations necessary to rule out progressive deficit Birth trauma ▪ Floppy infant with nonprogressive neurologic lesion Toddlers and young children ▪ Cervicothoracic junction injury ▪ Most severe deficit but best potential for recovery Adolescents ▪ Thoracolumbar fractures ▪ Incomplete neurologic deficits	Spinal canal stenosis a risk factor for neurologic impairment ▪ 35% at T11-T12 ▪ 45% at L1 ▪ 55% at L2 MRI demonstrates characteristic findings (Table 12.1-5)

(continued)

TABLE 12.1-4 (continued)

Injury	Clinical Features	Radiologic Features
SCIWORA	Spinal column 4 times more elastic than spinal cord Proposed mechanisms: ■ Longitudinal distraction ■ Hyperextension ■ Flexion ■ Spinal cord ischemia May have delayed onset of neurologic loss Relatively high rate at thoracolumbar junction	Findings absent on plain radiographs MRI findings: ■ Hemorrhage and edema from occult end-plate fracture ■ Widening of disc space following spontaneous reduction
Compression fracture (lumbar apophyseal injury)	Injury to posterior lumbar end plate in adolescents Portion of disc, apophysis, ± body retropulsed into canal Usually L4-5, L5-S1 Acute onset of low back pain with strenuous activities, athletics Shoveling, gymnastics, weight lifting Positive straight leg raise Variable motor, sensory loss Often not seen on plain films	CT scan diagnostic study of choice ■ Fragment size, extent of canal compromise Four types described (Table 12.1-6)
Flexion injuries	Hyperflexion injuries with compression are common Intact discs more resistant than vertebral body to axial load ■ Body collapses before disc fails Older children more susceptible to adult-type burst fracture	Usually less than 20% compression Multiple contiguous level injury common Posterior column involvement rare
Flexion–distraction (pediatric Chance fracture equivalents)	Lap belt injury (check for seat belt sign) High likelihood of associated neurologic, spinal, and visceral injuries Flexion–distraction mechanism ■ Anterior compression, posterior column distraction	Four types (Fig. 12.1-3)
Distraction and shear injuries	High-energy injuries ■ Pedestrian vs. auto ■ Crush by falling objects	Fracture through end-plate apophyses

CT, computed tomography; MRI, magnetic resonance imaging; SAC, space available for the cord; SCIWORA, spinal cord injury without radiographic abnormality.

TABLE 12.1-5 MAGNETIC RESONANCE IMAGING PATTERNS ON T2-WEIGHTED IMAGES OF ACUTE SPINAL CORD INJURIES

Type	Findings
I	Decreased signal due to intraspinal hemorrhage
II	Bright signal due to spinal cord edema
III	Mixed signal: central hypointensity and peripheral hyperintensity due to contusion

Adapted from Bondurant FJ, Cotler HB, Kulkarni MV, et al. Acute spinal cord injury: a study using physical examination and magnetic resonance imaging. Spine 1990;15:161–168.

TABLE 12.1-6 RADIOGRAPHIC CLASSIFICATION OF LUMBAR APOPHYSEAL INJURY

Type	Age Group (yr)	Radiographic Findings
I	11–13	Separation of the posterior vertebral rim. Arcuate fragment without osseous defect
II	13–18	Avulsion fracture of vertebral body, annular rim, and cartilage
III	≥18	Localized fracture posterior to end-plate irregularity
IV	≥18	Defect spans entire length and breadth of posterior vertebral margin between end plates

Adapted from Epstein N, Epstein J, Mauri T. Treatment of fractures of the vertebral limbus and spinal stenosis in five adolescents and five adults. Neurosurgery 1989;24:595–604 and Takata K, Inoue S-I, Takahashi K, et al. Fracture of the posterior margin of a lumbar vertebral body. J Bone Joint Surg 1988;70:589–594.

Pediatric Chance Fracture Equivalents (Fig. 12.1-3)

- Closed reduction, hyperextension casting for pure bony injuries
  - Restore lordosis
- Open reduction, posterior fusion for ligamentous injury
  - Spinous process wiring with casting for small children
  - Compression instrumentation in adolescents

Vertebral End-Plate Fractures

- Surgical excision of retropulsed disc, end-plate and bone fragments
  - Prevents healing of lesion to posterior vertebral body
  - Avoids subsequent spinal stenosis

Surgical Indications and Contraindications

Spine fractures heal better in children than in adults. Significant potential for remodeling exists. The majority of

BOX 12.1-5 CONSIDERATIONS FOR HALO RING APPLICATION IN CHILDREN

- Obtain CT to assess skull thickness in children less than 6 years of age.
- The ring should sit below the widest skull diameter, about 1 cm above the top of the ear.
- A 1-cm separation between the halo ring and patient's head should be present.
- Use 6 to 8 pins at low insertion torque (2 to 5 ft/lb).
  - Avoid thin bone at temporal region and frontal sinuses
  - Safe zone anteriorly: 1 cm above orbital rim, lateral two thirds of the orbit
- Insert anterior pins with patient's eyes closed to avoid trapping eyelids open.
- Tighten opposing pins simultaneously to minimize shifting of the ring.
- Pins can be retightened once and only if resistance is felt.
- Remove loose pins after placing a new pin in an adjacent location.

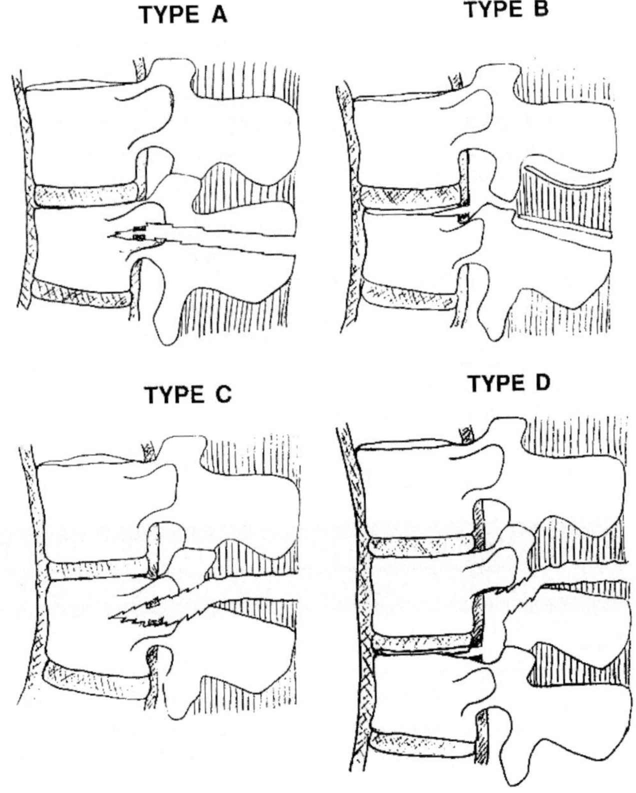

Figure 12.1-3 Pediatric Chance fractures. Type A: Bony disruption of the posterior column with minimal extension into the middle column. Type B: Avulsion of posterior elements with facet joint disruption or fracture and extension into vertebral body apophysis. Type C: Posterior ligamentous disruption with fracture entering vertebra close to pars interarticularis and extending into middle column. Type D: Posterior ligamentous disruption with fracture traversing lamina and extending into apophysis of adjacent vertebral body. (Adapted from Rumball K, Jarvis J. Seat-belt injuries of the spine in young children. J Bone Joint Surg [Br] 1992;74:571–574.)

TABLE 12.1-7 DENIS CLASSIFICATION OF SPINAL COLUMN INSTABILITY

Type	Instability Pattern	Example	Risk	Treatment
First degree	Mechanical	Severe compression fracture	Progressive kyphosis	Brace in extension
Second degree	Neurologic instability	Ligamentously stable burst fracture susceptible to collapse from axial load	Neurologic injury	Operative stabilization
Third degree	Mechanical and neurologic	Unstable burst fracture, fracture–dislocation	Progressive displacement and neurologic injury	Operative stabilization, decompression

Adapted from Denis F. Spinal instability as defined by the three-column spine concept in acute spinal trauma. Clin Orthop 1984;189:65–76.

pediatric spinal trauma can be treated nonoperatively; however, three primary factors need to be considered in determining if operative intervention is required.

- Fundamental considerations
  - Alignment
  - Stability
  - Canal compromise
- Alignment
  - Cervical spine
    - Radiographic criteria (see Table 12.1-3)
  - Thoracolumbar spine
    - Initial kyphosis less than 20 degrees
- Stability of the fracture pattern
  - Majority of spine fractures in children are stable
  - Cervical spine
    - Depends on specific injury
  - Thoracolumbar spine
    - Denis classification (Table 12.1-7)
- Canal Compromise
  - Insufficient space available for cord
  - Encroachment by retropulsed disc, bone fragments
- General surgical indications:
  - Unstable, purely ligamentous injuries
  - Unstable fractures that cannot be safely braced
  - Fracture with neurologic injury
- Incomplete neurologic loss with canal compromise
- Progressive neurologic deficit

SUGGESTED READING

Aufdermaur M. Spinal injuries in juveniles: necropsy findings in 12 cases. J Bone Joint Surg 1974;56:513–519.

Bondurant FJ, Cotler HB, Kulkarni MV, et al. Acute spinal imaging. Spine 1990;15:161–168.

Botte MJ, Byrne TP, Abrams RA, et al. Halo skeletal fixation: techniques of application and prevention of complications. J (Am) Acad Orthop Surg 1996;4:44–53.

Cattell HS, Filtzer DL. Pseudosubluxation and other normal variations in the cervical spine in children. J Bone Joint Surg (Am) 1965;47:1295–1309.

Copley LA, Dormans JP. Cervical spine disorders in infants and children. J Am Acad Orthop Surg 1998;6:204–214.

Denis F. Spinal instability as defined by the three-column spine concept in acute spinal trauma. Clin Orthop 1984;189:65–76.

Epstein N, Epstein J, Mauri T. Treatment of fractures of the vertebral limbus and spinal stenosis in five adolescents and five adults. Neurosurgery 1989;24:595–604.

Hadley M, Zabramski JM, Browner C, et al. Pediatric spinal trauma: review of 122 cases of spinal cord and vertebral column injuries. J Neurosurg 1988;68:18–24.

Herzenberg J, Hensinger R, Dedrick D, et al. Emergency transport and positioning of young children who have an injury of the cervical spine: the standard backboard may be hazardous. J Bone Joint Surg (Am) 1989;71:15–22.

Pang D, Wilberger JJ. Spinal cord injury without radiographic abnormalities in children. J Neurosurg 1982;57:114–129.

Rumball K, Jarvis J. Seat-belt injuries of the spine in young children. J Bone Joint Surg (Br) 1992;74:571–574.

Swischuk LE. Anterior displacement of C2 in children: physiologic or pathologic? Radiology 1977;122:759–763.

Takata K, Inoue S-I, Takahashi K, et al. Fracture of the posterior margin of a lumbar vertebral body. J Bone Joint Surg (Am) 1988;70:589–594.

12.2 ARM AND SHOULDER

JEFFREY R. WARMAN

FRACTURES OF THE HUMERAL SHAFT

PATHOGENESIS

Etiology

Fractures of the humeral shaft may occur secondary to a direct blow to the arm or, more commonly in children, though indirect twisting injuries. In neonates they may be associated with breech deliveries or child abuse.

Epidemiology

- Most common in children under 3 and over 12 years of age
- Represent about 2% of all children's fractures

Classification

There is no classification specific to humeral shaft fractures in children. The fracture may be described by separation into proximal, middle, or distal thirds of the shaft, or more commonly by the fracture pattern (e.g., transverse, spiral, oblique).

DIAGNOSIS

History and Physical Examination

- A newborn child will present with inability to move the arm and localized swelling, crepitance, or deformity of the arm.
  - A septic shoulder or brachial plexus palsy must also be considered.
- In older children, the history of injury is important, especially to rule out child abuse.
  - On physical exam, the extremity will usually be held against the body by the opposite hand.
  - Localized swelling, tenderness, and deformity may be noted.
  - A good neurologic exam is essential.

RADIOGRAPHIC FEATURES

Plain radiographs are diagnostic in all age groups. Look for evidence of bone cysts or other pathologic fractures.

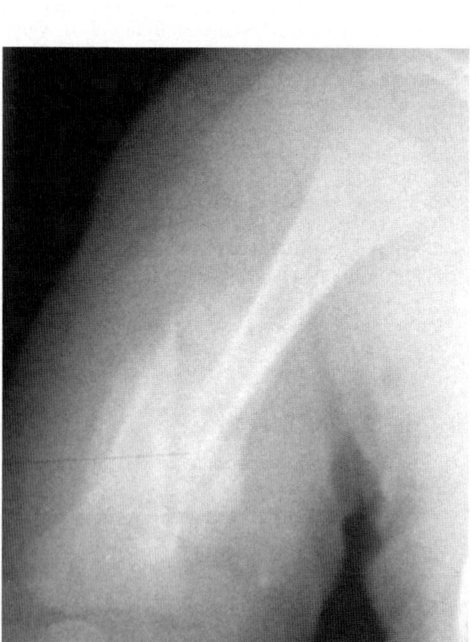

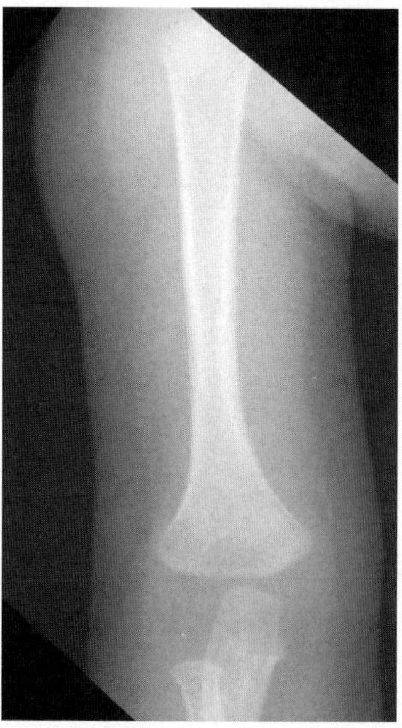

A B

Figure 12.2-1 (**A**) Anteroposterior radiograph of a humerus fracture sustained at delivery in a 4-week-old girl. (**B**) Complete remodeling seen at 10 months of age.

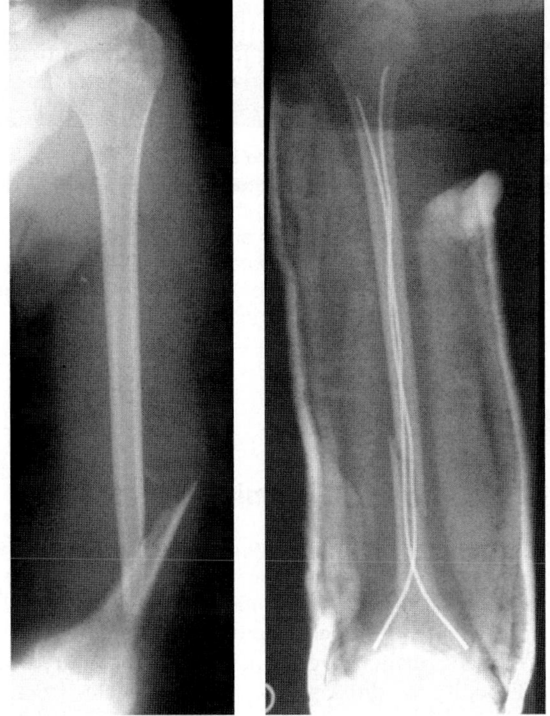

Figure 12.2-2 (**A**) Anteroposterior radiograph of a humeral diaphyseal fracture in a 15-year-old girl. (**B**) Postoperative radiograph after retrograde flexible intramedullary nailing.

TREATMENT

Nonoperative Treatment

- Most humeral shaft fractures can be treated nonoperatively.
- Neonates with humeral shaft fractures can be treated by pinning the cuff of the sleeve to the shirt or by splinting the arm in extension.
  - Angulation of up to 45 degrees can remodel in infants (Fig. 12.2-1).
- In older children, minimally displaced fractures can be treated in a shoulder immobilizer or Velpeau dressing.
  - Displaced or unstable fractures can be immobilized with a coaptation splint or hanging arm cast, using sedation if necessary for fracture reduction.
  - After early callus forms, a functional fracture brace offers protection and early mobilization for the patient.

Operative Treatment

- Operative treatment is rarely necessary in children but should be considered for open fractures, in patients with multiple injuries, and in older patients with unacceptable reductions.
- The method of choice for fixation of humeral shaft fractures in children is retrograde flexible intramedullary nailing (Fig. 12.2-2).
- For very distal shaft fractures, a crossed pinning technique may be performed, as with supracondylar humerus fractures (Fig. 12.2-3).

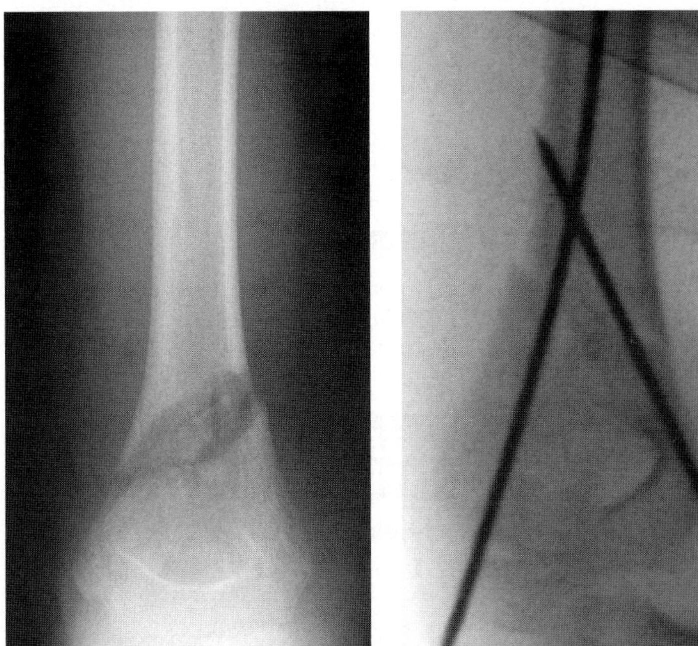

Figure 12.3-3 (**A**) Anteroposterior radiograph of a fracture at the distal diaphyseal/metaphyseal junction in a 9-year-old boy. (**B**) The fracture was treated with cross pins, using 0.062-inch K-wires.

- Plating a humeral shaft fracture is acceptable, but stress risers will be present at the ends of the plate, and empty screw holes after hardware removal can increase risk of refracture.
- External fixation is useful with comminuted or open fractures.

Results

- Humeral shaft fractures in children usually do very well; the vast majority may be treated nonoperatively.
- Malunion is unusual and nonunion is rare.
- Nerve palsies should be observed for 2 to 3 months for signs of recovery prior to further investigation or exploration, as most recover.

FRACTURES OF THE PROXIMAL HUMERUS

PATHOGENESIS

Etiology

- Occur in all age groups.
- In neonates, usually secondary to shoulder dystocia or birth trauma.
- In older children, the mechanism may be direct or indirect trauma.
- Pathologic fractures are also common in the proximal humerus secondary to unicameral bone cysts or other benign lesions.

Epidemiology

- Proximal humeral fractures are most common at 11 to 15 years of age.
- Boys are injured up to three times as frequently as girls.

Pathophysiology

- The forces generated by the shoulder girdle musculature displace fracture fragments in a characteristic fashion.
  - The rotator cuff flexes, abducts, and externally rotates the proximal fragment.
  - The distal fragment is adducted and anteriorly translated by the pull of the pectoralis muscles and latissimus dorsi.

Classification

The Salter-Harris classification is used to describe those fractures that involve the proximal humeral growth plate (Table 12.2-1). The Neer and Horowitz classification is based on the amount of fracture displacement (Table 12.2-2).

Fractures of the greater and lesser tuberosities are rare in children.

TABLE 12.2-1 SALTER-HARRIS CLASSIFICATION OF THE FRACTURES OF THE PROXIMAL HUMERUS

Type	Location of Fracture Line
I	Entirely through the physis
II	Traverses the physis and metaphysis
III	Traverses the physis and proximal epiphysis
IV	Extends across the proximal epiphysis, through the growth plate, and into the metaphysis

DIAGNOSIS

History and Physical Examination

- A neonate with a proximal humerus fracture will present with the arm held at the side.
  - Decreased or no active motion of the extremity will be noted and swelling of the proximal arm may be present.
  - Without further diagnostic studies, this injury will be difficult to differentiate from clavicle fractures, brachial plexus injuries, septic arthritis, or the rare shoulder dislocation.
- In an older child, making the diagnosis is easier.
  - The patient will usually recount a history of trauma and describe pain in the proximal arm.
  - The affected extremity will be held against the body, with swelling and tenderness noted in the proximal arm.

Radiographic Features

- In neonates, the proximal humeral epiphysis does not ossify until 6 months of age and an ultrasound or arthrogram will easily demonstrate the fracture.
- In older children, plain radiographs should be diagnostic.

TREATMENT

Nonoperative Treatment

The neonate with a proximal humerus fracture may be treated by pinning the cuff of the sleeve to the shirt. The fracture should be clinically healed in about 2 weeks.

TABLE 12.2-2 NEER AND HOROWITZ CLASSIFICATION OF FRACTURES OF THE PROXIMAL HUMERUS

Grade	Displacement
I	≤5 mm
II	5 mm to ⅓ of shaft width
III	⅓ to ⅔ shaft width
IV	>⅔ shaft width (includes complete displacement)

Sling, Shoulder Immobilizer (Velpeau)

In any age group, Neer grade I and II fractures may be treated by simple immobilization in a sling or shoulder immobilizer, whichever is more comfortable for the patient. In children less than 8 years of age, even significant displaced grade III and IV fractures should remodel, allowing for most all fractures in this age group to be treated with simple immobilization.

Closed Reduction and Casting

Unstable, displaced fractures of the proximal humerus, in need of reduction, are difficult to maintain by simple immobilization. Casting in a salute or Statue of Liberty position is mentioned for historical reasons only. These casts are difficult to apply and are associated with shoulder stiffness, nerve palsies, and cast sores. If fracture reduction is necessary, percutaneous pin fixation may be a better alternative.

Operative Treatment

Closed Reduction and Percutaneous Pinning

The need for reduction and fixation of displaced proximal humerus fractures is debated as similar functional outcomes have been documented in both operative and nonoperative treatment regardless of displacement. The remodeling capacity of the proximal humeral physis is significant and symptomatic malunion is unusual. Consideration for closed reduction and percutaneous pinning should be given for those children with Neer and Horowitz Grade III and IV fractures who are within two years of skeletal maturity. In this group, full remodeling of physeal fractures may not occur, which can result in limited range of motion at the shoulder.

Open Reduction and Internal Fixation

Proximal humerus fractures rarely require open reduction. Indications include open fractures, displaced intraarticular fractures, displaced tuberosity fractures, or fractures irreducible by closed methods. Failure of closed reduction is often due to entrapment of the periosteum or biceps tendon at the fracture site, which is easily removed surgically.

Results

As a general rule, fractures of the proximal humerus do quite well due to their excellent remodeling potential.

FRACTURES OF THE CLAVICLE

PATHOGENESIS

Etiology

- Occur through both direct and indirect trauma
- Only bony constraint between the upper extremity and axial skeleton
- In the newborn, pressure exerted on the shoulder during delivery can lead to fracture
- In older children, fractures may occur after a fall on an outstretched arm
- Direct trauma resulting in fractures is commonly due to the prominent and subcutaneous position of the clavicle

Epidemiology

- Occur in about 5 per 1,000 births
- Associated with high birth weight and shoulder dystocia
- Represent up to 15% of all children's fractures in older children

Pathophysiology

- Medial fragment is pulled proximally by the sternocleidomastoid.
- Distal fragment is pulled inferiorly by the pectoralis minor.
- Shortening occurs due to the pull of the subclavius and pectoralis muscles.
- Fractures of the medial or distal end of the clavicle usually occur through the physis.
- Lateral physis does not close until 19 years of age; medial physis does not close until 22 to 25 years of age.
- These fractures differ from those of adults, where there is associated ligament disruption of either the sternoclavicular or acromioclavicular joints.
- In children, disruption of the thick periosteal sleeve allows for displacement of the clavicle. The periosteum remains in its bed with its associated ligaments still intact. As remodeling occurs through this periosteum, the healed clavicle reforms in its anatomic bed and is stable. Often the displaced portion of the clavicle will resorb.
- Children over 13 years of age are more at risk for ligament disruption and may need to be treated as adults.

Classification

- Fractures of the clavicle are classified as involving the shaft, medial end, or distal end of the clavicle.
- True dislocations of the sternoclavicular joint or acromioclavicular joint are rare in children, as the physis will fail prior to joint dislocation.
- Fractures of the medial end of the clavicle may be classified by the direction of displacement, anterior or posterior, or by the Salter-Harris classification of physeal injuries.
- Fractures of the lateral end of the clavicle may be classified as shown in Table 12.2-3.

DIAGNOSIS

History and Physical Examination

- A newborn presents with the affected extremity held to the side.
- Swelling or crepitance may be present over the clavicle.
- Callus formation at the fracture site is palpable about 1 week postinjury.
- An older child with a clavicle fracture presents with pain, swelling, tenderness, and often a palpable step off at the fracture site.

TABLE 12.2-3 CLASSIFICATION OF FRACTURES OF THE LATERAL END OF THE CLAVICLE

Type	Description
I	Mild sprain of the acromioclavicular ligaments with no disruption of the periosteal sleeve
II	Partial disruption of the periosteal sleeve with mild widening of the acromioclavicular joint
III	Complete disruption of the periosteal sleeve with superior displacement of the clavicle; coracoclavicular interval 25%–100% normal
IV	Complete disruption of the periosteal sleeve with posterior displacement of the clavicle through the trapezius
V	Complete disruption of the periosteal sleeve with superior displacement of the clavicle; >100% widening of the coracoclavicular interval

- No active motion is noted.
- Anteriorly displaced medial clavicular injuries are more obvious than those with posterior displacement.
- Posteriorly displaced fractures may cause airway compromise or other mediastinal injuries.

Radiographic Features

- Fractures of the medial end of the clavicle may not be obvious radiographically.
  - A cephalically directed tangential radiograph can show subtle asymmetry between the sternoclavicular joints.
  - Computed tomography (CT) scan is the study of choice to visualize the fracture and diagnose mediastinal impingement.
- Displaced fractures of the midshaft of the clavicle are easily demonstrated radiographically.
- Incomplete or nondisplaced fractures in infants and young children may not be visualized until callus formation is radiographically evident, about 7 to 10 days after injury.
- Displaced fractures of the lateral clavicle are usually well-visualized radiographically.
- Imaging of both acromioclavicular joints on the same radiograph can demonstrate subtle differences, but stress views, with weights suspended from both wrists, are needed to reveal suspected injuries not otherwise evident.

TREATMENT

Nonoperative Treatment

- In the newborn, clavicle fractures may be treated by pinning the cuff off the sleeve to the shirt for about 10 days.
- Midshaft clavicle fractures in older children can be treated conservatively by a sling or figure-of-eight dressing with excellent functional results.
- Medial clavicle fractures in children do well with nonoperative care.
- Fractures with anterior displacement can be treated symptomatically as the reduction frequently is unstable.
- Moderate residual deformity in younger children will remodel and despite any residual deformity, older children will do well functionally.
- Mild posterior displacement of the medial clavicle without mediastinal impingement may be treated conservatively.
- Displacement causing mediastinal impingement needs to be urgently or emergently reduced by placing the patient supine with a bolster between the scapulae and applying longitudinal traction to the arm.
  - If traction alone does not affect the reduction, a towel clip may be used, under sterile conditions, to grasp the clavicle and manually pull it forward.
  - A vascular or thoracic surgeon should be on hand, even for closed reductions, as manipulation could start mediastinal bleeding.
  - Operative reduction may be needed if this is also unsuccessful.
- Lateral clavicular fractures in children less than 14 years should do well with simple sling immobilization.
  - Full functional recovery can be expected.

Operative Treatment

- Open fractures and fractures with impingement of underlying structures are indications for operative treatment of clavicle fractures.
- Closed fractures with displaced bone fragments endangering the integrity of the overlying skin, may also need to be treated operatively.
- Midshaft fractures of the clavicle requiring open reduction can be treated with a plate and screws or intramedullary fixation.
- When operative treatment is indicated for medial or lateral clavicle fractures, suture repair of the thick periosteal tube may provide sufficient stabilization.
  - For medial fractures, this avoids the potential of hardware migration into the mediastinum, which increases with transfixation of the sternoclavicular joint.

- Internal fixation of these injuries should be avoided if possible.

Results

Functional results of clavicle fractures in children are usually excellent, irrespective of the treatment selected.

FRACTURES OF THE SCAPULA

PATHOGENESIS

Etiology

Fractures of the scapula in children are rare and usually secondary to high-energy injuries, such as motor vehicle accidents. The more superficial and prominent parts of the scapula however, such as the acromion, may sustain a fracture during sports activities or falls. If a plausible history for a scapula fracture is not given, consider the possibility of child abuse.

Classification

- Scapula fractures can be classified by the anatomic location of the fracture:
- Body of the scapula
- Spine of the scapula
- Glenoid fossa or neck
- Acromion and the coracoid processes.

DIAGNOSIS

History and Physical Examination

On examination, there will be localized swelling and tenderness. Look for injury to structures in proximity to the scapula, including the ribs, lungs, and brachial plexus. This is especially true for high-energy injuries.

Radiographic Features

Three views of the scapula, a true anteroposterior (AP) view, a lateral scapula view, and an axillary view are needed for a complete radiographic examination of scapula injuries. A CT scan is often necessary for the evaluation and treatment of glenoid fractures.

TREATMENT

Nonoperative Treatment

Most scapula fractures can be treated nonoperatively, using a sling for comfort. Fractures of the scapula body are usually only minimally displaced because of the overlying muscular envelope.

Operative Treatment

Displaced fractures of the glenoid body or rim in older children may require operative intervention. These are intraarticular fractures and reduction is necessary for stability and function of the shoulder joint. Displaced fractures of the glenoid neck may require operative treatment, especially when associated with ipsilateral clavicle fractures. Operative intervention for acromion or coracoid fractures is rare in children.

GLENOHUMERAL DISLOCATIONS

PATHOGENESIS

Etiology

- Shoulder dislocations in children are uncommon.
- Usually secondary to indirect forces transmitted to the shoulder through a twisting of the arm.
- Direct trauma to the proximal humerus and shoulder area can also result in glenohumeral dislocation.
- Most occur during sports activity.
- Neonatal shoulder dislocations are rare.

Pathophysiology

- To accommodate its wide range of motion, the shoulder joint has minimal bony constraint.
- Ligamentous thickenings of the joint capsule are the primary stabilizers of the shoulder joint and the rotator cuff acts as a secondary stabilizer.
- Disruption of these capsular ligaments or their labral attachment (a Bankart lesion) is the mechanism of failure leading to dislocation.
- Shoulder dislocations are uncommon in young children, as the proximal humeral physis will often fail prior to failure of these thick ligaments.

Classification

- Shoulder dislocations can be classified by the direction of dislocation, including anterior, posterior, inferior (luxatio erecta), and superior dislocations.
- In children, anterior or anteroinferior dislocations are by far the most common and occur secondary to abduction and external rotation of the arm.
- Multidirectional instability is also possible.
- Dislocations can also be classified as traumatic or atraumatic.
  - Atraumatic dislocations are often seen in habitual dislocators, or in those with conditions associated with joint laxity (e.g., Larsen syndrome or Ehlers-Danlos syndrome).
  - Also found in patients with neuromuscular disease, such as cerebral palsy or brachial plexus injuries, due

to long-standing chronic muscular imbalance about the shoulder.
- Shoulder dislocations can also be classified as acute, recurrent, or chronic.

DIAGNOSIS

History and Physical Examination

- The patient with a traumatic shoulder dislocation presents with a painful deformity to the shoulder.
- If anteriorly dislocated, the arm is usually slightly abducted and externally rotated.
- The acromion will be prominent, and hollowness will be noted beneath it.
- The humeral head may be palpable anterior to the glenoid.
- The less common posterior dislocation will cause the arm to be held in adduction and internal rotation, with a posterior shoulder prominence.
- The axillary nerve is at risk of injury after shoulder dislocations and should be examined as part of a full neurovascular exam prior to initiating treatment.

Radiographic Features

- A shoulder dislocation can be visualized with plain radiographs which include an AP view of the shoulder, a lateral scapula view, and an axillary view.
- Note any associated proximal humeral fracture that could displace during reduction.
- After reduction, a compression fracture of the humeral head, called a Hill-Sachs lesion, can be visualized on an AP view with internal rotation of the arm.

TREATMENT

Nonoperative Treatment

The reduction of a glenohumeral dislocation may be accomplished under sedation. For both anterior and posterior dislocations, a traction/countertraction maneuver is effective for the reduction, using a sheet placed under the axilla. Postreduction radiographs are compulsory. Once a patient is comfortable, aggressive physical therapy should be instituted to strengthen the rotator cuff and shoulder girdle musculature. The family and patient should be made aware that there is a high risk of recurrence in children necessitating operative intervention.

Operative Treatment

Most patients will have a recurrence, and surgical stabilization is then recommended. The surgical procedure will depend upon the type of dislocation, whether there is a Bankart lesion, and the preference of the surgeon. Surgical intervention may not be recommended for habitual dislocators due to the high postoperative recurrence rate.

Results

The results of treating shoulder dislocations in children should be similar to the treatment results in adults.

SUGGESTED READING

Beringer D, Weiner DS, Noble JS, et al. Severely displaced proximal humeral epiphyseal fracture: a follow up study. J Pediatr Orthop 1998;18:31–37.

De Jong KP, Sukul DMKS. Anterior sternoclavicular dislocation: a long-term follow-up study. J Orthop Trauma 1990;4:420–423.

Eidman DK, Siff SJ, Tullos HS. Acromioclavicular lesions in children. Am J Sports Med 1981;9:150–154.

Larsen CF, Kiaer T, Lindequist S. Fractures of the proximal humerus in children: nine year follow-up of 64 unoperated cases. Acta Orthop Scand 1990;61:255–257.

Lewonowski K, Bassett GS. Complete posterior sternoclavicular epiphyseal separation: a case report and review of the literature. Clin Orthop 1992;281:84–88.

Marans HJ, Angel KR, Schemitsch EH, et al. The fate of traumatic anterior dislocation of the shoulder in children. J Bone Joint Surg (Am) 1992;74A:1242–1244.

Neer CS, Horowitz BS. Fractures of the proximal humeral epiphyseal plate. Clin Orthop 1965;41:24–31.

Oppenheim WL, Davis A, Growdon WA, et al. Clavicle fractures in the newborn. Clin Orthop 1990;250:176–180.

Rockwood CA. Dislocations of the sternoclavicular joint. AAOS Instr Course Lect 1975;24:144–159.

Young K, Sarwark JF. Proximal humerus, scapula, and clavicle. In: Beaty JH, Kassar JR, eds. Rockwood and Wilkins' fractures in children, 5th ed. Philadelphia: Lippincott Williams & Wilkins, 2001: 741–806.

12.3 ELBOW

EDWARD ABRAHAM

The elbow region includes the distal humeral metaphysis, epiphysis, radial head and neck, and ulnar olecranon process. The proximity of the radial, median, and ulnar nerves and the brachial artery to the elbow trauma can be a major source of apprehension and urgency for the physician.

ANATOMY

There are two well-known mnemonics used to remember the sequential appearance of the ossification centers: "CRITOE" and "Come rub my tree of life"—**c**apitellum, **r**adius, **i**nternal (*m*edial) epicondyle, **t**rochlea, **o**lecranon, and external (*lateral*) epicondyle (Fig. 12.3-1). On a lateral radiograph, the capitellar center is located anteriorly and tilts downward. Its posterior unossified epiphysis is wider posteriorly than it is anteriorly. A line drawn down the anterior surface of the humeral cortex passes through the middle to posterior half of the capitellum on a lateral roentgenogram (Fig. 12.3-2).

SUPRACONDYLAR FRACTURE

PATHOGENESIS

Etiology

- Usually caused from a fall on an outstretched extremity with the elbow in full extension.
- Child abuse must be suspected if child is less than 2 years of age.

Epidemiology

- The rate of occurrence between boys and girls is 3 to 2.
- Average age is 7 years.
- Nerve injury occurs in about 10% of cases (median and radial nerves).
- Distal radius fracture is the most common associated skeletal injury.

DIAGNOSIS

Physical Examination and History

Clinical Features

- Elbow swelling, tenderness, and diminished active movement of extremity.

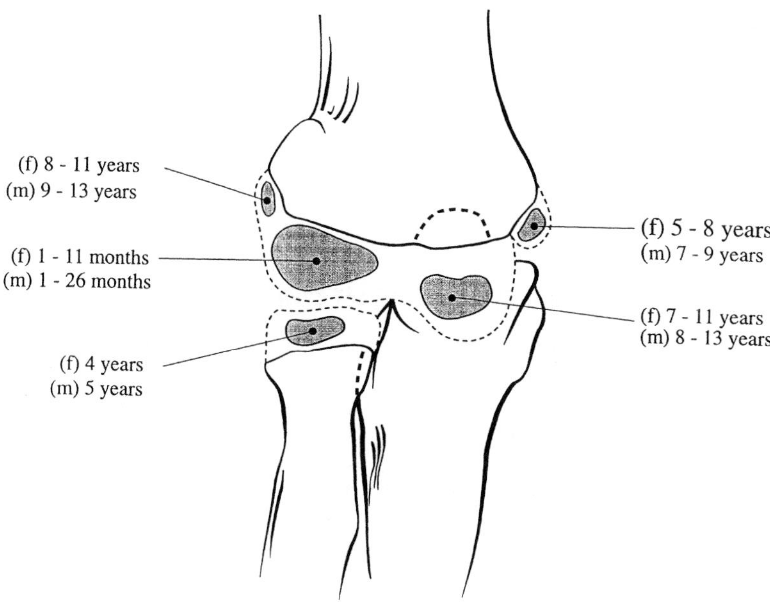

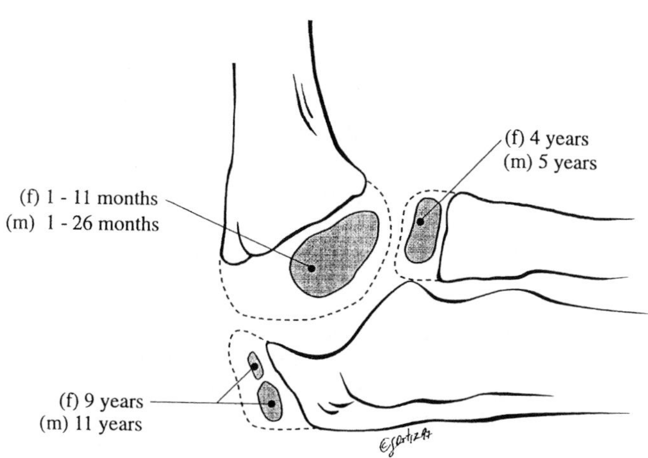

Figure 12.3-1 Chronologic appearance of the centers of ossification as seen on radiographs.

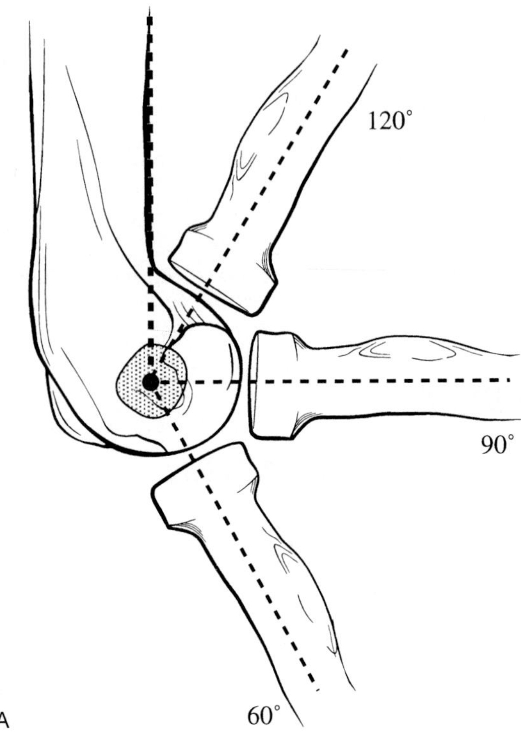

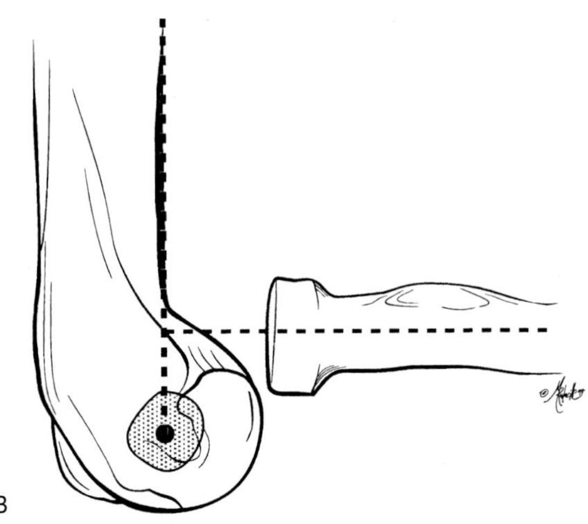

Figure 12.3-2 (**A**) The normal anterior humeral cortical line transecting the center of the capitellum as seen on a lateral radiograph. (**B**) Anterior radial head dislocation.

- Anterior Pucker sign occurs when the proximal bone spike penetrates into the subcutaneous tissue.
- Evaluate humerus, forearm, wrist and hand for associated injuries.
- Sensory loss is more difficult to assess in young children.
- Vascular examination: check for pulses, capillary refilling, skin temperature, and forearm compartment tenseness.
- Painful passive finger extension and flexion may indicate increased forearm compartment pressures.

Radiologic Features

- Get good quality x-rays of entire extremity.
- Contralateral radiographs are controversial and should only be obtained if the diagnosis is unclear.

TREATMENT

Reduction Technique (Fig. 12.3-3 and Table 12.3-1)

- Definitive reduction of the fracture is carried out under general anesthesia with C-arm fluoroscopic control.
- Apply longitudinal traction to reduce the proximal displacement and any varus or valgus angulation (see Fig. 12.3-3A).
- Reduce medial or lateral displacement (see Fig. 12.3-3B).
- Internally rotate the forearm if needed to correct external rotation of distal fragment (see Fig. 12.3-3C).
- Reduce the posterior displacement by applying pressure on the olecranon process while maintaining traction (see Fig. 12.3-3D).
- Flex elbow acutely with forearm in pronation for both medial and lateral displacement of distal fragment (see Fig. 12.3-3E).

Adolescent T-Condylar Fractures

- Open reduction and internal fixation for the unstable displaced fractures.
- Use the same treatment principles that apply to adult fractures.
- Open reduction indicated if vascular compromise exists or soft tissue interposition prevents adequate fracture reduction.
- Openly reduced fracture can be fixed with percutaneously placed pins.

Complications

Brachial Artery Injury

- Immediate fracture reduction is the treatment of choice for a distal pulseless extremity.
- An absent pulse with the following conditions warrants brachial artery exploration:
  - ☐ Abnormally high forearm compartment pressures and clinical findings of a development of compartment syndrome
  - ☐ Loss of pulse after closed reduction

Compartment Syndrome

- Early clinical findings are worsening forearm pain at rest or with passive finger movement.

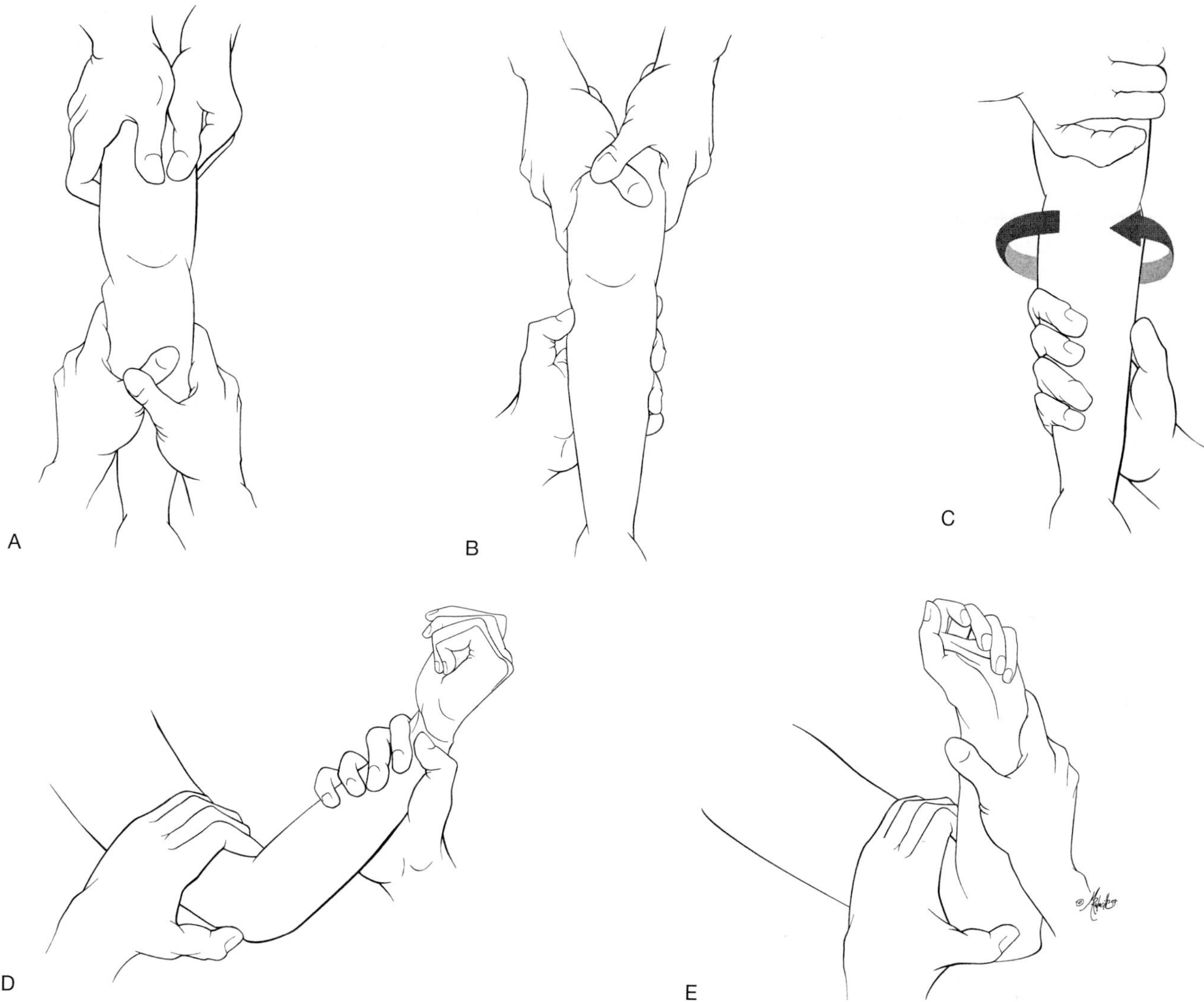

Figure 12.3-3 Reduction of supracondylar fractures. (**A**) Traction. (**B**) Correction of displacement. (**C**) Rotation correction. (**D**) Reduction. (**E**) Pronation.

- Compartment syndrome can exist in the presence of a palpable pulse.
- Forearm compartment pressures greater than 30 mm Hg and the presence of clinical findings warrant fasciotomy.
- Median nerve injury can mask the pain associated with Compartment syndrome.

Nerve Injury
- Occurs in about 15% of cases.
- The anterior interosseous branch of the median nerve is commonly involved.
- Nerve recovery usually occurs within 3 months

Malunion
- Cubitus varus is most common.
- Lateral downward tilt of the medial side of the fracture is the main cause of cubitus varus

Myositis Ossificans
- This rare condition is known to resolve within 2 years.
- Surgery is rarely indicated.

Avascular Necrosis of Trochlea
- An asymptomatic fishtail deformity may develop.
- Best treated conservatively.

Elbow Stiffness
- Loss of elbow flexion and increased hyperextension is associated with residual posterior tilt of the distal fragment.
- Anterior impingement by a medially rotated distal fragment can restrict elbow flexion.
- The combination of some bone remodeling with growth and therapy usually restores functional range of motion.

TABLE 12.3-1 CLASSIFICATION AND TREATMENT OF EXTENSION SUPRACONDYLAR FRACTURES

Type	Characteristics	Treatment
I	Hyperextension of distal fragment up to 30 degrees of angulation No displacement Detached but intact anterior periosteum Stable transverse fracture line through medial and lateral epicondylar columns and olecranon fossa	Reduction not needed Long arm splint for 1 week Convert to long arm cast, elbow flexed to 90 degrees with forearm in neutral rotation X-rays, then remove immobilization at 3–4 wk Rehabilitation: home program adequate
II	Hyperextension of distal fragment beyond 30 degrees of angulation No displacement Potentially unstable Anterior periosteum detached and partially torn	Closed reduction in ER under i.v. sedation. Long arm splint or cast with the elbow in 100–110 degrees of flexion and the forearm pronated *Or* closed reduction in OR under general anesthesia and immobilization as above or two lateral parallel or cross-fixing Kirschner pins (0.062 inch or 1.6 mm) Long arm splint for 1 week with the elbow in 70 degrees of flexion and the forearm in neutral rotation Convert to long arm cast for a total of 3–4 wk Pin removal in office Start exercise program at home
III	Distal fragment posterior and proximal displacement Unstable Anterior periosteum completely torn Circumferential detachment of posterior periosteum No lateral or medial periosteal hinges exist Distal anterior periosteal hem and retracted anterior proximal periosteum are characteristic findings	Closed reduction under general anesthesia[a] Two lateral parallel or cross-fixing Kirschner wires Long arm splint for 1 week with the elbow in 70 degrees of flexion and the forearm in neutral rotation Long arm cast for 2–3 more wk Pin removal in office Physical therapy consultation for supervised home rehabilitation
IV	Vertical extension fracture line that is usually medial but can be lateral Usually completely displaced Unstable if displaced There are three sub types: ▪ Type I early childhood—distal extension ▪ Type II preadolescent–distal and proximal extension ▪ Type III adolescent—T-condylar fracture	Closed reduction under general anesthesia Stabilize main fragment first Two to four cross-fixing Kirschner wires Long arm splint for 1 wk with the elbow in 70 degrees of flexion and the forearm in neutral rotation Replace splint with long arm cast for up to 4 wk. The elbow is in 70 degrees of flexion and the forearm in neutral rotation Pin removal in office Physical therapy consultation Treat T-condylar type as adult fracture

[a]Caution: Check both for arterial circulation and ulnar nerve function before and immediately after fracture reduction and fixation.
ER, emergency room; OR, operating room.

FLEXION-TYPE SUPRACONDYLAR FRACTURE

PATHOGENESIS

Etiology and Pathophysiology

- Accounts for less than 2% of all supracondylar fractures.
- The mechanism of injury in a direct blow on a flexed elbow.
- The periosteum is torn posteriorly so that the reduced fracture is unstable in flexion.
- The ulnar nerve is prone to injury.

Classification

- Similar to extension-type fractures
  - ☐ Type I: nondisplaced
  - ☐ Type II: mild angulation
  - ☐ Type III: displaced

DIAGNOSIS

- Swelling and tenderness about elbow.
- Radiographically, the distal humerus fragment is anteriorly angulated or displaced.

TREATMENT

Type I

- Long arm cast with elbow flex for comfort, neutral forearm rotation
- Home therapy program

Type II

- Closed reduction under general anesthesia by extending elbow
- Unstable fracture requires percutaneous Kirschner pin fixation
- Apply a long arm cast with elbow extended and forearm in neutral rotation

Type III

- Closed reduction under general anesthesia
- Percutaneous pin fixation with elbow in extension or 30-degree flexion
- Immobilize in a splint or cast with elbow in flexion or extension
- Remove Kirschner wires (K-wires) in 3 to 4 weeks

PHYSEAL FRACTURES

Physeal injuries about the elbow rank third in frequency for all physeal fractures after phalanx and wrist. The physis fracture type depends mainly on skeletal age and injury mechanism (Table 12.3-2).

TABLE 12.3-2 THE ROLE OF AGE IN PHYSEAL FRACTURE TYPES

Fracture Type	Age (yr)
Total separation of physis (Salter-Harris type I)	0–3
Lateral condylar physis fractures (Salter-Harris type IV)	3–8
Medial epicondylar apophysis	11–15

Lateral Condylar Physeal Fractures

Pathogenesis

- Account for 20% of distal humerus fractures.
- Likely mechanism of injury is elbow extension, forearm adduction, and supination.
- The commonest fracture line travels from the posterior lateral metaphysis, along the physis, and into the trochlea (Milch type II) (Fig.12.3-4).
- The rare fracture line type starts from the posterolateral metaphysis, through the physis and body of the capitellum (Milch type I) (see Fig. 12.3-4).
- Elbow arthrogram under general anesthesia and magnetic resonance imaging (MRI) are good for accessing lateral displacement of elbow if not obvious on radiographs.

DIAGNOSIS

History and Physical Examination

- History of mechanism is variable.
- Outer elbow swelling and tenderness with pain on elbow motion.

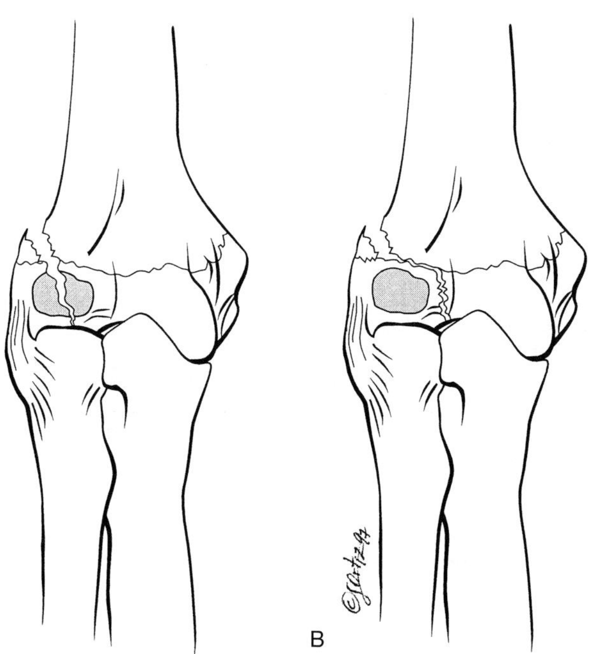

Figure 12.3-4 Classification of lateral condyle fractures. (A) Milch type I, lateral view (Salter-Harris type IV). (B) Milch type II, lateral view (Salter-Harris type II).

- Plain radiographs of elbow must include anteroposterior, lateral, and oblique views.
- MRI or arthrogram recommended if diagnosis unclear.

CLASSIFICATION AND TREATMENT

Lateral condylar physeal fractures are classified by, and treatment is based on, stage (Table 12.3-3 and Fig. 12.3-5).

Complications

Delayed Union

- Seen more frequently in patients treated with cast immobilization.
- For minimally displaced fractures (≈2 mm) keep immobilization for 2 months if necessary.
- Delayed *in situ* pinning is an option.
- Open reduction after 3 weeks of injury is controversial.

Nonunion

- Results from inadequate treatment.
- Untreated nonunion may lead to cubitus valgus and ulnar nerve dysfunction.
- Specific treatment is controversial—the best goal is prevention.

Pseudovarus

- Lateral spur formation most common deformity associated with this fracture.
- Cubitus varus may result secondary to condylar physeal overgrowth or inadequate fracture reduction.

Fishtail Deformity

- The sharp angle wedge type is caused by a bony bar from inadequate fracture reduction between the lateral condyle ossification center and that of the trochlea.
- The smooth curved wedge type is associated with osteonecrosis of the lateral part of the medial crista of the trochlea.
- Not associated with any significant elbow function deficiency.

Osteonecrosis

- May be caused by extensive dissection needed for late reduction of fracture.
- Regeneration of the condyle is likely to occur if union occurs.
- Loss of joint motion may result.

Myositis Ossificans

- Rare complication with resulting loss of elbow motion.

Physeal Arrest

- Premature closure of the physis can occur in conjunction with premature fusion of the secondary centers of ossification in the epiphysis.
- Limited growth potential of the distal humeral physis and the non-weightbearing status of the humerus decreases the adverse effects of a physeal arrest.

TABLE 12.3-3 STAGES AND TREATMENT OF LATERAL CONDYLAR PHYSEAL FRACTURES

Stage	Characteristics	Treatment
I	Condylar changes ■ ≤2 mm of downward displacement ■ Articular surface intact ■ No lateral shift	*Initial* ■ Long arm splint with elbow in 90-degree flexion and forearm in neutral rotation *Definitive* ■ Long arm cast in above position for 4 wk ■ Weekly radiographs for first 2 wk ■ Home physical therapy
II	Nondisplaced articular surface ■ 2–5 mm of downward displacement ■ Articular surface broken ■ Lateral shift possible	*Initial* ■ Same as stage I *Definitive* ■ Closed or open reduction with two Kirschner wire (1.6 mm) fixation ■ Long arm cast at stage I with wire removal in 3–4 wk
	Displaced articular surface	*Definitive* ■ Open reduction and wire fixation, rest same as for nondisplaced
III	Total displacement ■ Lateral displacement with break of capitellar line ■ Rotated (long axis of ossification center is vertical instead of horizontal) ■ Olecranon and radial translation possible with Milch I fractures	*Initial* ■ Same as stage I *Definitive* ■ Open reduction and Kirschner wire fixation

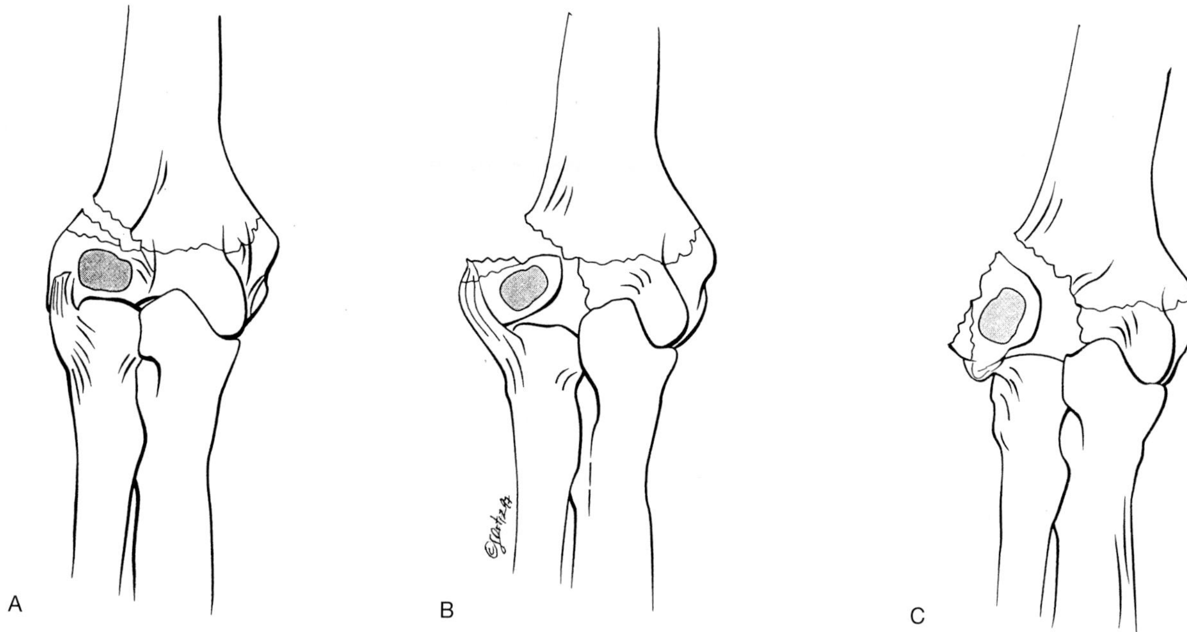

Figure 12.3-5 Rutherford classification of lateral condyle. (A) Type I. (B) Type II. (C) Type III.

CAPITELLAR FRACTURES

Fractures of the capitellum are intraarticular epiphyseal fractures of the lateral condyle and occasionally the lateral crista of the trochlea.

PATHOGENESIS

- Usually caused by the impaction of the radial head on the capitellum
- Rare injury, seen mainly in children older than 12 years
- Difficult to diagnose in the younger child
- Radial head fractures seen in one-third of patients

Classification

- Hahn-Steinthal type: includes the capitellum and cancellous bone from the lateral condyle and lateral crista of the trochlea.
- Kocher-Lorenz type: articular fracture seen mainly in adults.
- The Rutherford classification.

DIAGNOSIS

Clinical Features

- Elbow flexion is restricted.
- Swelling is limited in isolated injuries.

Radiologic Features

- Routine radiographs with oblique views to detect small bone fragments.
- Computed tomography (CT), arthrogram, and MRI are useful diagnostic tools.
- Look for associated radial head fractures.

TREATMENT

- Surgery is indicated in most cases because of intraarticular involvement.
- Excision of the fragment is recommended for comminuted or neglected fractures.
- Reattachment of large bone fragments with compression screw fixation gives better results than K-wire fixation.
- Avascular necrosis of the fragment is a potential complication.

FRACTURES OF THE MEDIAL CONDYLAR PHYSIS

PATHOGENESIS

- Isolated medial condylar fractures are rare, accounting for less than 1% of all elbow fractures in children between 8 and 14 years.
- Occasionally seen in association with supracondylar fractures of the humerus, olecranon process fractures, and posterolateral elbow dislocations.
- The most likely mechanism is a fall on an outstretched arm with a valgus strain or a direct fall on the flexed elbow.

DIAGNOSIS

- Swelling and pain on inner side of elbow.
- Joint instability on valgus stress.
- Diagnosis is based on radiograph findings.
- Before the age of 8 years extraarticular medial epicondylar apophyseal fractures may be confused with medial condylar fractures. An MRI or arthrogram may be helpful.
- A posterior fat pad sign is suggestive of intraarticular involvement.

CLASSIFICATION AND TREATMENT

The Kilfoyle classification and recommended treatment are given in Table 12.3-4.

Complications

- Cubitus varus: associated with failure to reduce a displaced fracture, nonunion, or avascular necrosis of the medial condyle.
- Avascular necrosis of the medial crista of the trochlea may follow open reduction of the fracture.
- Cubitus valgus can occur secondary to overgrowth.

DISTAL PHYSIS SEPARATION

PATHOGENESIS

- Primarily cartilaginous epiphysis makes diagnosis difficult.
- Fracture separation of entire physis usually occurs before 6 years of age.
- The medial epicondyle apophysis shares a common physeal line with the distal epiphysis until about 6 years of age in girls and 8 years of age in boys.
- It is believed that the horizontal line of the physis and its close proximity to the olecranon fossa are responsible for this fracture pattern.

Classification

Delee and colleagues' classification is given in Table 12.3-5.

DIAGNOSIS

- High index of suspicion is key.
- Often the result of abuse in non-ambulatory children.

Clinical Features

- Swelling may be minimal in the newborn
- Swollen elbow in an infant or toddler
- Crepitus with elbow motion

Radiologic Features

- Relationship between the radial head and lateral condylar center of ossification is maintained.
- Intact proximal radius and ulna displaces posterior and medial; with elbow dislocations the displacement is posterolateral.
- Arthrography, ultrasound, and MRI are helpful in differentiating the fractures.

TREATMENT

- Closed reduction is attempted in all cases under sedation. Medial displacement corrected in extension and elbow, then flexed and pronated.

TABLE 12.3-4 KILFOYLE CLASSIFICATION AND TREATMENT OF MEDIAL CONDYLAR FRACTURES

Type	Description	Treatment
I	Starts in the medial epicondylar column and ends between the capitellum and trochlea	Long arm splint or cast with elbow flexed to 90 degrees and forearm in neutral rotation
II	Fracture line extends into joint; potentially unstable	Same as type I if nondisplaced or same as type III if displaced
III	Medial condyle and epicondyle displaces and rotates	Open reduction and Kirschner pin or screw fixation

TABLE 12.3-5 CLASSIFICATION OF DISTAL PHYSIS SEPARATION

Classification	Age	Description
Group A (Salter-Harris type I)	Newborn–12 mo	Epiphysis is mainly cartilaginous tissue
Group B (Salter-Harris type I)	12 mos–3 yr	Possible metaphyseal bony flakes with epiphysis
Group C	3–7 yr	Large metaphyseal fragment, usually from the lateral side

- Two percutaneous K-wires can be used to fix the fracture in older children.
- For neglected fractures (more than 5 days) immobilize and expect sufficient remodeling with time.

Complications

- Malunion:
  - Most frequent complication
  - Seen mainly in untreated patients
- Rare: traumatic osteonecrosis of the trochlea, nonunion

MEDIAL EPICONDYLAR APOPHYSEAL FRACTURES

PATHOGENESIS

Epidemiology

- Male-to-female ratio of 4:1
- Associated with elbow dislocation in 50% of cases
- Peak age of incidence is 9 to 12 years.

Anatomy

- A traction apophysis that does not contribute to longitudinal humeral growth
- Common origin for forearm flexion muscle mass and medial capsular attachment
- Becomes an extraarticular structure at age 8 years

Mechanism of Injury

- Indirect:
  - Acute hyperextension of elbow with forced elbow valgus stress. Associated with anterior and distal displacement of apophysis greater than 5 mm.
  - Chronic repetitive or dominant overuse of extremity (e.g., Little League pitchers)
- Direct:
  - Direct posterior blow to the epicondyle

DIAGNOSIS

Clinical Features

- Pain, tenderness, and swelling localized medially.
- Increased pain with resistive wrist flexion or valgus stress to elbow.
- Loss of elbow motion.
- Other injuries may complicate the clinical findings (i.e., elbow dislocation, olecranon, or coronoid fractures).

Radiographic Features

- Standard anteroposterior, lateral, and oblique views of the elbow joint are required.
- In children younger than 5 years, MRI or arthrograms are useful.
- Look for widening of the physis, distal and anterior migration of apophysis.

CLASSIFICATION AND TREATMENT

Types of medial epicondylar apophyseal fractures, and their characteristics and treatment are shown in Table 12.3-6 and Figure 12.3-6.

Complications

Nonunion or Fibrous Union

- Seen in 60% of cases treated conservatively
- Elbow function rarely compromised
- Treatment necessary if pain or tenderness persists

Ulnar Nerve Dysfunction

- Associated with severe displacement or incarceration of the epicondyle in the elbow joint
- Necessitates exploration of the ulnar nerve and reduction of fracture

Elbow Stiffness

- Seen in 10% of cases

Myositis Ossification

- Rare
- Conservative measures recommended since lesions may spontaneously resolve

TABLE 12.3-6 TREATMENT OF MEDIAL EPICONDYLAR APOPHYSEAL FRACTURES

Type	Description	Treatment
Minimal	Less than 10 mm of displacement	Conservative measures only Long arm splint with elbow flexed at 90 degrees and wrist in neutral rotation for up to 2 wk Replace with splint Ace wrap and sling until patient is asymptomatic Start elbow motion exercises
Moderate	Greater than 10 mm	Conservative treatment as minimally displaced fracture ORIF controversial Gross elbow instability Ulnar nerve dysfunction
Severe	Incarcerated fragment in elbow	Requires ORIF

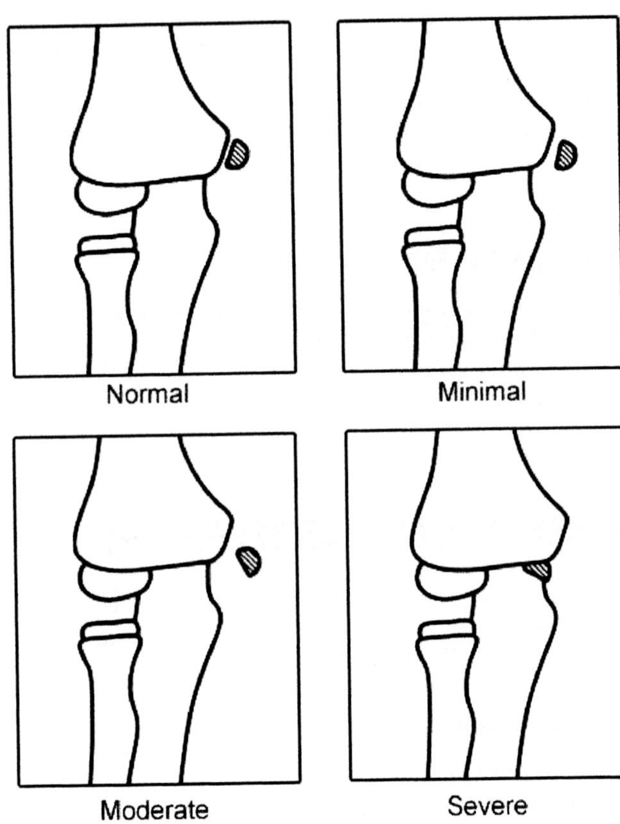

Figure 12.3-6 Degrees of medial epicondylar apophyseal fractures.

LATERAL EPICONDYLAR APOPHYSIS FRACTURES

Lateral apophyseal epicondylar fractures are rare and the natural appearance of this center is frequently confused for a fracture.

PATHOGENESIS

Anatomy

- Ossification center appears at about 10 years of age.
- The early bony sliver is normally separated from the metaphysis and epiphysis by 2 to 3 mm.
- The ossifying epicondylar epiphysis fuses first with the capitellum then the humeral metaphysis.

PATHOPHYSIOLOGY

- Violent contraction of the common extension muscles of the forearm causes isolated avulsion fractures.

DIAGNOSIS

Clinical Features

- Local pain and swelling over outer elbow
- Elbow joint stiffness

Radiologic Features

- Lateral separation of the ossification center from the metaphysis and capitellum is a normal finding.
- An avulsion fracture is diagnosed when the ossification center lies distal to the osteochondral epiphysis.

TREATMENT

- Immobilization of extremity in a sling or splint for comfort
- An incarcerated fragment in the elbow requires open reduction and wire fixation.

Complications

- Nonunion: usually asymptomatic

ELBOW DISLOCATIONS

PATHOGENESIS

Etiology

- Usually caused by an indirect hyperextension and valgus force to elbow with supination of forearm.
- Uncommon anterior elbow dislocation is caused by a direct force on the flexed joint.

Epidemiology

- Accounts for 3% of all joint dislocations
- Usually occur at age 13 to 14 years
- Associated elbow fractures in about 50% of cases
- Boy-to-girl ratio is 3:1
- Left-to-right-side ratio is 3:2

Pathophysiology

- Elbow hyperextension is the cause in over 90% of cases.

Classification

- Based on the position of the proximal radioulnar joint with regard to the distal humerus:
  - Proximal radius and ulna usually displace as a unit.
  - Disassociation of the proximal radioulnar joint rarely occurs.
  - Divergence of radius and ulna is rare.

DIAGNOSIS

Radiographic Features

- Routine anteroposterior and lateral radiographs are not always possible and multiple views and
- Comparison radiographs of the contralateral elbow may be helpful.

TREATMENT

- Prompt reduction is necessary to relieve pain, and prevent or minimize neurovascular complications.
- Check neurovascular status before and after reduction.
- Radiographs are necessary before and after reduction.
- Sedation and analgesia are recommended.

Posterolateral Dislocation

Closed Reduction Technique

- Hypersupinate forearm and apply traction
- Apply downward force along the distal arm and proximal forearm while using counter traction

COMPLICATIONS

- Loss of elbow motion:
  - Most common complication
  - Terminal extension loss of 15 degrees is commonplace
- Neurologic injuries:
  - Usually transient
  - Ulna nerve most commonly affected
- Arterial insufficiency:
  - Can be caused by thrombosis, rupture, or entrapment
  - Collateral arterial flow may be sufficient to permit a weak Doppler radial pulse or a good nailbed capillary flow in the finger in the presence of an obstructed proximal radial or brachial artery
- Myositis ossificans and heterotopic ossifications
- Recurrent posterior dislocation rare, but occurs more commonly in children than adults
- **Anterior elbow dislocation:**
  - Incidence 1%
  - Elbow held in extension and a fullness in the articubital fossa is felt
  - Treated by closed reduction: elbow is partially flexed with traction and a downward force on the distal arm
- **Medial and lateral elbow dislocations:**
  - Only lateral elbow dislocations are reported in children
  - Lateral subluxation may not be obvious as a complete dislocation on radiographs
- **Divergent elbow dislocations:**
  - Rare injury associated with excessive compressive forces of the elbow
  - Usually associated with radial head, neck, and proximal ulnar fractures
  - Proximal radius displaced posteriorly and radially

Results

Closed reduction with general anesthesia is usually successful and prognosis for elbow function is very good.

RADIAL HEAD DISLOCATION

- Isolated traumatic dislocations of the radial head are considered a variant of Monteggia fracture, type I.
- Partial or complete anterior displacement of the radial head and subtle anterior bowing of the ulnar shaft on lateral radiographs (ulna bow sign) are diagnostic.
- Other possible causes of anterior radial head dislocations: cubitus varus after supracondylar fractures, osteochondritis dissecans of the capitellum, and birth trauma.
- The mechanism of injury is the same as that for Monteggia injuries but without obvious ulna fracture.

- Unlike acute traumatic dislocations, long-standing traumatic dislocation may mimic congenital dislocations on radiographs.

TREATMENT

- Acute anterior dislocation: closed reduction with flexion and supination
- Chronic (more than 3 weeks) anterior dislocation: open reduction is controversial but may be recommended up to 3 years after injury.

SUBLUXATION OF RADIAL HEAD (NURSEMAID'S ELBOW)

PATHOGENESIS

Etiology

- Annular ligament slips proximally because of weak distal attachments of the annular ligament to the radial head.

Epidemiology

- Common injury under age 5 years (mean age, 2.5 years)
- Girls: 65% of the time
- Left elbow: 70% of the time
- Mechanism of injury: longitudinal pull on a straight elbow with forearm in pronation

Pathophysiology

- In forearm pronation, the lateral head surface is narrower and rounder, but it is wider and squarer in supination.

DIAGNOSIS

- History may not be readily obtainable.
- Child stops using the extremity.
- Forearm supination is more painful than pronation.
- Radiography is often normal.
- Look for other occult fractures (i.e., supracondylar, lateral condyle, or radial head and neck fractures)

TREATMENT

- Closed reduction by flexion and supination.
- Spontaneous reductions may occur before patient is seen by physician.

RADIAL HEAD AND NECK FRACTURES AND DISLOCATIONS

PATHOGENESIS

- Acute injury:
  - Usually a combination of forces, compression, angulation, and rotation on a hyperextended valgus elbow
  - May be isolated to the radius or in association with elbow dislocation, where the radius fracture may be caused as the elbow dislocates or when the joint reduces
- Chronic injury:
  - Seen in athletes who stress the elbow in a repetitive fashion (i.e., Little League pitcher)

Epidemiology

- 7% of elbow fractures
- Fractures seen at all ages (median age 9.5 years)
- Equal incidence between sexes

Pathophysiology

- Most common fracture pattern is through the less dense neck and physis.
- Radial head fracture likely to occur in older child.

DIAGNOSIS

Physical Examination and History

Clinical Features

- Isolated injury: outer elbow pain, swelling, and tenderness associated with loss of forearm rotation and elbow flexion and extension
- Associated with other injuries: elbow dislocation, olecranon process and ulnar shaft fractures (Monteggia), medial epicondyle injury, or distal radioulnar joint
- Elbow pain, swelling, and tenderness are more severe.
- Joint mobility severely restricted due to greater involvement of other elbow structures and hemarthrosis.
- Wrist and forearm pain may be present.
- Weak wrist extension with radial deviation occurs if posterior interosseous nerve function is compromised.

TREATMENT

The following treatment plan applies to the majority of fractures, where the articular surface of the radial head is intact and the fracture line is through the neck. The two important factors dictating treatment outcomes are radial head angulation and displacement.

TABLE 12.3-7 COMPARISON OF TWO CLOSED REDUCTION TECHNIQUES FOR RADIAL HEAD AND NECK FRACTURES

Patterson	Kaufman
Sedation or general anesthesia required	Same
Elbow extended	Flex elbow 90 degrees
Rotate forearm to bring head radially (use thumb palpation or fluoroscopy)	Place thumb anteriorly and over radial head, apply steady pressure
Apply distal traction and apply a varus force to increase radiocapitellar space	Pronate forearm fully
Check radiographs for quality of reduction	Same
Apply long arm cast with elbow at 90 degrees and forearm in pronation	Same

- Radial head—angulation ≤30 degrees and displacement ≤3 mm:
  - ☐ Stable fracture pattern
  - ☐ No reduction necessary
  - ☐ Immobilization with long arm splint or cast with elbow flexed at 90 degrees and forearm in neutral rotation
  - ☐ Discontinue immobilization in 2 to 3 weeks
  - ☐ Protected physical therapy in tally
  - ☐ Note: a minimally displaced articular fracture of the radial head usually seen in older child with closed physis is treated in a similar fashion
  - ☐ Fracture reduction required to guarantee acceptable elbow function
- Radial head angulation ≥30 degrees and displacement ≥3 mm
  - ☐ Closed reduction *only*
  - ☐ Patterson or Kaufman manipulation (Table 12.3-7)
  - ☐ Long arm cast with elbow at 90 degrees and forearm pronated
  - ☐ Remove cast at 3 weeks
- Percutaneous pin reduction or intramedullary pin reduction may be indicated if closed methods fail
- Open reduction indicated for a residual angulation ≥40 and displacement ≥3 mm or when there is failure to regain forearm supination 50% and pronation

Complications

- Elbow stiffness: associated with severe trauma or open reduction
- Hypertrophic changes of radial head:
  - ☐ Seen in about 30% of cases
  - ☐ Associated with a clicking sound with forearm rotation
  - ☐ No treatment needed
- Avascular necrosis of radial head:
  - ☐ Seen in about 15% of cases
  - ☐ Associated with surgical reduction
  - ☐ Expect unsatisfactory functional results
- Premature physeal closure:
  - ☐ Can potentially produce cubitus valgus
  - ☐ Elbow function not significantly affected
- Nonunion of radial neck: rare; treat conservatively
- Radioulnar synostosis: associated with severe trauma; open reduction and delay fracture treatment
- Malunion: predisposes the radiocapitellar joint to arthritis
- Nerve injury: posterior interosseous nerve injury is usually iatrogenic
- Myositis ossificans:
  - ☐ Common (30% of cases in one series)
  - ☐ Supinator muscle usually involved

APOPHYSEAL FRACTURES OF THE PROXIMAL ULNA

The proximal ulna's secondary center of ossification appears after 10 years of age and fuses at 14 years of age.

PATHOGENESIS

- Olecranon fracture accounts for 5% of elbow injuries and results from an avulsion force acting across a flexed elbow
- Triceps muscle insertion extends into the metaphysis, offering some protection to the epiphysis and physis

Classification

Classification of apophyseal fractures is given in Table 12.3-8.

DIAGNOSIS

Clinical Features

- Palpable defect can be felt between the apophysis and metaphysis with displaced fractures
- Tenderness and local soft tissue swelling present

TABLE 12.3-8 CLASSIFICATION OF APOPHYSEAL FRACTURES OF THE PROXIMAL ULNA

Type	Name	Description
I	Apophysitis	Abnormal development of the secondary ossification center with or without widening of the apophyseal line incompletely
II	Shen fracture	Occurs along the apophyseal line Usually associated with the overuse of the elbow (i.e., baseball pitcher)
III	Complete fractures	Two types: ■ Pure apophyseal avulsion ■ Apophyseal–metaphyseal fracture (Salter-Harris type II physeal injury)

Radiographic Features

- Obvious in the older child after the appearance of ossification centers
- Elbow arthrogram or MRI useful in the younger child

TREATMENT

- Open reduction and internal fixation with axial pins and figure-of-eight tension—band wiring for displaced fractures
- Rest for most stress fractures and avoidance of the offending elbow motion
- Nonunion requires compression screw fixation with bone graft

Complications

- Apophyseal arrest may occur but is not associated with functional loss

METAPHYSEAL FRACTURES OF THE PROXIMAL ULNA

PATHOGENESIS

Etiology

- Indirect traction forces with the elbow flexed
- Valgus or varus forces with elbow extended
- A direct blow to the olecranon

Epidemiology

- Seen at all ages, with peak incidence at age 5 to 10 years
- 20% associated with other elbow injuries

Classification

- By Chambers:
  - ☐ Group A: flexion injuries
  - ☐ Group B: extension injuries
    - ☐ Valgus pattern
    - ☐ Varus pattern
  - ☐ Group C: shear injuries
- By Papavasilouetted:
  - ☐ Group A: extraarticular
  - ☐ Group B: intraarticular

DIAGNOSIS

Clinical Features

- Local swelling over the olecranon
- Skin abrasions
- Palpable defect
- Weakness in elbow extension

Radiographic Features

- Get routine radiographs of entire elbow
- Look for perpendicular fracture lines
- Residual physeal line is oblique and runs proximal and anterior
- Look for associated injuries involving medial epicondyle, radial head and neck, and lateral condyle

TREATMENT

- Extension type, minimally displaced:
  - ☐ Long arm cast or splint immobilization for 3 weeks
  - ☐ Elbow may be flexed at 80 degrees or 10 degrees
  - ☐ Supervised rehabilitation
- Extension type, displaced more than 2 mm: open reduction
- Shear type:
  - ☐ Closed reduction if angulated more than 10 degrees with immobilization in a long arm cast for 3 weeks

- Screw or pin fixation for unstable fractures
- Long arm cast or splint with elbow flexed to 90 degrees for nondisplaced or minimally displaced fracture

Complications

- Uncommon
- Loss of elbow function associated with failure to correct alignment or loss of reduction
- Other uncommon complications include elongation of olecranon process, ulnar nerve transient neuropraxia, compartment syndrome, delayed unions, and nonunions

SUGGESTED READING

Abraham E, Powers T, Wit P, et al. Experimental hyperextension supracondylar fractures in monkeys. Clin Orthop 1982;171:309–318.

Beady JH, Kasser JA. Rockwood and Wilkins' fractures in children, 5th ed. Philadelphia: Lippincott Williams & Wilkins, 2001: 483–739.

Brodeur AE, Silberstein MJ, Graviss ER. Radiology of the pediatric elbow. MA: GK Hall Medical Publishers, 1981.

Delee J, Wilkins K, Rogers L, et al. Fracture separation of the distal numeral epiphysis. J Bone Joint Surg (Am) 1980;62:46–51.

Haraldsson S. On osteochondrosis deformans juvenilis capituli humeri including investigation of intra-osseous vasculature in distal humerus. Acta Orthop Scand [Suppl] 1959;38:81–93.

Jakob R, Fowels, JV, Rang M, et al. Observations concerning fractures of the lateral humeral condyle in children. J Bone Joint Surg Br 1975;57:430–436.

Lincoln TL, Mubarak SH. "Isolated traumatic radial-head dislocation." J Pediatr Orthop 1994;14:455.

Perry CR, Elstrom JA. Handbook of fractures, 2nd ed. New York: McGraw-Hill, 2000:98–130.

Silberstein MJ, Brodeur AE Craviss ER. Some vagaries of the lateral epicondyle. J Bone Joint Surg (Am) 1982;64:444–448.

Steele JA, Graham HK. Angulated radial neck fractures in children: a prospective study of percutaneous reduction. J Bone Joint Surg (Br) 1992;74:760–764.

12.4 FOREARM

TWEE DO

Radius and ulna fractures account for nearly half of all skeletal injuries in the pediatric population. The mechanism is usually an axial load, such as a FOOSH (fall onto an outstretched hand), with varying degrees of rotation. Depending on the amount of force at the time of impact, the fracture can occur at any location within the forearm. The distal one-third radius is usually the most common site of injury. Although most metaphyseal forearm fractures can be conservatively treated without sequelae in skeletally immature patients due to remodeling, some fractures at the midshaft and proximal one-third forearm may need operative intervention to avoid the occasional poor results. A thorough understanding of forearm fractures and an awareness of the potential pitfalls that may occur in some of these can ward off potential complications and assure a more clinically satisfactory result at the completion of fracture healing.

PATHOGENESIS

Etiology

Forearm fractures usually occur as a part of normal child's play. Tripping while running or a resisted fall during sports are probably the more common causes of fracture, followed closely by a fall from short heights, such as the monkey bars or trees. Higher energy trauma, such as from auto–pedestrian or motor vehicle accidents result in more dissipation of energy and more comminution, as well as fractures that are located more at the distal metaphysis or epiphysis.

Epidemiology

- Forearm fractures tend to occur during seasons of active play, such as spring and summer, or with changes in the temperature.
- Boys are affected more often than girls, in a 2.9:1 ratio.
- Both sexes tend to fracture the nondominant arm most frequently, as it is the free arm available to break a fall.
- The average age for forearm fractures tends to be 10.5 years for girls and 12.8 years for boys, although boys can tend to follow a bimodal peak.
- The first peak occurs around 9 years, with the second peak happening around 13 to 14 years. The distal third of the forearm is the most common location for fractures overall, as well as the most common site in the older child.
- The midshaft region is more commonly fractured in younger children. This is a reflection of their inherent anatomy, which includes more cancellous bone extending beyond the metaphysis into the diaphysis.
- Distal metaphyseal and epiphyseal fractures occur in the older child (most commonly in boys between 13 and 15 years, and girls between 12 and 13 years). This difference reflects the difference in the average age of skeletal maturation between the two genders. Near skeletal maturity, the amount of cortical bone at the dia-

physis increases and the metaphyseal area decreases, making the distal radius the weaker portion of forearm bone.

Anatomy and Pathophysiology

The radius is a gently bowed bone with a semilunar proximal end that articulates with a relatively straight ulna during forearm rotation. Muscles that attach to the forearm and act as potential deforming forces in fractures include, proximally, the biceps and supinator and, more distally, the pronators teres and quadratus.

Fracture at the level of the supinator leads to a supinated proximal fragment and the position of reduction should place the distal fragment into supination. Fracture at the midshaft should be reduced and stabilized in neutral. Fractures of the distal third of the radius need to be stabilized in neutral to slight pronation due to the activity of the pronators on the proximal fragment (Fig. 12.4-1)

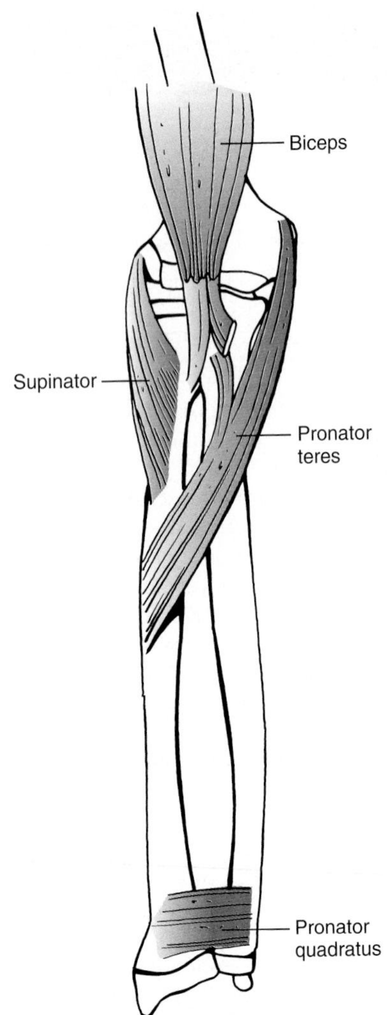

Figure 12.4-1 Musculature of the forearm.

Classification

Classification of forearm fractures includes the location of the fractures and the type of fractures (Boxes 12.4-1 and 12.4-2).

DIAGNOSIS

History, Physical Examination, and Diagnostic Workup

A history of a fall onto an outstretched hand with pain and ecchymosis at the forearm is fairly diagnostic. Gross displacement and angulation will enhance the deformity further and make the fracture more obvious on clinical examination. Swelling, crepitus, and gross motion can usually be elicited at the site of the fracture, which is associated with pain. Check for any lacerations or areas of fatty blood to rule out an open fracture (which may necessitate an operative irrigation and débridement).

- Examination of the wrist, elbow, and shoulder on the ipsilateral side should also be performed to rule out other associated fractures or dislocations [e.g., the radial head in Monteggia fractures, or distal radioulnar joint (DRUJ) disruption in Galeazzi fractures]. Supracondylar humeral fractures can occur in up to 5% of forearm fractures. Although rare, the most common ipsilateral carpal injury is the scaphoid fracture.

BOX 12.4-1 CLASSIFICATION OF FOREARM FRACTURES BY LOCATION

Distal Third
- Radius only
- Both bones
- Galeazzi fracture (distal radius fracture with disruption of the distal radioulnar joint)

Midshaft
- Radius only
- Both bones
- Night stick (midshaft transverse ulna fracture)
- Plastic deformation (failure of elastic limit leading to bowing)

Proximal Third
- Radius only
- Both bones
- Monteggia fracture (proximal ulna with radial head dislocation)

Classification for Monteggia Fractures

I Anterior radial head dislocation with apex anterior ulna fracture (Fig. 12.4-2)

II Posterior radial head dislocation with apex posterior ulna fracture

III Lateral radial head dislocation with apex lateral ulna fracture

IV Anterior radial head dislocation with fracture of both radius and ulna

Monteggia variant: dislocation of the radial head with plastic deformation of the ulna or radius

BOX 12.4-2 CLASSIFICATION OF FOREARM FRACTURES BY TYPE

Closed or Open Fracture
- Maintenance or loss of skin integrity over the fracture

Torus, or Buckle, Fracture (Fig. 12.4-3)
- Failure of one cortex in compression with preservation of other cortex, which leads to "buckling" of bone

Greenstick (Fig. 12.4-4)
- Failure of one cortex in compression and the other in bending/rotation
- Unstable fracture and may continue to angulate

Complete (Fig. 12.4-5)
- Cortical disruption through all cortices

Comminuted
- High-energy injury with multiple fragments and usually displaced or unstable

- The fingers should be checked for color and capillary refill.
- The hand should be checked for warmth of the distal limb and the presence of a good radial pulse.
- Neurovascular exam should include motor and sensory testing in the radial, ulnar, and median nerves (RUM) distribution (i.e., radial [motor—thumbs up/sensation—first web space dorsally], ulnar (motor—spread fingers against resistance/sensation—little finger), and median distributions [motor—cross index and middle finger/sensation—tips of index and middle finger]), including the anterior interosseous branch of the median nerves (primarily a motor branch to the Hexor indicisproprius (FIP), Hexor pollicis longus (FPL), and pronator quadratus/okay sign).
- Radiographs should include orthogonal visews of the entire forearm to include the wrist and elbow in order to determine rotational alignment and to rule out involvement of the joints above and below the fracture.

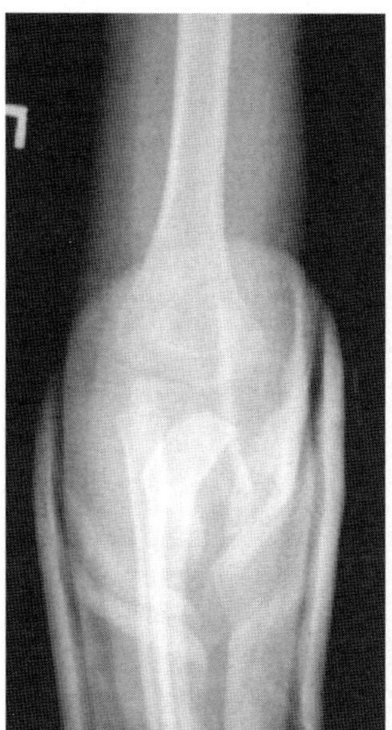
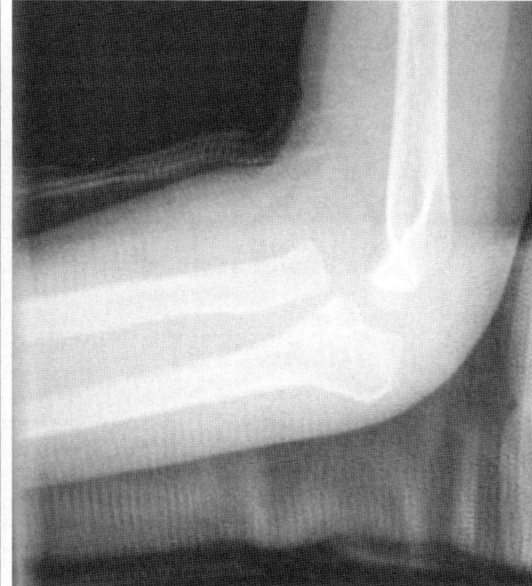

Figure 12.4-2 Anterior radial head dislocation with apex anterior ulna fracture.

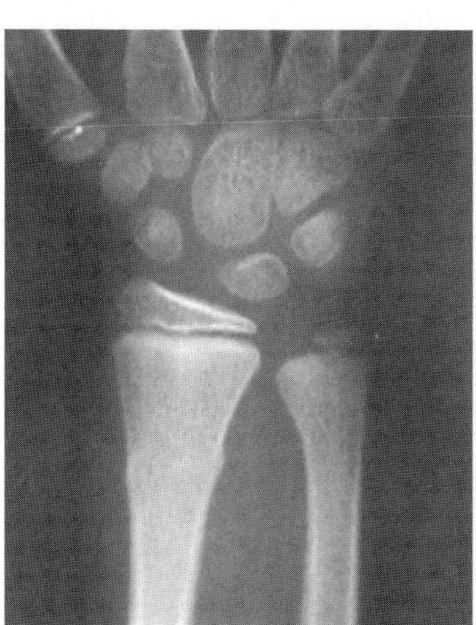
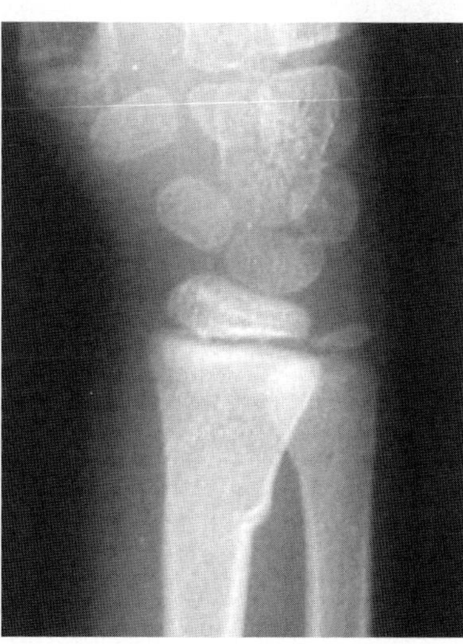

Figure 12.4-3 Torus, or buckle, fracture.

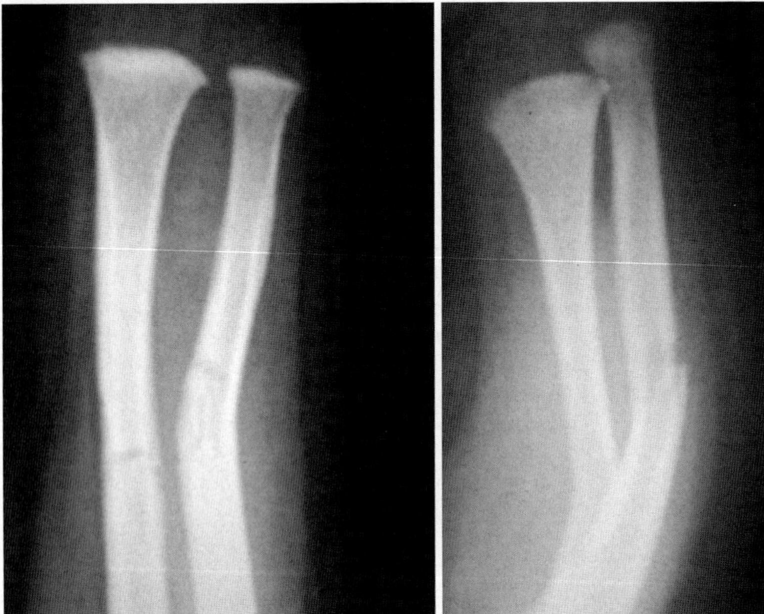

Figure 12.4-4 Greenstick fracture.

Rotational alignment is gauged by evaluation of the cortical thickness and contour of the fractured ends. This can sometimes be difficult in comminuted fractures. Other means of checking for fracture alignment include evaluation of the radial tuberosity relationship to the radial styloid in the coronal plane. They are usually 180 degrees apart. Other anatomic landmarks include the coronoid process and styloid on the ulna, which are not visible on the anteroposterior radiograph, but could be seen on the lateral x-ray. In this view, the coronoid process faces anteriorly and the styloid points posteriorly. The fracture is reduced by appropriately rotating the distal fragment to reestablish these normal anatomic landmarks.

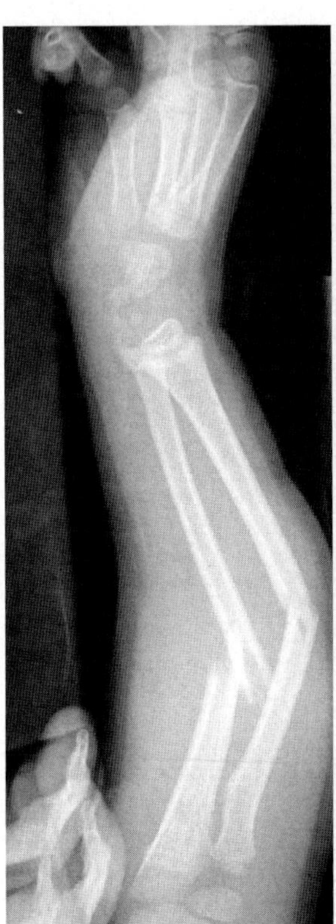

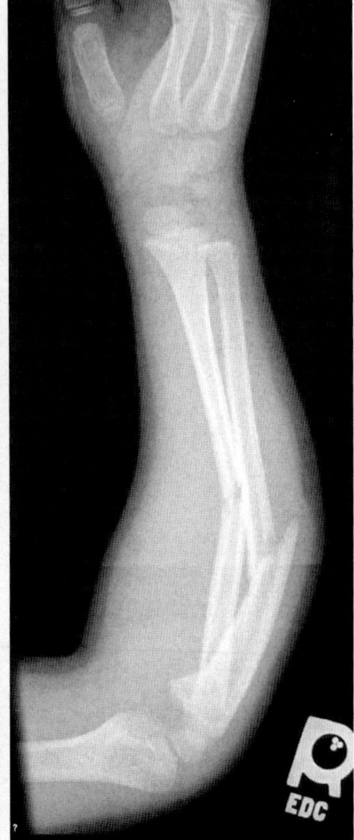

Figure 12.4-5 Complete fracture.

TREATMENT

Because of the unique potential of remodeling that can occur in skeletally immature individuals, most fractures tend to heal without sequelae. The goals of treatment are to initially obtain an acceptable alignment and maintain this alignment until the completion of healing.

Reduction

- Initial immobilization with a sugar tong splint (U-shaped splint around the wrist and elbow) in the emergency room (or cast if minimally swollen) is sufficient for buckle or minimally angulated greenstick fractures of the distal metaphysis.
- In badly angulated greenstick fractures, complete and displaced fractures or comminuted fractures, a provisional reduction is attempted under fentanyl/midazolem, or nitrous oxide conscious sedation in the emergency department, followed by application of a sugar tong splint.
- The reduction is achieved by first obtaining gentle traction through the fingers (manually or in finger traps), followed by exaggeration of the deforming force under traction to clear any intervening periosteum and reestablish length.
- The arm is then forcefully manipulated to achieve reduction.

- A three-point mold is placed into the splint with a good anteroposterior interosseous squeeze. Postreduction radiographs are always obtained to check the position of the reduction and to document the institution of treatment.

Occasionally, it is necessary to complete a greenstick fracture in order to obtain the reduction. Another benefit of completing a greenstick fracture is to avoid the stress of refracture.

In metaphyseal fractures of the forearm of children under 10 years of age, angulations up to 20 degrees, rotation up to 45 degrees, and shortening up to 1 cm will heal without clinical or functional sequelae (Table 12.4-1). This is because of the significant amount of longitudinal growth of the distal forearm, which varies between 75% to 81%. This allows overgrowth to occur at a rate of almost 6 mm on average in length and 0.8 degrees of angulation per month of remaining growth. Beyond these limits, and in more mature individuals, the amount of correction is limited and malalignment may not completely remodel. This may eventually lead to limitations of motion. Thus, in children over age 10 or those with less than 2 years of growth remaining, the acceptable range of angulation is less than 10 degrees and that of malrotation is less than 30 degrees.

Proximal fractures of the forearm tend to be more unstable, partially because of deforming muscular forces, and partially because of the muscle bulk that limits direct molding of the fracture fragments. Fractures associated with dislocations of the radial head need complete reduction and immobilization in supination. Closer monitoring of these fractures is necessary since less angulation, less rotation, and no joint dislocation can be accepted without clinical sequelae. As in the older child with more distal fractures, the limits of acceptability of proximal forearm fractures include 10 degrees of angulation, 30 degrees of rotation, and complete joint reduction.

Plastic deformation deformities do not demonstrate obvious fracturing, but there is an increase in the natural bow of the forearm. These "fractures" need to be manipulated in the operating room under pressure to restore the natural alignment as plastic deformation will not remodel over time.

Results and Outcome

Most fractures of the forearm in children heal well. This is due to their thicker periosteum, which may help contain fractures and limit their displacement as well as enhance the speed of healing and remodeling. The remodeling potential of the younger child allows acceptance of a greater degree of displacement, but not all perfectly aligned fractures will result in normal functioning limbs. Although Fuller and colleagues demonstrated a direct correlation with malrotation and the resulting range of motion, others have noted minor to moderate losses of rotation even in perfectly aligned limbs. In these cases, it is hypothesized that contractures of the soft tissue or interosseous membranes occurred, either from the injury or the subsequent immobilization (especially in pronation where the fibers are tightened).

As a general rule, it is advisable to obtain as near anatomic alignment as possible, with acceptance of only what has been previously outlined as these are well supported by the literature. As soon as fractures are radiographically healed, gentle range of motion should be initiated. Refracture at the site of previous injury may occur

TABLE 12.4-1 CLINICAL AND RADIOGRAPHIC CRITERIA FOR TREATMENT OF PEDIATRIC FOREARM FRACTURES

	Acceptable Range Age <10 (Age >10)					
Location/Type	**Angulation**	**Rotation**	**Position of Shortening**	**Immobilization**	**Time in a Cast**	**Potential Problems**
Distal						
Buckle	20 (15)	45 (30)	1 cm	Neutral	3–4 wk	
Greenstick	30 (15)	45 (30)	1 cm		4–6 wk	Angulation
Complete	30 (15)	45 (30)	1 cm		6–8 wk	Angulation
Galeazzi	30 (15)			Supination	6 wk	Ulnar prominence
Midshaft						
Supinator	15 (10)	45 (30)	1 cm	Supination	6–8 wk	Refracture
Between supinator and pronator	15 (10)	45 (30)	1 cm	Neutral	6–8 wk	Refracture
Distal pronator	15 (10)	45 (30)	1 cm	Slight pronation	6–8 wk	Refracture
Proximal						
Shaft	15 (0)	45 (30)	1 cm	(0) Neutral to slight supination	6 wk	
Monteggia	0 (0)	10 (0)	0	(0) Supination	6 wk	Posterior interosseus nerve injury stiffness

TABLE 12.4-2 OPERATIVE OPTIONS FOR THE TREATMENT OF FOREARM FRACTURES

Option	Advantages	Disadvantages
Pins and plaster	Maintains traction	Pin tract infection Loosening as swelling decreases
Closed reduction with Nancy nail	Minimizes scarring Minimizes soft tissue violation	Need for hardware removal Prominent insertion site
Closed reduction with PCP	Minimizes scarring Minimizes soft tissue violation	Infection Difficult to place (useful only in distal ⅓) Hardware removal
Open reduction and internal fixation	Stable fixation Early ROM No cast	Synostosis Nerve injury (PIN) Hardware removal Refracture Scar

PCP, percutanesus pinning; PIN, posterior interosseous nerve; ROM, range of motion.

in up to 30% of patients within the first 6 months of healing. This is most likely due to weakened bone structure from incomplete corticalization of a diaphyseal fracture. Patients and parents need to be forewarned at the time of cast removal that this potential complication may occur and early protective mobilization, such as a forearm splint, may be beneficial.

Surgical Indications

- Open fractures
- Neurovascularly compromised fractures
- Compartment syndrome of the forearm
- Displaced fractures in patients nearing skeletal maturity
- Floating elbow (ipsilateral supracondylar elbow fracture)
- Unstable fracture losing alignment on follow-up

Operative options are given in Table 12.4-2.

Postoperative Management

- Follow-up closely.
- Pins are removed when the bone appears healed on radiographs.
- After surgery, the arm is usually in a long cast for 4 to 6 weeks, followed by initiation of range-of-motion, depending on the type of fracture.

SUGGESTED READING

Blount W. Forearm fracture in children. Clin Orthop Rel Res 1967; 51:93–107.

Creasman C, Zaleske D, Erhlich M. Analyzing forearm fractures in children. The more subtle signs of impending problems. CORR 1984;188:40–53.

Davis D, Green D. Forearm fractures in children: pitfalls and complications. Clin Orthop Rel Res 1976;120: 172–184.

Do T, Strub W, Foad S, Mehlman C, Crawford A. Reduction vs. remodeling in pediatric distal forearm fractures: a preliminary cost analysis. J Pediatr Orthop B 2003;12(2):109–15.

Friberg KS. Remodeling after distal forearm fractures in children. The effects of residual angulation on spatial orientation of the epiphyseal plates. Acta Orthop Scand 1979;50:527–546.

Fuller D, McCullough C. Md united fractures of the forearm in children. JBJS (Br) 1982:64(3):364–7.

Hogshom H, Nilsson B, Willner S. Correction with growth following diaphyseal forearm fractures. Acta Orthop Scand 1976;47: 299–303.

Jones K, Weiner D. The management of forearm fractures in children: a plea for conservatism. J Pediatr Orthop 1999;19:811–815.

Keenan W, Clegg J. Intraoperative wedging of casts: correction of residual angulation after manipulation. J Pediatr Orthop 1995;15: 826–829.

Noonan K, Price C. Forearm and distal radius fracture in children. JAAOS 1998;6:146–156.

Younger A, Tredwell S, Mackenzie W. Factors affecting fracture position at cast removal after pediatric forearm fracture. J Pediatr Orthop 1997;17:332–336.

Younger A, Tredwell S, Mackenzie W, et al. Accurate prediction of outcome after pediatric forearm fracture. J Pediatr Orthop 1994;14: 200–206.

12.5 HAND

LAWRENCE L. HABER

Fractures involving the hand are common injuries in children. They account for 25% of all pediatric fractures, and many go unrecognized. Hand fractures have a bimodal distribution. The major peak occurs in adolescents due to sports injuries. There is a smaller peak in toddlers due to crush injuries of the distal phalanx. Anytime a child or adolescent "jams" a finger; this usually results in a fracture. This is evident by swelling, ecchymoses, and tenderness over the bone that lasts for 2 to 3 weeks. Fortunately, most of these fractures have a benign course and heal uneventfully. Most will be nondisplaced fractures. However, there are specific fractures that without proper treatment can lead to certain morbidity. This chapter discusses how to treat simple fractures, as well as how to identify more serious injuries and understand their treatments.

CARPAL FRACTURES

PATHOPHYSIOLOGY

- Carpal fractures occur in children less commonly than in adults and may be difficult to diagnose due to a lack of ossification.
- Many of these fractures result from axial loading with the wrist dorsiflexed or from direct impact.
- The scaphoid is the most commonly fractured carpal bone, with a peak incidence around 15 years of age.
- A direct impact mechanism usually causes a distal pole fracture.
  - More common in younger children
  - Rarely displaced; usually heal without complications
- In adolescents, hyperdorsiflexion injuries cause the more adultlike waist fracture, carrying an increased risk for nonunion and avascular necrosis.

DIAGNOSIS

- Scaphoid fractures are frequently occult injuries with normal initial radiographs.
- Radiographs should include anteroposterior, lateral, scaphoid, and pronated oblique views.
- Mid-body or "waist" fractures can usually be seen on all views.
- Pronated oblique radiograph is valuable for distal fractures.
- When an occult fracture is suspected, magnetic resonance imaging or computed tomography may be useful.

TREATMENT

- Tenderness over the scaphoid and normal radiographs indicate treatment with a short arm–thumb spica cast.
  - At 3 weeks, anteroposterior, lateral, and scaphoid views of the wrist are repeated.
  - In children with normal clinical and radiographic exams, casting is discontinued.
- If a fracture exists, the child will still be tender and radiographs may be positive.
  - These children are treated for 3 more weeks in a cast.
- Nondisplaced fractures, obvious on radiographs, are treated in a short arm–thumb spica cast for 6 weeks and then reassessed.
- Displaced fractures are treated operatively, as they are in adults.
- Any child with a scaphoid fracture should have a final radiographic exam 3 to 6 months after the injury is healed to avoid undetected late displacement.

OTHER CARPAL FRACTURES

- Other carpal fractures occur, but are rare and are usually a result of direct impact.
- The most common is the hook of the hamate fracture, which is treated with immobilization in a short arm cast.
- Rare painful nonunions may be treated with excision.

LIGAMENTOUS INJURIES

- Ligamentous carpal injuries are unusual in young children and occur rarely in adolescents via a dorsiflexion loading mechanism.
- The most common injury is a scapholunate ligament sprain, diagnosed by tenderness in this region.
- Without displacement, these patients are treated in a short arm–thumb spica cast for 4 to 6 weeks.
- Injuries with carpal displacement or instability are rare and should be treated as in adults.

METACARPAL FRACTURES

- Metacarpal fractures are common in children and most occur through the metacarpal neck proximal to the physis. Fractures through the shaft and base also occur.

Metacarpals II Through IV

- Fractures at the metaphyseal base of the second through fourth metacarpals occur as the result of a direct blow or axial load. Due to the ligament stability of the carpometacarpal (CMC) joint, significant displacement is rare.

- These fractures can be treated in a gutter splint or short arm cast for 3 to 4 weeks.
- If displaced, closed reduction with longitudinal traction and downward pressure is performed.
- Many of these will be unstable and require pin fixation across the base of the adjacent metacarpals or down the shaft of the involved metacarpal.
- Open reduction is rarely needed.

Metacarpal I

- Classified as A through D (Fig. 12.5-1).
  - Type A fractures are usually treated with closed reduction and immobilization in a thumb spica cast or splint.
  - Type B and C fractures are Salter-Harris type II fractures and are treated with closed reduction and immobilization. Unstable reductions may require pin fixation.
  - Open reduction is sometimes needed, especially in type C fractures, as the medial fragment may buttonhole the periosteum.
  - Type D fractures are more of an adult injury and when displaced require open reduction and internal fixation.

Metacarpal Shaft Fractures

- Occur mostly in older children.
- A twist, bend, or crush can result in an oblique or spiral fracture pattern.
- Careful clinical examination of alignment is important; special attention should be paid to rotational malalignment.
- In the absence of rotational malalignment, most of these can be handled by closed reduction and splinting with pressure on the apex and a three-point mold.
- If the reduction is unstable, pinning will hold the reduction.

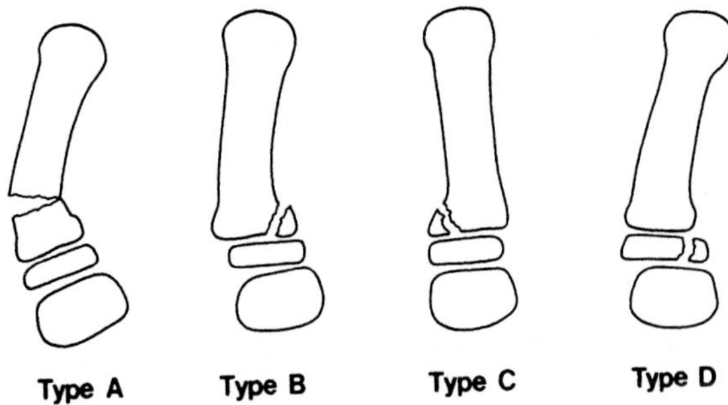

Figure 12.5-1 Classification of thumb metacarpal fractures. Type A is a metaphyseal fracture. Types B and C are Salter-Harris type II physeal fractures with lateral (type B) or medial (type C) angulation. Type D is a Salter-Harris type II fracture (pediatric Bennett fracture). (Adapted from Graham TJ, Waters PM. Fractures and dislocations of the hand and carpus in children. In: Beaty JH, Kasser JR, eds. Rockwood and Wilkins' fractures in children, 5th ed. Philadelphia: Lippincott Williams & Wilkins, 2001:269–379.)

- Any significant angulation will leave a bump on the back of the hand, but is of little functional significance.
- After adequate reduction, most metacarpal shaft fractures require 3 to 4 weeks of immobilization followed by only motion.

Metacarpal Neck Fractures

- Common in children and usually result from a direct blow or punch.
- Frequently volarly angulated.
- Closed reduction with flexion of the metacarpophalangeal (MCP) and proximal interphalangeal (PIP) joints to 90 degrees is usually successful.
- A gutter splint with 60 to 90 degrees of MCP joint flexion and the PIP joint in extension is applied.
- Angulation of less than 40 degrees is well tolerated in the fourth and fifth digits
  - No more than 20 degrees of angulation should be accepted in the second or third digits.
- Occasionally an unstable fracture will require pin fixation.
- Intraarticular head fractures are rare but require open reduction and pin fixation when displaced.
- Some remodeling will occur in younger children with open physes.

PHALANGEAL METAPHYSEAL FRACTURES

- Common in children, can involve any area.
- Salter-Harris I and II fractures and metaphyseal fractures at the bases of the proximal and middle phalanges are common.
- Fractures of the proximal phalanx are most common and result from axial loading, hyperextension, or a twisting mechanism.
- Nondisplaced fractures are splinted in a position of comfort for 2 to 3 weeks.
- Fractures with more than 10 degrees of angulation in the coronal plane usually appear deviated clinically and reduction is recommended.
- Angulation of up to 25 degrees in the plane of motion in a digit with open physes is well tolerated and will usually remodel.
- Digital block with longitudinal traction and a reversal of the mechanism will reduce displaced fractures.
- Coronal malalignment may require a fulcrum or bolster in the web space of the finger and is incorporated into the splint for 2 to 3 weeks.
- In the event of an unstable fracture, pinning with smooth Kirschner wires (K-wires) will achieve stability.
- Need for open reduction is rare.

PHALANGEAL SHAFT FRACTURES

- Can occur from bending, hyperextension, rotation, or crush injuries.

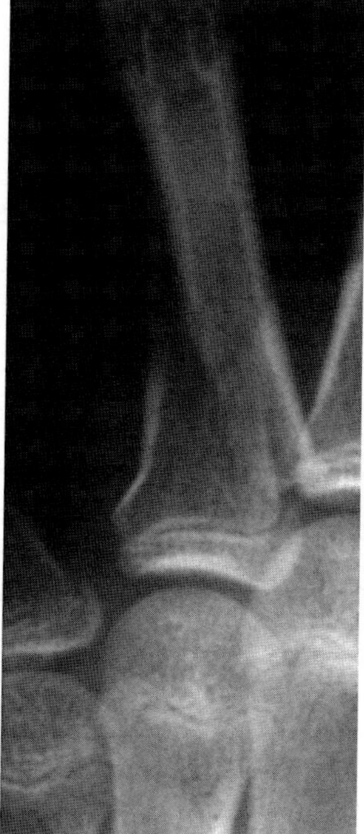

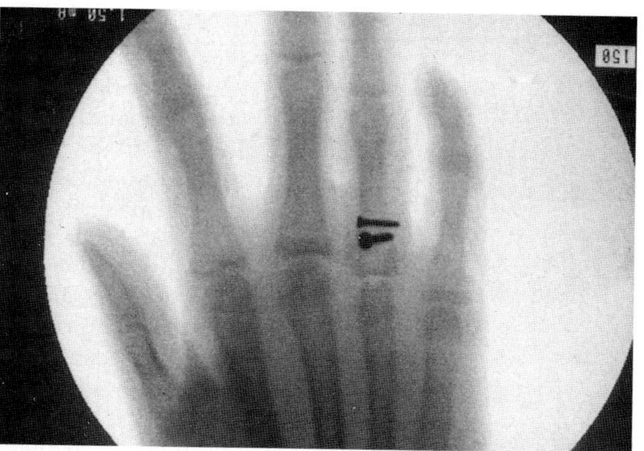

Figure 12.5-2 (A) Irreducible proximal phalangeal shaft fracture. (B) After open reduction and internal fixation through a dorsal approach.

- Fractures with more than 10 degrees of coronal deformity, 20 degrees of sagittal deformity, or any significant rotational deformity should be reduced.
  - ☐ Remember to check for rotational deformity. Clinically, it will not be visible on x-ray.
- Flexion at the PIP joint is sometimes needed for proximal phalanx fractures and extension is usually used for middle phalanx fractures.
  - ☐ The fracture force is reversed. If the reduction is unstable, percutaneous pinning is required.
- If closed reduction is not possible, open reduction is performed.
- This occurs in spiral fractures with rotational displacement and oblique fractures with shortening.
  - ☐ The dorsal approach is preferred, though some use a midlateral approach.
  - ☐ Fixation can be with smooth pins; however, mini-fragment screws afford earlier mobilization and improved stability in older children (Fig. 12.5-2).
  - ☐ Fractures undergoing reduction should be splinted for 3 weeks.
  - ☐ As soon as callus is seen, the pins are removed and motion is begun.

SALTER-HARRIS TYPE III FRACTURES

- Occur at the proximal, middle, and distal phalanx.
- In the proximal phalanx, they are the result of a bending motion.
  - ☐ The collateral ligament is avulsed with a fragment of bone.
  - ☐ This results in a Salter-Harris III or IV fracture.
  - ☐ May involve a significant part of the articular surface.
  - ☐ If the fracture is nondisplaced, treatment is conservative with splinting for 3 to 4 weeks.
  - ☐ If more than 25% of the joint is involved and there is more than 2.0 mm of displacement, open reduction is recommended.
  - ☐ Any widely displaced fracture should be reduced.
  - ☐ Fixation is with smooth pins in younger children.
  - ☐ In older children, mini-fragment screws may be used.
- Fractures in the middle and distal phalanges are usually a result of an avulsion of the central slip of the extensor at the base of the middle phalanx and the terminal extensor over the distal phalanx.
  - ☐ Rarely these avulsions will present as a Salter-Harris I or II fracture.
- There are four mallet finger equivalent fractures (Fig. 12.5-3).
  - ☐ These occur from forced flexion, usually during a ball sport.
  - ☐ A terminal extensor avulsion leads to a mallet finger.
  - ☐ Closed reduction is attempted with longitudinal traction and pressure over the displaced fragment.
    - ☐ If successful the finger can be splinted in extension for 3 weeks.
    - ☐ If significant displacement persists, greater than 2 mm, open reduction should be performed.
- Displaced fragments of greater than 25% of the joint surface area may lead to instability in addition to incongruity.
- In the distal phalanx, the fracture is approached dorsally.

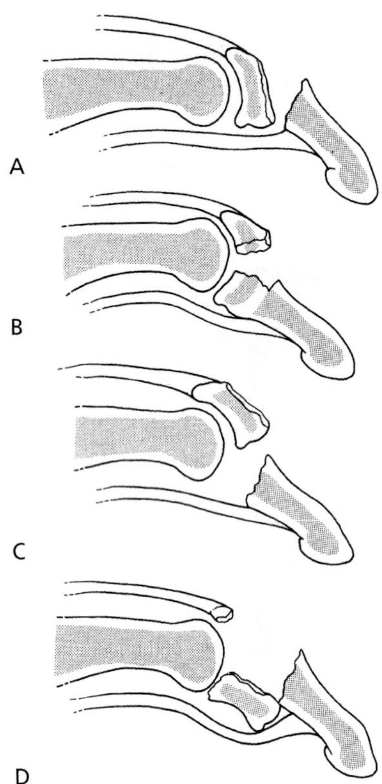

Figure 12.5-3 Mallet equivalent fractures. (Adapted from Graham TJ, Waters PM. Fractures and dislocations of the hand and carpus in children. In: Beaty JH, Kasser JR, eds. Rockwood and Wilkins' fractures in children, 5th ed. Philadelphia: Lippincott Williams & Wilkins, 2001:269–379.)

- If small, the fragment is excised and the tendon is reattached.
- When significant, it is repaired with pins or a mini-fragment screw.

- A flexor digitorum profundus (FDP) avulsion may cause a volar Salter-Harris type III, IV, or simple avulsion fracture.
  - These are rare in comparison to the dorsal injuries.
  - This is known as a reverse mallet or a jersey finger.
  - It is analogous to the adult type 2 or 3 FDP avulsion.
  - Repair is with open reduction and a pullout suture or other fixation.
  - Treated with open reduction when displaced.
- Fractures through the phalangeal necks of the proximal and middle phalanx are particularly bad actors.
  - When nondisplaced, treatment consists of splinting and careful follow-up.
    - These heal slowly and may require 4 weeks of immobilization.
  - When displaced, they are highly unstable.
    - Their juxtaposition to the joint and tendency to malrotate cause severe deformity (Fig. 12.5-4).
    - Closed reduction and cross-pinning can be attempted in minimally displaced fractures, but most will require open reduction and pinning.
    - It is almost impossible to judge rotation without a direct reduction.
    - A dorsal approach used, incising between the central slip and lateral band. Cross-pinning of the fragment with 0.45 K-wires (Fig.12.5-5).

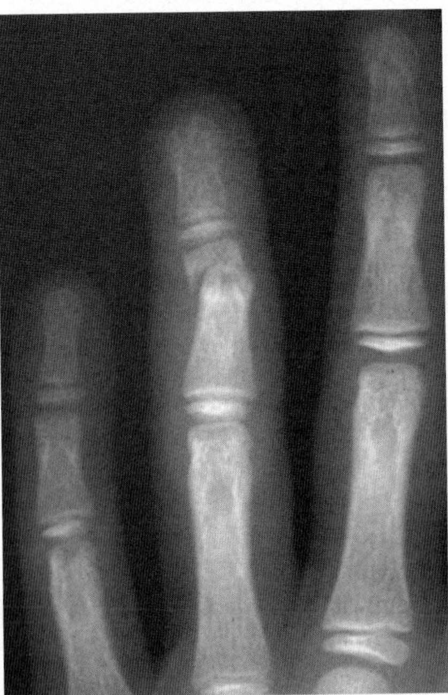

Figure 12.5-4 Angulated middle phalanx condylar neck fracture.

- A transverse incision within the distal creases with a proximal and distal limb is useful.
- Avoiding the germinal matrix of the nailbed is important.
- This incision leaves a minimal scar.
- The extensor apparatus will be retracted with the avulsed fragment.
- The fracture is reduced and fixed with K-wires or a pull out suture.
- The distal interphalangeal (DIP) joint is splinted in extension for 3 weeks.
- A smooth pin across the joint can be used to protect the repair.
- At 3 to 4 weeks, the splint is removed to begin motion, but should be left on for all other activities for 6 weeks.
- Prolonged splinting, without motion, will lead to a stiff DIP joint.

- Left displaced and untreated, a central slip avulsion may lead to a boutonniere deformity or incongruity of the joint surface.
  - Open reduction of middle phalanx fractures consists of a dorsal approach, incising between the central slip and lateral band.

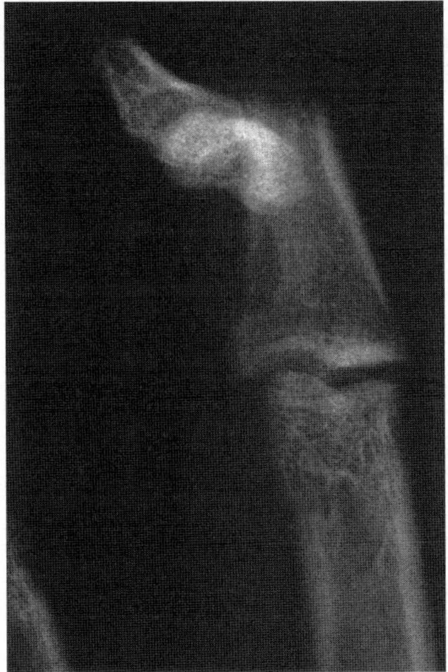

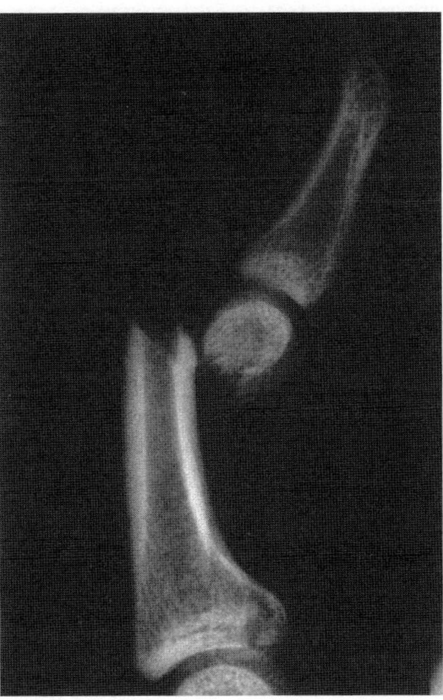

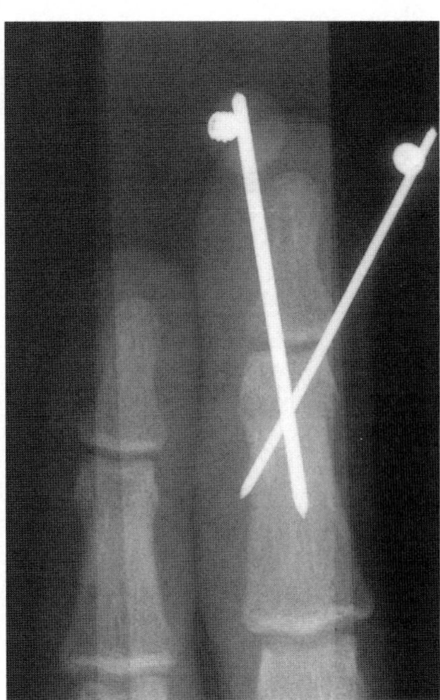

A,B C

Figure 12.5-5 Anteroposterior (**A**) and lateral (**B**) views of a displaced condylar neck fracture. (**C**) After open reduction and pin fixation through a dorsal approach.

  - ☐ The finger is immobilized for 4 weeks, at which time the pins are removed and motion begun.
  - ☐ Stiffness is common, necessitating early occupational therapy.
- ☐ Intraarticular fractures of the distal end of the proximal and middle phalanges are uncommon.
  - ☐ Except in minimally displaced fractures, open reduction and fixation is required.
  - ☐ Treatment is similar to condylar neck fractures.
  - ☐ Fixation is best with mini-fragment screws, which allows for early motion.
- ☐ Tuft fractures of the distal phalanx represent more of a soft tissue injury involving the distal pulp of the finger and the nailbed.
  - ☐ These are usually from a crush mechanism.
  - ☐ When the nail is avulsed from the fold, the nailbed must be explored and repaired.
  - ☐ The nail is then sewn back into the fold.
  - ☐ Some controversy exists about exploring a nailbed due to the presence of hematoma alone.
  - ☐ The most recent literature suggests these fingers can be treated with trephination of the hematoma by placing a hole in the nail.
  - ☐ Outcomes were equal to children undergoing exploration and repair.
- ☐ The nail is then sewn back into the eponychial fold. Splinting is of the middle and distal phalanges only and is discontinued when pain is gone, usually at 2 weeks.

SUGGESTED READING

Al-Quattan M. Phalangeal neck fractures in children: classification and outcome in 66 cases. J Hand Surg (Br) 1999;26112–121.

Beatty E, Light TR, Belsole RJ, et al. Wrist and hand skeletal injuries in children. Hand Clin 1990;6:723–738.

Compson JP. Transcarpal injuries associated with distal radial fractures in children: a series of three cases. J Hand Surg (Br) 1992; 17:311–314.

Coonrad RW, Pohlman MH. Impacted fractures of the proximal phalanx of the finger. J Bone Joint Surg (Am) 1969;51:129–1296.

D'Arienso M. Scaphoid fractures in children. J Hand Surg (Br) 2002; 27:424–426.

Greene WB, Anderson WJ. Simultaneous fracture of the scaphoid and radius in a child. J Pediatr Orthop 1982;2:191–194.

Hastings H II, Simmons BP. Hand fractures in children. Clin Orthop 1984;188:120–130.

Jahss SA. Fractures of the metacarpals: a new method of reduction and immobilization. J Bone Joint Surg 1938;20:178–186.

Leclerc C, Korn W. Articular fractures of the fingers in children. Hand Clin 2000;16:523–534.

Linscheid RL, Dobyns JH, Beabout W, et al. Traumatic instability of the wrist: diagnosis, classification, and pathomechanics. J Bone Joint Surg (Am) 1972;54:1612–1632.

Meek S, White M. Subungual hematomas: is simple trephining enough? Accident Emerg Med 1998;15:269–271.

Nafie SAA. Fractures of the carpal bones in children. Injury 1987;18: 117–119.

Simmons BP, Lovallo JL. Hand and wrist injuries in children. Clin Sports Med 1988;7:495–511.

Wood VE. Fractures of the hand in children. Orthop Clin North Am 1976;7: 527–542.

Worlock PH, Stower MJ. The incidence and pattern of hand fractures in children. J Hand Surg (Br) 1986;11:198–200.

12.6 PELVIS

MARTIN J. HERMAN

Pediatric pelvic fractures are rare, accounting for only 1% to 2% of all fractures in children. In most cases, these fractures are the result of high-energy trauma. Identification of a fracture of the pelvis in a pediatric trauma patient mandates a thorough search for concomitant, potentially more life-threatening injuries of the brain, abdominal viscera, and genitourinary system. As opposed to the adult trauma patient with a pelvic fracture, fatalities rarely occur in children with pelvic fractures as a direct result of their pelvic injury, but rather as the result of associated injuries.

MECHANISM OF INJURY

Most pediatric pelvic fractures result from pedestrian or cyclist/motor vehicle accidents, falls from heights, and other high-energy mechanisms. A subgroup of pelvic injuries—avulsion fractures—occur during sports activities such as soccer, gymnastics, and track and field.

CLASSIFICATION

Fracture patterns vary depending on the level of skeletal maturity:

- Children whose triradiate cartilage is open most commonly sustain fractures of the pubic rami and iliac wings; the triradiate cartilage of the acetabulum closes at approximately 14 years of age in boys and 12 years of age in girls.
  - The elasticity of the ligaments of the pubic symphysis and the sacroiliac joints, and the plasticity of the bony pelvis, are most likely responsible for the rare occurrence of unstable pelvic ring disruptions seen in adults.
- Adolescents approaching skeletal maturity, whose triradiate cartilage is closed, sustain pelvic injuries similar to those seen in adults.
- Older children and adolescents are more likely to require surgical treatment, with morbidity and mortality related to their pelvic injuries
- Avulsion injuries of the anterior superior and inferior iliac spines, ilium, and ischium most commonly occur in adolescent and young adult athletes.

Application of adult classification schemes to children's pelvic injuries is not ideal. The Torode and Zieg classification of pediatric pelvic fractures is the most widely used (Fig. 12.6-1 and Table 12.6-1). Bucholz and colleagues observed different patterns of physeal disturbance associated with triradiate cartilage injuries based on the Salter-Harris classification of these triradiate injuries (Fig. 12.6-2).

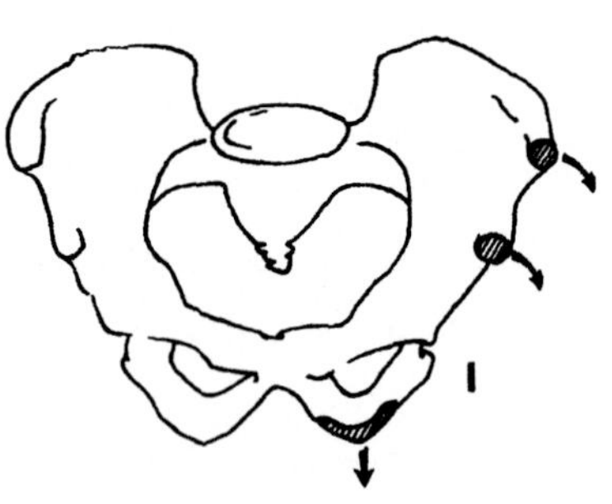

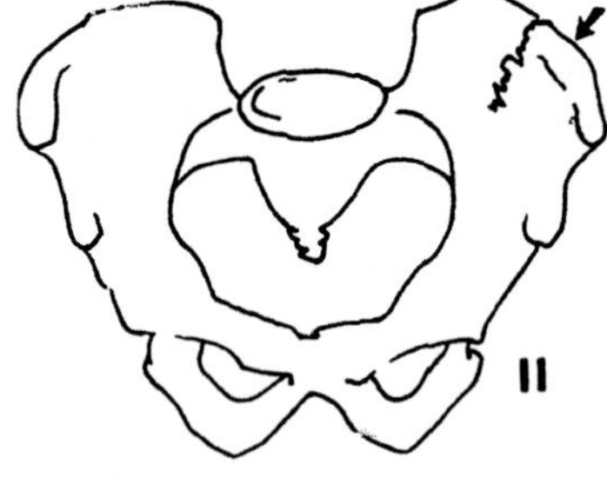

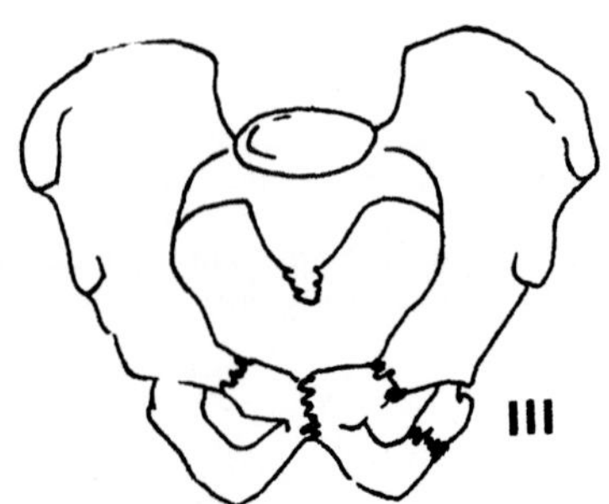

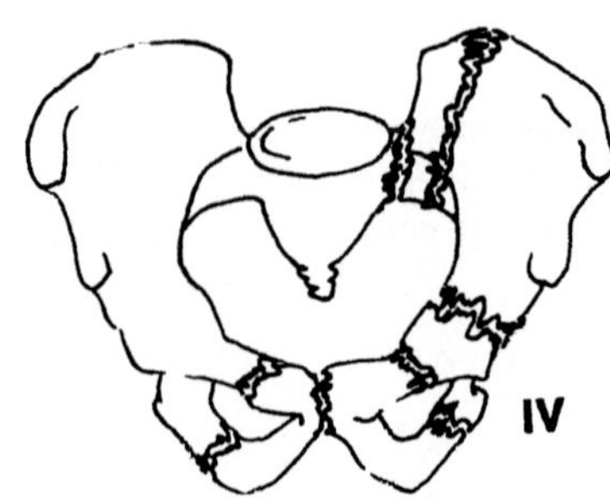

Figure 12.6-1 Torode and Zieg classification. Type I, avulsion fractures; type II, iliac wing fractures; type III, simple ring fractures (stable pelvic ring); type IV, ring disruption fractures (unstable pelvic ring). (From Canale ST, Beaty JH. Fractures of the pelvis. In: Beaty JH, Kasser JR, eds. Rockwood and Wilkins' fractures in children, 5th ed. Philadelphia, Lippincott Williams & Wilkins, 2001:883–911.)

TABLE 12.6-1 TORODE AND ZIEG CLASSIFICATION OF PELVIC FRACTURES IN CHILDREN

Type	Description
I	Avulsion fractures
II	Iliac wing fractures
IIa	Separation of the iliac apophysis
IIb	Fracture of the bony iliac wing
III	Simple ring fractures (stable pelvic ring)
IIIa	Fractures of the pubis and separation of the pubic symphysis; the posterior structures remain intact
IIIb	Fractures involving the acetabulum, without a pelvic ring fracture
IV	Fractures producing an unstable segment (unstable pelvic ring)
IVa	"Straddle" fractures (i.e., bilateral inferior and superior pubic rami fractures)
IVb	Fractures involving the anterior pubic rami or pubic symphysis and the posterior structures
IVc	Fractures that result in an unstable segment between the anterior ring of the pelvis and the acetabulum

DIAGNOSIS

History

Evaluation of the child with a suspected pelvic fracture begins with a thorough history of the traumatic events, as well as past medical and surgical history. The best effort must be made to gather this information from emergency personnel at the scene of an accident, emergency room staff, and family members. In a polytraumatized child, often the pelvic injury is a lower priority. The airway, breathing, circulation (ABC's) must be assessed and established as a first priority. Injuries of the head and spine, chest, and abdominal viscera, as well as the pelvis, must be carefully evaluated as potential sources of life-threatening injuries.

Physical Examination

- Visual inspection of the pelvis and perineum for lacerations, ecchymosis, hematoma, blood at the urethral meatus, and vaginal or scrotal injury is indicated.
- The anterior superior iliac spines, iliac crests, sacroiliac joints, and pubic symphysis are palpated.
- With hands placed on the iliac crests, apply posteriorly directed forces with gentle side-to-side rocking.
- Pain, crepitus, or excessive mobility is indicative of a potentially serious pelvic injury.
- Rectal examination is necessary to identify bony fragments, or a superiorly displaced prostate secondary to a urethral injury in older males.
- Hip range of motion must be evaluated, with pain or limits of mobility suggestive of a joint dislocation or associated acetabular fracture.
- Neurovascular examination of the lower extremities is documented.
  - Injuries of the lumbosacral plexus, femoral and sciatic nerves, as well as vascular injuries, may occur as the result of severe pelvic trauma.

Radiologic Findings

A standard component of the initial assessment of the polytraumatized patient is an anteroposterior radiograph of the pelvis in the emergency room. While this information is rarely necessary to effectively resuscitate and stabilize the child, early recognition of an unstable pelvic injury may be critical in the survival of the older child and adolescent. After the child is initially stabilized, rapid sequence spiral

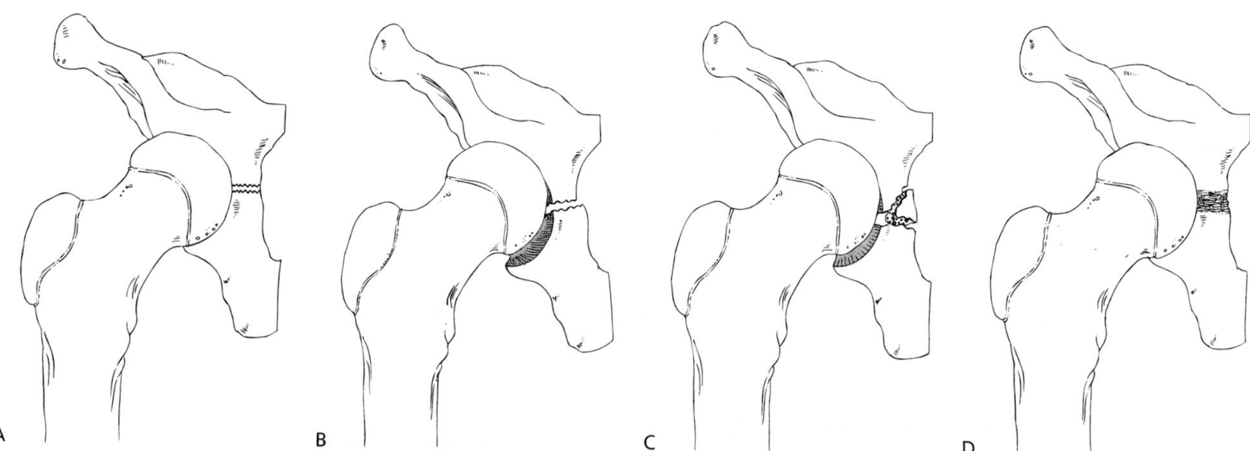

Figure 12.6-2 Triradiate cartilage injuries. (**A**) Normal. (**B**) Salter-Harris type I fracture. (**C**) Salter-Harris type II fracture. (**D**) Salter-Harris type V fracture. Growth disturbance, most commonly seen after type V injuries (compression), results in acetabular dysplasia. (From Scuderi G, Bronson MJ. Triradiate cartilage injury: report of two cases and review of the literature. Clin Orthop 1987;217:179–189.)

computed tomography (CT) scanning of the pelvis is the most effective method to fully evaluate the extent of pelvic injury. Often more serious concomitant injuries of the head and abdomen warrant evaluation by CT scan. Inclusion of the pelvis in the initial series of imaging studies allows for a more complete and efficient injury assessment.

Inlet, outlet, and oblique radiographic views of the pelvis may be useful for preoperative planning. Magnetic resonance imaging and bone scan have no role in acute evaluation of pelvic injuries. However, these modalities may be helpful in the analysis of soft tissue injury, cartilaginous injuries, and occult fractures.

TREATMENT

Most pelvic fractures in children are treated nonoperatively.

- Avulsion fractures (type I) are treated symptomatically with protected weightbearing for 2 to 4 weeks, followed by a stretching and strengthening program.
  - Return to sports may be expected within 6 to 8 weeks.
- Fractures of the iliac wing and iliac apophyseal separations (type II) are treated in a similar fashion.
- Simple ring fractures (type III) are stable fractures of the pelvis with intact posterior structures.
  - Cooperative patients without acetabular involvement may be treated with protected weightbearing with progression to full weightbearing over a 6-week period.
  - Bed rest or bed-to-chair activities are indicated for the noncompliant or very young child.
  - Type III fractures with nondisplaced fracture of the acetabulum may be treated with non-weightbearing ambulation or spica cast immobilization.
  - Distal femoral skeletal traction may be useful to improve alignment of minimally displaced fractures or to prevent premature weightbearing.
  - Intraarticular and triradiate cartilage displacement greater than 2 mm warrants open reduction and internal fixation.
- Type IV pelvic fractures are unstable ring disruptions.
  - A pelvic binder may be used as a temporary measure to assist in resuscitating the hemodynamically unstable child.
  - Emergent external fixation is indicated to control hemorrhage and to grossly align and stabilize the pelvis.
  - Pelvic arteriography and embolization are indicated if blood loss persists despite external fixation.
  - In a hemodynamically stable child, unstable pelvic disruptions may be treated with bed rest with or without skeletal traction, or in a spica cast. Progressive weightbearing and rehabilitation may be started within 6 weeks of injury.
  - Open reduction with internal fixation is indicated for acetabular and triradiate cartilage fractures with more than 2 mm of displacement.
  - Reduction and fixation of pelvic ring displacement, beyond the use of external fixation, is rarely indicated in children.
  - Displacement of up to 2 cm is acceptable, since rapid healing and significant remodeling of extraarticular fractures of the pelvis can be expected in children with more than 2 years of growth remaining.

COMPLICATIONS

Most pelvic injuries in children heal without complications. Nonunion and ligamentous instability of pediatric pelvic ring injuries do not occur. Malunion of the pelvic ring is well-tolerated because of the remodeling potential of the pediatric pelvis; leg length inequality may occur after an unstable fracture if residual vertical displacement of the hemipelvis exceeds 2 cm. Fractures involving the triradiate cartilage, especially in children younger than 10 years of age, may lead to growth disturbance of the acetabulum secondary to premature physeal closure. Manifestations of this abnormal growth include acetabular dysplasia, hip subluxation, and hip joint incongruity. Displaced acetabular fractures, despite anatomic realignment, may develop premature degenerative joint disease of the hip. Avascular necrosis of the femoral head may develop after fractures of the acetabulum associated with hip dislocation.

Other complications of fractures of the pediatric pelvis include myositis ossificans and permanent neurologic deficits of the lower extremity secondary to associated lumbosacral plexus, sciatic, and femoral nerve injuries. Death, as direct result of hemorrhage due to pelvic fracture, occurs in less than 0.5% of children. Nonskeletal injuries occurring in association with pelvic fractures in children, however, result in death of the child 10 times more frequently.

SUGGESTED READING

Bryan WJ, Tullos HS. Pediatric pelvic fractures: review of 52 patients. J Trauma 1979;19:799–805.

Bucholz RW, Ezaki M. Ogen JA. Injury to the acetabular triradiate physeal cartilage. J Bone Joint Surg (Am) 1982;64:600–609.

Canale ST, Beaty JH. Fractures of the pelvis. In: Beaty JH, Kasser JR, eds. Rockwood and Wilkins' fractures in children, 5th ed. Philadelphia: Lippincott Williams & Wilkins, 2001:883–911

Ismail N, Bellamare JF, Mollit DL, et al. Death from pelvic fracture: children are different. J Pediatr Surg 1996;31:82–85.

McIntyre RC Jr, Bensard DD, Moore EE, et al. Pelvic fracture geometry predicts risk of life-threatening hemorrhage in children. J Trauma 1993;35:423–429.

Quinby WC. Fractures of the pelvis and associated injuries in children. J Pediatr Surg 1966;1:353–364.

Silber JS, Flynn, JM. Changing patterns of pediatric pelvic fractures with skeletal maturation: implications for classification and management. J Pediatr Orthop 2002;22:22–26.

Torode I, Zeig D. Pelvic fractures in children. J Pediatr Orthop 1985; 5:76–84.

12.7 HIP

D. RAYMOND KNAPP, JR.

Hip fractures in children vary in several important aspects from those in adults. The bone is generally stronger and therefore significant trauma is usually required for fracture. The periosteum is thicker, thus making it possible for a fracture to be nondisplaced and relatively stable. This, however, does not protect the tendency for coxa vara if treated without fixation. The presence of the proximal femoral physis provides a weakened point for potential fracture. Damage to the physis can cause subsequent deformity of growth of the proximal femur. This group of fractures, although relatively rare, provides a significant challenge to the treating orthopedist, due to the frequency of potential complications including avascular necrosis, coxa vara, nonunion, premature physeal closure, and subsequent leg length discrepancy.

PATHOGENESIS

Etiology

Most proximal femur fractures occur as a result of severe trauma. Causes include motor vehicle accidents, pedestrian or cyclist/motor vehicle accidents, falls from heights, and child abuse. Occasionally, fractures may occur through pathologic bone such as a cyst or fibrous dysplasia.

Classification

These fractures are classified by the four-part classification system of Delbet (Table 12.7-1 and Fig. 12.7-1).

Epidemiology

The prevalence of pediatric hip fractures is less than 1% of that in adults. They account for 1% of all pediatric fractures.

- Type II fractures are most common—45% to 50%
- Type III—approximately 35%
- Type IV—12%
- Type I—8%

TABLE 12.7-1 HIP INJURY CLASSIFICATION SYSTEM OF DELBET

Type	Description
I	Transepiphyseal separation, with or without dislocation of the femoral head
II	Transcervical fracture
III	Cervicotrochanteric fracture (base of neck)
IV	Intertrochanteric fracture

Pathophysiology

The pertinent pathophysiology of proximal femoral fractures involves the blood supply to the capital femoral epiphysis and the manner in which complications are caused by its disruption. The blood supply to the femoral head from birth to 2 to 3 years of age comes from the medial and lateral circumflex vessels. This anastomotic ring courses along the intertrochanteric notch and is extracapsular. Transphyseal vessels exist up to 18 months of age.

After age 3 the entire femoral head is supplied by branches of the medial circumflex artery, and the posterosuperior and posteroinferior arteries, which course along the femoral neck and are vulnerable to injury from fracture. The posterosuperior artery supplies the lateral and anterior head, and the posteroinferior artery supplies the medial head.

Most of the metaphyseal circulation is supplied by the lateral circumflex artery. This limited vascular supply

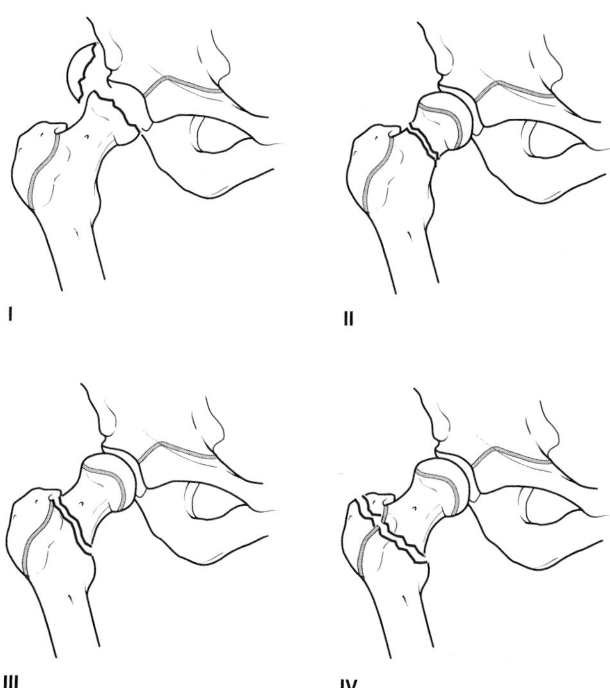

Figure 12.7-1 Delbet classification for proximal femur fractures. Type I is a transepiphyseal fracture. Type II is a transcervical fracture. Type III is a cervicotrochanteric fracture (basicervical). Type IV is an intertrochanteric fracture. (From Blasier RD, Hughes LO. Fractures and traumatic dislocations of the hip in children. In: Beaty JH, Kasser JR, eds. Rockwood and Wilkins' fractures in children, 5th ed. Philadelphia: Lippincott Williams & Wilkins, 2001:913–939.)

accounts for the frequent occurrence of avascular necrosis after fracture of the hip in children.

DIAGNOSIS

Physical Examination and History

Since these injuries occur in association with significant trauma, a thorough physical and radiologic exam is necessary to rule out other injuries. With displaced fractures, the leg is usually shortened and externally rotated. A thorough motor, sensory, and vascular exam of the extremity should be performed.

Nondisplaced fractures may present a diagnostic dilemma. Comparison radiographs may be helpful. Magnetic resonance imaging (MRI) has become increasingly useful to confirm the presence of a fracture. Also, a hip aspiration can be performed with a bloody aspirate being diagnostic.

In infants, a type I fracture may be difficult to diagnose and often is associated with child abuse. Aspiration, ultrasound, or MRI also can be useful to confirm the diagnosis.

TREATMENT

General Principles

- Accurate reduction must be obtained. If closed reduction fails, then open reduction should be performed.
- Stable fixation must be obtained.
  - Fracture stability takes precedence over physis sparing.
- Type I, II, and III fractures should be taken to the operating room emergently, preferably in less than 12 to 24 hours.
- Hip decompression should be performed with either open arthrotomy or aspiration for all type I, II, and III injuries.
- Spica cast should be used in younger children or if necessary to supplement internal fixation.

Type I Fractures

- Less than 2.5 years of age: closed reduction and spica cast if a stable reduction is obtained. Insertion of smooth pins if unstable
- Less than 9 years of age: closed or open reduction and smooth pins with hip decompression. Spica cast immediately
- More than 9 years of age: closed or open reduction and screw fixation with hip decompression

About half of these fractures are associated with a dislocation of the epiphysis. If the femoral head is dislocated, an attempt at closed reduction can be performed. If unsuccessful, this should be followed by immediate open reduction and pinning. The open reduction is performed on the side of the dislocated head [i.e., posterior approach of a posterior dislocation and an anterior (Watson-Jones) approach for an anterior dislocation].

Between 80% and 100% of those with a dislocation will develop avascular necrosis and premature physeal closure. Avascular necrosis is less often a problem in the under 2.5-year-old age group, since these are usually not associated with a dislocation, and remodeling of a severe varus malunion will occur if a growth arrest does not develop.

Type II Fractures

- Nondisplaced: screw fixation short of the physis if possible. Perform hip decompression.
- Displaced: closed or open reduction (anterior Watson-Jones) and screw fixation short of the physis. Hip decompression should also be performed.

Do not compromise fixation. If necessary, place fixation across the physis.

Consideration should be given for smooth pins in children under 9 years of age, if it is necessary to cross the physis

Type III Fractures

- Nondisplaced: screw fixation short of the physis and hip decompression
- Displaced: closed or open reduction (anterior Watson-Jones) with screw fixation short of the physis and hip decompression

Type IV Fractures

- Nondisplaced:
  - Children under 8 years of age may be treated with spica casting.
- Displaced:
  - Children under 8 years of age can be treated in 90–90 traction for 2 to 3 weeks followed by an abduction spica cast. Most are preferably treated with closed or open reduction, internal fixation, and spica casting.
  - For children older than 8 years of age, treatment should be similar to that of an adult, with open reduction and internal fixation.

COMPLICATIONS

Avascular Necrosis

Avascular necrosis is the most common and devastating complication of pediatric hip fractures. The incidence of avascular necrosis is directly related to the amount of fracture displacement and type of fracture.

- Type I fractures with associated dislocation have an 80% to 100% incidence, whereas without dislocation, the incidence is less than 25%.
- Displaced type II fractures—40% to 50% incidence
- Displaced type III fractures—approximately 25%
- Type IV fractures—avascular necrosis occurs rarely

Ratliff divided avascular necrosis into three types (Table 12.7-2 and Fig. 12.7-2). Avascular necrosis can be detected

TABLE 12.7-2 THREE TYPES OF AVASCULAR NECROSIS ACCORDING TO RATLIFF

Type	Involvement	Prognosis
I	Whole head	Worst
II	Partial head	Slightly better than type I
III	From the fracture line to the physis	Best

as early as 6 weeks after injury and usually develops by 1 year after injury. The risk of avascular necrosis can be markedly decreased in displaced fractures by immediate reduction in less than 24 hours, along with stable internal fixation and evacuation of the intracapsular hematoma. Recent studies show rates of 0% to 8% incidence of avascular necrosis with displaced fractures using this approach. Once avascular necrosis occurs there is no proven effective treatment. The internal fixation should be removed once the fracture heals.

Coxa Vara

Coxa vara resulting from malunion has essentially been eliminated with the routine use of stable internal fixation and spica casting. However, it may occur as a result of asymmetric physeal closure. This can be corrected by subtrochanteric valgus osteotomy.

Premature Physeal Closure

This complication usually occurs secondary to avascular necrosis or internal fixation crossing the physis. The proximal femoral physis provides 13% of the length of the leg. Therefore, growth arrest usually does not create significant (more than 2 cm) shortening except in very young children.

Nonunion

Historically, the rate of nonunion has been reported to be as high as 10%. Current recommended treatment has reduced this rate in most studies to 0% to 4%. If nonunion occurs, it should be treated as soon as it is recognized and usually by subtrochanteric valgus osteotomy and bone grafting, with internal fixation and spica casting.

Chondrolysis

This complication has been reported in one series and was always associated with avascular necrosis. Three of seven had pin penetration in the joint. All had a poor result.

Stress Fractures

Stress fractures can occur in children and adolescents, but less commonly than adults. All reported cases have involved the femoral neck.

Two types exist:

- Fatigue fracture: usually a result of overuse in children who have rapidly increased their activities.
- Insufficiency fractures: these occur in deficient bone in children with underlying disease processes.

Most stress fractures appear as compressive injuries with callus present along the inferior neck. A bone scan may be needed for diagnosis if there is no apparent radiographic abnormality. These can be treated with non-weightbearing on crutches or in a cast. If the fracture site widens or is displaced initially, then internal fixation is necessary.

HIP DISLOCATION

Hip dislocations are uncommon in childhood, but do occur more frequently than hip fractures and with less severe trauma. Prompt knowledgeable treatment is important to avoid potentially devastating complications. Specific treatment guidelines should be followed, thus avoiding the pitfalls of treating this rare injury.

PATHOGENESIS

Etiology

Hip dislocations are more likely to occur in children under 10 years of age from relatively minor trauma, such as a fall. This is thought to be due to the increased amount of cartilage in the joint, and the more generalized ligamentous laxity present in children. For children older than 10 years of age, a more forceful injury such as that sustained in a

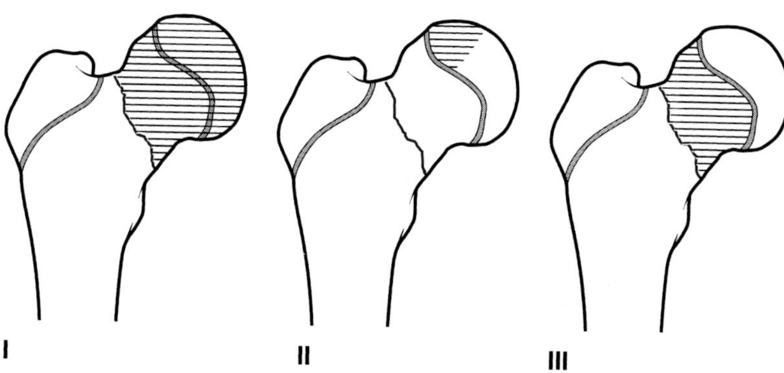

Figure 12.7-2 Three types of avascular necrosis. (Adapted from Ratliff AHC. Fractures of the neck of the femur in children. J Bone Joint Surg 1962;44B:528.)

motor vehicle accident or from contact sports is more likely.

Epidemiology

Hip dislocations can occur at any age with no specific peak incidence. They are more common in males than in females.

Pathophysiology

The femoral head can dislocate in any direction with 90% being posterior. These occur bilaterally 1% of the time. An associated fracture about the hip occurs approximately 15% to 20% of the time and is less frequent in younger children.

Classification

No formal classification of pediatric hip dislocations has been published. Each hip is described by its direction of dislocation:

- Anterior: the femoral head lies medial to the acetabulum.
- Anteroinferior: the femoral head lies in the region of the obturator foramen.
- Inferior: the femoral head lies inferior to the acetabulum and lateral to the ischial tuberosity.
- Posterior: the femoral head lies superior and lateral to the acetabulum.

DIAGNOSIS

History and Physical Examination

The history of mechanism of injury may range from a minor fall to a major high-energy accident. Approximately 65% are due to lower velocity injuries. Complaints of groin and hip pain will be evident.

Clinical Fractures

A thorough multisystem examination should be performed to determine associated injuries. An exam of the position of the limb will usually indicate the direction of dislocation. The leg is flexed, adducted, and internally rotated with a posterior dislocation, or extended, abducted, and externally rotated with an anterior dislocation. With an inferior dislocation, the hip is hyperflexed. A thorough neurologic examination of the lower extremity is mandatory, since sciatic nerve injury occasionally occurs. Pulses should be palpated, since femoral artery injuries have been reported. An associated femoral fracture may cause the lower extremity to be externally rotated.

Radiologic Features

A dislocated hip is evident on an anteroposterior (AP) pelvis x-ray. The entire involved femur should be imaged to exclude fracture. Careful viewing of the hip x-rays should occur and further films taken, if necessary, to rule out femoral head, acetabular, femoral neck, or transphyseal fractures. Judet (45-degree oblique) views may help to delineate a suspected acetabular fracture. Prereduction computed tomography (CT) scan may also be useful if fractures are suspected about the femoral head and acetabulum, as long as this doesn't significantly delay reduction.

TREATMENT

Prompt reduction of the dislocation should occur within the first 6 hours following injury to decrease the likelihood of avascular necrosis. An initial attempt under conscious sedation can be performed in the emergency department. If this fails, the next attempt should be performed under general anesthesia in the operating room. A posterior dislocation is reduced with the hip and knee flexed with countertraction to the pelvis applied by an assistant. An anterior dislocation is reduced with the hip extended and the knee flexed. If, after several attempts, reduction cannot be achieved, an open reduction should be performed. Failed reduction can occur secondary to interposed capsule, inverted labrum, and osteocartilagenous fragments. An anterior dislocation should be opened anteriorly and posterior dislocations should be opened posteriorly.

If there is an associated hip fracture, stabilization should be performed prior to reduction. If the femoral neck fracture is displaced, open reduction is performed.

After reduction, an AP pelvis x-ray should be taken to assess symmetry of the hip joints. If the joint spaces are not symmetric following reduction, a CT scan should be performed. If there is evidence of interposed soft tissue or bony fragments, an open reduction with removal of the interposed tissue should be performed.

Old Dislocations

Old traumatic dislocations are rare but can be treated initially by 1 to 2 weeks of skeletal traction. If this fails, open reduction is indicated.

Recurrent Dislocation

Recurrent traumatic dislocations usually occur in children under 8 years of age and are rare. The first recurrence should be treated with closed reduction and spica casting. Further recurrences should be treated with an open reduction, capsular repair, and spica casting.

Postoperative Management

There is no consensus regarding postoperative care. Most would recommend a spica cast for 6 weeks after reduction in children less than 6 to 8 years of age. A 6-week period of protected weightbearing is recommended in older children.

Outcome

Most children do well following an appropriately treated hip dislocation with functional outcomes being very good in 95%. Complications include avascular necrosis, sciatic nerve injury, recurrent dislocations, and osteoarthritis.

Avascular necrosis is associated with delay in reduction greater than 6 hours. The incidence ranges from 5% to 58% with most estimates between 8% and 10%. The risk of avascular necrosis is also related to the severity of the injury and age greater than 5 years. This can usually be detected by 6 months after injury, but children should be followed for up to 4 years.

Sciatic nerve injury occurs approximately 5% to 20% of the time and is usually a transient neuropraxia. Osteoarthritis is usually associated with the development of avascular necrosis.

SUGGESTED READING

Canale ST. Fractures of the hip in children and adolescents. Orthop Clin North Am 1990;21:341–352.

Canale ST, Bourland WL. Fracture of the neck and intertrochanteric region of the femur in children. J Bone Joint Surg (Br) 1977;59:431–443.

Flynn JM, Wong KL, Yeh GL, et al. Displaced fractures of the hip in children: management by early operation and immobilisation in a hip spica cast. J Bone Joint Surg (Br) 2002;84:108–112.

Hughes LO, Beaty JH. Fractures of the head and neck of the femur in children. J Bone Joint Surg (Am) 1994;76:283–292.

Mehlman CT, Hubbard GW, Crawford AH, et al. Traumatic hip dislocation in children: long-term follow-up of 42 children. Clin Orthop Rel Res 2000;376: 68–79.

Ng GPK, Cole WG. Effect of early hip decompression on the frequency of avascular necrosis in children with fractures of the neck of the femur. Injury 1996;27:419–421.

Ratliff AHC. Fractures of the neck of the femur in children. J Bone Joint Surg (Br) 1962;44:528–542.

Salisbury RD, Eastwood DM. Traumatic dislocation of the hip in children. Clin Orthop Rel Res 2000;377:106–111.

St Pierre P, Staheli LT, Smith JB, et al. Femoral neck stress fractures in children and adolescents. J Pediatr Orthop 1995;15:470–473.

Swiontkowski MF. Complications of hip fractures in children. Complications Orthop 1989;Mar/Apr:58–63.

12.8 FEMUR

R. DALE BLASIER

Femoral shaft fractures in children are common and usually result from moderate to high-energy injury. Fractures after trivial trauma should prompt a search for weakened bone. Nonoperative treatment methods are tried and true, but may be best suited for young children who are unable to walk with crutches. Operative stabilization is best suited for those who can be taught to ambulate without bearing weight. The prognosis for healing is excellent. Some overgrowth is to be expected and should be considered in the treatment plan. Overtreatment should be avoided.

PATHOGENESIS

Etiology

The femur may fracture as a result of a strong axial load, twisting force, three-point bend, or a direct blow. Motor vehicle accidents, recreational vehicle accidents, sports injuries, and falls are common causes. Rarely stress fractures or pathologic bone lesions may progress to overt fracture.

Epidemiology

Femur fracture is very common in childhood. About 1 in 2,000 children sustains a femur fracture each year. Up to 40% of boys and 25% of girls sustain a femur fracture in childhood.

Pathophysiology

The child's femur can be mildly deformed and will elastically recoil. Larger amounts of applied energy will cause the bone to fracture. The more energy applied to the bone, the more comminution and soft tissue disruption should be expected. Muscles that span the length of the thigh will tend to shorten the fractured femur. For this reason, traction—either skeletal or skin—is often applied to prevent shortening prior to definitive management. These fractures always heal unless open or operated. Hyperemic overgrowth is to be expected and should be considered in the treatment plan.

Classification

Three types of classification are useful (Box 12.8-1).

BOX 12.8-1 THREE METHODS OF CLASSIFYING FEMORAL SHAFT FRACTURES IN CHILDREN

Integrity of Soft Tissues
- Open fracture
- Closed fracture

Associated Injury Status
- Polytrauma
- Isolated injury

Fracture Pattern
- Stable—not prone to shortening
  - Short oblique fracture
  - Transverse fracture
- Unstable—prone to shortening
  - Comminuted
  - Long oblique
  - Segmental

DIAGNOSIS

Physical Examination and History

- A history of significant trauma is usual.
- The diagnosis is usually obvious in displaced fractures.
- Undisplaced fractures occur. Get an x-ray after a history of significant injury.
- Look for associated injuries.

Clinical Features

- Swelling and deformity are immediate findings. Ecchymosis occurs later.
- Tense swelling or unremitting pain should prompt compartment pressure measurement. Thigh compartment syndrome is rare, but significant.
- Check and document pulses. Vascular injury is rare.
- Check and document distal nerve status. Nerve palsy is presumed to be due to treatment unless clearly documented before treatment.
- Look for associated injuries in relation to the history of injury. Check the hip after an axial loading injury. Check the knee after a direct blow to the limb.

Radiologic Features

- Make sure the hip and knee joints are visible.
- Look for undisplaced (ghost) fracture lines which may affect choice of fixation.
- If there is considerable comminution or bone loss, an x-ray of the uninjured femur will provide an estimate of original bone length.
- If intramedullary fixation is contemplated, the size of the canal and bone length should be estimated.

TREATMENT

Algorithm 12.8-1 covers treatment decisions.

- Patient age is important:
  - Patients under 6 years of age should generally be treated with a spica cast as the fractures tend to heal quickly
  - Children older than 6 years will benefit from fixation of the femur, which allows ambulation with crutches.
- The presence of growth plates mitigates against treatment with a standard reamed nail placed through the piriform fossa.
  - Damage to the ascending vessels of the femoral neck may cause avascular necrosis, for which there is no satisfactory treatment.
  - Skeletally mature patients can be treated with a standard, reamed locked nail.
- The fracture pattern is important.
  - Fractures prone to shortening due to comminution or segmentation should be treated with an external fixator or locked nail to maintain length.

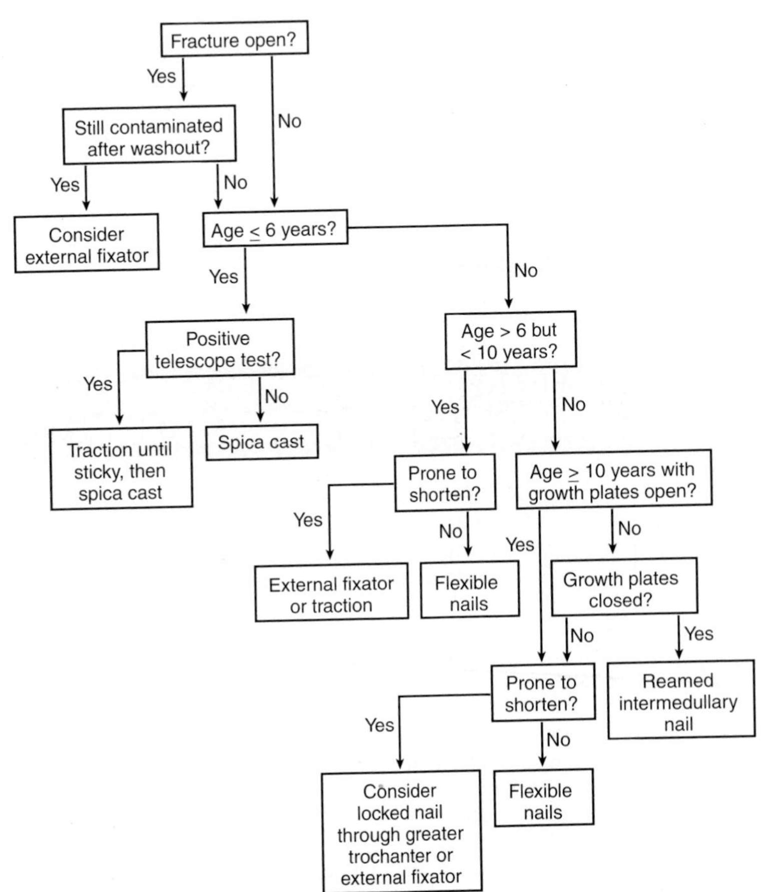

Algorithm 12.8-1 Treatment decision algorithm for femur fractures.

- Short oblique or transverse fractures are excellent candidates for flexible nails.
- Femur fractures in polytrauma patients will benefit from stabilization to facilitate patient care and mobility or to permit wound or skin care.

Nonoperative Treatment

Spica Casting

- Casting is the mainstay of treatment for the young.
- Reduction and casting are performed under sedation or anesthesia
- Positive piston test (fracture can be overlapped more than 2.5 cm) indicates preoperative traction until sticky to prevent shortening in cast.
- The cast can be wedged up to 1 to 2 weeks after application to correct angulation.
- Two weeks is long enough to heal in infants. Healing takes up to 6 weeks in older children.

Traction

- Safe and effective
- Prolonged recumbency is a drawback.
- Skin traction is useful for young children. Larger children will benefit from a distal femoral traction pin as the skin will not tolerate large shear forces from skin traction.
- Periodic x-rays needed to check alignment and length. Make corrections.
- Traction is maintained until fracture is sticky. Spica cast is then applied and maintained until healing.

Operative Treatment

- Open reduction and internal fixation with plate and screws (Fig. 12.8-1):
  - ☐ Relatively safe and effective
  - ☐ Easily placed by direct lateral approach, elevating the vastus lateralis.

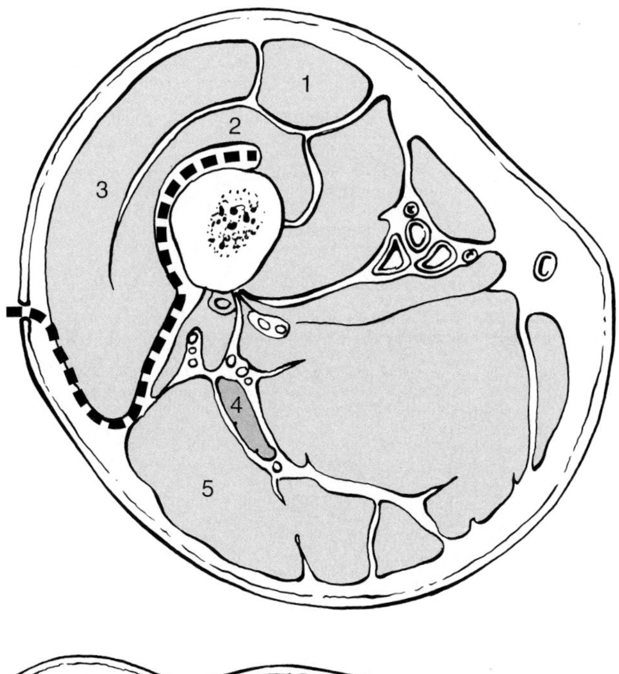

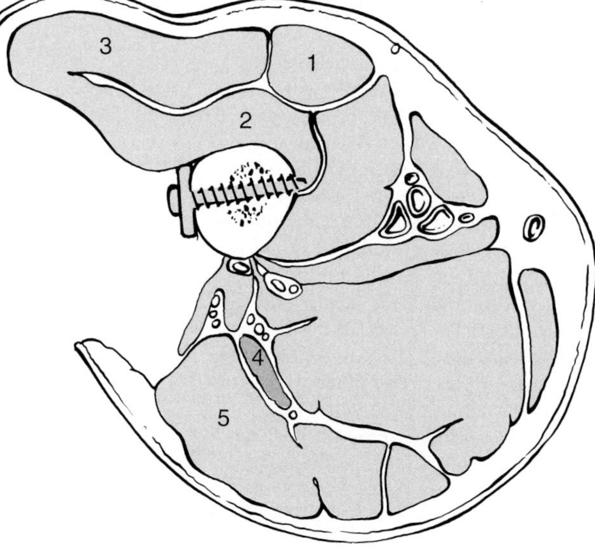

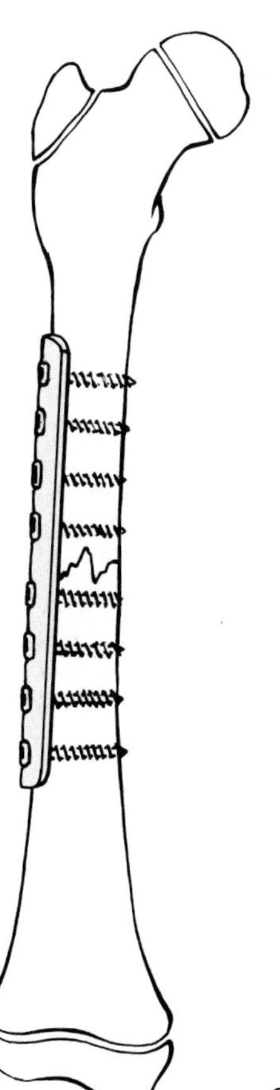

Figure 12.8-1 Lateral approach to the femur for open reduction and internal fixation. *1,* rectus femoris; *2,* vastus intermedius; *3,* vastus lateralis; *4,* sciatic nerve; *5,* biceps femoris (long head). **(A)** A direct lateral skin incision is made. The fascia is sharply incised. Vastus lateralis muscle (3) will be elevated off the intramuscular membrane. **(B)** With the vastus lateralis elevated, a plate can easily be placed along the lateral femoral cortex. **(C)** The plate should span the fracture site and screws should engage six to eight cortices on either side of the fracture to provide adequate purchase.

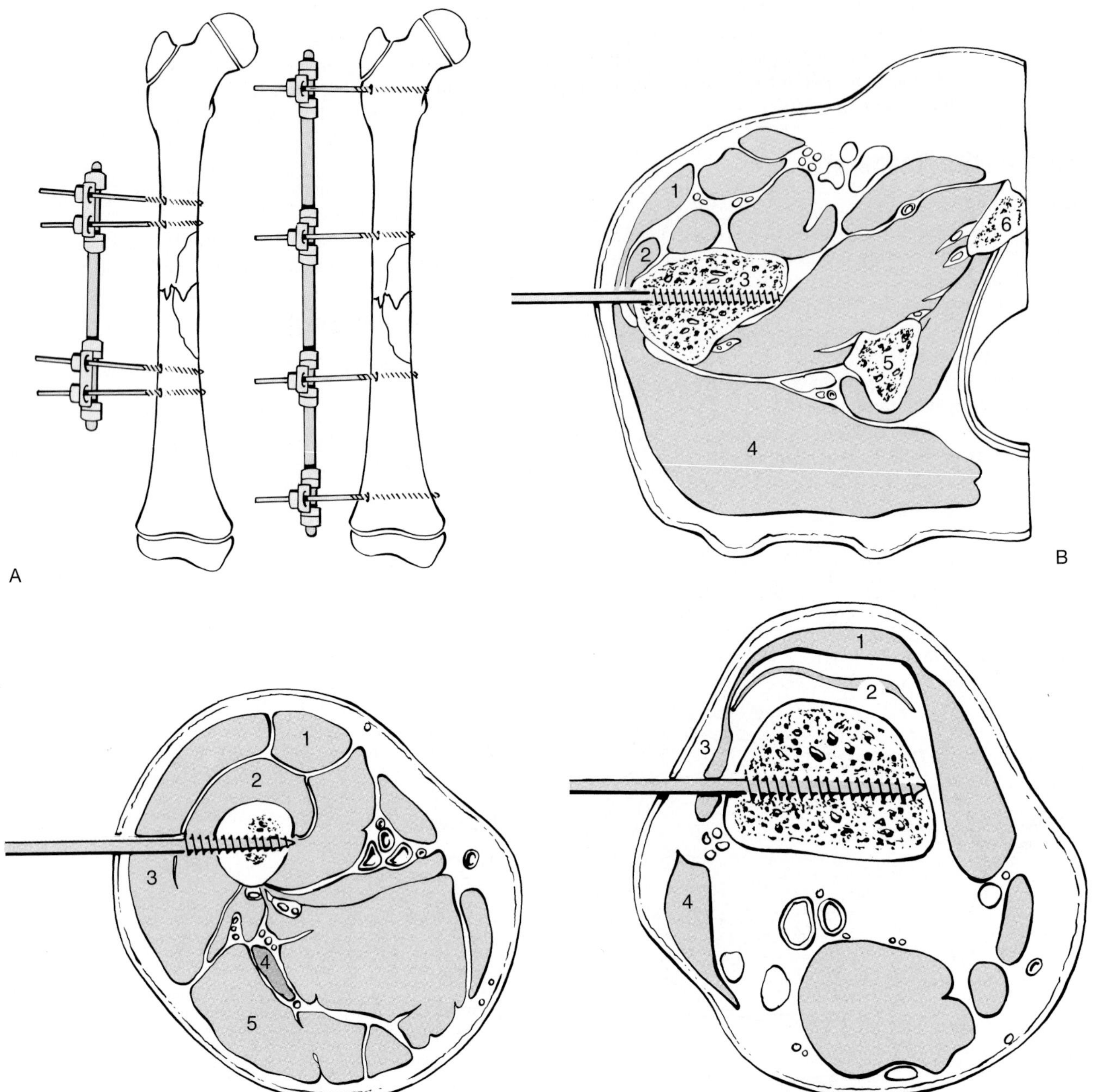

Figure 12.8-2 (**A**) Fixator pin placement. Placing pins too close to the fracture (**left**) provides poor control of fracture alignment. Pins in diaphyseal bone will act as stress risers. Try to limit the number of diaphyseal pins. Keeping the pins spread out (**right**) will provide better mechanical advantage in controlling fracture alignment. Try to place the proximal pin as proximal as possible and the distal pin as distal as possible without violating the physes. The intermediate pins should be close to but not violate the fracture site. (**B**) Cross-section of proximal thigh. *1*, tensor fascia lata; *2*, vastus lateralis; *3*, femoral neck; *4*, gluteus maximus; *5*, ischium; *6*, pubis. The most proximal pin should be in the intertrochanteric region, which is largely cancellous bone. Cancellous bone is less likely to fracture through pin tracts than is cortical bone. Because there is considerable motion of the soft tissues over the greater trochanter, some irritation is to be expected at this pin tract. (**C**) Cross-section of midthigh. *1*, rectus femoris; *2*, vastus intermedius; *3*, vastus lateralis; *4*, sciatic nerve; *5*, biceps femoris (long head). The diaphyseal pins will be in cortical bone. Here, they have significant stress riser effect. There will always be a risk of fracture through a pin tract until the pin has been removed and the hole refills with bone. The pins will transfix the vastus lateralis muscle. Few children will want to bend the knee as long as these pins are in place. (**D**) Cross-section of distal thigh, just above the distal femoral epiphysis. *1*, quadriceps tendon; *2*, suprapatellar pouch; *3*, vastus lateralis; *4*, biceps femoris. The most distal fixator pin should be in metaphyseal bone. Fracture through a pin tract here is virtually unheard of. The pin will transfix the iliotibial band, thereby precluding painless knee flexion.

- ☐ Requires a large incision and surgical dissection.
- ☐ There are stress risers while the hardware is in place and after removal.
- ☐ May be a good choice for patients who cannot be placed on a fracture table or subject to vigorous manipulation.
- ☐ Requires non-weightbearing until fracture callus is seen.

■ External fixation (Fig. 12.8-2):
- ☐ Usually quite effective; there is occasional delayed healing or refracture.
- ☐ Pin tracts require daily cleansing and still may drain or become infected.
- ☐ Pins should be spread out to allow control of fracture and limit stress risers.
- ☐ Pins through the iliotibial band cause pain. Expect limited knee motion until the fixator is removed.
- ☐ Weightbearing must be encouraged to strengthen fracture callus.
- ☐ The knee can be manipulated under anesthesia when the fixator is removed at about 3 months after implantation.
- ☐ May be a good choice in children (a) who are too young for a locked nail with fractures prone to shortening, (b) who have a deformed canal that will not accommodate flexible nails, and (c) who are too sick to tolerate prolonged anesthesia or vigorous manipulation.

■ Flexible intramedullary nails (Fig. 12.8-3):
- ☐ Excellent for fractures in juveniles with short oblique or transverse fracture patterns.
- ☐ The fracture must be reducible in order to pass the nails. If the fracture is not reducible under anesthesia, open reduction or another method of stabilization should be considered.
- ☐ Usually placed retrograde from distal femoral metaphyseal portals.
- ☐ Must be prebent to provide three-point fixation.
- ☐ Must be sized to fit in canal—larger is stronger. The two nails should be the same size, and should fill 80% of the canal at the isthmus.
- ☐ Should be cut just outside femoral cortex to allow later removal. If they protrude, there will be irritation with knee motion.
- ☐ Non-weightbearing should be maintained until callus is seen, usually 3 to 4 weeks after implantation.
- ☐ Nails should be removed after solid fracture healing.

■ Locked intramedullary nail through the piriformis fossa (Fig. 12.8-4A):
- ☐ May damage the ascending cervical vessels so this procedure is contraindicated in the skeletally immature. There is no satisfactory treatment for avascular necrosis of the capital femoral epiphysis.
- ☐ Reaming of the isthmus allow placement of a larger diameter nail.
- ☐ Should be the standard treatment for femur fracture in the skeletally mature.

■ Locked intramedullary nail through the greater trochanter (see Fig. 12.8-4B):
- ☐ Avoids damage to the ascending cervical vessels.
- ☐ Passing a small diameter nail prevents obliteration of the greater trochanteric apophysis.

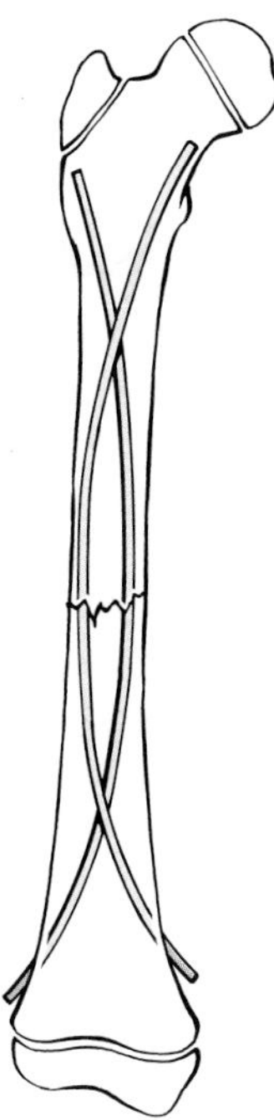

Figure 12.8-3 Retrograde placement of flexible nails for femoral shaft fracture. Small incisions just proximal to the knee allow creation of entry holes into the distal metaphyseal flare. Nails should be prebent with a long, gentle C-curve, which will provide three-point fixation of the fracture. Two nails are inserted—one from each side. The prebends oppose each other. The distal nail tips should be cut just outside the distal femoral cortex. They should be left long enough to enable future removal and short enough to prevent irritation of the mobile soft tissues around the knee—approximately 1 cm outside the bone.

- ☐ Allows passage of the nail from the greater trochanter into the intramuscular canal, which is not collinear with the greater trochanter.
- ☐ May not fill the canal, so may not be as strong a construct as a standard reamed nail.
- ☐ Requires non-weightbearing until callus is seen.

■ Débridement of open fractures:
- ☐ Open fractures always need prompt débridement.
- ☐ The traumatic wound should be extended to allow visualization and curettage of bone ends. The surgical wound should be closed and the traumatic wound left open.
- ☐ Open fracture is not a contraindication to internal fixation. If there is gross contamination, consider use of an external fixator and repeated débridement.

■ Antibiotics should be given.
- ☐ A cephalosporin is indicated for clean wounds.
- ☐ Add an aminoglycoside for contaminated wounds and penicillin for barnyard wounds.

Surgical Anatomy and Biomechanics

The intramedullary canal is narrowest at its isthmus. The isthmus must be scrutinized prior to any planned intramedullary fixation to make sure it is large enough to

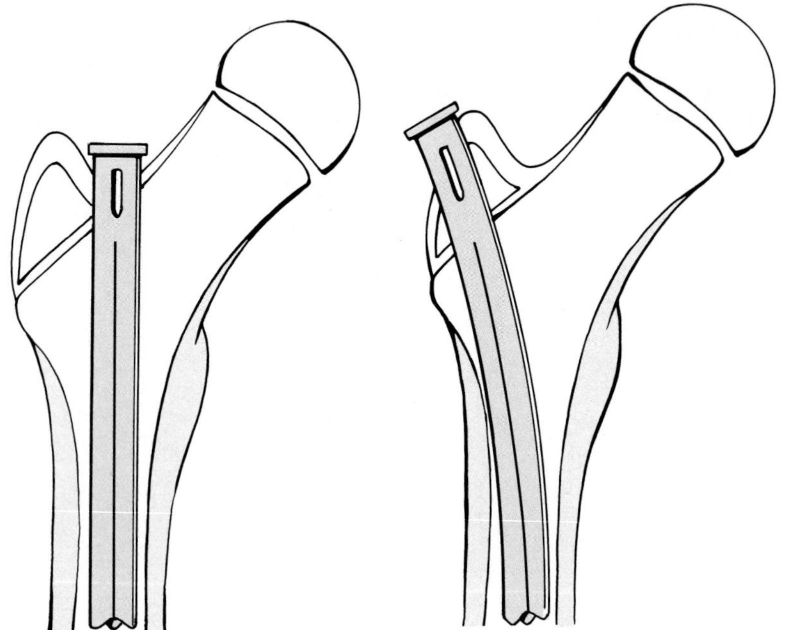

Figure 12.8-4 (A) Placement of intramedullary through the piriform fossa. This starting point is ideal for placing a reamed antegrade nail as it is coaxial with the intramedullary canal. Its use must be avoided in the skeletally immature patient due to the risk of damage to the ascending vessels, which supply the capital femoral epiphysis. (B) Placement of intramedullary through the greater trochanteric apophysis. This starting point is not ideal for placing an antegrade nail as it is not coaxial with the intramedullary canal. A smaller diameter nail will be used than with a standard piriform fossa approach to be able to "get around the corner" from the trochanter into the femoral canal and to eliminate the need to ream a very large hole in the trochanteric apophysis.

allow passage on the implant. The distal femur gradually expands into a metaphyseal flare which is much wider from medial to lateral than front to back. There is a gradual transition from cortical to cancellous bone.

Postoperative Management

- Routine wound surveillance is indicated.
- Non-weightbearing should be maintained until callus is seen.
- Crutches should be used until bridging callus is seen on anteroposterior and lateral radiographs.
- Hardware should be removed after fracture healing and remodeling.

Complications

Infection

- Superficial infection (cellulitis) can sometimes be managed with antibiotics.
- Deep infections need open débridement.
- Antibiotics should be tailored to the culture organism.
- Loose hardware should be removed and an external fixator can provide stability.
- Stable hardware should be maintained in place.

Delayed Union

- Unusual in children
- Weightbearing, bone stimulators, and bone grafting can be effective.

Nonunion

- Extremely rare in the absence of an open fracture or surgical treatment.
- Fractures tend to heal in children even if the bone ends are not apposed.
- Treatment is the same as for delayed union.
- Repeat or more secure fixation may be required.

Leg Length Discrepancy

- Fractures not reduced out to length can heal shortened.
- 1 cm of overgrowth can be expected in children between 4 and 10 years.
- The treatment plan should take this into account.
- The process of overgrowth should be complete 6 to 12 months after injury.
- Discrepancies of less than 2 cm can generally be treated with shoe modifications.
- Discrepancies predicted to be from 2 to 4 cm can be managed by epiphysiodesis.
- Greater discrepancies may require lengthening procedure.

Angular Deformity

- Should be prevented.
- Infants have impressive remodeling potential.
- Up to 15 degrees of angulation can be accepted in younger children and less angulation can be accepted near skeletal maturity.
- In general, valgus is better tolerated than varus and procurvatum is better tolerated than recurvatum.
- Persistently symptomatic angulation, which is not likely to remodel should be treated with osteotomy.

Rotational Deformity

- Should be prevented.
- No more than 20 degrees should be accepted.
- If there is any doubt as to whether rotation is correct, simultaneous radiographs should be taken of femurs to include hips and knees in an effort to match version prior to surgical fixation.
- Persistently symptomatic rotation, which is not likely to remodel should be treated with osteotomy.

PEARLS

- Parents should be warned about the possibility of late leg length discrepancy. A few words of early warning are worth more than volumes of late explanation.
- After cast removal, a limp is to be expected. Parents should be warned. The limp is not permanent.
- 1 cm of overgrowth can be expected in children between 4 and 10 years. The treatment plan should take this into account.

SUGGESTED READING

Beaty JH. Femoral-shaft fractures in children and adolescents. J Am Acad Orthop Surg 1995;3:207–217.

Berbeek HO, Bender J, Sawidis K. Rotational deformities after fractures of the femoral shaft in childhood. Injury 1976;8:43–48.

Blasier RD, Aronson J, Tursky EA. External fixation of pediatric femur fractures. J Pediatr Orthop 1997;17:342–346.

Buckley SL. Current trends in the treatment of femoral shaft fractures in children and adolescents. Clin Orthop 1997;338:60–73.

Canale ST, Tolo VT. Fractures of the femur in children. IIOS Instr Course Lect 1995;44:255–273.

Gregory P, Pevny T, Teague D. Early complications with external fixation of pediatric femoral shaft fractures. J Orthop Trauma 1996; 10:191–198.

Heinrich SD, Drvaric DM, Darr K, et al. The operative stabilization of pediatric diaphyseal femur fractures with flexible intramedullary nails: a prospective analysis. J Pediatr Orthop 1994;14:501–507.

Hughes BF, Sponseller PD, Thompson JD. Pediatric femur fractures: effects of spica cast treatment on family and community. J Pediatr Orthop 1995;15:457–460.

Hutchins CM, Sponseller PD, Sturm P, et al. Open femur fractures in children: treatment, complications, and results. J Pediatr Orthop 2000;20:183–188.

Kregor PJ, Song KM, Routt ML, et al. Plate fixation of femoral shaft fractures in multiply injured children. J Bone Joint Surg (Am)1993;75:1774–1780.

Parsch KD. Modern trends in internal fixation of femoral shaft fractures in children: a critical review. J Pediatr Orthop (Part B) 1997; 6:117–125.

Skaggs DL, Leet AI, Money MD, et al. Secondary fractures associated with external fixation in pediatric femur fractures. J Pediatr Orthop 1999;19:582–586.

Thompson JD, Buehler KC, Sponseller PD, et al. Shortening in femoral shaft fractures in children treated with spica cast. Clin Orthop 1997;338:74–78.

Townsend DR, Hoffinger S. Intramedullary nailing of femoral shaft fractures in children via the trochanter tip. Clin Orthop 2000;376: 113–118.

12.9 KNEE

JULIA E. LOU ■ JEVERE HOWELL ■ JOHN M. FLYNN ■ THEODORE J. GANLEY

Most knee injuries in children occur as a result of sports-related injuries, motor vehicles accidents, or falls. Fractures may disrupt the extensor mechanism, create knee instability, or injure the physes. Therefore, diagnosis and treatment measures are critical to the future function and development of the child with a knee fracture.

PATELLA FRACTURE

PATHOGENESIS

Direct trauma, sudden forceful contraction of the quadriceps, or a combination of the two may result in patella fracture. Linear or comminuted fractures are characteristic patterns that result from direct impact to the knee and patella subluxation or dislocation may result in an osteochondral fracture. Patella fractures can be classified according to location (Table 12.9-1).

DIAGNOSIS

Patella fractures may be difficult to diagnosis due to existing knee joint anomalies such as bipartite patella, Osgood-Schlatter disease, or Sinding-Larsen-Johansson (SLJ) disease. Additionally, small fracture fragments associated with patella fractures are easily missed on radiographs.

TABLE 12.9-1 FRACTURES OF THE PATELLA

Type	Location	Radiograph	Characteristics	Mechanism of Injury
Superior	Proximal patellar pole	Least common		
Sleeve (inferior)	Distal patellar pole	Small fragment Large cartilaginous component	8–12 yrs of age	Acute, sudden forceful contraction of quadriceps following extension of knee
Lateral	Superolateral margin	Vertically oriented, traverse entire patella, crescent-shaped line	Bipartite patella 0.2%–6% incidence Male > female Fragment edges are sclerotic in chronic conditions	
Medial	Medial margin		Fragment edges are sclerotic in chronic conditions	Acute lateral patellar dislocation
Osteochondral fracture	Patellar margin	May be difficult to see radiographically	Associated with large amount of cartilage	Lateral patellar dislocation (occurs in 5%)

Physical Examination and History

Clinical Features

- Effusion, hemarthrosis
- Refusal to bear weight
- Point tenderness
- Patella alta
- Inability to fully extend knee
- Palpable defect (sleeve fracture)

In patients with distal pole avulsions, the patella moves proximally with voluntary contraction of the quadriceps while the patellar ligament remains relaxed. Patients with stable, nondisplaced fractures will be able to perform straight leg raises. Osteochondral fractures may result from patellar dislocations which have spontaneously reduced prior to presentation. A patient who has had a dislocated patella will resist passive manipulation by contracting the quadriceps or by physically grabbing the examiner to prevent further manipulation (positive apprehension test).

Radiologic Features

- Fragmentation
- Fracture lines
- Patella alta
- Knee effusion

TABLE 12.9-2 RADIOGRAPHIC GUIDELINES FOR IMAGING PATELLA FRACTURES

Fracture Type	Radiographic Studies
Transverse	Lateral x-ray with knee flexed 30 degrees
Marginal (longitudinal)	Anteroposterior, axial, or merchant x-ray

Some fracture patterns are best seen on a specific radiographic view (Table 12.9-2). In patients with large knee effusions who have sustained significant injury, magnetic resonance imaging (MRI) scans may be valuable to visualize cartilage damage or fracture fragments.

TREATMENT

Surgical Indications

Fractures with more than 3 mm of displacement or articular step-off require open reduction and fixation, followed by 4 to 6 weeks of immobilization in a cylinder cast. A torn retinaculum and other functionally debilitating cartilage or ligament injuries should be surgically treated.

Contraindications

Nondisplaced fractures are treated conservatively with 4 to 6 weeks of immobilization with the knee held in extension in a cylinder cast.

Results and Outcome

Adequate surgical repair of patella fractures generally achieves acceptable results. Overall, patients with nondisplaced fractures have good results while patients with comminuted, displaced fractures experience more complications.

Complications

- Decreased range of motion
- Patella deformity
- Patella alta
- Osteochondral defects

- Quadriceps weakness
- Posttraumatic osteoarthritis
- Extensor lag
- Osteonecrosis

Postoperative Management

Following cast removal, patients should be assigned a physical therapy program for range of motion and continued muscle strengthening.

PATELLA SLEEVE FRACTURE

PATHOGENESIS

Although rare, patella sleeve fractures are the most commonly reported patella fracture in children. A small fragment of bone attached to a sleeve of cartilage avulses from the lower pole of the patella.

DIAGNOSIS

Physical Examination and History

Clinical Features

- Severe knee pain
- Inability to fully extend the knee
- Point tenderness
- Palpable gap
- Inability to bear weight
- High-riding patella
- Effusion
- No history of direct blow to knee

It is important to differentiate patella sleeve fractures from SLJ disease. Unlike SLJ disease, patella sleeve fractures are an acute injury with intense pain. The palpable gap at the distal pole of the patella is an important clinical sign characteristic of patella sleeve fractures.

Radiologic Features

- Effusion
- Small fragment avulsed from distal patellar pole
- Patella alta

The fragment may be so small that it is difficult to see radiographically. Sagittal MRI views along the axis of the patellar tendon are helpful in diagnosis.

TREATMENT

This injury must be accurately reduced to ensure proper healing and return to function.

Surgical Indications

The majority of patellar sleeve fractures should be treated with open reduction and fixation in order to realign the articular surfaces. Patients treated by cast immobilization have a higher rate of complications than those treated surgically.

Results and Outcome

Normal range of motion and return to normal function generally occurs following successful surgery.

Complications

- Loss of full knee extension
- Subchondral articular defect
- Patellar deformity
- Loss of reduction
- Loss of motion
- Ossification of patellar tendon

Postoperative Management

After surgery, the knee should be immobilized for 4 to 6 weeks in a cylinder cast. Following casting, physical therapy for range of motion and strengthening is helpful.

OSTEOCHONDRAL FRACTURES

PATHOGENESIS

Osteochondral fractures in children often occur in association with lateral patellar dislocations. Dislocation may cause a fragment of the medial patella or lateral femoral condyle to break away from the bone. Osteochondral fractures can be classified by location and mechanism of injury.

DIAGNOSIS

Physical Examination and History

Clinical Features

- Effusion
- Knee held in slight flexion
- Knee pain
- Inability to bear weight
- Resist movement
- Point tenderness

Radiologic Features

Osteochondral fractures (Table 12.9-1) are often difficult to see on plain films, as the fragment size may be very small or hidden from view. Anteroposterior and lateral as well as sunrise and tunnel views should be obtained. Arthrography, computed tomography (CT) scan, or MRI can be useful in visualizing the cartilaginous nature of the injury, which may be extensive.

TREATMENT

Surgical Indications

Acute osteochondral fractures with large fragments (≥2 cm) should be treated surgically with pins or screws. The knee is then immobilized in flexion for 4 to 6 weeks following surgery. Small fragments (≤1 cm) may be removed arthroscopically.

Results and Outcome

Smaller fragments in non-weightbearing areas produce better outcomes than large fragments in weightbearing areas.

Complications

- Loss of motion
- Femoral condyle deformity
- Patellar deformity
- Late osteoarthritis changes

FRACTURE OF THE DISTAL FEMORAL PHYSIS

PATHOGENESIS

- Blow to the knee with a planted foot
- Fall on a bent knee
- A birth injury may occur with a breech presentation
- Hyperextension of the knee
- Other factors may also predispose patients to physeal injury:
  - Osteomyelitis
  - Myelomeningocele
  - Leukemia
  - Osteosarcoma
  - Hemophilia
- Account for about 1% to 6% of all physeal injuries
- Occur in adolescents between 12 and 16 years of age
- Associated pathology: ligament, popliteal artery, and peroneal nerve injury possible
- Classified according to the Salter-Harris classification

DIAGNOSIS

Physical Examination and History

Clinical Features

- Swelling and effusion
- Report hearing a pop at the time of injury
- Tenderness about the physis
- Inability to bear weight

Because of the potential risk to nerve and vessels, a complete neurovascular assessment is necessary.

Radiologic Features

Anteroposterior, lateral, and oblique views are valuable. MRI, ultrasound, or arthrography may aid in the diagnosis of physeal fractures in infants. Arteriography should be performed when vascular injury is suspected.

Radiographs demonstrate:

- The patella and femoral condyles in line with the proximal tibia, ruling out knee dislocation
- Fracture line
- Degree of displacement

TREATMENT

Surgical Indications

Surgery consists of reduction and internal fixation for all displaced distal femoral physeal fractures. The joint may be aspirated prior to manipulation and traction should be applied to minimize cartilage damage. Closed reduction should be performed under general anesthesia to prevent muscle spasm, which may cause grinding of the physis.

Closed reduction alone (without internal fixation) risks loss of reduction.

Smooth pins or wires should be used if the physis must be crossed. Many type II fractures can be fixed with interfragmentary screw fixation through the Thurston-Holland fragment and type III fractures can be reduced with pins or screws placed transversely through the epiphysis. Similarly, pins or screws should be placed transversely through the epiphysis or metaphysis when reducing type IV fractures.

Nondisplaced fractures can be immobilized. After aspiration of tense effusions, the patient should be placed in a long leg or hip spica cast with 15 to 20 degrees of knee flexion.

Results and Outcomes

The prognosis for these fractures is generally good with a greater potential for leg length discrepancy and angular deformity secondary to physeal arrest in younger children.

Complications

- Popliteal artery impairment
- Angular deformity
- Compartment syndrome
- Partial/complete physeal arrest
- Peroneal nerve palsy
- Leg length discrepancy
- Recurrent displacement
- Knee stiffness
- Ligamentous injury

Postoperative Management

After surgery, the patient is placed in a long leg cast with slight flexion and allowed to ambulate on crutches.

Straight leg raises are initiated within 1 week and at 4 weeks; range of motion and muscle strengthening exercises are begun.

FRACTURE OF THE PROXIMAL TIBIAL PHYSIS

PATHOGENESIS

Fracture of the proximal tibial physis is extremely rare in children and its mechanisms are similar to those of distal femoral fractures. Fractures of the proximal tibial physis account for approximately 0.8% of all physeal injuries and occur most commonly in adolescent boys.

Associated injuries include injury to the popliteal artery, damage to the collateral ligaments, and proximal fibular fracture.

The Salter-Harris classification is also used to describe proximal tibial fractures.

DIAGNOSIS

Physical Examination and History

Clinical Features

A thorough neurovascular examination should be performed to assess the status of the peroneal nerve and popliteal artery. Compartment syndrome must be ruled out:

- Tense joint with hemarthrosis
- Tenderness over the physis 1.0 to 1.5 cm below the joint line
- Fibular tenderness

Radiologic Features

- Fracture line
- Effusion
- Associated injuries

Associated ligamentous or knee injury may be present but difficult to appreciate on plain radiographs alone. CT scanning or MRI may provide additional information. Arteriography should be performed when vascular injury is suspected.

TREATMENT

Surgical Indications

Unstable reductions and Salter-Harris type II, III, and IV fractures are candidates for operative treatment. Unstable Salter-Harris type I fractures may be fixed with percutaneous pins that cross distal to the physis. The wires should be removed 4 to 6 weeks after surgery. Open reduction and internal fixation is indicated for displaced type III and type IV fractures and pins or screws may be placed horizontally parallel to the physis. Ligamentous and meniscal injuries should be repaired.

Contraindications

- Nondisplaced fractures treated in a long leg cast with 30 degrees of flexion for 4 to 6 weeks.

Results and Outcome

- Similar to those of patients with distal femur physeal fractures.

Complications

- Popliteal artery impairment
- Angular deformity
- Compartment syndrome
- Partial/complete physeal arrest
- Peroneal nerve palsy
- Leg length discrepancy
- Recurrent displacement
- Knee stiffness
- Ligamentous injury

Postoperative Management

Patients placed in a long leg cast with 30 degrees of flexion should be immobilized for 6 to 8 weeks. After removal of the cast, range of motion and quadriceps strengthening exercises should be initiated.

TIBIAL SPINE (TIBIAL EMINENCE) FRACTURES

PATHOGENESIS

Tibial spine fractures result when a force causes a bony fragment of the anterior or posterior aspect of the tibial eminence to avulse. The more common anterior tibial spine injuries result in a bony fragment with an attached (anterior cruciate ligament) ligament.

Tibial spine fractures are relatively uncommon, with an estimated incidence of 3 per 100,000 each year. They are thought to result from a combination of rotational, hyperextension, and valgus force. Children often sustain this injury after falling from a bicycle, during athletic activity, or rarely as a result of trauma. The classification for this injury is based on fragment displacement (Fig. 12.9-1).

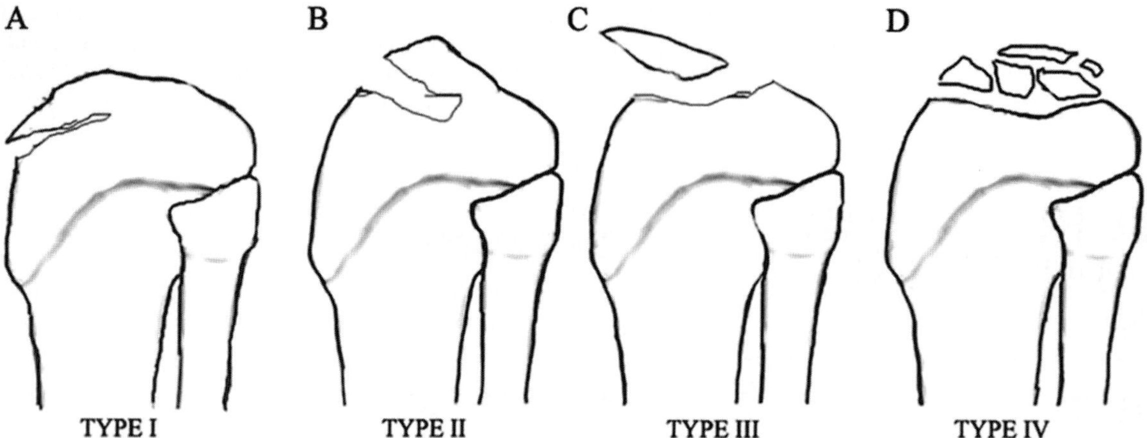

Figure 12.9-1 (A-D) Meyers and McKeever classification of tibial eminence fractures.

DIAGNOSIS

Physical Examination and History

Clinical Features

- Pain
- Hemarthrosis
- Inability to bear weight
- Painful and limited range of motion

The ligaments should be assessed for stability and associated injury using:

- Lachman test
- Drawer test
- Pivot shift test

Radiologic Features

Anteroposterior and lateral radiographs should be obtained and examined for the presence of a bony fragment. Tunnel or stress views may also be helpful. The lesion is frequently larger than it appears radiographically due to cartilaginous involvement not visible on plain radiographs.

TREATMENT

Surgical Indications

Type III and IV fractures are most often treated with open reduction and internal fixation with sutures, pins, screws, or Kirschner wires. These injuries have poor outcomes when treated nonoperatively.

Contraindications

Type I and II fractures are most often treated with closed reduction in a splint or a cast for 4 to 6 weeks. The knee should be immobilized in slight flexion (10 to 20 degrees).

Results and Outcome

Proper treatment generally achieves good results, although complications are associated with inappropriate treatment.

Complications

- Anteroposterior laxity
- Loss of extension due to bony block
- Late sequelae meniscal injury as a result of cruciate laxity
- Extensor lag
- Quadriceps weakness

Postoperative Management

Whether the patient undergoes surgery followed by immobilization or closed reduction through cast immobilization for 4 to 6 weeks, all patients should be assigned range of motion therapy and muscle strengthening training following cast removal.

AVULSION FRACTURE OF THE TIBIAL TUBERCLE

PATHOGENESIS

Tibial tubercle avulsions typically result from jumping or landing during a sporting event. Associated pathology may include meniscal tear or patellar fractures. This injury represents 1% to 3% of all physeal injuries and is seen most commonly in athletic adolescent males. Predisposing factors include:

- Patella baja
- Osgood-Schlatter disease
- Tight hamstrings
- Physeal abnormalities

The Watson-Jones classification is used to describe this injury (Fig. 12.9-2).

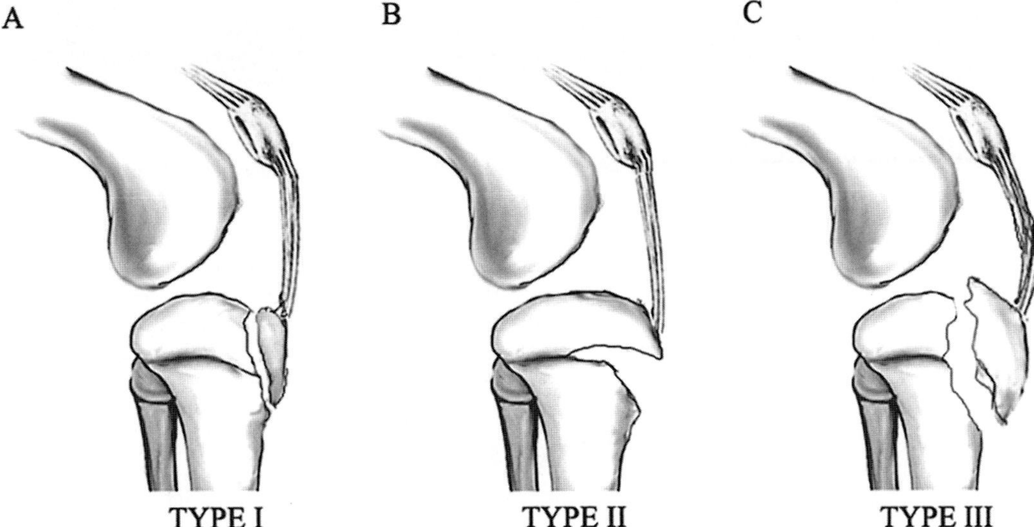

Figure 12.9-2 (A-C) Watson-Jones classification of tibial tubercle avulsions.

DIAGNOSIS

Physical Examination and History

Clinical Features

- Swelling and tenderness
- Lack of full extension (type II and III fractures)
- Palpable fracture fragment
- Patella alta
- Effusion
- Hemarthrosis

Radiologic Features

Lateral plain radiographs with slight internal rotation are optimal imaging studies to view this injury.

- Patella alta
- Fracture fragment
- Effusion

TREATMENT

Surgical Indications

Surgery is indicated for type IB and higher grade fractures. Fixation is achieved by smooth pins or small wires if the patient is more than 3 years from skeletal maturity or if the fracture fragment is small. Large fragments or older children can have fracture fixation with screws, threaded Steinmann pins, or tension holding sutures.

Contraindications

Typically, minimally displaced type I fractures are treated by reduction with the knee in extension and casting.

Results and Outcome

Patients with completely reduced fractures of the tibial tubercle tend to have a favorable outcome and usually return to normal activities.

Complications

- Compartment syndrome
- Loss of flexion or extension
- Meniscal tear
- Patella alta
- Genu recurvatum

Postoperative Management

Patient should be placed in a long leg cast with the knee in extension for 4 to 6 weeks. Physical therapy for quadriceps strengthening and range of motion exercises are instituted at cast removal.

SUGGESTED READING

Flynn JM, Hresko T, Reynolds RA, et al. Titanium elastic nails for pediatric femur fractures: a multicenter study of early results with analysis of complications. J Pediatr Orthop 2001;21:4–8.

Flynn JM, Luedtke L, Ganley TJ, et al. Titanium elastic nails for pediatric femur fractures: lessons from the learning curve. Am J Orthop 2002;31:71–74.

Ganley TJ, Pill SG, Flynn FM, et al. Pediatric and adolescent sports medicine. Curr Opin Orthop 2001;12:456–461.

Houghton GR, Ackroyd CE. Sleeve fractures of the patella in children: a report of three cases. J Bone Joint Surg (Br) 1979:61:165–168.

Insall JN, Windsor RE, Scott WN, et al, eds. Surgery of the knee, 2nd ed. New York: Churchill Livingstone, 1993.

Micheli LJ, Foster TE. Acute knee injuries in the immature athlete. In Heckman JD, ed. Instructional Course Lectures 42. Rosemont, IL: American Academy of Orthopaedic Surgeons, 1993:473–481.

Ogden JA, Tross RB, Murphy MJ. Fracture of the tibial tuberosity in adolescents. J Bone Joint Surg (Am) 1980;62A;205–215.

Pasque CB, McGinnis DW. Knee. In: Sullivan JA, Anderson SJ, eds. Care of the young athlete. Rosemont, IL: American Academy of Orthopaedic Surgeons, 2000:377–404.

Smith AD, Tao SS. Knee injuries in young athletes. Clin Sports Med 1995;14:629–650.

Sponseller PD, Stanitski CL. Fractures and dislocations about the knee. In JH Beaty, JR Kasser, eds. Rockwood and Wilkins' fractures in children, 5th ed. Philadelphia: Lippincott Williams & Wilkins, 2001:981–1076.

12.10 TIBIA AND FIBULA

MICHAEL C. ALBERT ■ GURPAL S. AHLUWALIA

FRACTURES OF THE TIBIAL TUBEROSITY

- The postnatal development of the tibial tubercle can be divided into four stages (Table 12.10-1).
- Fractures of the tibial tuberosity can occur during any of the first three stages of development.

PATHOGENESIS

Etiology

- Most fractures occur while a child or adolescent is involved in athletics, especially in those that involve jumping and landing.
- Basketball, track and field, and gymnastics are the three sports in which these injuries most commonly occur.
- The mechanism of these fractures is an avulsion most often caused by sudden acceleration or deceleration of the knee extensor mechanism.

Epidemiology

- Fractures of the tibial tuberosity only occur in children and adolescents in whom the ossification centers are still open or incompletely closed.
- Some studies suggest that acute disruptions of the tibial tuberosity occur with increased incidence in knees with preexisting Osgood-Schlatter disease.
- Despite the considerable force exerted upon the insertion of the quadriceps muscle when it contracts, especially when jumping or landing, fractures of the tibial tuberosity are relatively rare.

Pathophysiology

- These avulsion-type fractures occur when the patellar tendon pulls hard enough to overcome the combined strength of the growth plate underlying the tubercle, the surrounding perichondrium, and the adjacent periosteum.
- There are two ways in which this mechanism can occur:
  - Violent contraction of the quadriceps muscle against a fixed tibia.
  - action occurs when an athlete springs off to jump, as in a basketball game or a track and field event.
- Acute passive flexion of the knee is strong enough to override the contracted quadriceps.
  - This variation of the mechanism can occur, for example, when an athlete makes a bad landing at the end of the jump or fall, as in a gymnastic event or in the long jump.

Classification

Watson-Jones classified the three types of injury to the tibial tuberosity (Table 12.10-2). In general, the difference between the subtypes is in the degree of separation from the metaphysis and in comminution of the avulsed fragment.

TABLE 12.10-1 STAGES OF DEVELOPMENT OF THE TIBIAL TUBERCLE

Stage	Description
Cartilaginous	Occurs before the secondary ossification center appears and persists until approximately age 11 yr in girls and approximately age 13 yr in boys
Apophyseal	The ossification center appears in the tongue of cartilage and occurs in girls between 8–12 yrs and in boys between 9–14 yr
Epiphyseal	The secondary ossification centers coalesces to form a tongue of bone continuous with the proximal tibial epiphysis. This stage occurs in girls between ages 10–15 yr and in boys between the ages of 11–17 yr.
Bony	Defined as the point at which the epiphyseal line is closed between the fully ossified tuberosity and the tibial metaphysis

TABLE 12.10-2 CLASSIFICATION OF INJURY TO THE TIBIAL TUBEROSITY

Type	Description
I	Fracture across secondary ossification center
II	Fracture of junction of primary and secondary ossification centers
III	Fracture extends into knee joint through proximal tibial epiphysis

DIAGNOSIS

Physical Examination and History

Clinical Features

- Patients with a fracture of the tibial tuberosity will present with a history of an acute injury, most often during participation in an athletic event involving jumping.
- They describe immediate marked pain and swelling at the time of injury, and are often unable to stand or walk.
- These fractures can be distinguished from Osgood-Schlatter disease because in the latter, onset of symptoms is often insidious rather than acute. In addition, the symptoms in Osgood-Schlatter disease are usually mild and intermittent, the patients have only partial disability as opposed to the inability to stand or walk, and treatment is only symptomatic and supportive.

Radiologic Features

- The tibial tuberosity lies just laterally to the midline of the tibia.
- The best radiologic view to evaluate this injury is a lateral radiograph with the tibia rotated slightly medially. Findings will vary depending upon the type of injury.

TREATMENT

Surgical Indications

There are two primary indications for surgery in fractures involving the tibial tuberosity:

- Anterosuperior displacement of one or more fragments of the tuberosity
- Extension of the fracture through the proximal tibial ossification center into the joint with disruption of the joint surface

Surgical Contraindications

- In general, the only type of tibial tuberosity fracture that should be managed without surgery is a type I fracture that involves small fragments that are either nondisplaced or only minimally displaced.
- Type II and III fractures are treated with open reduction and internal fixation.
- In cases of displaced fractures, a periosteal flap may be folded under the avulsed fragments.
  - The fracture bed should be cleared of any debris and any such periosteal flaps should be extracted and spread out during reduction of the fragment with the knee extended.
  - Fixation of the fragment should be reinforced by repair of the torn periosteum.

Results and Outcome

- The outcome of properly reduced or surgically treated fractures of the tibial tuberosity is good.
- Nearly all patients are able to return to full activity, including participation in athletics.

Postoperative Management

- After reduction or repair, a cylinder or long leg cast should be applied for 4 weeks.
- Rehabilitation should focus on active range of motion and quadriceps strengthening exercises.
- The patient can return to full participation in athletics after the mass and strength of the quadriceps on the affected side is equal to that on the opposite side.
- Patients should be followed for any loss of range of motion of the knee, atrophy of the quadriceps muscles, persistent prominence of the tuberosity, the possibility of patella alta in an inadequately reduced displaced tuberosity, and the possibility of infection following open reduction.

PROXIMAL TIBIAL METAPHYSEAL FRACTURES

PATHOGENESIS

- Usually occur in younger children between the ages of 3 and 6 years
- Result from a valgus stress applied to an extended knee.
- May be nondisplaced and incomplete versus displaced with valgus opening of the medial cortex

DIAGNOSIS

- Present with swelling and tenderness of the proximal tibia
- Significant displacement requires a thorough neurovascular exam to rule out compartment syndrome. Most patients will have a nondisplaced buckle fracture or valgus greenstick fracture by radiographs.

TREATMENT

- An acute valgus deformity requires a closed reduction under conscious sedation and placement of a long leg cast in extension.
- If correction cannot be achieved by closed techniques, an open reduction with removal of interposed soft tissue should be performed.
- The most common complication of proximal metaphyseal tibial fractures, even in anatomically reduced injuries, is valgus deformity. Most practitioners believe that asymmetric growth occurs.
- Parents should be informed about the possibilities of valgus overgrowth occurring the first year after injury; bracing is ineffective and corrective osteotomies should not be performed until skeletal maturity. Most patients will correct the valgus deformity with continued growth.

TIBIA AND FIBULAR SHAFT FRACTURES

- Common injuries to the lower extremities.
- Closed injuries heal faster and have fewer complications than similar adult injuries.

PATHOGENESIS

Etiology

- *Indirect* means through a rotational twisting force, presenting as a spiral or oblique fracture pattern.
- A direct force presents as a transverse or butterfly-type fracture pattern.

Classification

Tibia Fractures

- Tibial and fibular fractures can be categorized according to which bone is fractured.
- The most common type of fracture is an isolated tibia fracture in the distal third of the tibia.
- The intact fibula prevents shortening but varus angulation can occur secondary to deforming force of the toe flexors and posterior tibialis tendon.

Tibia and Fibula Fractures

- The second type of fracture pattern involves both the tibia and fibular shafts.
- The most common angular problem is valgus malalignment secondary to deforming forces of the anterior extensor muscles.
- Maintaining length can be a problem.

Fibula Fractures

- The third type involves an isolated fibula fracture, which usually occurs from direct trauma to the lateral aspect of the leg. One must rule out an associated distal tibial physeal injury.

DIAGNOSIS

- Pain with local swelling and tenderness will be present.
- Radiographs should include anteroposterior and lateral views to include the knee and ankle joint.
- Most will have a nondisplaced buckle fracture or valgus greenstick fracture by radiographs.

TREATMENT

- Most closed tibial and fibular shaft fractures can be treated with closed reduction and long leg casting.
- There is minimal overgrowth of the tibia so shortening of more than 1 cm is unacceptable.
- In younger children angulation of up to 10 degrees is acceptable, however angulation of more than 5 degrees in adolescents may not remodel.

Surgical Indications

- Unstable or open tibial fractures that cannot be adequately reduced and held in a cast can be treated by a variety of techniques including external fixation, pins and plaster, lag screws, plating and flexible intramedullary nails, taking care to avoid the growth plates at the insertion sites of the nails.
- All open tibia and fibular fractures are treated with emergent irrigation and débridement and antibiotics.
- Gustillo and Anderson grade 1 fractures can be treated with long leg casting.
- Grade 2 and 3 open fractures can be treated with various techniques previously mentioned, depending on the soft tissue injury and wound contamination.

Results and Outcomes

- Complications such as angulatory deformity, leg length discrepancy, and malrotation can occur. Adherence to acceptable amounts of angulation and shortening will prevent these complications.
- Malrotation will not remodel with growth and should not be accepted.
- Delayed union and nonunion is unusual in closed tibial shaft fractures.
- Delayed union and osteomyelitis can occur in open fractures; however, current treatment techniques can achieve good results in these types of fractures.
- Compartment syndrome can occur in tibial shaft fractures and a high index of suspicion must be present when a child has pain out of proportion to the injury and has pain of passive stretch of the toes.

TIBIAL STRESS FRACTURES

PATHOGENESIS

- Stress fractures must be considered in the differential diagnosis of leg pain.
- Generally tibial stress fractures occur between 10 and 15 years of age without a history of specific injury.

DIAGNOSIS

- Most children have a painful limp and have local bone tenderness usually occurring on the upper tibia.
- Radiographs may be normal in the first 10 to 14 days, but subsequent radiographs will show periosteal reaction.
  - □ The proximal posterior medial tibia is the most common site.
- Magnetic resonance imaging or bone scan may aid in diagnosis if early plain radiographs are normal.
- Differential diagnosis includes Ewing sarcoma and osteomyelitis.

TREATMENT

- The treatment of tibial stress fractures is relative rest.
- If there is significant pain on weightbearing, crutches and a long leg cast may be used for 4 weeks followed by gradual increase in activity.
- Nonunion of tibial stress fractures has been reported but is extremely rare.

TODDLER'S FRACTURE

PATHOGENESIS

Etiology

- "Toddler's fracture" is a spiral fracture of the tibia without a concomitant fibular fracture.
- Mechanism of injury is usually a rotational force through the tibia, namely internal rotation of the proximal leg, with the foot and ankle in a fixed position. It most often occurs when a toddler stumbles while running or walking.

Epidemiology

- The majority of these fractures occur in children less than 2.5 years of age.

Pathophysiology

- The most common site of this fracture is the distal metaphysis of the tibia.
- Spiral fractures of the midshaft of the tibia can also occur, but are more often associated with child abuse rather than an accidental twisting or tripping injury.

Classification

Toddler's fractures can simply be classified as either displaced or nondisplaced.

DIAGNOSIS

Physical Examination and History

Clinical Features

- The inability to bear weight and focal tenderness are the most common presenting features in a child with a toddler fracture. History of an acute twisting or tripping injury may be elicited, but more commonly the injury mechanism is not obvious.

Radiologic Features

- Radiographs of the tibia and fibula should be obtained in both anteroposterior and lateral projections.
- An internal oblique view can help in recognition of nondisplaced toddler's fractures and sometimes may be the only view that identifies this type of fracture.
- Follow-up films at 10 to 14 days will usually demonstrate callus formation.

TREATMENT

- A long leg cast, bent knee, is applied for about 3 weeks.

Results and Outcome

- Most patients with these fractures recover full preinjury activity and normal growth following immobilization.

SUGGESTED READING

Dunbar JS, Owen HF, Nogrady MB, et al. Obscure tibial fracture of infants: the toddler's fracture. J Can Assoc Radiol 1964;25:136–144.

Halsey MF, Finzel KC, Carrion WV, et al. Toddler's fracture: presumptive diagnosis and treatment. J Pediatr Orthop 2001;21:152–156.

Ogden JA, Tross RB, Murphy MJ. Fractures of the tibial tuberosity in adolescents. J Bone Joint Surg (Am) 1980;62A:205–215.

Tenenbein M, Reed MH, Black GB. The toddler's fracture revisited. Am J Emerg Med 1990;8:208–211.

Tuten HR, Keeler KA, Gabos PG, et al. Posttraumatic tibia valga in children: a long term follow up note. J Bone Joint Surg (Am) 1999;81:799–810.

Yang JP, Letts RM. Isolated fractures of the tibia with intact fibula in children: a review of 95 patients. J Pediatr Orthop 1997;17:347–351.

12.11 ANKLE

ANDREW W. HOWARD ■ ANDREW M. WAINWRIGHT

Ankle fractures are fractures of the distal tibia, or distal fibula, distal to the metaphysis. This may affect the ankle joint by entering the articular cartilage or disrupting the tibiofibular syndesmosis, thus widening the space between the tibia and fibula.

These injuries are different in children than they are in adults, although the mechanism may be similar. The differences are attributed to the presence of the growth plates, which are weaker than the ligaments and adjacent bones. These physes also close slowly resulting in a stress riser at the point where the unossified growth plate meets the ossified growth plate. Many of these fractures may be treated nonoperatively. However, it is important to identify, assess, and operate on those fractures that require open reduction and internal fixation to prevent complications.

PATHOGENESIS

Anatomy

Growth Plates

- Tibial and fibular growth plates are most important features that make these injuries different from adult injuries.
- Damage to the growth plate may lead to angular or longitudinal growth problems.
- Tibial growth plate is proximal to the joint line and to the fibular growth plate.
- Fibular growth plate is level with the ankle joint line.
- The growth plate is weaker than adjacent ligaments.
- Distal tibial growth plate closes over a period of 18 months.
- Order of closure: central, medial, lateral, posterior, anterior.

Ligaments

- Medial: deltoid ligaments—superficial and deep
- Lateral:
  - □ Anterior talofibular ligament
  - □ Posterior talofibular ligament
  - □ Calcaneofibular ligament
- Central—syndesmosis:
  - □ Anterior inferior tibiofibular ligament
  - □ Posterior inferior tibiofibular ligament
  - □ Interosseous membrane

Epidemiology

- Annual incidence:
  - □ 0.1% of children sustain ankle fractures
  - □ Constitute 10% to 25% of all physeal injuries
  - □ Second most common fracture after distal radius
- Sex ratio: boys more than girls by 2:1
- Especially common at age 10 to 15 years (during which time physes are closing)

Pathomechanism

- The ankle joint transmits the whole body weight to the ground through the foot.
- Resists torsion in all three planes.
- Indirect mechanism: with a fixed foot, the body is forced into internal rotation/external rotation, eversion/inversion, plantarflexion/dorsiflexion
- Direct mechanism: vehicle crash, falls, sports

Classification

Anatomy of Fracture

- The Salter-Harris classification describes the fracture anatomically relative to the growth plate and joint line (Figs. 12.11-1 and 12.11-2 and Table 12.11-1).
- Higher grades represent increasing risks of growth complications.
- Type of fracture can be correlated with patient age.

Mechanism

- Understanding the injury mechanism facilitates planning closed or open reduction maneuvers. In general, this is done by reversing the injury mechanism.
- Dias-Tachdjian system (Fig. 12.11-3):
  - □ Modified Lauge-Hansen classification system of adult ankle fractures.
  - □ Used with descriptors from the Salter-Harris classification system.

DIAGNOSIS

Differential Diagnosis

Acute

- Fracture of adjacent bone:
  - □ Distal tibia proximal to metaphysis
  - □ Proximal fibula fracture
  - □ Hindfoot, especially the talus and base of fifth metatarsal
- Septic arthritis, osteomyelitis

Chronic

- Osteochondritis dissecans of talus
- Tarsal coalition
- Chronic ankle instability
- Tendinitis
- Juvenile chronic arthritis
- Tumor, osteoid osteoma, osteosarcoma, Ewing sarcoma

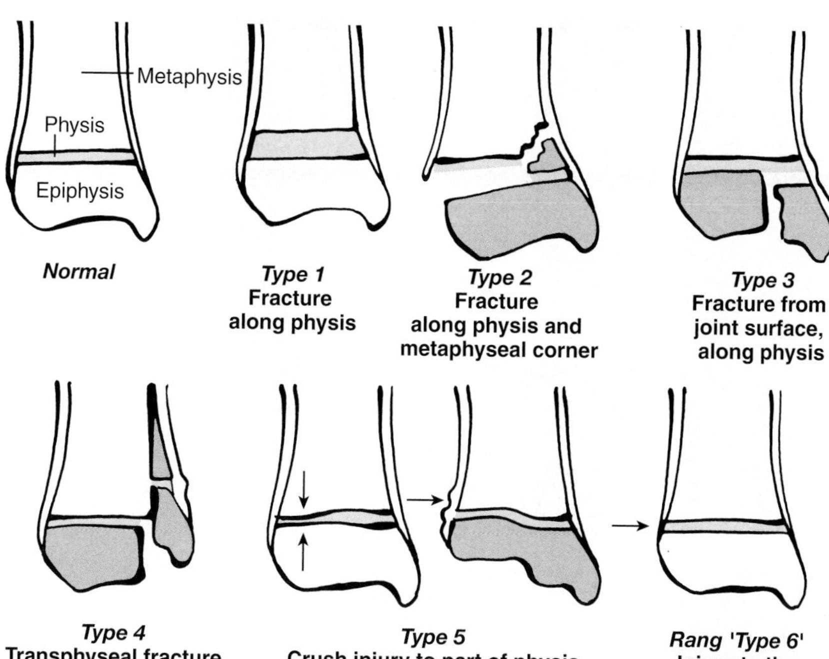

Figure 12.11-1 Salter-Harris classification system for growth plate fractures. (Adapted from Salter RB, Harris WR. Injuries involving the epiphyseal plate. J Bone Joint Surg 1963;45A:587–622.)

TABLE 12.11-1 SALTER-HARRIS CLASSIFICATION SYSTEM

Grade	Description	Comments
I	Complete separation of the epiphysis from the metaphysis (without a fracture through bone)	Fibula—common Tibia—less common, seen in younger children
II	Fracture through the physeal plate and cuts through portion of metaphysis	Triangular piece of metaphyseal bone is called the Thurston-Holland fragment
III	Intraarticular fracture that extends from the joint surface to the deep zone of the growth plate and along the plate to the periphery	Special type: juvenile Tillaux (named after Paul Jules Tillaux)—avulsion fracture of distal tibia; anterolateral epiphysis is avulsed by anterior talofibular ligament
IV	Intraarticular fracture that extends from the joint surface across all of the growth plate and through a portion of the metaphysis	Special type: triplane fracture—fracture of the distal tibia that runs in three perpendicular planes: ▪ Sagital plane from the joint surface to the growth plate ▪ Axial plane along the growth plate ▪ Coronal plane from the growth plate through part of the metaphysis
V	Crush injury to one area of the physeal plate	Uncommon fracture Difficult to diagnose at time of injury, but often diagnosed retrospectively (on review of initial radiographs after growth arrest has occurred)
Additions to Original Salter-Harris Classification		
VI[a]	Injury to the perichondrial ring of LaCroix	Leads to scarring/bridge across the growth plate and angular deformity
VII[b]	Avulsion fractures of the medial malleolus	

[a]Added by Mercer Rang.
[b]Added by John Ogden.

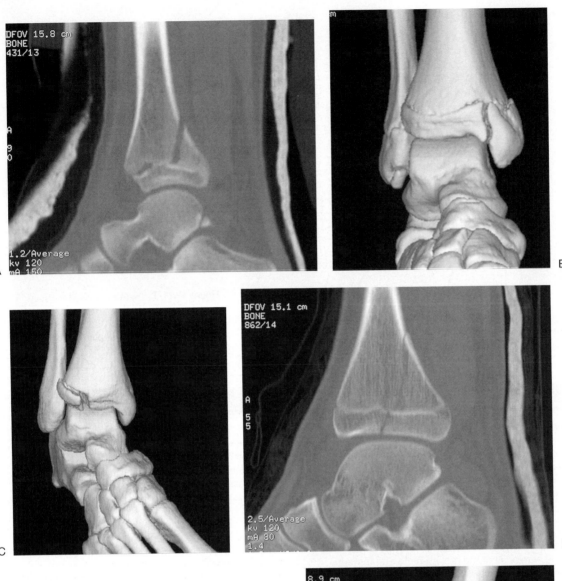

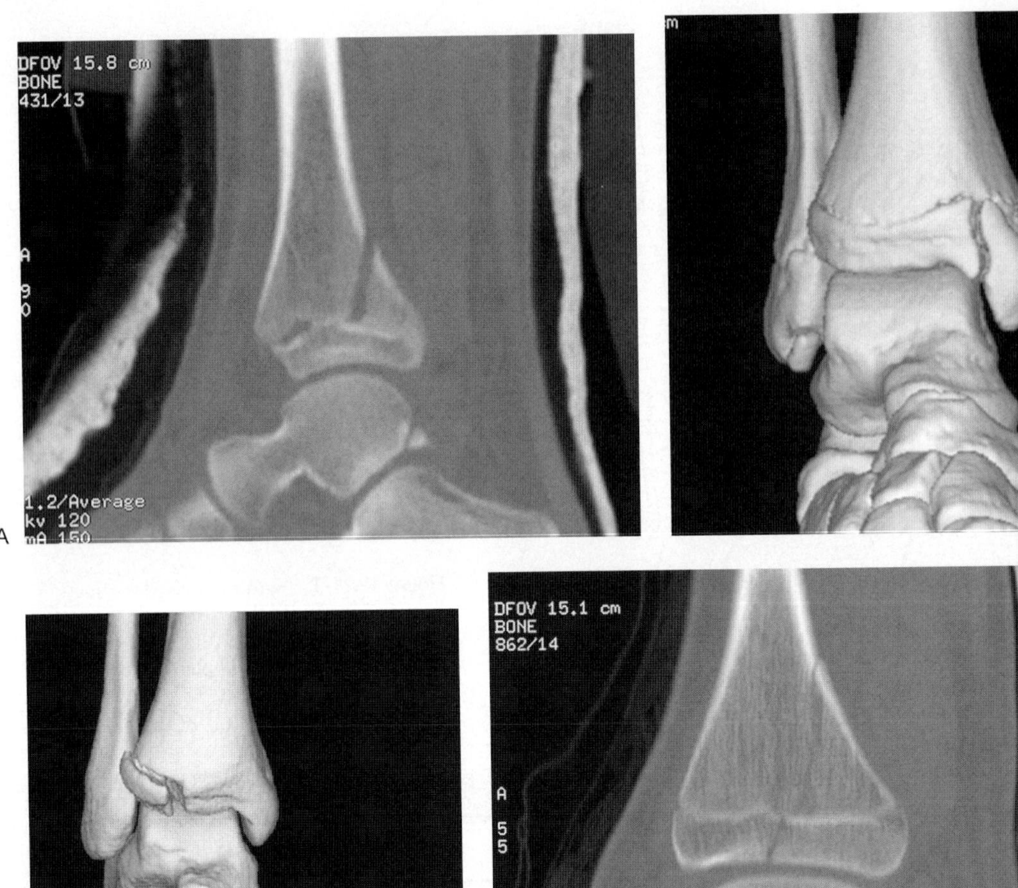

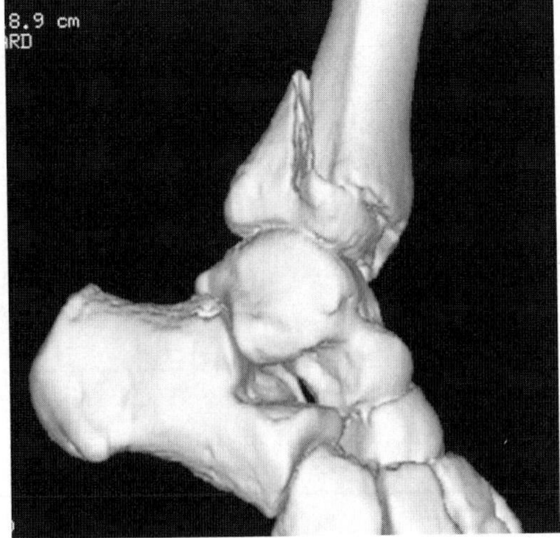

Figure 12.11-2 Ankle fractures. (**A**) Sagittal reconstruction of computed tomography (CT) scan of a Salter-Harris type II fracture. (**B**) Three-dimensional (3D) rendering of CT scan reconstruction of Salter-Harris type III fracture. (**C**) 3D rendering of CT scan reconstruction of Tillaux fracture. (**D**) Sagittal reconstruction of CT scan of Salter-Harris type IV fracture. (**E**) 3D rendering of CT scan reconstruction of triplane fracture. (The fibula has been digitally removed for easier appreciation.)

Physical Examination and History

History

- Trauma usually not witnessed and details poorly described
- Important to exclude from history:
  - ☐ Nonaccidental injury
  - ☐ Pathologic fracture
  - ☐ Differential diagnosis (chronic ankle pain)

Clinical Features

- Inspection:
  - ☐ Open/closed
  - ☐ Impending skin breakdown
  - ☐ Bruising, swelling, deformity
  - ☐ Foot perfusion, capillary refill
- Palpation:
  - ☐ Local tenderness over fracture (may have tenderness anteriorly only with a Tillaux fracture, not along medial or lateral malleoli)
  - ☐ Salter-Harris type I fibula fracture: localized tenderness over bone rather than ligaments distinguishes this from sprain
  - ☐ Pedal pulses
  - ☐ Crepitus
- Movement:
  - ☐ Range of motion
- Special tests:
  - ☐ Neurologic assessment of sensation and foot intrinsic muscle function
  - ☐ Joint instability (ankle anterior drawer)

Radiologic Features

Imaging is not required (i.e., low risk of significant fracture being missed) if there is isolated pain and tenderness, edema, and swelling over distal fibula and adjacent ligament below level of joint line.

Radiographs

- Standard views: anteroposterior, lateral, mortise view (15- to 20-degree internal rotation oblique)
- Special views:
  - ☐ Oblique view in adolescents to exclude lateral fracture distal tibia (that would otherwise be overshadowed by fibula)
  - ☐ Stress views: occult joint instability

Computed Tomography

- To determine displacement in Tillaux, triplane fracture
- Best to do this after initial closed reduction to assess success

TREATMENT

- Aims:
  - ☐ To obtain and maintain a satisfactory reduction
  - ☐ To avoid joint incongruity or instability
  - ☐ To avoid growth plate incongruity and growth plate arrest

By Type

Salter-Harris Type I Fibula Fracture

- Below-knee walking cast for 3 weeks

Salter-Harris Type II Tibia Fracture

- May be more rotated than appears on anteroposterior and lateral view: consider oblique and assess clinically
- Closed reduction; hold reduction in molded cast for 3 weeks with weekly x-rays
- Can accept less than full reduction if no soft tissue interposition (less than 5 degrees varus, less than 10 degree valgus acceptable)
- If full reduction not possible because of periosteal interposition, open procedure required to remove periosteum

Salter-Harris Type III Tibia or Tillaux Fracture

- Intraarticular fracture requires reduction if displaced 2 mm or more
- Stabilize with Kirschner wire or screw directed parallel to physis and joint line
- Avoid crossing physis unless very near complete growth plate closure

Salter-Harris Type IV Tibia Fracture

- Intraarticular fracture and transphyseal fracture
- Requires accurate open reduction and internal fixation
- Thurston-Holland fragment can be used to stabilize fracture if large

Salter-Harris Type IV Triplane Fracture

- Intraarticular fracture and transphyseal fracture
- Computed tomography (CT) scan required to plan approach, reduction, and fixation
- Requires accurate open reduction and internal fixation
- Operation is difficult because of fragmentation and soft tissue swelling
- Many anatomic variants
- Order of reduction: posteromedial fragment → fibula fracture → anterolateral fragment

Salter-Harris Type V Tibia Fracture

- If recognized at time of injury, patient should be maintained non-weightbearing for 3 weeks to avoid further damage to the crushed part of the physis, although no intervention is known to reduce risk of partial growth arrest.

Ankle Dislocation

- Requires urgent closed reduction because soft tissues and neurovascular structures at risk.
- Often associated with open injuries.
- Should not delay initial manipulation to correct severe deformity to obtain a radiograph.
- Once reduced, radiographs or special imaging (e.g., CT scans) can be performed.

Summary of Treatment

Closed

- Indications: usually Salter-Harris type I or II fractures of tibia and fibula can be reduced.

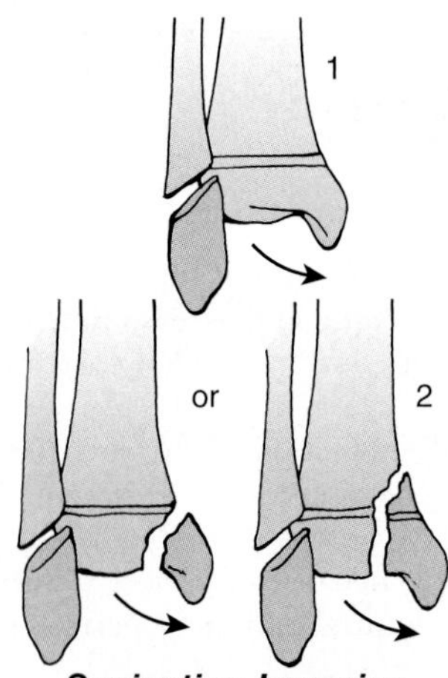

Supination-Inversion
Fully supinated foot sustains an inversion force

Grade 1: Traction produces SH I or II fracture of distal fibula (rarely ligament or avulsion fracture of tip of lateral malleolus)

Grade 2: Medial impaction causes SH III or IV fracture of medial tibia

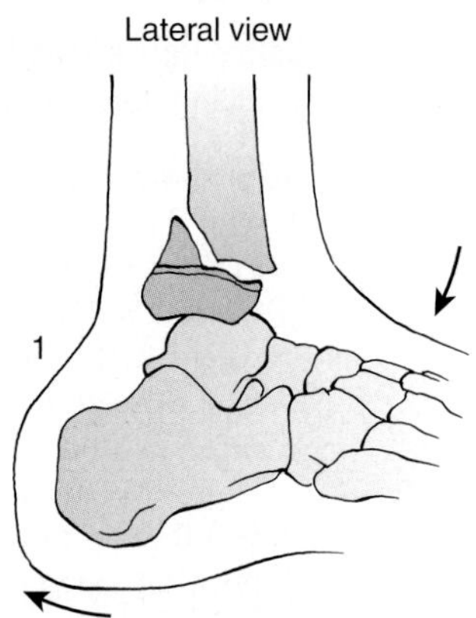

Supination-Plantarflexion
Fully supinated foot sustains a plantarflexion force

Grade 1: SH II (occasionally SH I) fracture of distal tibia best seen on lateral radiograph
- Metaphyseal fragment and displacement is posterior.

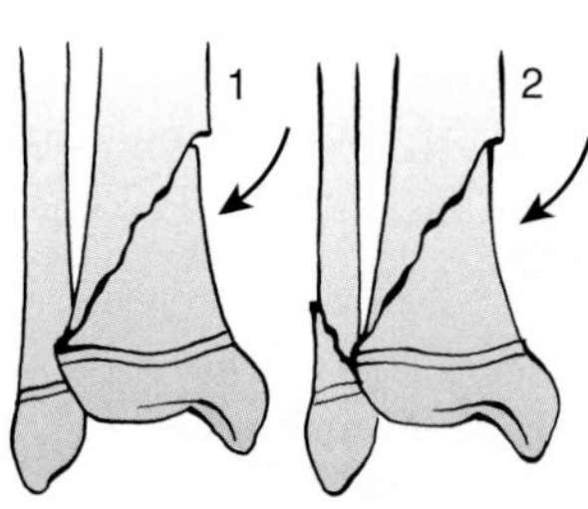

Supination-External Rotation
Fully supinated foot sustains an external rotation force

Grade 1: SH II fracture distal tibial epiphysis with a long spiral fracture of distal tibia:
- Starts laterally at the distal tibial growth plate
- Metaphyseal fragment and displacement posterior
- Similar to supination-plantarflexion injury, but in AP view fracture goes proximomedially

Grade 2: Additional spiral fracture fibula (medial superior to posterior).

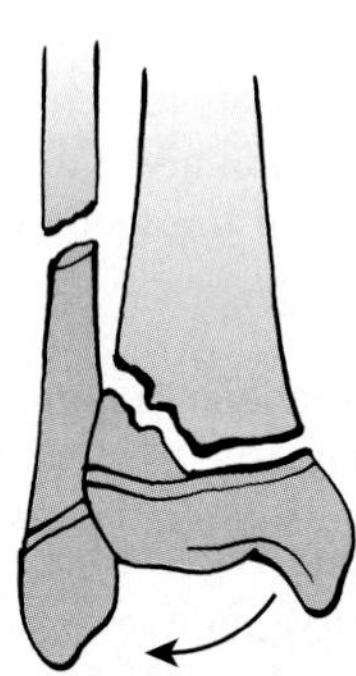

Pronation-Eversion-External Rotation
Pronated foot sustains an eversion-external rotation force

- Tibial fracture (usually SHII) and fibula fracture (short, oblique, 4 to 7 cm from tip of lateral malleolus)
- Metaphyseal fragment and displacement lateral or posterolateral

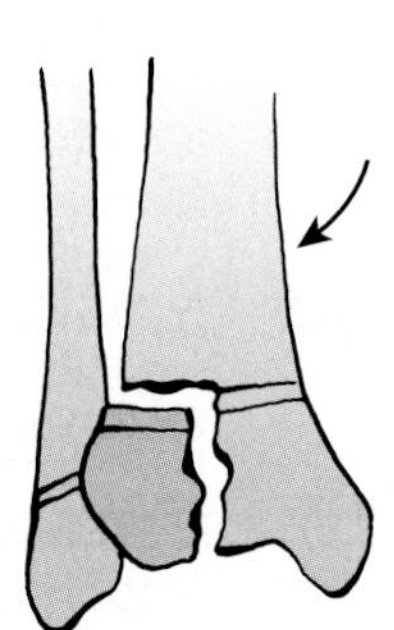

Salter-Harris III (Tillaux)
Effect of an external rotation force with a variable foot position

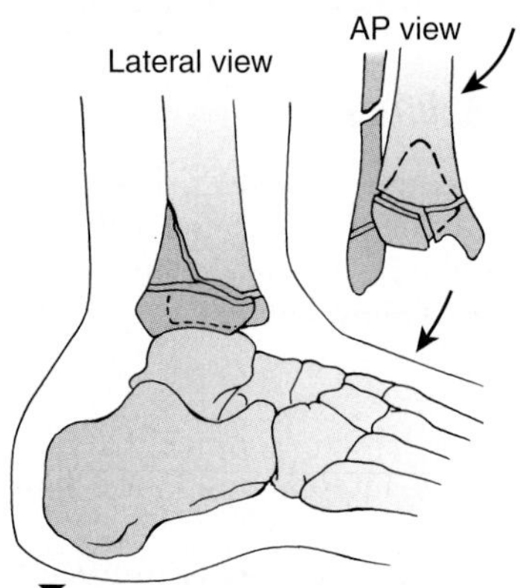

Triplane (Salter-Harris IV)
External rotation force with a variable foot position

Grade 1: SH III tibia on AP view and SH II metaphysis on lateral view

Grade 2: Additional high fracture of fibula

Figure 12-11.3 Dias and Tachdjian classification system of pediatric ankle fractures. *SH,* Salter-Harris. (Adapted from Dias LS, Tachdjian MO. Physeal injuries of the ankle in children. Clin Orthop Rel Res 1978;136:230–233.)

Open

- Indications:
  - □ Inability to obtain and maintain a closed reduction
  - □ Displaced intraarticular fracture (Salter-Harris type III or IV)
  - □ Displaced transphyseal fracture
  - □ Open fractures
- CT to plan approach
- Delay definitive open reduction until severe swelling of soft tissue has diminished (this may be up to 7 days)

Follow-Up

- For 2 years; growth arrest may occur at any time from 6 to 18 months
- Clinical and radiologic assessment for:
  - □ Angular deformity
  - □ Harris lines (nonparallel, closer together on side of growth arrest)
  - □ Leg length discrepancy: distal tibia contributes 2 to 3 mm of growth per year.

Complications

- Inability to obtain reduction
- Growth plate arrest:
  - □ In general, risk of growth arrest is higher with higher class of fracture in the Salter-Harris fracture classification system.
  - □ Salter-Harris types I and II: central arrest common. Early closure of growth plate compared with opposite ankle
  - □ Salter-Harris types III, IV, V, and VI: peripheral arrest/bone bridge leading to angulation:
    - □ Often varus deformity with supination inversion injury
    - □ Consider completing epiphysiodesis to prevent angulation
- Postoperative: wound complication, infection
- Medial malleolar ossicle
- Malunion, avascular necrosis, and nonunion—rare
- Talar dome osteochondral lesion: may become symptomatic after associated fracture is healed

Prognosis

- Depends on:
  - □ Skeletal age: bone, ligament, physis
  - □ Amount of soft tissue injury
  - □ Involvement of physis
  - □ Involvement of articular surface
  - □ Amount of fragmentation

SUGGESTED READING

Boutis K, Komar L, Jaramillo D, et al. Sensitivity of a clinical examination to predict need for radiography in children with ankle injuries: a prospective study. Lancet 2001;358:2118–2121.

Crawford A. Fractures and dislocations of the foot and ankle. In: Green NE, Swiontkowski MF, eds. Skeletal trauma in children, 2nd ed. Vol 3. Philadelphia: WB Saunders, 1998.

Dias LS, Tachdjian MO. Physeal injuries of the ankle in children. Clin Orthop Rel Res 1978;136:230–233.

Salter RB, Harris WR. Injuries involving the epiphyseal plate. J Bone Joint Surg (Am) 1963;45:587–622.

12.12 FOOT

JUAN A. REALYVASQUEZ

The ossification of a child's foot varies with age and influences fracture patterns, making recognition of injury more difficult. The calcaneus is the first bone to ossify, followed by the talus. The major mechanism of injury is direct force from a fall, being crushed by a heavy object, or indirect injury from a lawn mower or forceful rotation. Fortunately, the cartilage anlage gives the foot more resilience to injury.

FRACTURES OF THE TALUS

- Fractures of the talus are rare in children, and the pattern varies with age.
- In the very young child, an incompletely ossified talus is able to absorb more energy before disruption.
- Magnetic resonance imaging (MRI) and computed tomography (CT) scanning may be necessary to appreciate damage to the cartilaginous body.
- The mechanism of injury is usually forced dorsiflexion or dorsiflexion and rotation.

VASCULAR SUPPLY

- The main blood supply is provided by an anastomosis between the laterally arising artery of the sinus tarsi and medial artery of the tarsal canal.
- Both enter the talus inferiorly at the junction of the neck with the body.

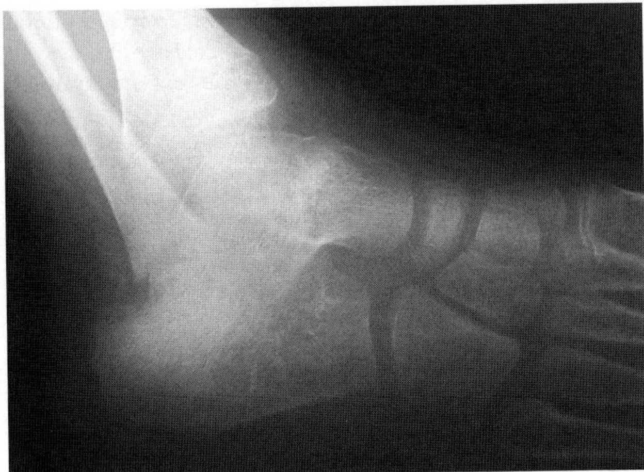

Figure 12.12-1 Hawkins sign.

- Hawkins sign, the presence of subchondral lucency, indicates an intact blood supply, resulting in osteopenia (Fig. 12.12-1).
- Marti classifies fractures of the talus by their potential to develop avascular necrosis (Table 12.12-1).

TREATMENT

Nondisplaced fractures of the talar neck are immobilized in a long leg cast with the knee bent to prevent weightbearing. Displaced fractures require open reduction and internal fixation and weightbearing is not allowed for 6 to 8 weeks.

Fractures of the body, especially if associated with dislocation, require immediate reduction. The posterior approach does not disturb the medial blood supply. An anteromedial approach combined with a medial malleolar osteotomy can be used.

Forceful supination and pronation on a dorsiflexed foot can lead to fractures of the medial and lateral process of the talus. These are often confused with ankle sprains and are common in snowboarders. A high index of suspicion is necessary and oblique views of the foot and ankle and CT are useful. Treatment for large or displaced fragments is open reduction.

TABLE 12.12-2 CLASSIFICATION OF OSTEOCHONDRAL FRACTURES OF THE TALUS

Type	Description
I	Trabecular compression that can only be seen by magnetic resonance imaging
IIA	An incomplete separation
IIB	A subchondral cyst
III	An unattached and nondisplaced fragment
IV	An unattached displaced fragment

Adapted from Anderson JF, Crichton KJ, Gratten-Smith T, et al. Osteochondral fractures of the dome of the talus. J Bone Joint Surg (Am) 1989;71:1143–1152.

Osteochondral fractures of the talus (Table 12.2-2 and Fig. 12.12-2) are the result of torsional impaction. Forceful plantar flexion and inversion combined with external rotation of the foot produces the medial lesion. Inversion and dorsiflexion produces an anterolateral lesion that can be accompanied by injury to the lateral ankle ligaments.

Treatment is directed at preservation of ankle joint congruity. Removal of a displaced fragment through medial malleolar osteotomy is reported and arthroscopic treatment may also be considered.

FRACTURES OF THE CALCANEUS

Calcaneal fractures are more common in children than talar fractures and are usually the result of a fall from a significant height. Most fractures involve the body and the subtalar joint. In the younger child, incomplete ossification makes diagnosis more difficult and an MRI may be indi-

TABLE 12.12-1 CLASSIFICATION OF TALAR FRACTURES

Type	Fracture Location	Blood Supply to Body	Necrosis
I	Distal talar neck	Intact	None
II	Proximal talar neck or body; nondisplaced	Largely intact	Rare
III	Fracture–dislocation of proximal neck or body	Interosseous intact; maxillary disrupted	Frequent
IV	Proximal neck fracture with body located out of mortise	Interosseus and auxiliary disrupted	Always

Adapted from Marti R. Fractures of the talus and calcaneus. In: Weber BG, Brunner CH, Freuler F, eds. Treatment of fractures in children and adolescents. New York: Springer-Verlag, 1980.

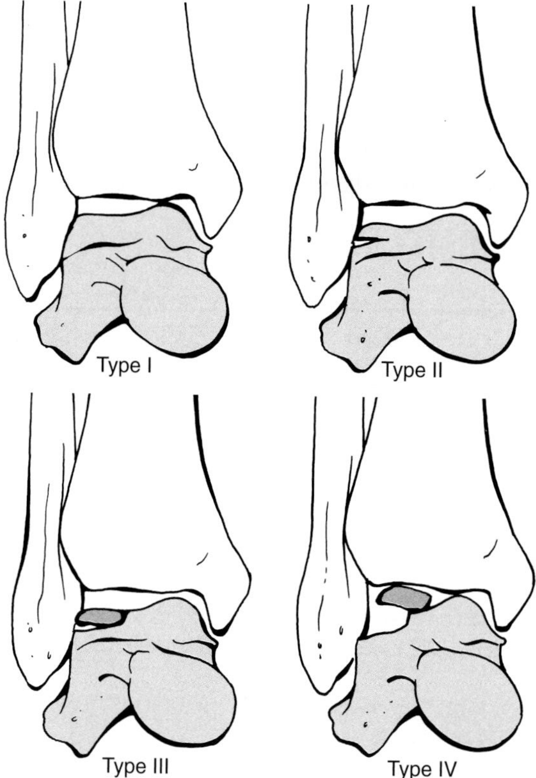

Figure 12.12-2 Osteochondral fractures of the talus. (Adapted from Marti R. Fractures of the talus and calcaneus. In: Weber BG, Brunner CH, Freuler F, eds. Treatment of fractures in children and adolescents. New York: Springer-Verlag, 1980.)

cated. Wiley's classification is most applicable to children and CT is helpful for visualization:

- Type I fractures involve the subtalar joint.
- Type II fractures do not involve the joint. Open reduction and restoration of the articular surface in intraarticular fractures is recommended.

FRACTURES OF THE ANTERIOR PROCESS OF THE TALUS

These can present as chronic foot pain with peroneal spasm and may be confused with ankle sprains. Accurate diagnosis requires an oblique x-ray or CT scan. Cast immobilization is usually successful in acute injuries, but excision of a loose fragment may be necessary in chronic problems.

CALCANEAL STRESS FRACTURES

These may be confused with Achilles tendonitis, plantar fasciitis, or other causes of heel pain. Diagnosis is made by clinical examination and confirmed by bone scan. A swollen painful heel without a history of trauma should raise suspicion. Tenderness is localized to the posterosuperior aspect and the medial and lateral aspect of the calcaneus. Radiographs are usually negative for up to 3 weeks; however bone scan or MRI may be useful in establishing an early diagnosis. Treatment is rest and limited weight-bearing and resumption of activities is not recommended before 4 to 6 weeks.

OCCULT FRACTURES

An occult fracture of the calcaneus has been found in young children resulting from minor trauma. Pain is elicited by medial and lateral compression and scintigraphy can confirm the diagnosis. Treatment is immobilization with follow-up radiographs showing the fracture and callus.

FRACTURES OF THE MIDFOOT

Fractures of the midfoot are rare and the result of direct trauma from a falling object or indirect force from a fall applied on a plantarflexed foot. Fractures of the tarsal navicular are rare and are classified into three anatomic sites (tuberosity, dorsal lip, body) plus stress fractures, which are seen in runners.

FRACTURES OF THE TUBEROSITY

These are the result of an acute eversion force. The fragment is usually not displaced. Treatment is cast immobilization with molding of the medial longitudinal arch. Nonunion can occur and if associated with recurrent symptoms, excision of the fragment is recommended. Differentiation from an accessory navicular is made by smooth contour of the line of separation in the latter.

FRACTURES OF THE DORSAL LIP

These are the most common type of navicular fractures. They are associated with sprains occurring in the inverted, plantarflexed foot. Treatment is similar to an ankle sprain. If a significant portion of the joint is involved, open reduction is necessary to preserve the integrity of the medial longitudinal arch.

FRACTURES OF THE BODY

These are the least common of all navicular injuries (Table 12.12-3). A direct force will cause comminuted nondisplaced fractures, whereas force from a fall on the hyperplantar flexed foot will result in dislocation and injury to

TABLE 12.12-3 CLASSIFICATION OF NAVICULAR BODY FRACTURES

Type	Description
I	Fracture line in plane of foot resulting in dorsal and plantar fragments
II	Fracture line passes dorsolateral to plantar medial resulting in medial and lateral fragment
III	Severe comminution of the body of the navicular

the head of the talus and other tarsal bones. Marked displacements will disrupt the subtalar and midtarsal joints and lead to degenerative arthritis. Treatment is restoration of the joint surface by closed or open methods. Severely comminuted type III fractures may require primary arthrodesis.

STRESS FRACTURES OF THE NAVICULAR

These have been described in children who perform high-impact sports or activities. They are associated with the tight heel cords limiting dorsiflexion of the foot, a short first metatarsal or metatarsus adductus, or limited subtalar motion. The presenting symptom is pain in the medial longitudinal arch with tenderness on compression of the tarsal navicular. The fracture is best visualized by a true anteroposterior radiograph of the foot centered on the navicular. Treatment is a cast immobilization and non-weightbearing for at least 6 weeks. Surgery is recommended if there is delay in healing and the fracture extends through two cortices.

FRACTURES OF THE METATARSALS

- Metatarsal fractures are usually nondisplaced. Lisfranc injuries mimic adult patterns.
- Mechanisms of injury as listed in Box 12.12-1.
- Multiple fractures occur proximally in the first metatarsal and distally in the lateral four rays.

BOX 12.12-1 MECHANISM OF INJURY IN TARSOMETATARSAL INJURIES

- Striking an object while in tiptoe position (jumping from a height to the ground)
- Heel-to-toe compression (foot crushed while kneeling)
- Foot fixed in plantarflexion while falling backward

- Fracture of the first metatarsal is more common before the age of 5 years and often goes unrecognized at the initial evaluation.
- Cuneiform fractures can also occur and these usually heal uneventfully unless the fracture involves the physis.
- Accurate reduction is necessary to prevent growth disturbance from early physeal closure.

TUBEROSITY

- In children, the apophysis of the fifth metatarsal does not appear until age 8 and is seen as a line parallel to the shaft.
- Fractures of the tuberosity are avulsion fractures and have a better prognosis.
- Avulsion fractures are transverse and are treated in a short leg cast.

SHAFT

- Usually the result of a crash injury.
- Treated with compression dressing, casting, and elevation.
- Reduction is necessary if the metatarsal heads are displaced or plantarflexed.

STRESS FRACTURES

- Common in ballet dancers, runners, and gymnasts.
- Second metatarsal is most commonly involved, followed closely by the third.
- Predisposing factors include overtraining, delayed menarche, and poor nutrition.
- Treatment is a short leg cast for 6 to 8 weeks.

JONES FRACTURE

- Fracture of the proximal fifth metatarsal is the most common metatarsal fracture and is common in children over the age of 10.
- It is a transverse fracture at the junction of the metaphysis and diaphysis (Fig. 12.12-3).

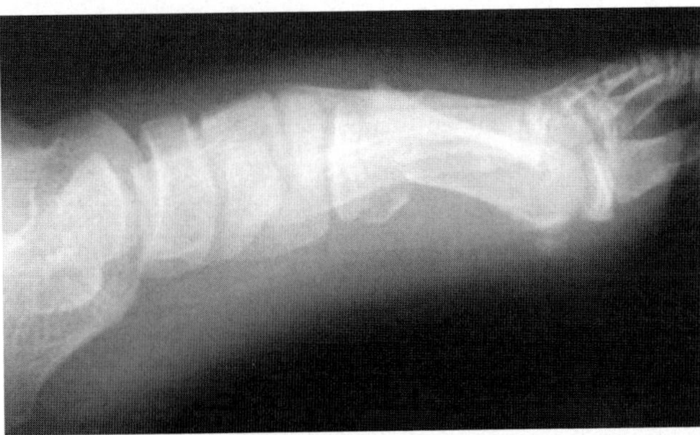

Figure 12.12-3 Jones fracture.

BOX 12.12-2 CLINICAL FEATURES OF COMPRESSION SYNDROME

- Pain that is progressive, not relieved by narcotics, and out of proportion to examination
- Pain with passive range of motion of the toes
- Parasthesias: decreased pin, light touch, or two-point discrimination
- Pulselessness: absent palpable or Doppler pulses
- Cool, tense foot
- Motor deficit

- Treatment is difficult because of poor blood supply.
- The presence of previous injury, such as sclerosis or pre-install reaction, often leads to delayed union, nonunion, and refractors.
- Acute injury is treated with a short leg cast for 6 weeks or until the fracture is healed radiographically.
- Surgery is recommended for fracture with evidence of chronic injury.
- Grafting can be done in delayed unions.
- Return to full activity before complete healing is often associated with treatment failure.

COMPARTMENT SYNDROME

- Evaluation for compartment syndrome must be considered in all injuries to the foot.
- It is most common in crush injuries of the foot with fractures of the metatarsals, phalanges, and Lisfranc dislocation.
- Surgical decompression is required.
- Box 12.12-2 outlines clinical features.

FRACTURES OF THE PHALANGES

- Most common injury of the forefoot.
- May result from direct axial injury (striking the toe against an object) or a crush injury.
- Fractures of the proximal phalanx of the great toe require accurate reduction of displacement and angulations.
- Salter-Harris type III physeal injuries are common and require open reduction if displaced to restore the joint surface.
- Fractures of the distal phalanx, even if crushed, require alignment of the toe and nail should be preserved as it acts as splint.
- Phalanx fractures of the lesser toes can be treated less aggressively, however reduction is necessary for displaced plantarflexed fractures of the head as they can cause abnormal plantar pressure.

LESIONS THAT MAY BE CONFUSED WITH FRACTURES

Sever disease or calcaneal apophysitis is a common finding in the rapidly growing child athlete. The child presents with heel pain and tenderness is elicited on compression of the metaphysis and not the apophysis. Treatment is rest, physical therapy, and orthotics.

The accessory navicular is also often a source of foot pain. Its opposition and intimate association with the posterior tibial tendon can result in a tendonitis known as a prehallux syndrome. This is often associated with a pronated flat foot. Ogden describes three types of accessory navicular: ossicle in substance of posterior tendon, synchondrosis, and cornuate navicular. Treatment is rest and immobilization in a cast followed by orthotic support of the medial longitudinal arch. Persistent pain is relieved by excision of the accessory navicular. Advancement of the posterior tibial tendon does not restore the arch.

Freilberg's infraction is an avascular necrosis of the second metatarsal head and is often confused with a fracture. It is more common in adolescent girls and is associated with repetitive trauma. It can be symptomatic for up to 6 months before radiographic changes are visible. Hamilton describes four types (Table 12.2-4). Treatment of type I is cast immobilization, while surgery is indicated in types II and III. Each metatarsal is treated individually.

Köhler's disease is a clinical diagnosis presenting with a painful limp and tenderness of the tarsal navicular. It is more common in boys, presenting around the age of 5 years. In girls it presents at age 4 and is unilateral in the majority of cases. Köhler's disease is associated with x-ray changes of density and narrowing of the navicular.

Treatment of Köhler's disease is immobilization in a short leg walking cast for 8 weeks. Casting for a shorter period may result in recurrence of symptoms and prolonged recovery.

TABLE 12.12-4 VARIANTS OF FREIBERG INFARCTION

Type	Description
I	Avascular necrosis of head heals by "creeping substitution"
II	Head collapses during revascularization but articular surface remains intact
III	Head collapses and articular surface is disrupted
IV	Multiple heads involved (form of epiphyseal dysplasia)

Adapted from Hamilton WG. Foot and ankle injuries in dancers. In: Mann RA, Coughlin MJ, eds. Surgery of the foot and ankle. St Louis: Mosby, 1993.

SUGGESTED READING

Anderson JF, Crichton KJ, Gratten-Smith T, et al. Osteochondral fractures of the dome of the talus. J Bone Joint Surg (Am) 1989;71A: 1143–1152.

Berndt AL, Harty M. Transchondral fractures. J Pediatr Orthop 2001; 10B:68–72.

Bibbo C, Lin S, Cunningham FJ. Acute traumatic compartment syndrome of the foot in children. Pediatr Emerg Care 2000;16:244–248.

Hamilton WG. Foot and ankle injuries in dancers. In: Mann RA, Coughlin MJ, eds. Surgery of the foot and ankle. St Louis: Mosby, 1993.

Laliotis N, Pennie BH, Carty H, et al. Toddler's fracture of the calcaneus. Injury 1993;24:169–170.

Marti R. Fractures of the talus and calcaneus. In: Weber BG, Brunner CH, Freuler F, eds. Treatment of fractures in children and adolescents. New York: Springer-Verlag, 1980.

Owen RJ, Hickey FG, Finley DB. A study of metatarsal fractures in children. Injury 1995;26:537–538.

Spitz DJ, Newberg AH. Imaging of stress fractures in the athlete. Radiogr Clin North Am 2002;40:313–331.

Wiley JJ, Prifitt A. Fractures of the os calcis in children. Clin Orthop Rel Res 1984;188:131–138.

Williams GA, Cowell, Henry HR. Köhler's disease of the tarsal navicular. Clin Orthop Rel Res 1981;158:53–58.

POLYTRAUMA

R. DALE BLASIER

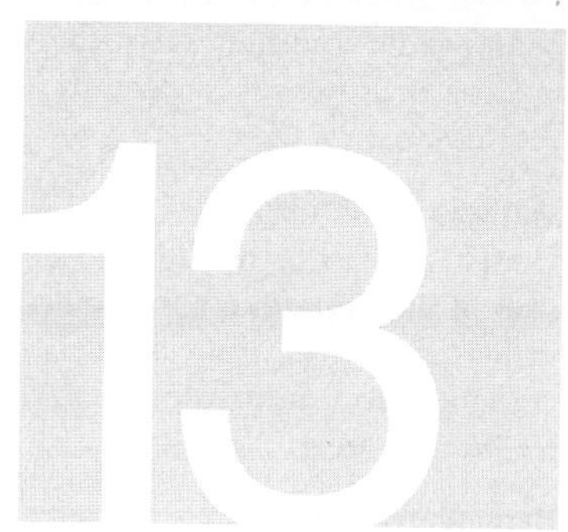

The treatment of fractures in children who have multiple injuries is often complex. Fractures that are complicated by truncal, burn, or head injuries may be especially challenging. These children may be *in extremis* or very unstable at the time of presentation and thus may be poor candidates for anesthesia. Nonorthopaedic injuries may take precedence and orthopaedic procedures postponed. However, because of the unique problems that occur in these patients both immediately after the injury and in the long term, operative stabilization of fractures often can provide great benefits. The sickest patients may benefit the most from surgery; however, unlike adults, children do not derive any significant protection from pulmonary complications as a result of long bone fracture stabilization.

PATHOGENESIS

Epidemiology

Injury is the leading cause of death and a major cause of disability in children. Only acute infection causes more morbidity than trauma. The estimated annual cost of pediatric injury is greater than 7.5 billion dollars, with estimates of loss of future productivity at greater than 8 billion dollars.

Etiology

Blunt trauma causes 65% to 90% of childhood injury although the incidence of penetrating injury is rising. Motor vehicle accidents, pedestrian injuries, recreational vehicle injuries, major falls, and physical abuse are common causes.

Pathophysiology

Third Spacing

Several factors contribute to massive soft tissue swelling and fluid accumulation, including the cycle of hypoperfusion and reperfusion, direct contusion, fluid and electrolyte imbalances, and sepsis. Increased interstitial fluid makes access to and evaluation of internal structures difficult. Surgery and wound closure are difficult in swollen tissues. Organ function is diminished by fluid accumulation and swelling, especially in the brain and lung. It often takes several days to resorb excess interstitial fluid after resolution of hemodynamic, metabolic, and septic derangements.

Head Injury

Head injury by itself is a serious problem and source of morbidity and mortality. This is worsened when there is polytrauma. Increased intracranial pressure is always a source of concern and usually requires intracranial pressure monitoring. Increased pressure may prevent or delay surgical repair of other internal or skeletal injuries. The brain injury itself may cause abnormal posturing, increased muscle tone, or agitated movements—all of which can make fracture management difficult. Injury-induced or medically induced coma will render the child immobile and require constant vigilance for contractures and bedsores. The search for additional injuries is more difficult in the child who is unresponsive. Special care must be taken to look for associated injuries which could otherwise be missed.

Respiratory Failure

Pulmonary contusion, sepsis, fluid–electrolyte imbalances, and multiple transfusions may all have an effect on fluid accumulation in the lung parenchyma that results in decreased oxygenation of the blood. Intubation and sedation are usually required. Hypoxemia will prevent prompt orthopaedic surgery. It may take several days for pulmonary problems to resolve.

Sepsis

Infection is not uncommon in the polytrauma patient within the first several days of injury. Frequently the lungs are the source of infection. Sepsis may contribute to multiple organ failure. It may require the use of multiple antibiotics—some with side effects. It complicates fluid and electrolyte management and provides an undesirable setting for the placement of internal orthopaedic implants.

Internal Injuries

Intraabdominal and intrathoracic injuries can be life-threatening. Their management nearly always takes priority over that of orthopaedic injury. Unless simultaneous orthopaedic and general surgery is possible (and it rarely is), the orthopaedic procedures must follow treatment of the internal injuries.

Multiple Transfusions

While isolated orthopaedic injuries rarely require transfusion of blood products, multiple injuries often do. Multiple transfusions will often be associated with interstitial fluid accumulation, impaired blood clotting, and decreased systemic immunity.

Hypoalimentation

Obviously, normal intake of fluids and nutrients is interrupted after severe trauma. Mobilized stores of nutrients will sustain the child for a few days. After that, alimentation must be provided either enterally or intravenously to provide substrates for healing and repair.

The Intensive Care Setting

The orthopaedist is rarely a master of the intensive care unit setting. Intensivists tend to make the important treatment decisions and often the orthopaedist must receive permission before initiating treatment for skeletal injuries. The orthopaedist is often not familiar with intensive care techniques and procedures. Likewise, intensivists and intensive care nurses are frequently unfamiliar with orthopaedic devices and casts. Parents are often distraught or restless. Patient and diligent communication must be maintained between medical professionals and with parents.

Classification

The Modified Injury Severity Scale (MISS) may be useful for children with multiple injuries (Table 13-1). Treatment decision must not be based on injury scale. Unless the child is clearly going to die, orthopaedic treatment must proceed as if the child is going to survive.

DIAGNOSIS

Physical Examination and History

Clinical Features

- Deformity: splints and clothing must be removed to really see deformity.
- Bleeding: watch for poke holes over fracture sites.

TABLE 13-1 MODIFIED INJURY SEVERITY SCALE FOR CHILDREN WITH MULTIPLE INJURIES

Region	1—Minor	2—Moderate	3—Severe; Not Life-Threatening	4—Severe; Life-Threatening	5—Critical; Survival Uncertain
CNS	GCS (Table 13-2) 13–14; abrasion or contusion of the eye or lid	GCS 9–12; undisplaced facial fracture	GCS 9–12; loss of eye; avulsion of optic nerve	GCS 5–8; bone or soft tissue injury with minor destruction	GCS 4 with airway obstruction
Neck and face	Vitreous or conjunctival hemorrhage	Laceration of the eye; disfiguring laceration	Displaced facial fracture; orbital blowout fracture		
Thorax	Muscle ache or chest wall stiffness	Simple rib or sternal fracture	Multiple rib fractures; hemothorax or pneumothorax; diaphragmatic rupture	Open chest wound; pneumomediastinum; cardiac contusion	Hemomediastinum; laceration to trachea, aorta, or heart; cardiac rupture
Abdomen	Muscle ache; seat belt abrasion	Major abdominal wall contusion	Visceral contusion; retroperitoneal hematoma; extraperitoneal bladder rupture; thoracic or spine fracture	Major visceral laceration; intraperitoneal bladder rupture; spine fracture with paraplegia	Rupture or laceration of vessel or viscus
Pelvis and extremities	Minor sprains; simple fractures or dislocations	Open fractures of digits; nondisplaced long bones or pelvic fracture	Displaced long bone fractures; multiple hand or foot fractures; displaced single long bone or pelvis fracture; major nerve or muscle injury	Multiple closed long fractures; amputation of limb	Multiple long bone fractures

CNS, central nervous system; GCS, Glasgow Coma Scale score (Table 13-2).
Adapted from Mayer T, Matlak ME, Johnson DG, Walker ML. The Modified Injury Severity Scale in pediatric trauma patients. J Pediatr Surg 1980;15:719–726.

- Swelling and ecchymosis: key to underlying injury but take some time to develop.
- Tenderness: pain on palpation is always key. Even unconscious patient may manifest a useful response.
- Abnormal motion: movement in the middle of a long bone or out of the plane of joint motion indicates radiography is necessary.
- Crepitus: common after displaced fracture and reminds examiner that a splint will be necessary.
- Pulses: important to document but not as important as perfusion status.
- Neurologic function: important to note before treatment is instituted. If a good neurologic examination isn't possible, write a note that explains why and remember to come back later and keep trying.

Radiologic Features

- Chest, cervical spine, and pelvis films should be ordered automatically.
- Spine and extremity films should be requested based on clinical evaluation.
- Computed tomography (CT) scanning of spine or pelvis is indicated by suspicious radiographic or clinical evaluation.
- In suspected abuse cases, a skeletal survey is medicolegally indicated. Multiple fractures in various stages of healing and metaphyseal corner fractures are highly suggestive of abuse. Spiral fractures are not.
- Technetium bone scanning will be helpful to locate skeletal injuries in victims who are very young or unable to manifest a pain response because of central nervous system injury.
- Magnetic resonance imaging to evaluate joint derangement is not a priority in the acute injury phase.

Diagnostic Workup

- The history is always important and leads the examiner to suspected areas of injury.
- It is useful to know what the emergency transport team perceived to be injured at the scene.
- Obviously life-threatening conditions take priority over orthopaedic injuries.
- Splinted limbs should be rechecked with the splint removed if possible.
- Obvious deformities should be noted. Open wounds must be noted.
- Assume spinal injury until proved otherwise.
- An inconsistent or changing history may suggest nonaccidental trauma. Be on the lookout.
- Get plain radiographs of suspicious areas.
- Ensure limb perfusion. If a problem, get help from the surgeons.
- Provisional splintage decreases pain and limits further soft tissue injury.
- Obtain special studies—CT scans, arteriograms, and so forth.
- Think about and look for compartment syndrome, especially in patients unable to feel or speak.

TABLE 13-2 GLASGOW COMA SCALE

Eyes Open	**Score**
Spontaneously	4
To verbal command	3
To pain	2
No response	1
Best Motor Response	
To verbal command:	
Obeys	6
To painful stimulus:	
Localizes pain	5
Flexion-withdrawal	4
Flexion-abnormal (decorticate rigidity)	3
Extension (decerebrate rigidity)	2
No response	1
Best Verbal Response	
Oriented and converses	5
Disoriented and converses	4
Inappropriate words	3
Incomprehensible sounds	2
No response	1
Total	3-15

The Glasgow coma scale, which is based upon eye opening, verbal, and motor responses is a practical means of monitoring changes in level of consciousness. If each response on the scale is given a number (high for normal and low for impaired responses), the responsiveness of the patient can be expressed by the summation of the figures. The lowest score is 3 and the highest is 15.

- Wash out open injuries as soon as it is safe for the patient.
- Make plans to fix each fracture that would require surgery as if it were an isolated injury as soon as possible.
- Consider stabilizing major bone fractures (i.e., femur, humerus, pelvis) to facilitate patient care.
- Work hard to stabilize fractures within limbs that will require frequent or painful manipulation, like those with traumatic wounds, skin loss, burns, or compartment syndromes.

TREATMENT

Surgical Anatomy and Biomechanics

- Treatment of the uncomplicated femur fracture in young children often includes the use of traction or a spica cast.
  - Polytraumatized children often need to be turned, transported, and scanned—all of which are made difficult by traction.
  - Spica casts limit access to the limbs and abdomen.
- Stabilization of long bone fractures enables transport and leaves the limbs and trunk free for examination or treatment.
- Stabilization of long bone fractures eliminates further damage to soft tissue by underlying mobile bone segments and may limit further bleeding.

- This is especially important in patients with head-injuries, who may be agitated or become spastic.
- Patients with traumatic wounds, burns, or compartment syndrome of limbs will likely need regular and repeated access to the extremities.
  - Circumferential casts make this difficult.
  - Without support, the fractured limb is painful and repeated manipulations for dressing changes would be cruel.
  - Stabilization of the skeleton makes wound management much easier.
- Bony spinal injuries may render the spine unstable and render the neurologic structures at risk.
  - Surgical stabilization lessens pain with movement and protects the neural elements from unstable segments.

Surgical Indications, Contraindications, and Nonoperative Options (Fig. 13-1)

- Simple closed fractures distal to the elbow or knee should be managed with reduction and splintage or casting.
- Open fractures need surgical irrigation and drainage.
  - Stable fractures can be splinted or casted.

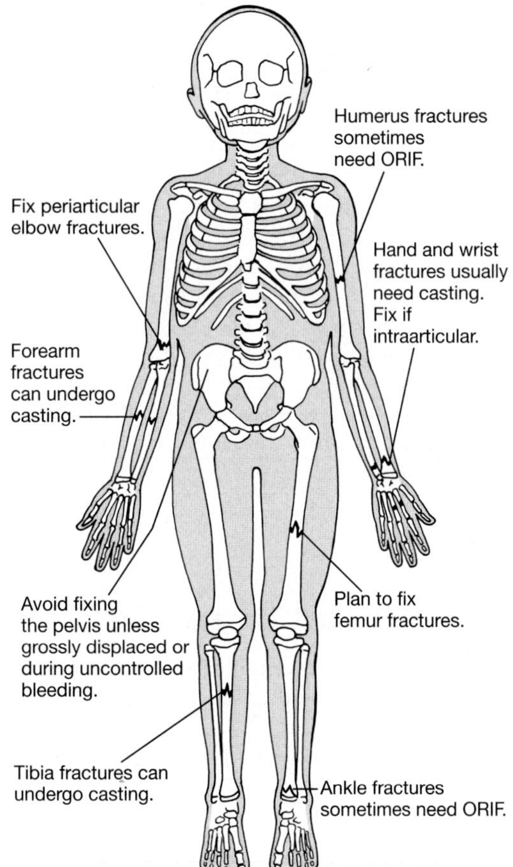
Humerus fractures sometimes need ORIF.
Fix periarticular elbow fractures.
Hand and wrist fractures usually need casting. Fix if intraarticular.
Forearm fractures can undergo casting.
Avoid fixing the pelvis unless grossly displaced or during uncontrolled bleeding.
Plan to fix femur fractures.
Tibia fractures can undergo casting.
Ankle fractures sometimes need ORIF.

Figure 13-1 Periarticular fractures should be fixed just as indicated in isolated injuries. Fractures distal to knee and elbow can generally be managed in a cast. The threshold should be lowered for fixing the pelvis, humerus, and femur in the polytrauma patient. ORIF, open reduction and internal fixation.

  - Unstable fractures or those that require frequent wound care will benefit from surgical stabilization.
- Fractures of the femoral shaft should be stabilized in multiply-injured children older than 6 years for the same reasons as they are in children with fracture only.
- Surgical stabilization should be considered for shaft fracture of the femur in polytraumatized children of any age for the following reasons:
  - Facilitate transport (i.e., in and out of scanners)
  - Facilitate hygiene
  - Facilitate wound, burn, or skin care
  - Facilitate rehabilitation
  - Obtain or maintain reasonable bony alignment which cannot be done by closed means
  - Control alignment and limit shortening and further soft tissue injury in patients with head injuries who are spastic or agitated
  - Aid in pain control
- Fractures of the pelvis should be stabilized if there is gross displacement, gross instability, or expanding hematoma that does not stabilize with transfusion.
- Fractures of humeral shaft do not generally require surgical fixation, but in general the threshold for surgical fixation can be lowered in the polytrauma setting.
- Reasons to consider surgical fixation include the following:
  - Inability to maintain alignment with usual splintage in a recumbent position
  - Difficulty with access to venous or arterial circulation due to splintage of upper arm
  - Multiple injuries in the same limb
  - Skin or wound problems of chest or upper arm
  - Agitation or spasticity in the patient with head injury
  - Proximate nerve or vascular injury
- Periarticular fractures that would be managed by surgery in otherwise normal patients should be managed by surgery.
  - Postponing surgery because the child has a head injury or truncal injury often leads to problems or a compromised result.
  - The following scenario must be avoided: The child is believed to be too sick to fix an orthopaedic injury and is likely to die. The child recovers, and the untreated orthopaedic injury becomes a major problem and a difficult reconstruction.
- Fractures under burns can be safely fixed up to 48 hours after injury.
  - Incision through or around burned skin is relatively safe.
  - After that, the skin must be considered to be colonized with bacteria and open reduction with internal fixation will be prone to infection.
  - Minimal or external fixation should be considered.
  - Otherwise, fixation should be delayed until skin healing or grafting.

Surgical Options and Preoperative Planning

- Intramedullary fixation is ideal for closed fractures of long bones (see sections on individual bone injuries).

- In patients unable to tolerate extreme positioning or vigorous pushing and pulling, external fixation and plating may be good solutions.
- External fixation is almost always the quickest and easiest solution for long bone fracture but commits the patient to daily pin care.
- Try to avoid operating on the pelvis.
  - Use an anterior external fixator if simple stabilization is needed.
  - Be prepared to place anterior plates and posterior sacroiliac screws for the unstable pelvis in older children.
- Periarticular fixation should be performed as in patients with isolated injury.

Surgical Goals

- Do not harm the patient. Unresponsive shock and severely elevated intracranial pressure are reasons to delay fracture treatment.
- Try to minimize blood loss and operative time in the sick patient.
- Try to achieve stability that obviates the need for cast or splintage, especially proximal to the elbow or knee.
- Goals for stabilization:
  - Pain control
  - Patient portability
  - Free access to trunk and circulation
  - Fracture alignment
  - Easy access to skin, burns, and traumatic wounds

Complications

Infection

- Infection is always a possibility in the trauma patient.
- The possibility of infection should not be a deterrent to skeletal stabilization, but active systemic sepsis should be.
- Treat wound infection in the trauma patient just as in any other patient.

Failed Fixation

- Unlike patients with isolated injuries, polytrauma patients are often manipulated by others who cannot feel the pain.
- Skeletal fixation should be strong enough to protect against the manipulations of caretakers.
- Head-injured or previously spastic patients may thrash about or have intense muscle spasms that can overcome weak fixation.
- Be prepared to use strong fixation devices in these patients.

Contracture

- Prevention is easier than treatment.
- Equinus contracture is ubiquitous in bedridden patients.
- Ankle–foot orthoses and daily manipulation are helpful.
- Flexion contractures of elbows, knees, and hips are not uncommon.
- Daily physical therapy and varied positioning are helpful.

Missed Injury

- Warn the parents about the possibility of missed injury in the obtunded patient.
- Check the patient at each visitation by palpating and tying to elicit tenderness.
- Have a low threshold for obtaining radiographs.

Heterotopic Ossification

- Not uncommon in the polytrauma patient, especially if there is head injury.
- Preventive treatment is not indicated.
- Symptomatic residuals of heterotopic ossification can be treated after the patient is stabilized.

Postoperative Management

- Positioning patients to maximize pulmonary care and social interaction is important.
- Mobilization of joints through active movement—in those who can—and passive movement—in those who cannot—is important to maintain function.
- Children who will need their upper limbs to provide mobility with either crutches or wheelchair after the acute phase of trauma should begin working on strength as soon as possible in the hospital.

PEARLS

- Survey and resurvey for injuries. Missed injuries in the polytrauma setting are an embarrassment for the physician and may be a cause for medicolegal action. Warn the parents of the obtunded child that some injuries are hard to find and may not be apparent at first.
- Fat embolism syndrome does occur in children and adolescents. Watch for mental status changes with tachycardia and decrease in arterial oxygenation after long bone fracture.
- Rib fractures are a danger sign. They generally occur in two clinical settings: high-energy trauma and abuse. Look for associated injuries.
- Always assume the child is going to recover.
- Try to operate before the child gets sick. Problems with fluid retention, sepsis, respiratory failure, and skin contamination with hospital flora are likely to worsen in the first few days after injury.
- Warn parents that recovery may not be full. Take the time to explain enough pathophysiology so that parents do not confuse neurologic residuals with bad fracture treatment.
- Don't lose track of the patient. Polytrauma patients often are transferred to rehabilitation units after the acute phase of treatment. It is important that they are followed for their fractures by an orthopaedic surgeon.

- Weightbearing should be encouraged as soon as callus is seen unless there are other mitigating factors.
- For larger children who are unable to transfer, consider the home use of a hospital bed, lift, and bedside commode.
- Let the lawyer know that it may be years before the permanent residuals of injury can be fully realized in the growing child.

SUGGESTED READING

Blasier RD. Treatment of fractures complicated by burn or head injuries in children. J Bone Joint Surg (Am) 1999;81:1038–1043.

Ciarallo L, Fleisher G. Femoral fractures: are children at risk for significant blood loss? Pediatr Emerg Care 1996;12:343–346.

Cramer KE. The pediatric polytrauma patient. Clin Orthop 1995;318: 125–135.

Dossett AB, Hunt JL, Purdue GF, et al. Early orthopaedic intervention in burn patients with major fractures. J Trauma 1991;31:888–893.

Garcia VF, Gotschall CS, Eichelberger MR, et al. Rib fractures in children: a marker of severe trauma. J Trauma 1990;30:695–700.

Hedequist D, Starr AJ, Wilson P, et al. Early versus delayed stabilization of pediatric femur fractures: analysis of 387 patients. J Orthop Trauma 1999;13:490–493.

Heinrich SD, Gallagher D, Harris M, et al. Undiagnosed fractures in severely injured children and young adults: identification with technetium imaging. J Bone Joint Surg (Am) 1994;76:561–572.

Loder RT. Pediatric polytrauma: orthopaedic care and hospital course. J Orthop Trauma 1987;1:48–54.

Loder RT, Gullahorn LJ, Yian EH, et al. Factors predictive of immobilization complications in pediatric polytrauma. J Orthop Trauma 2001;15:338–341.

Mendelson SA, Dominick T, Tyler-Kabara E, et al. Early versus late femoral fracture stabilization in multiply injured pediatric patients with closed head injury. J Pediatr Orthop 2001;21:594–599.

Porat S, Milgrom C, Nyska M, et al. Femoral fracture treatment in head-injured children: use of external fixation. J Trauma 1986;26:81–84.

Stauffer UG. Indications for operative treatment of fractures in childhood. Prog Pediatr Surg 1978;12:187–208.

Tolo VT. External fixation in multiply injured children. Orthop Clin North Am 1990;21:393–400.

Tolo VT. Orthopaedic treatment of fractures of the long bones and pelvis in children who have multiple injuries. J Bone Joint Surg (Am) 2000;82:272–282.

Ziv I, Rang M. Treatment of femoral fracture in the child with head injury. J Bone Joint Surg (Br) 1983;65:276–278.

OPEN FRACTURES

KATHRYN E. CRAMER

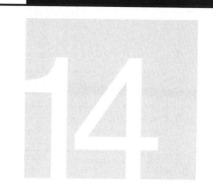

Open fractures in children are a heterogenous group of injuries. While the goals of treatment are similar to those in adults, the methods used to achieve these goals may differ. Children heal more quickly, have significant remodeling potential, and generally have fewer premorbid conditions than adults. However, open physes and size limitations preclude many of the fixation options available for adult fractures.

PATHOGENESIS

Etiology

- Occur as a result of higher energy injuries
- Associated injuries seen in 25% to 75% of children with open fractures
- Motor vehicle accidents, pedestrians/bicyclists hit by vehicles, and falls are common causes.
- 10% of all polytraumatized children have open fractures.

Epidemiology

- While pediatric fractures are extremely common, open fractures fortunately account for only 2% of the total.
- Higher energy trauma results in higher grade injuries.

Pathophysiology

- Higher energy required to cause an open fracture results in increased comminution and soft tissue stripping.
- Communication with the external environment allows foreign material and bacteria to contaminate the fracture site.
- Necrotic soft tissue and bone are easily infected and poor antibiotic penetration in these areas makes controlling any infection difficult.
- Fracture stabilization of unstable fractures prevents further soft tissue damage, and allows for neovascularization and healing.

Classification

Open fractures in children are classified by the same system used in adults (Gustilo classification) (Table 14-1).

DIAGNOSIS

Physical Examination and History

History

- Mechanism
- Time of injury
- Medical history
- Tetanus immunization

Physical Examination

- Head-to-toe evaluation of entire patient to rule out other injuries—remember your ABCs!
- Detailed evaluation of injured extremity, including skin condition
  - ☐ Neurologic exam
  - ☐ Vascular exam
  - ☐ Size and configuration of wound
  - ☐ Amount of contamination
  - ☐ Tissue pressure measurements if compartment syndrome suspected
- The diagnostic workup of open fractures is considered in Algorithm 14-1.

TABLE 14-1 CLASSIFICATION OF OPEN FRACTURES

Grade	Description
I	Open wound <1 cm with minimal muscle contusion
II	Open wound >1 cm with minimal comminution or moderate muscle contusion
III	Large open wound with extensive degloving, comminution, or contamination

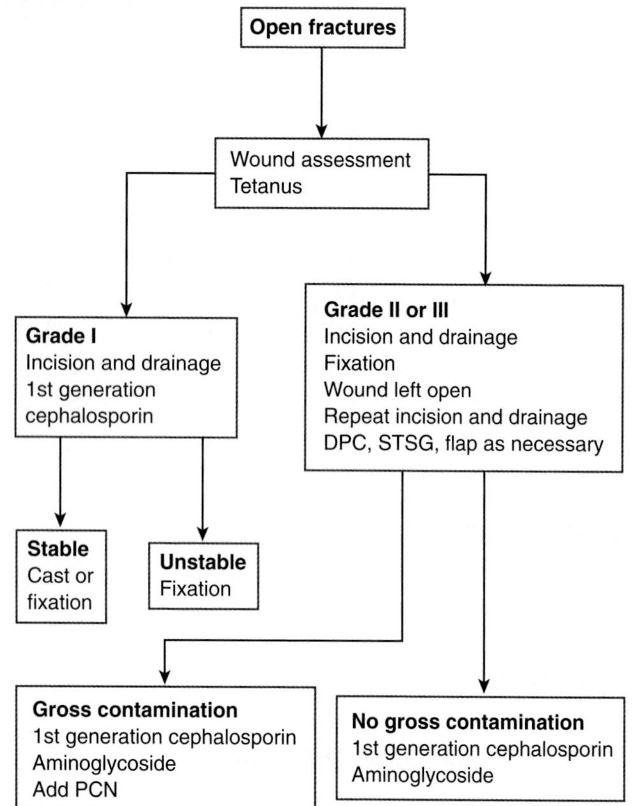

Algorithm 14-1 The diagnostic workup of open fractures in children.

Treatment

Treatment begins in the emergency department.

- Antibiotics:
  - Broad-spectrum cephalosporin for grade I and II injuries
  - Aminoglycoside added for Gram-negative coverage in grade III injuries
  - Penicillin or clindamycin added for severely contaminated injuries (i.e., farm injuries)
- Tetanus toxoid
- Wound coverage with sterile dressing to prevent further contamination
- Splinting of injured extremity to prevent further soft tissue damage

Surgical Indications and Contraindications

- An open fracture is a surgical emergency. However, life-threatening injuries must be evaluated and treated first. Operating room treatment is then considered.
- Wound margins are extended for visualization and débridement of all contaminated tissue.
- Contaminated and necrotic tissue is thoroughly débrided and irrigated, devitalized bone is removed and the wound is left open.
- Routine use of perioperative cultures has not been shown to be effective and is not recommended. Primary closure of open wounds and retention of devascularized fragments in children are controversial and data limited, therefore a conservative course is recommended.
- Stable fractures with minor soft tissue injury may be splinted or casted. However, unstable fractures or those with significant soft tissue injury benefit from operative stabilization.
- Because children are smaller and generally heal quickly, implants do not necessarily need to meet the biomechanical requirements of implants used in adults. Kirschner-wires, flexible intramedullary nails, external fixation, and small plates and screws are commonly used.
- Delayed primary closure, split thickness skin grafting, or free tissue transfers are performed once a stable, clean wound is obtained. Despite the increased technical challenge of smaller vessels in pediatric free tissue transfer, the general health status and lack of premorbid conditions make success more likely and excellent results have been reported.

Results and Outcome

- While good outcomes of lower grade injuries in most published studies dealing with open fractures in children have been reported, the risk of complications is increased with higher fracture grades.
- Delayed union, nonunion, infection, and compartment syndrome are all found with increasing frequency in higher grade injuries.
  - Delayed union is reported in 5% to 33% of all open tibia fractures in children and nonunion rates of 0% to 16% have been documented.
  - Bone healing complications in open forearm fractures in children have been reported in 22% of patients.
  - The effect of age on delayed union and nonunion is controversial, with some studies finding an increased rate of delayed union and nonunion in older children.
- Lawnmower injuries in children may be devastating. Shredding injuries are associated with a high risk of amputation and poor long-term results.
- Open physeal injuries frequently occur as a result of direct trauma and growth arrest is more likely.

Complications

- Compartment syndrome
- Delayed union
- Nonunion
- Infection
- Limb length discrepancy
- Angular deformity
- Motion loss

Postoperative Management

- The less rigid implants used and the usual activity levels of children dictate a period of immobilization and protection.

- ☐ Children are unlikely to develop permanent stiffness, and immobilization to allow fracture healing rarely compromises final range of motion.
- ☐ Implants are removed after fractures heal and before bony overgrowth occurs.

- While physical therapy may be required in older children or children with severe soft tissue injuries, it is often unnecessary in young children or children with lesser degrees of injury.
- The potential for overgrowth and limb length discrepancy in long bone fractures and growth arrest and deformity in physeal injuries requires long-term follow-up and regular radiographic review in children.

SUGGESTED READING

Buckley SL, Smith G, Sponseller PD, et al. Severe type III open fractures of the tibia in children. J Pediatr Orthop 1996;16:627–634.

Buckley SL, Smith G, Sponseller PD, et al. Open fractures of the tibia in children. J Bone Joint Surg 1990;72A:1462–1469.

Cramer KE, Limbird TJ, Green NE. Open fractures of the diaphysis of the lower extremity in children. J Bone Joint Surg (Am) 1992; 74:218–232.

Cullen MC, Roy DR, Crawford AH, et al. Open fracture of the tibia in children. J Bone Joint Surg (Am) 1996;78:1039–1047.

Dormans JP, Assoni M, Davidson RS, et al. Major lower extremity lawnmower injuries in children. J Pediatr Orthop 1995;15:78–82.

Greenbaum G, Zionts LE, Ebramzadeh R. Open fractures of the forearm in children. J Orthop Trauma 2001;15:111–118.

Haasbeek JF, Cole WG. Open fractures of the arm in children. J Bone Joint Surg (Br) 1995;77:576–581.

Hope PG, Cole WG. Open fractures of the tibia in children. J Bone Joint Surg (Br) 1992;74:546–553.

Kreder HJ, Armstrong P. The significance of peri-operative cultures in open pediatric lower extremity fractures. Clin Orthop 1994;302: 206–212.

Lewallen RP, Peterson HA. Nonunion of long bone fractures in children. J Pediatr Orthop 1985;5:135–142.

Shapiro J, Akbarnia BA, Hanel DP. Free tissue transfer in children. J Pediatr Orthop 1989;9:590–595.

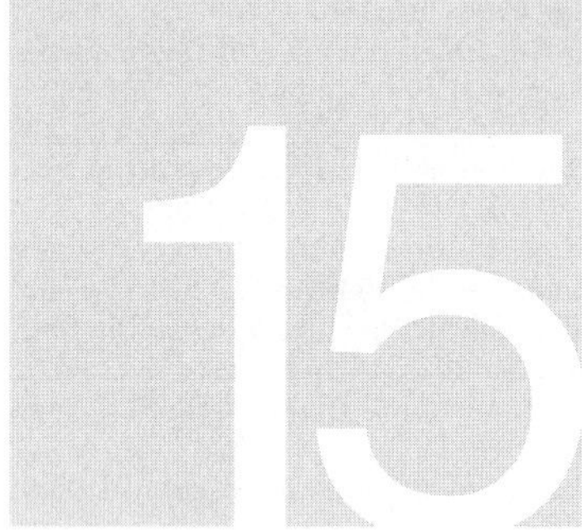

COMPARTMENT SYNDROME

HOWARD R. EPPS

Compartment syndrome is a potentially devastating condition that requires immediate attention. Elevated pressures, within the confined compartments of a limb, cause permanent injury to muscle and nerves. Early recognition and treatment can arrest the process before irreversible damage occurs. Prompt detection and treatment can result in excellent outcomes; delayed or missed diagnosis can cause significant disability. The challenge remains to make an early diagnosis, particularly in children.

PATHOGENESIS

Etiology

Compartment syndrome results from intrinsic causes, extrinsic causes, or both (Box 15-1).

BOX 15-1 CAUSES OF COMPARTMENT SYNDROMES

Intrinsic Causes
- Fracture (open or closed)
- Crush injury
- Vascular injury
- Burns
- Toxic venom
- Viral illness
- Intraosseous infusion
- Venous or arterial access
- Intramuscular hematoma
- Hemophilia
- Traction (skin or skeletal)
- Intraoperative positioning (lithotomy)
- Osteotomy or leg lengthening
- Osteomyelitis
- Prolonged tourniquet application

Extrinisic Causes
- Compressive cast or bandages
- Pneumatic antishock garment
- Prolonged external pressure

- Intrinsic factors increase the volume inside the limited space of a limb compartment, raising the internal pressure.
- Extrinsic causes elevate the intracompartmental pressure by external compression.

Pathophysiology

Intrinsic or extrinsic factors initiate a series of events that eventually cause a compartment syndrome:

- Bleeding within a compartment is a common etiology, but increased vascular permeability, or transient ischemia followed by reperfusion and cellular edema are commonly implicated as well.
- The insult raises the pressure inside the compartment.
- Once the pressure rises above venous pressure, outflow is obstructed.
- Decreased venous outflow, in turn, causes intracompartmental congestion and further elevation of tissue pressure.
- The pressure eventually exceeds arteriolar and capillary pressure, causing ischemia.
- Cellular swelling from ischemia further increases the volume and pressure within the compartment.
- Without decompression, the ischemia eventually causes irreversible damage to muscles and nerves.

DIAGNOSIS

Compartment syndrome is a clinical diagnosis. A high index of suspicion is critical, particularly in children. While compartment pressure measurement provides valuable information, when possible one should rely primarily on the clinical examination.

Physical Examination and History

Clinical Features

The clinical signs of a compartment syndrome result from the effects of increased pressure and subsequent ischemia. The primary features include:

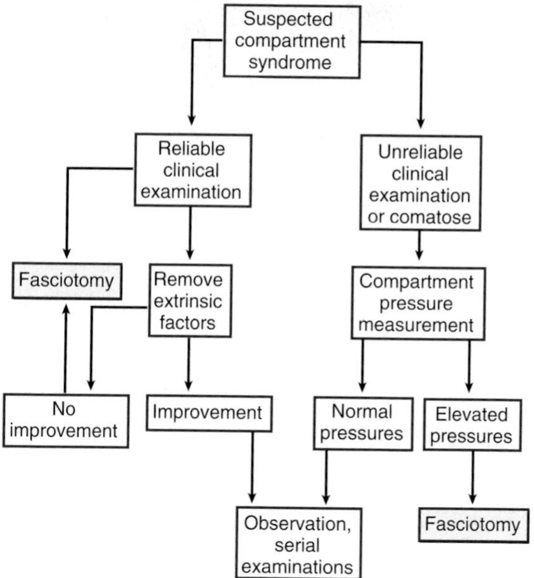

Algorithm 15-1 Algorithm for diagnosis and treatment of compartment syndrome.

- Pain (particularly with the characteristics listed below)
  - Out of proportion to clinical scenario
  - Progressive
  - Poorly controlled by analgesics
  - Persistent despite fracture stabilization
- Pain with passive stretch of muscles of compartment
- Tenseness of compartment
- Tenderness to palpation of compartment
- Paresthesias in distribution of involved nerves (late)
- Paralysis (late)

A noncommunicative, very young, or comatose patient deserves special attention. Sometimes the only signs of compartment syndrome are a child who is inconsolable or agitated, or one with an increasing analgesic requirement. A high index of suspicion is essential in this group of patients. One should have a low threshold for measuring compartment pressures to supplement the clinical findings.

The diagnostic workup of compartment syndrome is outlined in Algorithm 15-1.

TREATMENT

Any patient with suspected compartment syndrome requires immediate treatment. Sometimes the process can be halted by prompt removal of extrinsic factors like a constricting bandage or cast. Patients who do not respond to such measures require an urgent fasciotomy.

Surgical Indications

The indication for fasciotomy is a clinical examination consistent with compartment syndrome. In equivocal cases, compartment pressures can help clarify the clinical picture. Pressures are measured in all compartments with a commercial pressure-measuring device, slit catheter, wick catheter, or arterial line transducer. The value necessary for diagnosis varies; pressures over 30 mm Hg and pressures within 30 mm Hg of diastolic blood pressure have both been proposed as diagnostic. It must be emphasized that the entire clinical picture should be weighed. An examination suggestive of compartment syndrome outweighs nonsupportive pressure measurements. The morbidity of a missed compartment syndrome considerably exceeds the morbidity of a fasciotomy.

Surgical Approaches

- The standard fasciotomy in the leg is performed through two longitudinal incisions, one on each side.
  - The medial incision provides access to the posterior superficial and posterior deep compartments.
  - The lateral incision opens to the anterior and lateral compartments (Fig. 15-1).
  - Ideally, there should be a skin bridge of at least 6 cm between the incisions.
  - Careful dissection is necessary to avoid injury to the superficial peroneal nerve in the lateral incision, and both the saphenous nerve and vein in the medial incision.
- Another technique is the single incision or perifibular approach.
  - A single lateral incision is made on the lateral side of the leg extending from the fibular head to the lateral malleolus.

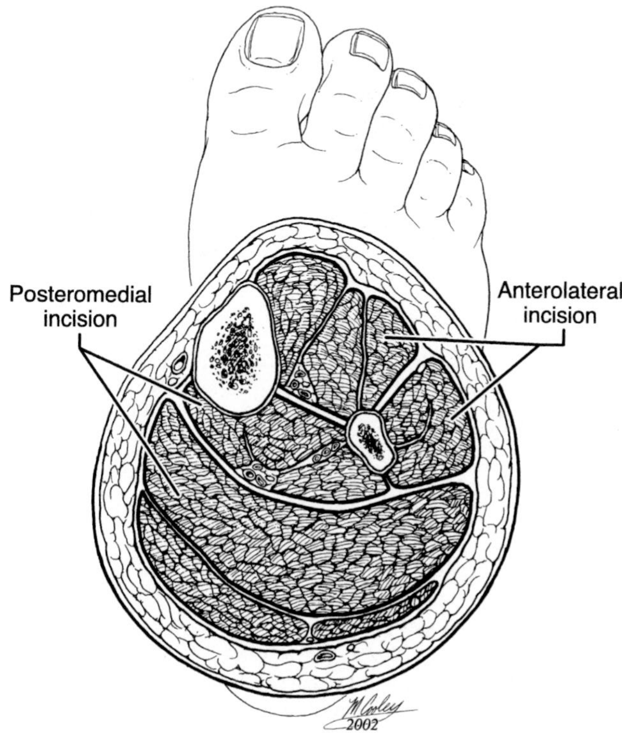

Figure 15-1 Surgical technique for two-incision fasciotomy of the leg. (Adapted from Green NE, Swiontkowski MF, eds. Skeletal trauma in children. Philadelphia: WB Saunders, 1994:84.)

- ☐ Dissection anteriorly allows release of the anterior and lateral compartments; posterior dissection exposes the posterior superficial compartment.
- ☐ The interval between the lateral and posterior superficial compartments provides access to the posterior deep compartment (Fig. 15-2).
- ☐ Proximally, the peroneal nerve is at risk for injury and should be avoided.

- The partial fibulectomy technique is contraindicated in children.
- In the forearm, a volar Henry approach is used to release the superficial and deep flexor compartments.
  - ☐ The incision can be extended into the hand if a carpal tunnel syndrome is suspected.
  - ☐ A midline incision is used dorsally (Fig. 15-3).
- The nine compartments of the foot are decompressed through a single medial incision and two dorsal incisions.
  - ☐ The medial incision extends from behind the medial malleolus to the first metatarsal neck.
  - ☐ The dorsal incisions are centered over the second and fourth metatarsals. Both approaches provide access to all nine compartments.
- If the compartment syndrome is diagnosed late, and myonecrosis is present, devitalized tissue is débrided.
  - ☐ The patient is returned to the operating room after 2 to 3 days for reexamination and further débridement if necessary.
  - ☐ Closure is attempted once all necrotic tissue has been removed and the wound is healthy.

Results and Outcome

With early diagnosis and treatment, the results after fasciotomy are excellent. If necrosis has occurred, the patient

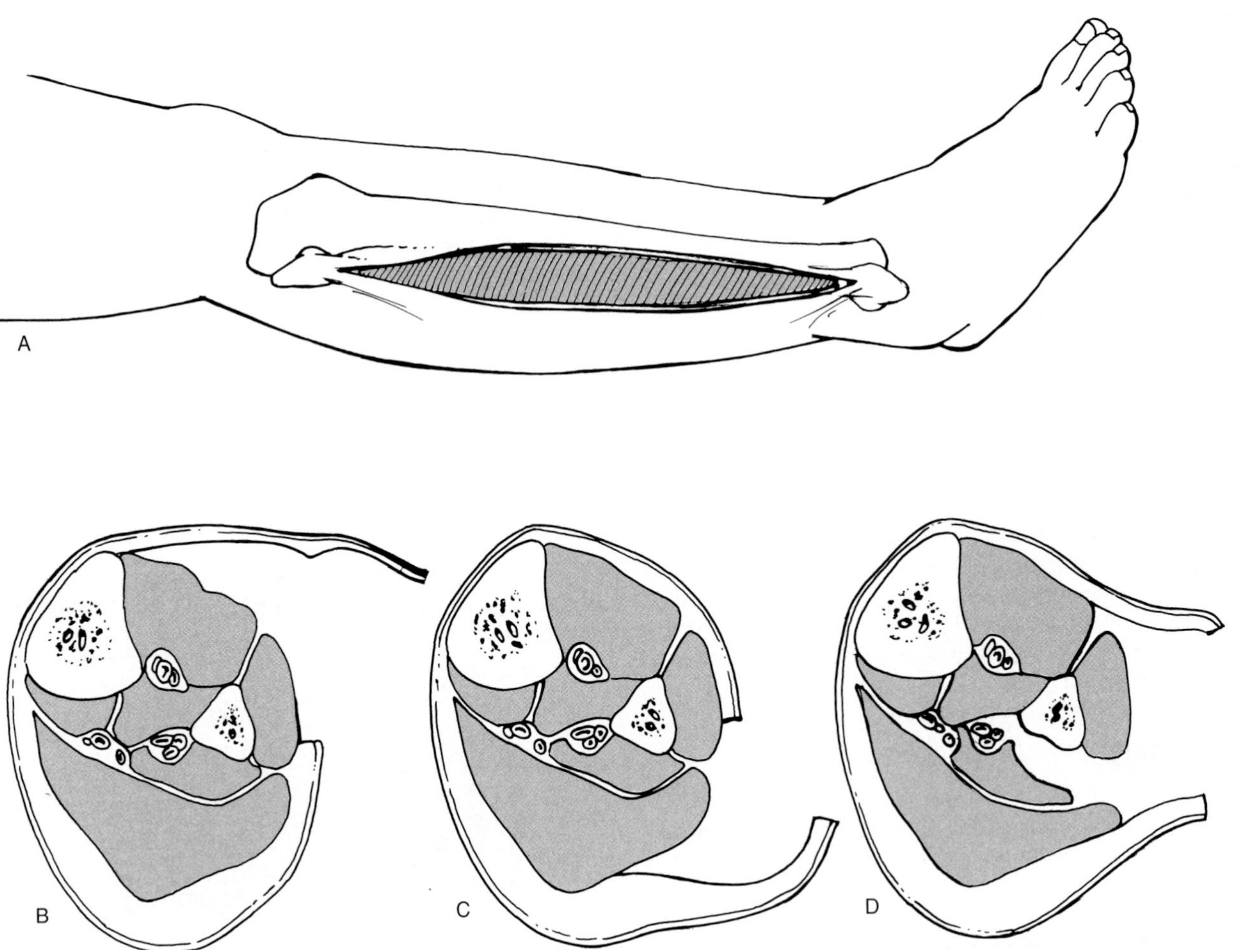

Figure 15-2 Technique of Davey, Rorabeck, and Fowler for decompression of leg compartments. **(A)** Lateral skin incision from fibular neck to 3 to 4 cm proximal to lateral malleolus. **(B)** Skin is undermined anteriorly, and fasciotomy of anterior and lateral compartments is performed. **(C)** Skin is undermined posteriorly, and fasciotomy of superficial posterior compartment is performed. **(D)** Interval between superficial posterior and lateral compartments is developed. Flexor hallicus longus muscle is dissected subperiosteally off fibula and retracted posteromedially. Fascial attachment of tibialis posterior muscle to fibula is incised to decompress muscle. (Adapted from Davey JR, Rorabeck CH, Fowler PJ. Am J Sports Med 1984;12:391.)

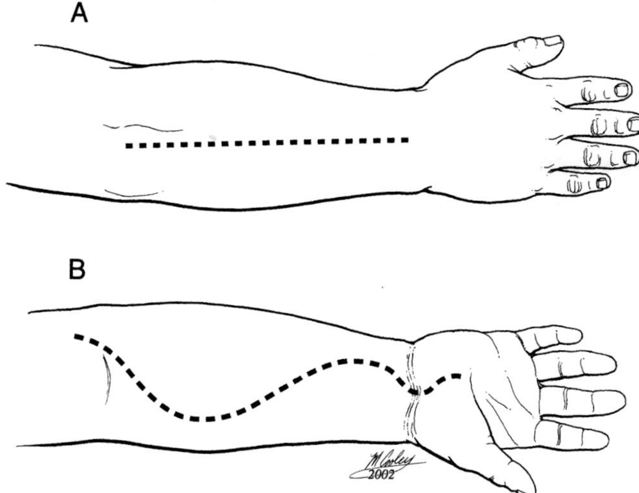

Figure 15-3 Surgical technique for fasciotomy of the forearm. (A) Dorsal incision. (B) Volar incision. (Adapted from Green NE, Swiontkowski MF, eds. Skeletal trauma in children. Philadelphia: WB Saunders, 1994:83.)

will have disability dependent on the extent of the muscle loss and nerve injury.

Postoperative Management

After uncomplicated fasciotomy, the limb is elevated for 5 to 7 days to decrease swelling. The child then returns to the operating room for delayed primary closure or skin grafting if necessary.

SUGGESTED READING

Bae DS, Kadiyala RK, Waters PM. Acute compartment syndrome in children: contemporary diagnosis, treatment, outcome. J Pediatr Orthop 2001;21:680–688.

Bourne RB, Rorabeck CH. Compartment syndromes of the lower leg. Clin Orthop 1989;240:97–104.

Heinrich SD. Fractures of the shaft of the tibia and fibula. In: Beaty JH, Kasser JR, eds. Rockwood and Wilkins' fractures in children, 5th ed. Philadelphia: Lippincott Williams & Wilkins, 2001: 1077–1119.

Kadiyala RK, Waters PM. Upper extremity pediatric compartment syndromes. Hand Clin 1998;14:467–475.

Mars M, Hadley GP. Raised compartmental pressure in children: a basis for management. Injury 1998;29:183–185.

Matsen FA III, Veith RB. Compartmental syndromes in children. J Pediatr Orthop 1981;1:33–41.

Mubarak SJ, Carroll NC. Volkmann's contracture in children: aetiology and prevention. J Bone Joint Surg (Br) 1979;61:285–293.

Silas SI, Herzenberg JE, Myerson MS, et al. Compartment syndrome of the foot in children. J Bone Joint Surg (Am) 1995;77:356–361.

Willis RB, Rorabeck CH. Treatment of compartment syndrome in children. Orthop Clin North Am 1990;21:401–412.

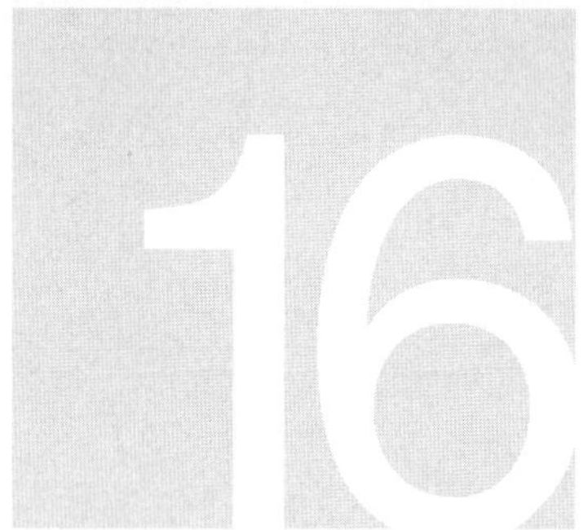

CHILD ABUSE

JOSHUA T. SNYDER
JEFFREY R. SAWYER

Child abuse has plagued humankind for centuries, but has been recognized in literature by the medical community only in the past 50 years. Dr. John Caffey, a pediatric radiologist, published the first contemporary medical report in 1946, and about 20 years later the term *battered child syndrome* was coined by Kempe and colleagues in 1962. Currently, the deliberate harm of children by the people who care for them is known as child abuse. Reports of child abuse are increasing as the medical profession gains experience recognizing the signs and symptoms of abuse. This increase demands significant attention from medical professionals to prevent and investigate abuse as well as to care for those children who are abused. Prevention of further episodes of abuse to the child is essential as the rate of reabuse if the initial event is missed is 35% with a mortality rate of 5%. It is important for orthopaedic surgeons and all other professionals in contact with children to have a clear understanding of what child abuse is, how it presents, and what steps can be taken to identify and treat it once it is identified.

PATHOGENESIS

Etiology

The U.S. Department of Health and Human Services defines four main types of child maltreatment:

- Neglect: 52% of reported cases
- Physical abuse: 24%
- Sexual abuse: 12%
- Emotional abuse: 6%

Many children fit into more than one category. Orthopaedic surgeons are more often consulted for cases of physical abuse and neglect rather than cases of sexual and emotional abuse.

Physical abuse involves inflicting a physical harm to a child, through beating, burning, choking, biting, shaking, pushing, restraining, kicking, or any other mechanism that may have been meant to hurt or punish the child. Signs of neglect are not as objective and often do not carry the same visual impact as signs of physical abuse. Neglect, however, defined as not meeting a child's basic needs of life, may aid in diagnosing cases of physical abuse. For example, caregivers delaying or not seeking medical attention for routine care in times of illness can alert suspicion and warrant further investigation. Physical abuse and chronic neglect of young children tend to be recurrent, and often result in permanent sequelae, such as skeletal deformities, brain injury, and even death.

Epidemiology

Children

It has been reported, in 1997, that within 45 states nearly 3 million children were alleged victims of maltreatment. This is a rate of 42 children per 1,000. Over 4,000 children die each year in the United States from abuse and neglect. Most abused children are white (53%), followed by African-American children (27%), Hispanic (11%), Native-American (2%), and Asian children (1%). There is a slightly higher rate of physical abuse in girls than boys (52% vs. 48%), and girls are three times more likely to be sexually abused. Boys suffer emotional abuse more frequently and also have a 24% higher risk for serious physical injury.

Perpetrators

Some 77% of perpetrators are parents, with relatives accounting for 11%. Most abusers are between the ages of 20 and 40, with women slightly more likely than men to be abusers.

Family

The family of an abused child is more likely to be a single-parent family and the incidence of abuse is higher if the children are living with the father than the mother. Children from larger families (more than four children) are more likely to be abused than children from families with less than three children. Other family risk factors are low socioeconomic status, low education, psychiatric disorders, drug or alcohol abuse, and poor social support systems.

TABLE 16-1 SEVEN-POINT SCALE FOR RATING THE CLINICAL LIKELIHOOD OF CHILD ABUSE

Classification	Description
Definite	Positive skeletal survey, eyewitness, multiple internal injuries, suggestive bruises, sibling also abused, suggestive injury with definite later abuse
Likely original	Doctors called injury abuse *and* history inconsistent or insufficient for injury Inappropriate delay in seeking care
Questionable	History inconsistent, not sufficient for injury *or* story of accident changes
Unknown cause	Insufficient information available in charts
Questionable accident	Isolated incident, social worker/physician had no suspicion of abuse, story somewhat inconsistent with the extent of injury, but consistent with type of injury
Likely accident	Consistent story, social worker/physician had no suspicion of abuse, isolated injury or aggressive or irresponsible behavior involved: however, injury not directly inflicted
Definite accident	Motor vehicle accident, multiple witnesses, pedestrian hit by automobile

Adapted from Levinthal JM, Thomas SA, Rosenfield NS, et al. Fractures in young children: distinguishing child abuse from unintentional injuries. Am J Dis Child 1993;147:87.

Classification

Given the complex nature of child abuse, it is difficult to objectively and accurately classify it. A seven-point scale has been developed to rate the clinical likelihood of abuse, which is helpful in both the clinical and research settings (Table 16-1).

DIAGNOSIS

History

Many details in the history must be documented; therefore, a uniform and stepwise approach is beneficial. The American Medical Association provided a set of recommendations that were modified by Jain to serve as guidelines for an adequate history. It is important to obtain an individual history from all sources separately including the child, caretakers, and any other witnesses at the scene of the injury. During the interview, a nonaccusatory, objective demeanor must be used at all times. After taking each history, the details should be compared to identify any discrepancies. Events related to the injury should also be documented such as activities immediately preceding the injury, was the injury observed or not, and were there any circumstances that could have precipitated an abusive event. It is also important to understand who the child's primary caregiver is and who else participates in that child's care. Box 16-1 provides a list of what to look for during an interview to suggest child abuse. Also in the history, certain risk factors can be identified to aid in the diagnosis (Boxes 16-2 and 16-3).

Physical Examination

Orthopaedic surgeons who are involved in the care of children should be able to recognize the common presentations of child abuse and to differentiate these from normal development and common injuries of childhood. It is important to examine the entire child when abuse is con-

BOX 16-1 WHAT TO LOOK FOR DURING HISTORY AND INTERVIEW

- Self-contradicting statements
- Irritability
- Unavailability
- Delays in seeking medical attention
- Overreaction or underreaction
- Frequent hospitalizations, often at different facilities
- Inconsistencies between all the histories obtained

BOX 16-2 AT-RISK PROFILES IN CHILDREN

- Children <3 yrs especially <1 yr
- Stepchildren
- Premature birth
- Firstborn children
- Children with complex medical problems
- Unplanned births (increased risk with increasing number of unplanned births)
- Unwanted children

BOX 16-3 AT-RISK PROFILES FOR PARENTS AND FAMILY

- Substance abuse
- Household crisis (job loss, marital separation or divorce, death in family)
- New additions to the family (boyfriends/girlfriends, stepparents, and babysitters)
- Older siblings caring for younger children
- Young, poor, and socially isolated parents
- Unmarried mothers
- History of abuse against the perpetrator

sidered, not just the location of pain. Often the child presents to the medical practitioner with nonspecific symptoms such as failure to thrive, feeding difficulties, irritability, or lethargy that may be related to recurrent brain injury. A pattern of physical findings, including bruises and fractures in areas unlikely to be accidentally injured, patterned bruises from objects, and circumferential burns or bruises in children not yet mobile should be viewed as suspicious for child abuse. Toddlers frequently have accidental bruising to the chin, brow, elbows, knees and shins, but bruises to other areas including the back of the head, genitals, abdomen, posterior calf, and thigh are suspicious for abuse.

Clinical Features

Young children are prone to accidental injuries during normal activities and recreation. These patterns of injury however can be distinguished from those injuries of nonaccidental causes. Even though child abuse injuries can affect any organ system and can mimic accidental trauma, certain patterns of soft tissue injury strongly suggest nonaccidental causes (Box 16-4).

- Head injury
  - ☐ Child abuse is the most common cause of serious head injury in infants and the most common cause of mortality in victims of child abuse.
  - ☐ Signs of head injury are usually nonspecific: irritability, lethargy, poor feeding, seizures, varying states of consciousness, bradycardia, apnea, and cardiorespiratory arrest.
  - ☐ Skull fractures from abuse are more likely to be bilateral, comminuted, depressed, wider than 1 mm, and involving nonparietal bone or crossing suture lines.
  - ☐ Subdural hematomas strongly suggest nonaccidental trauma.
- Abdominal trauma
  - ☐ Second most common cause of death
  - ☐ Tears, lacerations, and perforations of organs, including the spleen, small and large bowel, kidney, and pancreas
  - ☐ High mortality rate secondary to delay in seeking treatment
- Fractures
  - ☐ Long bone fractures in children less than 1 year of age
  - ☐ Rib fractures.
  - ☐ Metaphyseal "corner fractures"
  - ☐ Fractures of different ages

Radiologic Features

In addition to history and physical exam, a focused radiographic examination is helpful in making the diagnosis of child abuse. As with any musculoskeletal injury, the radiographic workup begins with plain radiographs of the affected area(s). If an injury is detected or the index of suspicion for abuse remains high, a skeletal survey should be obtained. Total body radiographs or "babygrams" should be avoided. It is important to estimate the age of the fracture(s) as well. In most children, periosteal reaction and new bone formation occurs within 7 to 14 days following fracture. Loss of resolution of fracture lines (3 weeks), dense callus formation (3 to 6 weeks), and remodeling (more than 6 weeks) are typically later findings. There is some variability between patients in the rate of bone healing, but these general guidelines can help with attempting to date fractures. If the first skeletal survey is negative and the index of suspicion for abuse is high, it may be necessary to repeat the skeletal survey in several weeks to attempt to find these later radiographic changes.

Bone scan may be helpful in evaluating the child for occult fractures. Bone scan is typically not helpful in evaluating injuries near the growth plate such as metaphyseal "corner fractures" due to the high rate of metabolic activity at the open growth plate which will cause a false-positive reading. Computed tomography (CT), magnetic resonance imaging (MRI), and ultrasound are useful in certain situations if the diagnosis remains unclear. CT and MRI may also be used to rule out brain or spinal cord injury but typically require sedation in this age group. Boxes 16-5 to 16-7 list radiologic features of the skeletal survey that are pathognomonic, that are highly suggestive, or that have low likelihood of child abuse.

Diagnostic Workup

Obtaining a complete history is the first objective in any medical visit. Unfortunately, with child abuse cases the frustration, anger, and apprehension of the parents or caretakers make a clear and focused history difficult to produce. Suspicion should be raised if the mechanism of injury is inconsistent with the history given or the child's developmental stage.

BOX 16-4 SOFT TISSUE INJURIES OFTEN SEEN IN CHILD ABUSE

- Ecchymosis, abrasions, burns, welts, lacerations, and scars
- Bruising of unusual areas such as buttocks, perineum, trunk, back of legs, head, and neck
- Circumferential immersion burns
- Unexplained retinal hemorrhages
- Bruises in the shape of instruments or objects
- Human hand marks or bite marks
- Multiple lesions at different stages of healing

BOX 16-5 RADIOLOGIC PATTERNS WITH HIGH SPECIFICITY FOR CHILD ABUSE

- Posterior rib fractures
- Costochondral junction fractures (associated with significant abdominal injury)
- Metaphyseal "corner" fractures most common: distal femur, tibia, and proximal humerus
- Scapular fractures
- Spinous process fractures
- Sternal fractures

BOX 16-6 RADIOLOGIC FEATURES HIGHLY SUGGESTIVE OF OR MODERATELY SPECIFIC FOR CHILD ABUSE

- Fractures of different ages
- Fracture of the lateral third of the clavicle
- Vertebral fractures
- Any vertebral body fractures or subluxations, especially C2-C3
- Digital injuries
- Diaphyseal injuries in children younger than 1yr or children not yet walking
- Epiphyseal separations
- Complex skull fractures

A complete physical examination of the entire child completely undressed must be performed, noting any skin or soft tissue injury. Signs of sexual abuse should also be noted. This should be followed by a thorough radiologic examination as previously mentioned.

If an unexplained injury is identified the possibility of underlying bone disease should be considered. Other conditions confused with nonaccidental injuries include:

- Normal variants
  - Spurring and cupping of the metaphysis
  - Periosteal reaction of the newborn
- Birth trauma
  - Clavicle, humerus, and long bone fractures may occur during traumatic birth.
  - Absence of callus formation at any fracture site found after 2 weeks after delivery strongly suggests abuse.
- Osteogenesis imperfecta
  - Fractures of the long bones
  - Osteopenia, thin cortices, and bowing or angulation of healed fractures
  - Blue sclerae, dentinogenesis imperfecta, deafness due to otosclerosis
- Rickets
  - Fraying of metaphysis
  - Widening of physis
  - Looser zones (transverse stress fractures in shafts of long bones)
- Congenital syphilis
  - Metaphyseal lucencies parallel to the physis of long bones
  - Periosteal reaction along the entire length of long bones
  - Osteolytic metaphyseal long bones
  - Lesions usually symmetric
- Congenital insensitivity to pain
  - Rare autosomal recessive trait with indifference to painful stimuli
  - Present with repeated unrecognized injuries to the growth plate
- Caffey disease
  - Infantile cortical hyperostosis in infants younger than 6 months
  - Painful periosteal reaction resulting in cortical thickening
  - Mandible, clavicle, and ulna
- Vitamin A intoxication
  - Thick periosteal reaction of the tubular bones: ulna and metatarsals
  - Widening of the cranial sutures
  - Metaphyseal and epiphyseal areas are normal radiographically
- Leukemia
  - Periosteal reaction with diffuse demineralization commonly occurs in association with multiple osteolytic lesions
  - Narrow radiolucent metaphyseal bands ("leukemic lines").
- Hemophilia
  - Multiple bruises with minimal/no trauma
  - Bruises at different stages of healing
  - Family history (X-linked recessive)
- Toddler fracture
  - Commonly occurs between ages of 1 and 3 years
  - Spiral fracture of distal tibia
  - Common without history of trauma
- Drug-induced bone changes
  - Periosteal reaction of the ribs and long bones with prostaglandin E1, used to maintain a patent ductus arteriosis.
  - Methotrexate and antiseizure medications can cause osteopenia and fractures.

BOX 16-7 RADIOLOGIC FEATURES WITH LOW LIKELIHOOD OF CHILD ABUSE OR THAT ARE SO COMMON AS TO BE OF LOW SPECIFICITY

- Clavicular fractures of the medial third
- Long bone shaft fracture[a]
- Linear skull fractures
- Subperiosteal new bone formation

[a]Studies have shown that single, transverse long bone fractures are the most common fractures in child abuse. These fractures however, are also common in accidental causes of injury and should be correlated with a suspicious history or other suggestive physical findings.

The information from the history, physical examination, and radiographic studies is then combined and the diagnosis of child abuse can be made. Once the diagnosis is made, physicians and other health care professionals are mandated reporters and are required to report suspected abuse to the appropriate child protection agencies. Health care professionals who report suspected cases of abuse and neglect in good faith are protected from both civil and criminal prosecution.

TREATMENT

Because of the enhanced healing capacity of a child's skeleton, most of the orthopaedic injuries associated with child abuse heal very rapidly. A child's ability of bone to remodel is high, therefore the potential of late residual skeletal deformity is low. The primary treatment of orthopaedic injuries from abuse is the same as for any musculoskeletal injury: immobilization of the injured areas with precise anatomic reduction of rotational deformities, angulation, or displaced intraarticular fractures. These injuries rarely require operative management with the exception of physeal injuries, particularly those to the proximal femur and distal humerus. Again, equally important to treating the musculoskeletal injury is preventing the child from sustaining further harm from the abuser.

SUGGESTED READING

Akbarnia BA, Campbell RM Jr. The role of the orthopaedic surgeon in child abuse. In: Morrissy RT, Weinstein SL, eds. Lovell and Winter's pediatric orthopaedics, 5th ed. Philadelphia: Lippincott Williams & Wilkins, 2000:1423–1445.

Council on Scientific Affairs. AMA diagnostic and treatment guidelines concerning child abuse and neglect. JAMA 1985;254:796–803.

Egami Y, Ford DE, Greenfield SF, et al: Psychiatric profile and demographic characteristics of adults who report physically abusing or neglecting children. Am J Psychiatry 1996;153:921–927.

Kempe CH, Silverman FN, Steele BF, et al. The battered child syndrome. J Bone Joint Surg (Am) 1960;40:407.

Kleinman PK. Skeletal trauma: general considerations. In: Kleinman PK, ed. Diagnostic imaging of child abuse. Baltimore: Williams and Wilkins, 1987:8–25.

Levinthal JM, Thomas SA, Rosenfield NS, et al. Fractures in young children: distinguishing child abuse from unintentional injuries. Am J Dis Child 1993;147:87.

US Department of Health and Human Services, Administration on Children, Youth and Families. Child maltreatment 1997: reports from the states to the National Child Abuse and Neglect Data System. Washington, DC: Government Printing Office, 1999.

INFECTION

JON R. SHERECK
RICHARD M. SCHWEND

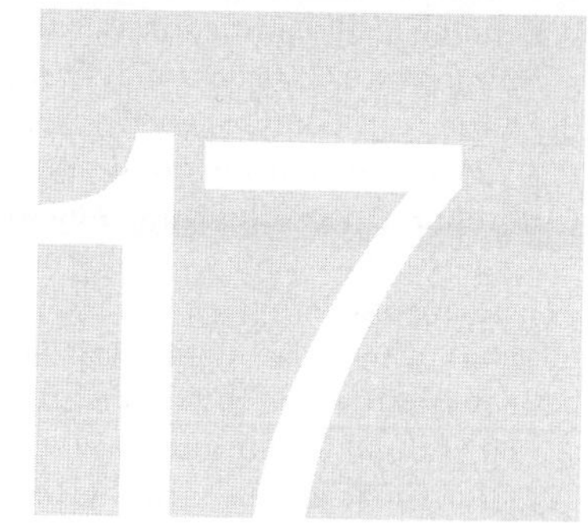

Musculoskeletal infections in children are common conditions likely to be encountered by all orthopaedic surgeons. The diagnosis of bone or joint sepsis is often difficult to make. The child can present with many different signs and symptoms (Box 17-1), and there are multiple conditions that can mimic infection (Box 17-2). Although evaluation and treatment of orthopaedic infections is sometimes controversial, by following basic principles, significant sequela can be prevented.

ACUTE HEMATOGENOUS OSTEOMYELITIS

PATHOGENESIS

Etiology

- *Staphylococcus aureus* (most common)
- Group A *Streptococcus*
- *Streptococcus pneumoniae*
- Group B β-hemolytic *Streptococcus* (usually in neonates)

BOX 17-1 MANIFESTATIONS OF ORTHOPAEDIC INFECTIONS IN CHILDREN

- Malaise
- Irritablility
- Fever
- Pain
- Pseudoparalysis
- Tenderness
- Limp
- Refusal to walk
- Stiff joint
- Joint effusion, if superficial joint
- Asymmetric positioning
- Erythema
- Swelling
- Warmth

Epidemiology

- Half of affected children are younger than 5 years of age, one-third are younger than 2 years of age.
- Male-to-female ratio is up to 4 to 1.
- Common in warmer climates; peak incidence in late summer or early fall
- Most common in metaphyseal region of lower extremity long bones. Seen in locations with the fastest growth rate, such as distal femur

Pathophysiology

- Trauma to the metaphysis and bacteremia have a combined role in initiating osteomyelitis.
- Blood-borne bacteria are deposited in metaphyseal venous sinusoids.
- Medullary vessels thrombose.
- This inhibits access of inflammatory cells for proper immune response.

BOX 17-2 DIFFERENTIAL DIAGNOSIS OF ORTHOPAEDIC INFECTIONS

Osteomyelitis
- Transient synovitis
- Soft tissue abscess
- Cellulitis
- Pyogenic arthritis
- Fracture
- Thrombophlebitis
- Rheumatic fever
- Bone infarction
- Gaucher disease
- Malignancy
  - Osteosarcoma
  - Ewing sarcoma
  - Leukemia
  - Neuroblastoma
  - Wilms tumor

Septic Arthritis
- Transient synovitis
- Rheumatic fever
- Leukemia
- Cellulitis
- Juvenile arthritis
- Osteomyelitis
- Hemophilia
- Lyme arthritis
- Henoch-Schönlein purpura
- Hemiarthrosis
- Viral or reactive arthritis
- Chondrolysis
- Sickle cell crisis
- Lillonodular synovitis
- Legg-Calvé-Perthes disease
- Slipped capital femoral ephiphysis

- Purulent material is produced. Infection spreads through Volkmann canals or the haversian bone system. Subperiosteal abscess may form.
- Due to the compromised vascularity of cortical bone, a sequestrum (loosely adherent piece of dead bone) may develop. An involucrum (new bone) may form over the sequestrum. Poor vascularity may lead to chronic osteomyelitis.
- Joints where the metaphysis lies within the capsule are at particular risk for septic arthritis:
  - Proximal femur and hip
  - Proximal humerus and glenohumeral joint
  - Lateral distal tibia and ankle
  - Radial neck in the elbow

DIAGNOSIS

Criteria for diagnosing osteomyelitis are outlined in Boxes 17-3 and 17-4.

History

- History of recent or concurrent infection in about 50% of patients
- Preceding trauma in up to 50%
- Duration of symptoms typically less than 2 weeks
- Continuous bone pain for at least 24 hours

Physical Examination

- Local signs of erythema, swelling, and warmth are seen with advanced infection. If cellulitis is present, this may indicate an underlying abscess.
- Pain is not well localized if the infection involves the spine or pelvis
- Signs are different for different ages.
  - Neonates: swelling at the affected site due to an easily penetrated thin periosteum. However, the only finding may be a systemically ill neonate, or one who is irritable and failing to thrive.
  - Toddler and young children: pain, usually point tenderness, is seen in 50%. A limp or inability to bear weight is commonly seen with infections of the lower extremity.
  - Adolescents: may be more locally tender because of more resilient and tense tissues.

BOX 17-3 MORREY AND PETERSON CRITERIA FOR THE DIAGNOSIS OF OSTEOMYELITIS

Definite: The pathogen is isolated from the bone or adjacent soft tissue, or there is histologic evidence of osteomyelitis.

Probable: A blood culture is positive in the setting of clinical and radiographic features of osteomyelitis.

Likely: Typical clinical findings and definite radiographic evidence of osteomyelitis are present, and there is a response to antibiotic therapy.

Adapted from Morrey BF, Peterson HA. Hematogenous pyogenic osteomyelitis in children. Orthop Clin North Am 1975;6:935–951.

BOX 17-4 PELTOLA AND VAHVANEN CRITERIA FOR THE DIAGNOSIS OF OSTEOMYELITIS

The diagnosis is established when two of the following four criteria are met:

- Pus is aspirated from bone.
- A bone or blood culture is positive.
- The classic symptoms of localized pain, swelling, warmth, and limited range of motion of the adjacent joint are present.
- Radiographic features characteristic of osteomyelitis are present.

Adapted from Peltola H, Vahvanen V. A comparative study of osteomyelitis and purulent arthritis with special reference to aetiology and recovery. Infection 1984;12:75–79.

Laboratory Features

- White blood cell (WBC) count may be normal in up to 70% of patients.
- Erythrocyte sedimentation rate (ESR):
  - Elevated in more than 90% of patients, but is nonspecific.
  - Levels rise slowly and peak in 3 to 5 days, so may be normal if child presents early in the course of the infection. The neonate, patient with sickle cell disease, or the child who is taking steroids may not have an elevated ESR.
- C-reactive protein (CRP):
  - Acute phase protein synthesized by the liver.
  - Elevated in as many as 97% of patients.
  - Levels rise rapidly and peak in 2 days. CRP is quick to decline (within 6 hours) after initiation of appropriate therapy.
- Blood cultures are positive in 30% to 60% of patients.
- Cultures taken from involved bone:
  - Have a higher yield of pathogens (positive in up to 75% of patients) and may be the only positive culture site in 28%.
  - Gram stain should be performed at same time.
  - Consider fine-needle biopsy to obtain material for histologic examination.
- Surgical biopsy should be sent for histopathology when débridement is clinically indicated.

Radiologic Features

- Plain radiographs
  - Do not accept incomplete or poor quality films. Need two orthogonal views of the involved area.
  - Soft-tissue swelling is evident within 48 hours of onset of infection; soft tissue planes may be poorly visualized. Always look for subtle evidence of free air

in the tissues to suggest an anaerobic, gas-producing infection.
  - ☐ Comparison views of the contralateral extremity may be helpful.
  - ☐ Periosteal new bone formation may be evident by 5 to 7 days.
  - ☐ Osteolytic changes require bone mineral loss of 30% to 50%. May not be apparent until 10 to 14 days after onset.
- Technetium-99m bone scintigraphy
  - ☐ Useful if of normal radiographs but still clinical suspicion of osteomyelitis.
  - ☐ Sensitivity: 84% to 100%. Specificity: 70% to 96%. Sensitivity is decreased in the neonate.
  - ☐ Prior aspiration does not give false-positive results.
  - ☐ "Cold" scans in late stages of infection.
    - ☐ Very worrisome for a severe infection or osteonecrosis.
    - ☐ Decreased uptake due to relative ischemia caused by increased pressure from purulent material: leads to vascular congestion and osteonecrosis
    - ☐ Positive predictive value of up to 100%
- Magnetic resonance imagine (MRI)
  - ☐ Sensitivity: 88% to 100%. Specificity: 75% to 100%
  - ☐ Very useful for suspected spinal and pelvic infections. Consider using if patient has not responded after 2 days of antibiotic therapy
  - ☐ Excellent imaging modality for planning surgical approaches
  - ☐ T1-weighted and short-tau inversion recovery (STIR) images are most useful for detection of acute osteomyelitis
- Computed tomography (CT)
  - ☐ Most useful in detection of gas in soft tissue infections and in identification of sequestra in chronic osteomyelitis
- Ultrasound
  - ☐ Detects fluid collections and soft tissue swelling
  - ☐ Advantages: low cost, relative availability, noninvasive, nonionizing radiation, no sedation required
  - ☐ Disadvantages: lack of specificity, operator dependent, inability to image marrow or show cortical detail

Diagnostic Workup

- A complete and thorough history and physical examination is performed. Be anatomically specific about the location of the pain.
- Laboratory and imaging studies as previously described
- Once an anatomic source is localized, aspiration is used to obtain the organism. Surgical biopsy can also be used to obtain the organism. The decision to use surgery requires clinical judgment. It usually is performed to drain pus, débride necrotic tissue, or when the patient has not responded to appropriate antibiotic therapy.

TREATMENT

Morrissey has advocated the following treatment principles for infection:

- Find the organism, which can generally be identified in 50% to 70% of cases.
- Use appropriate antibiotics.
- Deliver the antibiotic to the area of infection.
- Stop the tissue destruction: typically by surgical drainage and débridement.
- Once the diagnosis has been made and blood and tissue cultures obtained, begin empiric intravenous (i.v.) antibiotics. Since most infections are caused by *S. aureus*, group A *Streptococcus*, or *Pneumococcus*, Cefazolin (Kefzol) 50 mg per kg per dose, every 8 hours, maximum dose 12 g per day is a safe and reasonable initial choice.
- Nafcillin or oxacillin are reasonable initial alternatives.
- Consider the following special situations:
  - ☐ Neonates: add gentamicin or cefotaxime to the regimen.
  - ☐ Allergy to penicillin: cefazolin is the antibiotic of choice.
  - ☐ Allergy to both penicillin and cephalosporins: clindamycin or vancomycin.
  - ☐ Methicillin-resistant S. *aureus* is suspected: vancomycin.
  - ☐ Consider infectious disease consultation for these special situations.
- Aspiration or biopsy is indicated if no improvement after 36 to 48 hours of appropriate i.v. antibiotics.
- Switching to oral antibiotics: very subjective and clinical judgment is required. The patient should appear well, have a normal temperature and pulse, have a markedly improved clinical examination, and be able to take oral medication.
- Intravenous antibiotics may be continued longer if:
  - ☐ Initiation of therapy is markedly delayed and necrotic tissue is suspected.
  - ☐ Poor response, or no response, after empiric i.v. therapy.
  - ☐ Patient is unable to take oral medications.
  - ☐ There is no effective oral antibiotic for the identified organism or if there is a very unusual organism.
- Duration of therapy is determined by clinical improvement. Traditionally, antibiotics are used for 4 to 6 weeks. Follow clinical response and ESR.
- Indications for surgical débridement
  - ☐ Evidence of an intraarticular, subperiosteal, intramedullary, or soft-tissue abscess
  - ☐ Sequestrum
  - ☐ Contiguous focus of infection
  - ☐ Poor response to appropriate i.v. antibiotics
- Surgical management
  - ☐ Drain the soft tissue abscess
  - ☐ Incise the periosteum
  - ☐ Drill the cortex
  - ☐ Remove all dead bone
- Postoperative immobilization in a splint or cast, especially if at risk for a pathologic fracture.

SEPTIC ARTHRITIS

PATHOGENESIS

Etiology

- Neonates: group B *Streptococcus, S. aureus,* Gram-negative bacilli
- 1 month to adolescent: *S. aureus, S. pneumoniae, S. pyogenes*
- Adolescents: may also see *Neisseria gonorrheae*
- *Haemophilus influenzae* B rare unless child has not been immunized

Epidemiology

Septic Arthritis

- Most common in children less than age 2 years of age
- More common in boys than girls

Pathophysiology

- Hematogenous seeding of bacteria in the rich vascular network in the subsynovial layer is present, which then progresses into the joint.
- Other possible routes for septic arthritis to develop:
  - Local spread from a contiguous infection, such as an intraarticular osteomyelitis.
  - Penetrating trauma or surgical infection.
  - Percutaneous fixation pins that are intraarticular, such as in the knee.
- Acute inflammatory stage:
  - Polymorphonuclear cells (PMNs) rapidly enter the joint space.
  - Plasma proteins cross the synovial membrane, resulting in a tense effusion.
  - Leading to significant pain even at rest
- Articular cartilage can be destroyed in response to infection by two mechanisms:
  - Degradation by proteolytic enzymes (e.g., collagenase, proteinases).
  - Interleukin-1 from monocytes mediates the release of acid and neutral proteases by chondrocytes and synoviocytes.
- Early diagnosis and treatment is essential to limiting articular cartilage destruction. If treatment is delayed beyond 4 days, articular damage can be permanent.

DIAGNOSIS (BOX 17-5)

History

- May have a history of a recent upper respiratory infection or local soft tissue infection, preceding trauma, fever, malaise, and pain
- Pain at rest, limp, and limited spontaneous motion
- Fever, which may not be present if small joint involved
- Consider the possibility of an altered immune status.

Physical Examination

- Patients may appear more ill compared with osteomyelitis.
- Young children may be very irritable (see Box 17-1).
- Pain is present at rest and is increased with passive joint motion and axial loading.
- If the hip joint is involved, it is typically held in external rotation, abduction, and mild flexion to maximize the joint volume and decrease the resting pressure.
- The neonate may have mild or absent signs and symptoms.
- When a septic hip is suspected, consider adjacent sites as the primary cause of infection, including pelvic abscess, infection of any of the muscles about the hip and pelvis, pelvic osteomyelitis, or proximal femur osteomyelitis. The psoas sign of pain on extension and internal rotation of the hip is present in as many as 89% of patients with primary pyogenic psoas abscess.

Laboratory Features

- WBC count elevated in 30% to 60% of patients
  - PMNs elevated in 60% to 80%
- ESR elevated in more than 90% of patients, but not elevated early in the course of the infection. It is highly sensitive, but nonspecific.
- CRP
  - Helps detect associated septic arthritis in patients with acute hematogenous osteomyelitis
  - If CRP concentration by the third day is 1.5 times the level on admission, there is a high likelihood that associated septic arthritis is present.
- Blood cultures are positive in 40% to 50% of patients and are the only positive culture site in 12%. Up to 70% yield if both blood and joint cultures obtained.
- A large-bore (20-gauge or larger) needle aspiration should be obtained on all septic joints. There is little risk of seeding a bone or joint in an area of cellulites.
  - Hip joint aspiration: consider using arthrographic or ultrasound guidance. Patient should be sedated or under general anesthesia.
- Synovial fluid analysis:
  - WBC greater than 50,000/mL with 90% PMNs is indicative of bacterial infection.
  - Glucose level: synovial fluid/serum glucose ratio of less than 0.5, or synovial fluid glucose 40 mg/dL less than serum level.
  - Positive mucin clot test: assesses integrity of hyaluronic acid of joint fluid. Place a drop of glacial acetic acid into the fluid while stirring with a glass rod. In the presence of bacteria, the consistency of the fluid resembles that of curdled milk due to degraded hyaluronic acid.
  - Gram stain is positive in about 50% of cases.
- A Mantoux skin test, or purified protein derivative (PPD) skin test should be placed if tuberculosis is a possibility.

Radiologic Features

- Plain radiographs
  - Frequently normal
  - Changes are subtle and may include:

- Soft tissue edema, loss of tissue planes
- Joint space widening is seen with capsular distention, especially in the infant hip joint
- Subluxation or dislocation of the involved joint, particularly in the neonate
- Epiphyseal ischemic necrosis
- Associated metaphyseal or epiphyseal osteomyelitis

- Bone scan
  - Rarely useful to diagnose septic arthritis, but can be helpful when the exact location of the septic joint is difficult to identify.
  - A "cold bone scan" of the hip is particularly worrisome.
  - In a septic joint, the distribution of uptake is uniform within the joint capsule; asymmetric uptake indicates osteomyelitis.
- MRI
  - Used in patients with septic hip arthritis who have not responded to conventional therapy: useful in delineating areas of residual infection and defining associated osteomyelitis.
  - Very helpful for imaging the pelvis if an abscess is suspected.
- CT: no useful role in septic arthritis
- Ultrasound
  - More sensitive (almost 100%) than plain radiography in diagnosing an effusion. However, it is not specific in determining whether the effusion is infectious.
  - Very useful in evaluating suspected sepsis of the hips. Both hips should be imaged along the axis of the femoral neck. Affected hip will show asymmetry of the capsule-to-bone distance of 2 mm or more, indicating an intraarticular effusion. Echogenicity suggests a septic arthritis or clotted hemorrhagic collections, but is not very specific.
  - Results must be combined with clinical impression to determine need for hip aspiration.
  - Aspiration can be performed under guidance.

Diagnostic Workup

- A septic hip arthritis clinical practice guideline (CPG) algorithm has been proposed by Kocher and colleagues (Algorithm 17-1). It includes a thorough diagnostic workup protocol as well as the appropriate treatment.
  - Compared with previous standard practice, use of this CPG has resulted in:
    - Less frequent use of bone scan (13% vs. 40%)
    - Earlier conversion to oral antibiotics (3.9 vs. 6.9 days)
    - Lower use of inappropriate surgical drainage (53% vs. 87%)
    - Lower rate of nonrecommended antibiotic course (7% vs. 93%).
    - Shorter hospital stay (4.8 vs. 8.3 days)
  - Despite less extensive diagnosis and treatment, there was no less successful clinical outcome with use of the CPG.

BOX 17-5 MORREY AND PETERSON CRITERIA FOR THE DIAGNOSIS OF SEPTIC ARTHRITIS IN PATIENTS WITH NEGATIVE CULTURES

The diagnosis is established when five of the following six criteria are present:

- Temperature exceeds 38.3°C
- Swelling of the suspected joint is present. This is not always obvious for a deep joint such as the hip
- Pain that is exacerbated with movement
- Systemic symptoms
- No other pathologic processes are present
  - Satisfactory response to antibiotic therapy

Adapted from Morrey BF, Peterson HA. Hematogenous pyogenic osteomyelitis in children. Orthop Clin North Am 1975;6:935–951.

- If clinical suspicion is high after a thorough history and physical and is supported by initial lab values or radiographs, then aspiration of the involved joint is used to confirm the presence of infection.
  - CRP, ESR, complete blood count (CBC) with differential, Lyme titer, blood culture, throat culture/rapid strep, anti-strepolysin (ASLO).
  - Plain radiographs
  - If there is uncertainty about the presence of a septic effusion about the hip after the initial evaluation, ultrasonography is of diagnostic value to confirm the presence of an effusion. Confirmed hip effusion with a clinical picture suggestive of septic arthritis should receive diagnostic aspiration.
- Septic arthritis can still be present despite negative cultures (Box 17-5).

TREATMENT

- Blood and joint cultures should be obtained prior to administration of antibiotics.
- Open arthrotomy for patients with hip involvement.
- Septic knee arthritis does well with arthroscopic lavage.
- Empiric antibiotic therapy should be initiated. Cefazolin (Kefzol) 50 mg/kg per dose, every 8 hours, maximum dose 12 g/day. Nafcillin or oxacillin are reasonable initial alternatives.
- Special situations are similar to those described for osteomyelitis. Ceftriaxone for possible *H. influenzae* B or *N. gonorrhea* infection.
- Final antibiotic choice is directed by the culture and sensitivity results.
- Duration of i.v. antibiotics is based on the clinical response. The CPG typically averaged 4 days of i.v. antibiotic before switching to an oral antibiotic. Serum bactericidal levels are not routinely obtained.
- Total duration of antibiotics for septic arthritis is typically about 3 weeks. Follow clinical response and ESR.

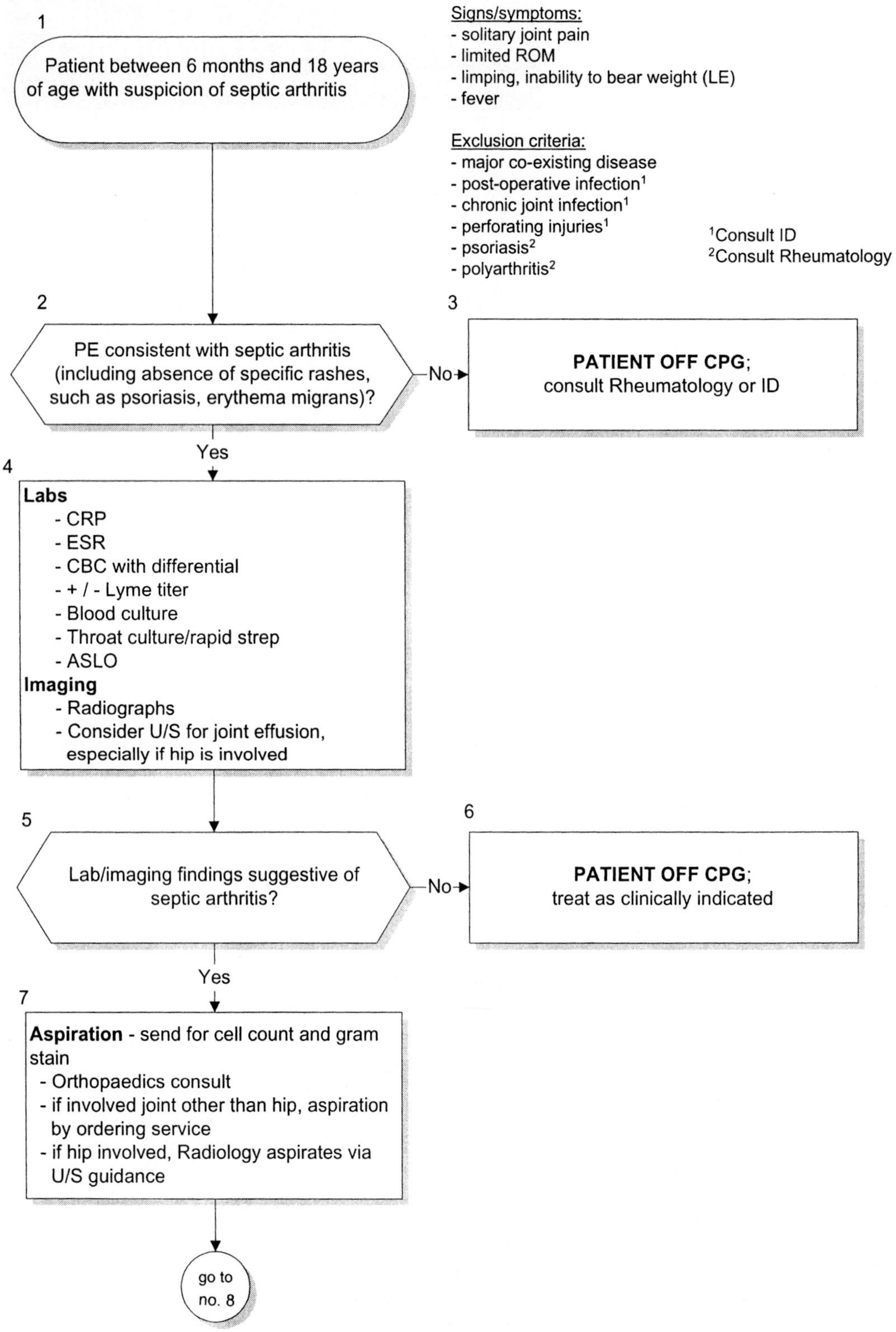

1

Patient between 6 months and 18 years of age with suspicion of septic arthritis

Signs/symptoms:
- solitary joint pain
- limited ROM
- limping, inability to bear weight (LE)
- fever

Exclusion criteria:
- major co-existing disease
- post-operative infection[1]
- chronic joint infection[1]
- perforating injuries[1]
- psoriasis[2]
- polyarthritis[2]

[1]Consult ID
[2]Consult Rheumatology

2

PE consistent with septic arthritis (including absence of specific rashes, such as psoriasis, erythema migrans)?

No → 3

PATIENT OFF CPG; consult Rheumatology or ID

Yes ↓

4

Labs
- CRP
- ESR
- CBC with differential
- + / - Lyme titer
- Blood culture
- Throat culture/rapid strep
- ASLO

Imaging
- Radiographs
- Consider U/S for joint effusion, especially if hip is involved

5

Lab/imaging findings suggestive of septic arthritis?

No → 6

PATIENT OFF CPG; treat as clinically indicated

Yes ↓

7

Aspiration - send for cell count and gram stain
- Orthopaedics consult
- if involved joint other than hip, aspiration by ordering service
- if hip involved, Radiology aspirates via U/S guidance

go to no. 8

Algorithm 17-1 Septic arthritis clinical practice guideline algorithm. (Copyright © 2001 by Children's Hospital, Boston.)

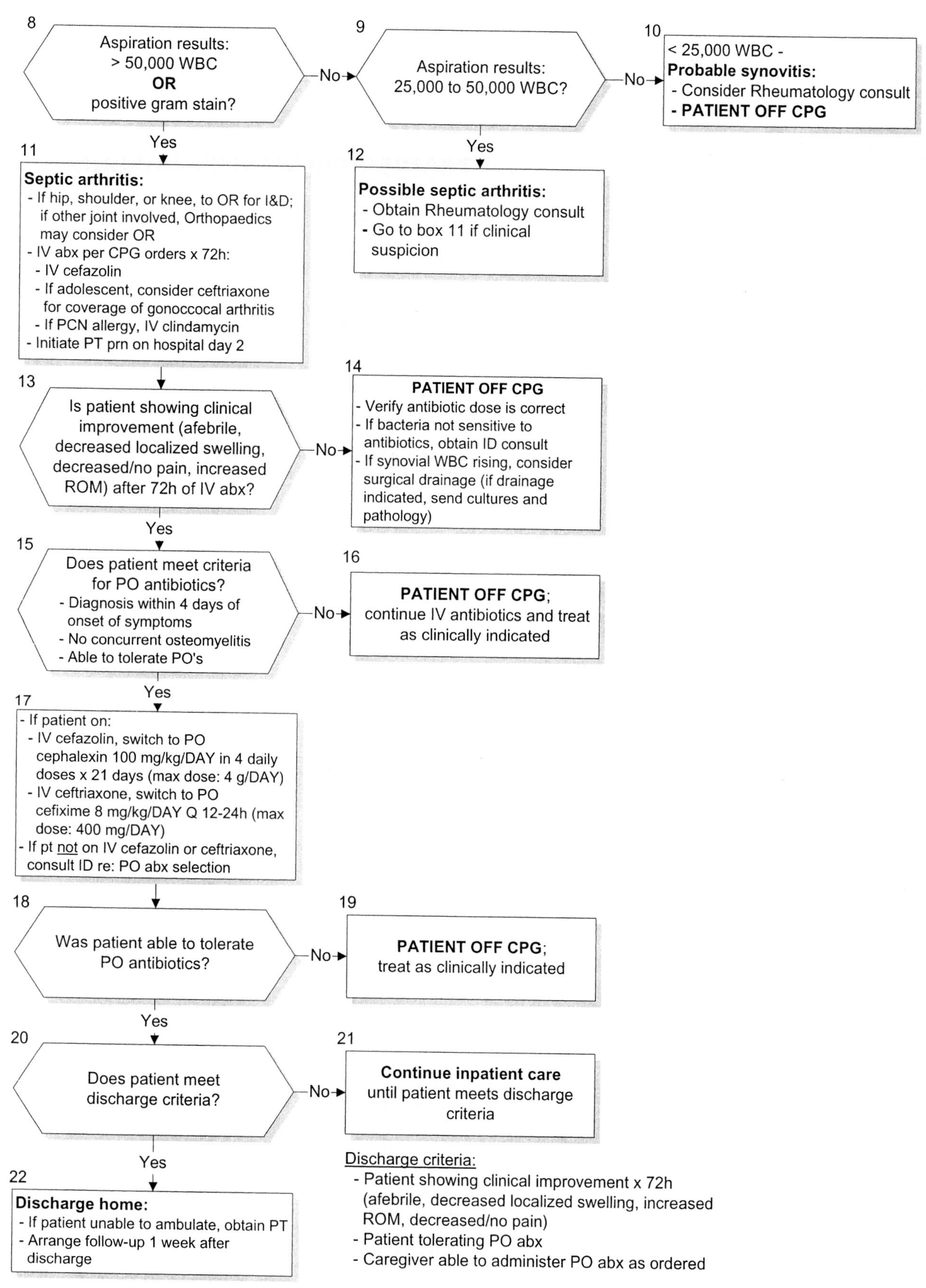
8
Aspiration results:
> 50,000 WBC
OR
positive gram stain?
No
9
Aspiration results:
25,000 to 50,000 WBC?
No
10
< 25,000 WBC -
Probable synovitis:
- Consider Rheumatology consult
- PATIENT OFF CPG
Yes
11
Septic arthritis:
- If hip, shoulder, or knee, to OR for I&D; if other joint involved, Orthopaedics may consider OR
- IV abx per CPG orders x 72h:
- IV cefazolin
- If adolescent, consider ceftriaxone for coverage of gonoccocal arthritis
- If PCN allergy, IV clindamycin
- Initiate PT prn on hospital day 2
Yes
12
Possible septic arthritis:
- Obtain Rheumatology consult
- Go to box 11 if clinical suspicion
13
Is patient showing clinical improvement (afebrile, decreased localized swelling, decreased/no pain, increased ROM) after 72h of IV abx?
No
14
PATIENT OFF CPG
- Verify antibiotic dose is correct
- If bacteria not sensitive to antibiotics, obtain ID consult
- If synovial WBC rising, consider surgical drainage (if drainage indicated, send cultures and pathology)
Yes
15
Does patient meet criteria for PO antibiotics?
- Diagnosis within 4 days of onset of symptoms
- No concurrent osteomyelitis
- Able to tolerate PO's
No
16
PATIENT OFF CPG; continue IV antibiotics and treat as clinically indicated
Yes
17
- If patient on:
- IV cefazolin, switch to PO cephalexin 100 mg/kg/DAY in 4 daily doses x 21 days (max dose: 4 g/DAY)
- IV ceftriaxone, switch to PO cefixime 8 mg/kg/DAY Q 12-24h (max dose: 400 mg/DAY)
- If pt not on IV cefazolin or ceftriaxone, consult ID re: PO abx selection
18
Was patient able to tolerate PO antibiotics?
No
19
PATIENT OFF CPG; treat as clinically indicated
Yes
20
Does patient meet discharge criteria?
No
21
Continue inpatient care until patient meets discharge criteria
Yes
22
Discharge home:
- If patient unable to ambulate, obtain PT
- Arrange follow-up 1 week after discharge
Discharge criteria:
- Patient showing clinical improvement x 72h (afebrile, decreased localized swelling, increased ROM, decreased/no pain)
- Patient tolerating PO abx
- Caregiver able to administer PO abx as ordered

Algorithm 17-1 *(continued)*

SPECIAL SITUATIONS

SUBACUTE HEMATOGENOUS OSTEOMYELITIS

- Slow, insidious onset. Commonly presents as a metaphyseal lesion such as a Brodie abscess or an epiphyseal lesion
- Can mimic other lesions such as chondroblastoma, eosinophilic granuloma, osteoid osteoma, or osteoblastoma
- Treat with i.v. antibiotics. Surgery if unresponsive.

CHRONIC RECURRENT MULTIFOCAL OSTEOMYELITIS

- Inflammatory process of the bone with no clear etiology
- Multiple lesions, normal WBC count. Nonspecific radiographs with poorly defined metaphyseal lesions
- Symptoms resolve, then recur, and can continue to recur for several years.
- Treat with nonsteroidal inflammatory drugs.

OSTEOMYELITIS AND SEPTIC HIP ARTHRITIS IN THE NEONATE

- Group B *Streptococcus* most common; however, many different organisms can be involved.
- Immature immune system. Infection can be extensive with multiple sites. Symptoms are often mild or minimal. In the septic newborn one should always suspect a bone or joint infection.
- Infections may be related to an indwelling i.v. catheter or may occur in the apparently healthy newborn after discharge.
- The hip is very susceptible to infection, ischemic necrosis, septic dislocation, and physeal injury. Aspiration of a suspected hip infection should always be performed and surgery provided whenever pus is found.
- Intravenous rather than oral antibiotics

TRANSIENT SYNOVITIS OF THE HIP

- Must always be differentiated from septic arthritis of the hip
- Considered to be an immune-mediated mechanism after a viral infection
- Less signs of systemic illness or joint inflammation. More comfortable at rest
- Kocher and colleagues looked at the following four predictors of septic arthritis versus transient synovitis:
  - History of fever
  - Non-weightbearing
  - ESR ≥40 mm/hour
  - WBC >12,000 cells/mm^3
- Probability of septic arthritis with positive predictors:
  - 1 of 4:2—5%
  - 2 of 4:33—62%
  - 3 of 4:93—97%
  - 4 of 4:99—99.8%

POSTGASTROENTERITIS ARTHRITIS

- Joint involvement after infection with intestinal pathogens: *Salmonella, Shigella, Yersinia, Campylobacter*
- Positive stool culture

REITER SYNDROME

- Oral and genital lesions. May have eye symptoms
- In the sexually active child, positive *Gonococcus* or *Chlamydia* cultures confirm the diagnosis.

SACROILIAC JOINT INFECTIONS

- Pain in gluteal region, abdomen, or lumbar region
- FABER (flexion, abduction, external rotation) test positive on physical examination
- Initially, radiographs are normal. MRI is very useful in the pelvic region and can detect an adjacent soft tissue abscess, particularly when the patient is not responding to antibiotic treatment.
- Blood and stool cultures are obtained and are positive in 60%. Usually *S. aureus,* but can be caused by *Salmonella.*
- Treatment: i.v. antibiotics to cover *S. aureus*

CULTURE-NEGATIVE AND GONOCOCCAL SEPTIC ARTHRITIS

- Rash, tenosynovitis especially on the dorsum of the hands and polyarticular arthritis are suspicious findings for *N. gonorrheae.*
- Culture all mucous membranes.
- Report to protective services if *N. gonorrheae* infection is confirmed in a young child.
- In future, polymerase chain reaction (PCR) may be useful for diagnosis.
- Ceftriaxone (50 mg/kg/day) is used for possible *H. influenzae* B or *N. gonorrhea* infection.

LYME ARTHRITIS

- History of documented tick bite in known endemic area
- Typical rash of erythema migrans
- Obtain Lyme titer if diagnosis considered.

VIRAL ARTHRITIS

- Multiple small joints
- May mimic septic arthritis, especially if caused by parvovirus

TUBERCULOSIS

- Bone or joint involvement is seen in 10% of tuberculosis cases.
- Systemic symptoms, and mild pain are often seen.
- The spine is the most common musculoskeletal site and is involved in 50%, with kyphosis the most common deformity.
- PPD
- Prolonged and monitored antimicrobial therapy is mainstay of treatment.

DISCITIS

- The pediatric disc receives its blood supply directly from the adjacent bone, which makes the disc susceptible to hematogenous infection.
- Findings include fever, systemic illness, refusal to walk, or abdominal pain in the younger child. Back pain, night pain, and stiffness in flexion are more common in the older child.
- Blood cultures are positive in 50%, CRP is markedly elevated, and ESR is moderately elevated.
- Plain radiographs show disc space narrowing and occasionally end-plate changes. Bone scan is more sensitive and can diagnose the infection about a week earlier than can plain radiographs.
- Initially treat with antistaphylococcal antibiotics. Casting or bracing is used for comfort.

SICKLE CELL DISEASE

- Patients are at risk for osteomyelitis due to microvascular disease and bony infarcts.
- Vasoocclusive pain crisis (infarction) more common than osteomyelitis. Symptoms resolve sooner.
- Osteomyelitis produces high fever and an ill patient. There is an elevated ESR and positive blood cultures. Aspiration is the best diagnostic test to confirm infection. Surgical drainage is usually necessary.
- *S. aureus* is still the most common organism in osteomyelitis in sicklers, but *salmonella* is more common in sicklers than in the general population.

PUNCTURE WOUNDS

- Classically, a nail through a dirty, old athletic shoe
- Small percentage develops osteomyelitis or septic arthritis by direct inoculation into the bone or joint. Typically caused by *Pseudomonas*.
- Confirmed deep infection with *Pseudomonas* requires surgical débridement and i.v. antibiotic coverage.

PEARLS

- Septic arthritis of the hip is a true surgical emergency, especially in the neonate.
- Ultrasound of the hip is very sensitive to confirm an effusion, which then needs to be explained.
- Beware of the "cold" bone scan: associated with worse prognosis and suggestive of ischemia.
- Obtain infectious disease consultation for:
  - Unusual organism: *S. pneumoniae, H. influenzae*, gram-negative
  - Unusual host: sickle cell, immunocompromised, malabsorption
  - Unusual site: multiple joints, bones, or multiple organs
- If patient unresponsive to antibiotic treatment consider:
  - Wrong diagnosis
  - Wrong antibiotic, dose, or route of administration
  - An abscess or undrained pus
  - Immune deficiency
- Pus should be drained surgically when:
  - Purulence on aspiration
  - Radiographic evidence of purulence/abscess: hole in bone, fluid collection
  - Unresponsive to appropriate antibiotics

SUGGESTED READING

Herring, JA. Tachdjian's pediatric orthopaedics, 3rd ed. Philadelphia: WB Saunders, 2002;1841–1877.

Kocher MS, et al. Efficacy of a clinical practice guideline on process and outcome for septic arthritis of the hip in children. Paper No. 74 presented at Annual Meeting POSNA; Salt Lake City; 2001.

Kocher MS, Zurakowski D, Kasser JR. Differentiating between septic arthritis and transient synovitis of the hip in children: an evidence-based clinical prediction algorithm. J Bone Joint Surg (Am), 1999; 81:1662–1670.

Morrey BF, Peterson HA. Hematogenous pyogenic osteomyelitis in children. Orthop Clin North Am 1975;6:935–951.

Morrissy RT, Weinstein SL. Lovell and Winter's pediatric orthopaedics, 5th ed. Philadelphia: Lippincott Williams & Wilkins, 2001: 459–505.

Peltola H, Vahvanen V. A comparative study of osteomyelitis and purulent arthritis with special reference to aetiology and recovery. Infection 1984;12:75–79.

Song KM, Sloboda JF. Acute hematogenous osteomyelitis in children. J Am Acad Orthop Surg 2001;9:166–175.

Sponseller PD. Orthopaedic knowledge update: pediatrics 2. Rosemont, IL: American Academy of Orthopaedic Surgeons, 2002: 27–41.

Sucato DJ, Schwend RM, Gillespie R. Septic arthritis of the hip in children. J Am Acad Orthop Surg 1997;5:249–260.

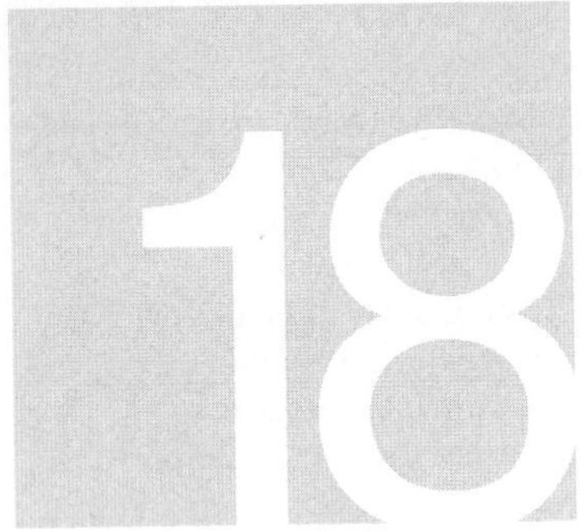

CEREBRAL PALSY

ARABELLA I. LEET

Cerebral palsy results in a wide spectrum of disease ranging from severely affected children who rely on wheelchairs for ambulation and who have low cognitive function to mildly involved children who are difficult to distinguish from idiopathic toe walkers. Cerebral palsy is a disorder of the central nervous system that causes neuromuscular derangements in a cascade from abnormality in muscle tone and strength that can, in turn, have secondary deleterious effects on bones and joints. Orthopaedic management cannot address the true location of pathology, which is in the brain, but instead focuses on making the child more independent with increased functional capacity.

Since cerebral palsy may encompass such a large spectrum of involvement, both physical and cognitive, treatment must be geared to the needs of the individual child. The first step is to try to estimate what might be the highest level of function achievable for a child, and next devise ways to reach this highest level of function whether through nonsurgical means (such as braces, medications, or therapy) or by surgical interventions that can lengthen muscles or correct bone deformity.

If the orthopaedist understands that what is most essential to adults with cerebral palsy is the ability to communicate, the neuromuscular issues become only a part of the management of cerebral palsy. Thus, a team approach involving therapists, physiatrists, orthotists, neurologists, developmental pediatricians, and social workers is often necessary in order to more completely address the complex needs of an individual patient.

PATHOGENESIS

Etiology

Cerebral palsy is caused by an injury to the developing brain. By definition the injury is nonprogressive and occurs before age 2, when glialization of the brain is still occurring. The brain injuries that cause cerebral palsy are diverse. Children with hemiplegia tend to have a fixed focal lesion in the brain caused by brain malformation, infection, or embolic event. The pattern of diplegia results from injury around the third ventricle where the corticospinal tracks descend from the motor cortex as the corona radiata en route to the internal capsule. Since the tracks for the legs are closest to the third ventricle, hemorrhage around the third ventricle leads to the pattern of injury seen in diplegia where both legs are involved. Bleeds around the third ventricle, diagnosed by ultrasound in the nursery can be a predictive sign of diplegia, as can periventricular leukomalacia (PVL).

Many causes can contribute to cerebral palsy, but almost 50% of children with cerebral palsy are born full term and 35% of the time the exact etiology remains unknown (Box 18-1).

Epidemiology

Cerebral palsy is thought to have an incidence of 1 to 3 per 1,000 live births. It affects over 700,000 children and adults in the United States. The incidence has remained unchanged over time, but there has been a shift in the last half century from children with ataxia (secondary to Rh incompatibility, which is now easily diagnosed and treated) to children with diplegia (occurring as lower birthweight children survive with better neonatal intensive care unit management). Cerebral palsy is associated with prematurity (less than 32 weeks gestation) and low birthweight (less than 1,500 g).

BOX 18-1 POSSIBLE CAUSES OF CEREBRAL PALSY

Prenatal
- Maternal toxemia
- Maternal epilepsy
- Third trimester bleeding

Perinatal
- Hypoxia (risk factors: placental abruption, nuchal cord)
- Intracranial hemorrhage
- Prematurity (low birthweight)

Pathophysiology

The mechanism of brain injury is not yet completely understood. Prematurity or endotoxins from maternal infection may increase the brain tissue sensitivity to injury from other sources such as hypoxia. After initial injury, there appears to be a cascade of cellular events that generate the release of cytokines causing further cellular damage by increasing apoptosis (programmed cell death). Research on the causes of brain injury is ongoing.

Classification

Children with cerebral palsy are classified both by the type of muscle tone exhibited and the location of the disease (Table 18-1). For example, a child whose leg involvement is greater than arm involvement and who is spastic would be classified as cerebral palsy subtype spastic diplegia.

DIAGNOSIS

Usually the diagnosis of cerebral palsy also is multidisciplinary involving the pediatrician, neurologist, orthopaedist, and physical therapist. Depending on the history, workup often includes:

- Computed tomography or magnetic resonance imaging or ultrasound of the brain
- Serology to rule out intrauterine infection
- Physical therapy evaluation for developmental assessment.
- Orthopaedic evaluation of the musculoskeletal system
- Other tests depending on the age and needs of the child and the presence of visual or hearing impairments, mental retardation, or medical problems (seizures or pneumonia)

Prognosis

- Life expectancy is variable and generally depends on the overall medical condition of the child, including history of recurrent pneumonias, seizures, and nutritional status.
- Parents often want to know whether their child will walk. Predictors of the ability to walk include:
  - ☐ Loss of primitive reflexes before 24 months:
    - ☐ Moro
    - ☐ Parachute
    - ☐ Asymmetric tonic neck reflex
    - ☐ Extensor thrust
    - ☐ Neck-righting reflex
  - ☐ Sitting by 2 years
  - ☐ Development of reciprocal activities (e.g., crawling)
  - ☐ In general, if walking is not achieved by 7 years, then it is unlikely that a child will develop the ability to walk in the future.

TABLE 18-1 CLASSIFICATION OF CEREBRAL PALSY

Type	Description
Tone	
Spastic	Increased stretch reflex, increased clonus
Dyskinetic	Abnormal motor involvement
Ataxic	Cerebellar involvement
Mixed	Combinations of above
Location	
Quadriparesis	All limbs involved
Diplegia	Legs involved to a greater extent than arms
Hemiplegia	One-sided involvement

Physical Examination and History

Physical Examination

- Observation of extraneous movements (i.e., athetoid motion)
- Muscle tone
  - ☐ Subjectively graded as high to low
- Selective control (ability to place limbs in a desired location in space)
- Sensibility
- Contracture
  - ☐ Fixed loss of motion to be distinguished from resistance secondary to high tone.
  - ☐ There can be a high degree of variability between exams based on the child's ability to relax. Tone will increase if the patient is upset, cold, or frightened.
- Torsional deformity (results in lever arm dysfunction)
  - ☐ Femoral anteversion
  - ☐ External tibial torsion
- Balance and equilibrium
- Gait evaluation
  - ☐ Observational gait analysis (Box 18-2)
  - ☐ Three-dimensional gait analysis
    - ☐ Computer-based evaluation including kinetics, kinematics, and electromyelograph (EMG) analysis
- Special physical exam tests used for cerebral palsy to test muscles that cross two joints that are often more specifically involved
  - ☐ Phelps test: tests if gracilis muscle is involved compared with hip adductors

BOX 18-2 FIVE COMPONENTS OF NORMAL GAIT

1. Conservation of energy
2. Stability in stance
3. Clearance in swing
4. Pre-positioning of the foot in swing
5. Adequate step length

Adapted from Gage JR. Gait analysis in cerebral palsy. Oxford: MacKeith Press, 1991.

- The patient is positioned prone with the knee flexed.
- As the knee is extended, the hip is observed for adduction.

- Silverskiöld test: used to distinguish involvement of gastrocnemius from the soleus.
  - With the patient supine, the ankle is dorsiflexed with the knee extended and then again with the knee flexed.
  - Since the gastrocnemius attaches at the distal femur it is relaxed with knee flexion, allowing the foot to dorsiflex if the soleus is not spastic or contracted.
- Duncan-Ely test: distinguishes whether the rectus femoris or iliopsoas is contracted by observing the pelvis rising with knee flexion when the patient is prone.
- Popliteal angle: determines the extent of hamstring involvement across the hip and knee joints (Fig. 18-1).

History

- Prematurity
- Low birthweight
- Maternal toxemia
- Placental complications: abruption or previa
- Medical history to identify seizure disorders, gastrointestinal reflux, pneumonias, and strabismus—disorders often seen in children with cerebral palsy
- Developmental milestones

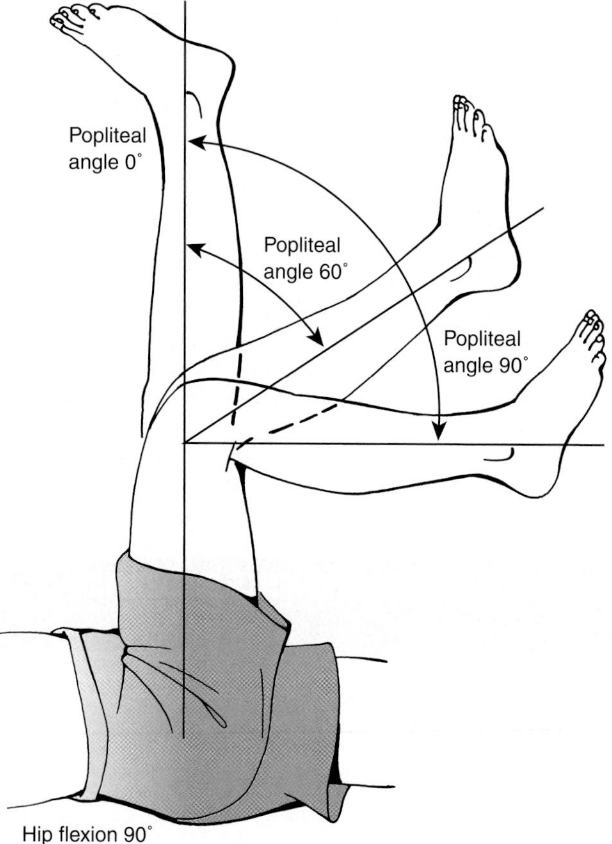

Figure 18-1 The popliteal angle is measured with the child supine and the hip flexed at 90 degrees.

- Handedness
  - Unusual to show hand dominance before 18 months
  - Suspect hemiplegia if child is not using both hands

Clinical Features

Children with severe involvement often have microcephaly apparent to observation, as are extraneous movements. Assessment of motor tone, by range of motion of joints, reveals increased tone, clonus, or contractures. Specific secondary orthopaedic developments from the brain injury include:

- Hip subluxation/dislocation
  - Children with cerebral palsy have structurally normal hips at birth, but muscle imbalance over time (especially increased adduction and flexion) can cause the hips to sublux and finally to dislocate completely causing hip pain and difficulty with seating and perineal care.
- Scoliosis
  - Curves tend to be long C-shaped or S-shaped curves that often include the pelvis.
- Foot deformity
  - Pes planovalgus in children with diplegia
  - Equinovarus feet develop more commonly in children with hemiplegia.
- Gait deviations
  - Caused by deformities to joints from contractures or spasticity
  - Proximal compensations are necessary to accommodate distal pathology.
  - Problems with balance
  - Gait analysis can be a useful tool to sort deformities (which can respond to surgical correction) from compensations (which will resolve without the need for intervention once the true pathology is resolved).
- Upper extremity involvement
  - Typically involves elbow flexion, forearm supination (from pronator spasticity), wrist volar flexion, and finger fisting or thumb-in-palm deformity
  - Sensibility may be lost, making eventual use of arm problematic because correcting the deformity may not make up for the fact that there is poor sensory information being relayed back to the brain.
  - The size of the involved arm has been shown to correlate well with the amount of sensibility:
    - If the involved arm is considerably smaller then the uninvolved side, much of the sensibility in the involved arm can be assumed to be decreased.
    - Hygiene problems can result from fisted hand position or from thumb in palm deformity.
- Pathologic fracture
  - Most children with cerebral palsy have a significant decrease in bone density. The etiology of low bone density includes the following:
    - Non-weightbearing
    - Seizure medications (Dilantin, Carbamazepine) can impede vitamin D absorption.
    - Poor nutrition leads to insufficient intake of calcium and vitamin D.
    - Casting after surgery leads to disuse osteopenia.

- Fractures can occur with transfers or spontaneously (no recognized event), and are managed by casting (which can be difficult secondary to shortening while in a cast caused by muscle spasticity) or alternatively operative strategies including external or internal fixation.

Differential Diagnosis

- Genetic syndromes
  - Familiar spastic paraplegia
  - Hereditary microcephaly
- Progressive neurologic disorders

Radiographic Features

- Anteroposterior pelvis: Check for hip subluxation using the Reimer Migration Index (Fig. 18-2).
- Spine films: Use the Cobb angle technique to measure the amount of scoliosis.

TREATMENT

Decreasing Spasticity

- Medical
  - Baclofen: GABA antagonist, given either orally or intrathecally through pump.
  - Botulinum toxin: temporary muscle paralysis.
  - Valium: given at 0.1 mg/kg, most effective of all agents as a muscle relaxant, but also leads to central nervous system effects
- Surgical
  - Selective dorsal rhizotomy usually performed by a neurosurgeon; dorsal nerve rootlets are identified, and 30% to 60% are divided from L1-S2. Candidate selection for rhizotomy must be done carefully. The procedure is best for ambulatory spastic diplegics. The most common complication of rhizotomy is weakness after the procedure.

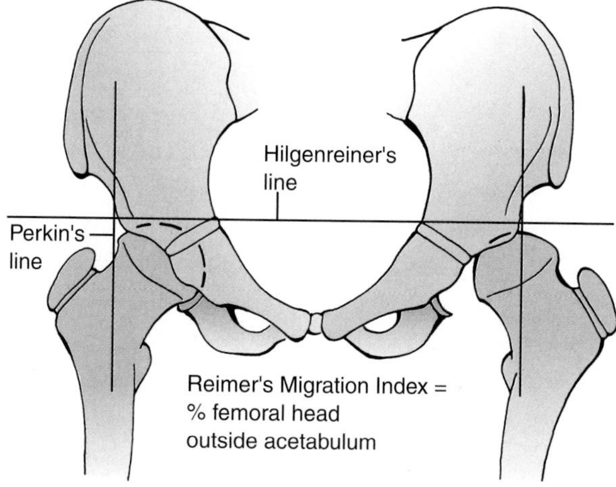

Figure 18-2 Reimer's Migration Index is a measure of the percentage of femoral head outside the acetabulum.

Maintaining Positioning

- Bracing upper and lower extremities to maintain functional positions
  - Ankle foot orthosis (AFO) made out of semi-rigid material
  - May be solid or articulated, depending on ambulatory status
- Seating system in nonambulatory children
  - Position the trunk upright, head forward, so children can interact with the world around them
  - Accommodate trunk and pelvic deformity in design of wheelchair
  - Use of tilt chairs prevents skin breakdown in children who cannot shift their weight while sitting
  - Use electric wheelchairs, if child capable of steering safely.
  - Traditional custom wheelchairs are often difficult to transport in a car, thus families also will need a stroller-type device that is more portable.

Managing Deformity

- Soft-tissue release: lengthening a muscle, whether at the musculotendinous junction or through the tendon, treats fixed contractures but also results in muscle weakness.
  - Adductor tenotomy
    - Indications: a Reimer Migration Index of more than 50 percent, or loss of more than 30 degrees of hip abduction in hip extension resulting in difficulty with diapering, or perineal hygiene
  - Gastrocnemius recession
    - Indication: for ankle equinus and a positive Silverskiöld test (soleus not contracted)
  - Tendo-Achilles lengthening
  - Reserved for equinus involving both gastrocnemius and soleus muscles
  - Must be careful not to over lengthen the tendo-Achilles, which will result in an iatrogenic crouch gait
  - Hamstring lengthening
    - Indications: popliteal angles greater than 45 to 60 degrees or difficulty with sitting secondary to extension of the pelvis from the proximal attachment of the hamstrings
    - Medial or medial and lateral depending on the amount of the popliteal angle preoperatively
- Tendon transfer: aimed to rebalance muscles around a joint
  - SPLATT/SPLOTT (split anterior or posterior tibialis tendon transfer)
    - Indications: hindfoot varus, passively correctable, and identification of spasticity (may require EMG) in either the posterior or anterior tibialis muscle
- Osteotomies: correction of bone for torsional correction or to address deficiency of structures (i.e., acetabulum)
  - Varus derotation osteotomy (VDO) of the proximal femur
    - Correction of valgus and anteversion of the proximal femur

        - □ Indication: for Reimer Migration Index of more than 50 degrees that cannot be corrected with adductor tenotomy
    - □ Pelvic osteotomy (Dega, Chiari)
        - □ Indications: acetabular deficiency
        - □ Acetabulum usually deficient in children with cerebral palsy posteriorly or laterally, as opposed to hip dysplasia where the deficiency tends to be anterior
    - □ May be performed in combination with VDO
    - □ Os calcis lengthening
        - □ Indications: for flexible pes planovalgus
        - □ Navicular is subluxed on the talar head
- Fusion
    - □ Spine
        - □ Indications: for scoliotic curves of greater than 50 degrees that are rigid. Traction films can help determine curve flexibility, as can clinical examination.
        - □ Add anterior release or fusion for excessively large curves (more than 70 to 80 degrees)
        - □ Fuse to include the pelvis if there is pelvic obliquity
        - □ Since fusions are long, allograft often used as bone graft
    - □ Subtalar joint
        - □ Indications: for pes planovalgus that is not passively correctable
    - □ Great toe for hallux valgus deformity
    - □ Routine bunion corrections less reliable
    - □ Must fuse in 20 to 30 degrees of dorsiflexion

SUGGESTED READING

Abel MF, Damiano DL, Pannunzio M, et al. Muscle-tendon surgery in diplegic cerebral palsy: functional and mechanical changes. J Pediatr Orthop 1999;19:366–375.

Bleck EE. Orthopedic management in cerebral palsy. Oxford: Blackwell Scientific Publications, 1987.

Comstock CP, Leach J, Wenger DR. Scoliosis in total-body involvement cerebral palsy. Analysis of surgical treatment and patient caregiver satisfaction. Spine 1998;23:1412–24.

Cosgrove AP, Graham HK. Botulinum toxin A prevents the development of contractures in the hereditary spastic mouse. Dev Med Child Neurol 1994;36:379–385.

Dolk H, Pattenden S, Johnson A. Cerebral palsy, low birthweight and socio-economic deprivation: inequalities as a major cause of childhood disability. Pediatr Perinatal Epidemiol 2001;15:359–363.

Gage JR. Gait analysis in cerebral palsy. Oxford: MacKeith Press, 1991.

Miller F, Cardoso Dias R, Dabney, KW, et al. Soft-tissue release for spastic hip subluxation. J Pediatr Orthop 1997;17:571–584.

Rang M, Douglas G, Benner GC, et al. Seating for children with cerebral palsy. J Pediatr Orthop 1981;1:279–286.

Sussman MD. The diplegic child. evaluation and management. Rosemont, IL: American Academy of Orthopedic Surgery, 1992.

Winters TF, Gage JR, Hicks R. Gait patterns in spastic hemiplegia in children and young adults. J Bone Joint Surg (Am) 1987;69: 437–441.

SPINA BIFIDA

LAURA LEMKE
LUCIANO DIAS

Spina bifida is a nonspecific term used to describe a broad spectrum of defects that occur during the formation of the neural tube. Spina bifida occulta is an asymptomatic localized defect in the formation of the vertebral arch that is present in 10% of normal adults. It is not associated with any defect of the spinal cord or meninges. Spina bifida cystica describes four types of defects that occur in the meninges and spinal cord. Myelocele is a protrusion of the spinal cord. Meningocele is a protrusion of the meninges of the spinal cord through a defect in the spinal column. Myelomeningocele is a protrusion of the meninges and spinal cord through a defect in the spinal column. Rachischisis is a congenital fissure of the spine at the level of a vertebral arch. The term spina bifida also includes anencephaly, absence of the brain, and encephalocele, a congenital gap in the skull with herniation of brain substance. Ninety percent of children described as having spina bifida will have myelomeningocele, so that will be the primary focus of this discussion.

PATHOGENESIS

Etiology

Defects causing spina bifida are a result of failure of closure of the neural tube, as opposed to reopening after closure. Closure of the neural tube occurs at various sites with each site controlled by a different gene. Environmental factors also play a role in closure of the neural tube. Maternal insulin-dependent diabetes, maternal hyperthermia, use of valproic acid, and folate deficiency have all been linked to myelodysplasia.

Prevention

Avoidance of hyperthermia (hot baths and saunas) and discontinuation of valproic acid can reduce the risk of myelodysplasia. Daily ingestion of 4 mg of folic acid supplement before and early in pregnancy reduces the risk of neural tube defect by 60% to 72%. High dietary intake of folic acid can also reduce risk. Screening programs such as maternal α-fetoprotein, ultrasound, and amniotic α-fetoprotein and cholinesterase can detect virtually all open spina bifida by 18 weeks of gestation.

Epidemiology

The most recent estimate of the incidence of neural tube defects is 0.6 to 0.9 per 1,000 live births. The incidence, however, has been decreasing over the last few decades, particularly with the discovery of the correlation with folic acid deficiency.

Classification

The best classification for myelomeningocele is based on the neurologic level of the lesion. Neurologic level can be correlated with function and predict likelihood of ambulation. See Table 19-1 for the classification of myelomeningocele.

ASSOCIATED NEUROLOGIC CONDITIONS

Hydrocephalus

Hydrocephalus is an excessive accumulation of fluid in the cerebral ventricles that causes thinning of the cerebral tissue and can cause separation of the cranial bones. In infants accumulation of fluid can also occur in the subarachnoid or subdural space. Cerebrospinal fluid shunting is required in 80% to 90% of children with myelomeningocele because of hydrocephalus. The incidence of hydrocephalus is related to the level of the lesion: 83% in thoracic and upper lumbar lesions, 60% in low lumbar and sacral lesions. Children who do not require shunting have a better prognosis than those who do require shunting. Those who do not require shunting have better upper extremity function and trunk balance as well as a lower incidence of hydromyelia and tethered cord. Infection and obstruction of the shunt are the two most common complications and have been negatively correlated with the child's motor and intellectual development.

TABLE 19-1 CLASSIFICATION OF MYELOMENINGOCELE

Group	Lesion Level	Function	Ambulation[a]
1	Thoracic and high lumbar	No quadriceps function	Minimal to age 13 with HKAFO or RGO 95%–99% wheelchair-bound as adults
2	Low lumbar	Quadriceps and medial hamstring function	Require AFO and crutches. Many (79%) community ambulators as adults. L4 level better chance for ambulation with proper musculoskeletal care
3	Sacral	Quadriceps and medial hamstring function	94% ambulatory as adults
	High sacral	No gastrocsoleus strength	Use AFO but no crutches. Gluteus lurch and excessive pelvic obliquity
	Low sacral	Good gastrocsoleus strength. Normal gluteus medius and maximus function	Walk without AFO or crutches. Gait close to normal

[a]Braces are described in Chapter 2.
AFO, ankle–foot orthosis; HKAFO, hip–knee–ankle–foot orthosis; RGO, reciprocating gait orthosis.

Arnold-Chiari Malformation

Arnold-Chiari malformation is a common clinical and anatomic finding in children with myelomeningocele. This is a displacement of the hindbrain into the foramen magnum. This occurs in three types. In type I, the cerebellum is displaced but the brainstem is not. This type often presents in adolescence with headaches, lower extremity spasticity, and upper extremity pain. Type II, which occurs in 90% of children with myelomeningocele, involves displacement of the brainstem commonly in association with hydrocephalus. This caudal displacement leads to dysfunction of the lower cranial nerves, causing weakness and paralysis of the vocal cords and difficulty feeding. These symptoms become apparent in infancy. Patients may also display ocular disturbance, apneic episodes, and progressive respiratory difficulty. Type III Arnold-Chiari malformation, is an encephalocele at the craniocervical junction.

Tethered Spinal Cord

During normal fetal development, the spinal cord ascends until it is at level L3 at birth. By the second month of life it has reached the adult level at approximately L1. In children with neural tube defects there is communication with the overlying ectoderm at birth. All children with myelomeningocele have a tethered cord at birth but with closure of the defect the spinal cord falls back within the canal. Scarring of the overlying tissues results in most children with myelomeningocele showing signs of tethering on magnetic resonance imaging (MRI) but only 15% to 30% of these children show clinical manifestations of tethered cord. Clinical signs can be variable but commonly involve:

- Loss of motor function
- Lower extremity spasticity, particularly in the medial hamstrings, ankle dorsiflexors, and ankle evertors
- Scoliosis before age 6 in the absence of congenital vertebral anomaly
- Back pain and increased lumbar lordosis in ambulatory children
- Changes in urologic function

When there is suspicion of tethered cord syndrome, MRI or computed tomography (CT)/myelogram can be used to evaluate the spinal cord. Shunt malfunction should also be ruled out.

Hydromyelia

Hydromyelia or syringomyelia of the spinal cord is a fluid-filled cavity within the spinal cord itself. This occurs in up to 54% of children with myelomeningocele. The presumed mechanism is that fluid in a hydrocephalic fourth ventricle enters the central canal. Pressure causes gradual expansion of the canal. This problem manifests as increasing spasticity, upper extremity weakness, back pain, and classically, as worsening spinal deformity. Evaluation should include CT or MRI. Treatment is controversial and includes shunt placement or revision, posterior fossa decompression, or direct shunting of the cavity itself. Treatment can lead to some scoliosis regression.

Cognition

Children who do not require shunting have normal intelligence. Of those who do require shunting, 70% to 80% will have IQs above 80; the remainder will have IQs below 80. Verbal skills are good but perceptual scores are low resulting in a social, verbal child with limited ability for rehabilitation.

RELATED CONCERNS

Urologic Considerations

Urologic dysfunction is common in children with myelomeningocele. Incomplete emptying is common due to bladder spasticity or flaccidity and predisposes these children to recurrent urinary tract infections. Vesicoureteral reflux is also common. Urinary diversion, intermittent catheterization, and suppressive antibiotics have decreased the percent of patients with renal dysfunction from 75% to 30%.

Latex Allergy

Latex allergy is a topic of great concern in patients with myelomeningocele. Reactions range from urticaria and bronchospasms to anaphylaxis and death. The reaction is immunoglobulin E–mediated. Patient screening with skin testing and radioallergosorbent (RAST) testing has shown that the incidence is 1% in adults in the general population, 7.5% in operating room personnel, and 18% to 89%, with both types of screening in various studies, in children with myelomeningocele. Multiple exposures early in life have been postulated to be a major risk factor in latex allergy. For children with myelomeningocele, a latex-free surgical environment is safest. Premedication with histamine-blocking agents and steroids is controversial and has not been proven to be beneficial.

Anesthesia Considerations

Malignant hyperthermia has been reported in patients with myelomeningocele. There is at best a weak association between the two conditions. Treatment is the same for all patients with malignant hyperthermia.

Infection Risks

Recurrent urinary tract infections can lead to a higher postsurgical infection rate for patients with myelomeningocele. Blood-borne bacteria are presumed to seed wounds but no correlation has been found between urine, blood, and wound infections. Infection rates have been found to decrease if preoperative antibiotics were based on preoperative urine cultures. Other important factors include poor skin in the area of sac closure, insensate skin, and nutrition.

ORTHOPAEDIC EVALUATION

Serial Muscle Test

This test is used to determine the neurologic level of function. It should be done at birth before closure, 10 to 14 days after closure, and then annually. If possible, the same therapist should always do this. The child may be 3 or 4 years old before the neurologic level is absolutely defined because gluteus medius and maximus strength can be accurately determined only around this age. The level should stay the same throughout the child's life. Any change can be a sign of neurologic dysfunction such as tethered cord.

Sitting Balance

The ability to sit without support is a good indicator of nearly normal central nervous system function. If support is required for sitting, walking ability with an orthosis or external support is limited.

Upper Extremity Function

Abnormalities in upper extremity function have been documented in 60% to 82% of patients with myelomeningocele. Gait training involves the use of crutches and walkers, making upper extremity function important for ambulation. Loss of grip strength and thenar atrophy are reliable signs of hydromyelia. Other risk factors for upper extremity dysfunction include thoracic or high lumbar involvement, upper extremity spasticity, and greater than three shunt revisions.

Spine Examination

Annual spine radiographs are recommended for patients with high-level lesions. The incidence of scoliosis is quite low in patients with low lumbar of sacral scoliosis. Any spinal curvature in patients with lesions at these levels suggests tethering of the spinal cord.

Hip Range of Motion

Hip contractures are very common, particularly in patients with high lumbar or thoracic-level lesions. Abduction or adduction contractures can cause infrapelvic obliquity that interferes with bracing and ambulation. Flexion contractures are also common. These can be measured with the Thomas test. Internal and external rotation deformities can interfere with gait. Internal and external rotation should always be accurately recorded. Internal rotation deformity during gait combined with external tibial torsion is a common cause of increased valgus stress at the knee.

Knee Alignment and Range of Motion

Knee flexion contracture is common. Contracture of greater than 20 degrees can interfere with bracing and lead to a crouched gait. Knee extension contractures are usually congenital. External tibial torsion with a thigh–foot angle of more than 20 degrees can lead to increased valgus stress at the knee. Internal tibial torsion is often associated with congenital clubfoot deformity.

Foot and Ankle Deformities

Ankle valgus is common and may cause pressure sores at the medial malleolus with orthotic wear. Alignment of the forefoot and hindfoot, and ankle range of motion are very important to record in patients with myelomeningocele. Approximately 90% of patients with myelomeningocele have some type of foot deformity. Subtle changes that occur with tethered cord should be recognized early.

Gait Analysis

Clinical Application

Gait analysis is commonly used in the treatment of patients with cerebral palsy. For patients with myelomeningocele, gait analysis is useful for two groups:

1. Patients with low lumbar lesions who walk with below-knee orthosis and external supports
2. Patients with sacral-level lesions who walk with ankle–foot orthoses and no support

The average walking velocity for low lumbar-level patients is 54% of normal. The average velocity for a patient with a sacral-level lesion is 70% of normal.

Kinetic Pattern

All patients with myelomeningocele show some form of compensatory movement with gait based on their level of muscle weakness. Weakness of the gluteus medius and maximus necessitate pelvic rotation and obliquity to facilitate forward progression and maintain independent ambulation. Increased stance-phase hip abduction, increased knee flexion, and increased ankle dorsiflexion also help to facilitate gait. The magnitude of compensatory movement at the pelvis is related to the level of motor deficit.

Gait analysis has been particularly helpful in understanding the gait patterns of those with hip pathology and those with valgus knee stress. The quality of crutch walking in children with hip subluxation and dislocation has been found to be much more effective than any attempts to correct these problems and have the children walk without supports. External tibial torsion can lead to significant valgus knee stress. When understood, correction of this problem is very beneficial to these patients.

PRINCIPLES OF ORTHOPAEDIC MANAGEMENT

Orthotic Management

Approximately 95% of patients with myelomeningocele require orthotic support to achieve ambulation. The goal of orthotic treatment is to achieve effective mobility with minimal restriction.

- A hip–knee–ankle–foot orthosis (HKAFO) is used for patients with high lumbar level lesions who can perform swing through ambulation with crutches.
- A knee–ankle–foot orthosis (KAFO) is used for patients with low lumbar-level paralysis to reduce valgus stress at the knee when the patient is too young for osteotomies.
- An ankle–foot orthosis (AFO) is used for patients with low lumbar- and high sacral-level lesions. They are usually made with a solid ankle and hold the ankle in neutral dorsiflexion (90 degrees) to minimize knee crouch.
    - Twister cables can be added to the AFOs when a child has rotational malalignment (in-toeing and out-toeing), which is frequently seen in patients with low lumbar- and high sacral-level lesions.
    - Surgical treatment is usually recommended for patients with rotational malalignment but is best done after 6 years of age. Therefore, twister cables can be used from 2 years of age until surgical correction is achieved.

Most high lumbar- and thoracic-level patients will not be ambulatory.

- The A-frame is a prefabricated brace that includes the trunk and lower extremities and allows the child to stand without hand support.
    - It can be used up to 3 hours per day in 20- to 30-minute intervals.
    - It can be started at age 12 to 18 months.
- The parapodium and reciprocating gait orthosis (RGO) are custom braces that also include the trunk and lower extremities.
    - These allow ambulation but are only indicated in high lumbar- and thoracic-level patients with good sitting/trunk balance and good upper extremity function.
    - These can be introduced around the age of 2 years.
- A wheelchair may allow independent mobility for the nonambulatory patient.
    - Seating is very important to prevent ulcers, the backrest should have trunk support when necessary, and the armrest should facilitate easy transfer in and out of the chair.
    - The chair should be fitted carefully to the specific need of the child.

Night splinting is used primarily as a preventive measure in both ambulatory and nonambulatory patients.

- A patient with a high-level lesion and complete lower extremity paralysis can benefit from a total body splint at night to prevent flexion contractures at the hips and knees and equinus deformity at the ankle.
- Careful fitting of splints is very important to prevent skin breakdown.

Physical Therapy

Development is dependent on a child's ability to move, explore, and experience the environment. These abilities are compromised in a patient with lower extremity paralysis and an abnormal central nervous system. Physical therapy plays a role in maintaining range of motion, preventing contractures, and gait training with the necessary aides. Strengthening and physical fitness are also important. Therapy is also used to monitor the child to assure that neurologic deterioration does not occur. Intensive, multifaceted therapy should lessen a child's disability.

Fractures and Physeal Injuries

Pathologic fractures of the long bones are common in patients with myelomeningocele. The incidence is higher in children with high-level lesions. Patients are particularly susceptible after the paralyzed limb has been further immobilized by casting. Fractures can occur with no history of trauma and are most common in the supracondylar femur and proximal tibial metaphysis. Symptoms usually include erythema, warmth, and swelling. Increased temperature, white blood cell count, and erythrocyte sedimentation rate can also be present. Because of this clinical presentation, fractures in patients with spina bifida can be mistaken for infection. These fractures generally heal rapidly and therefore rarely require surgery. Short periods of immobilization are recommended to prevent further osteopenia. Functional alignment and proper rotation in a well-padded cast are often enough to allow ambulation with an orthosis.

Physeal injuries are far less common and usually occur in the distal femur, proximal tibia, or distal tibia. These are usually caused by repetitive trauma similar to Charcot neuropathy. Immobilization and non-weightbearing are recommended until there is radiographic healing. When this is hard to determine clinically, loss of swelling and a normal anatomic contour compared to the other side are useful clinical determinates.

Spine Deformities

Spinal deformity is common in children with myelomeningocele. Congenital scoliosis occurs in 1% to 15% of patients. Kyphotic deformity occurs in 5% to 20% of patients, primarily those with thoracic-level lesions. A scoliotic curve of greater than 10 degrees occurs in 69% of patients with myelomeningocele. The prevalence of spinal deformity increases with higher levels of involvement.

Scoliosis

Paralytic scoliosis occurs in up to 100% of children with high-level lesions, 40% to 60% of children with low lumbar-level lesions, and 5% to 10% of children with sacral-level lesions. Curve development is gradual before the age of 10 and increases rapidly with the adolescent growth spurt. Factors that lead to progression are not well documented. Curve magnitude, Risser sign, menarchal status, and bone age are not closely linked to the likelihood of curve progression as they are in idiopathic scoliosis. Tethered cord, hydromyelia, and worsening hydrocephalus have been implicated as factors in worsening deformity. Correction of these problems may stop curve progression but a true cause-and-effect relationship has not been proven.

The frequency of spinal deformity necessitates yearly spinal radiographs beginning at about 5 years of age. If scoliosis is found, MRI is often necessary to rule out the possibility of hydromyelia or tethered cord. Any abnormalities of the spinal cord should be surgically corrected. Observation is the treatment of choice for curves less than 25 degrees. When curves are greater than 25 degrees, bracing is recommended. This is primarily a temporary measure that will delay, but not stop, curve progression. The Milwaukee brace or thoracolumbosacral orthosis (TLSO) is used. These are recommended for either daytime or 23-hour use. Pressure sores and worsening pulmonary status can occur and should be prevented. Surgical treatment is recommended for progressive curves greater than 40 degrees. For the most severe curves anterior and posterior fusion is recommended. Pseudoarthrosis rates of 40% to 75% and infection rates of 20% to 40% have been reported. Pseudoarthrosis has decreased to less than 20% with the use of anterior and posterior fusion. Infection occurs in 0% to 8% when prophylactic antibiotics are used. Fusion to the pelvis is often necessary, and up to 57% of patients will lose some ambulatory capacity after spinal fusion.

Kyphosis

Most myelomeningocele patients with kyphosis have high lumbar- and thoracic-level lesions. Kyphosis usually occurs at the thoracolumbar junction or in the lumbar spine. This deformity is usually present at birth and can progress to greater than 90 degrees by age 2 or 3 years. Congenital kyphosis is completely unresponsive to bracing and requires surgical treatment. Many techniques have been described for the kyphectomy. Each carries significant risk of complication including spinal fluid/pressure imbalance, pseudoarthrosis, and infection. Careful preoperative and postoperative care is imperative.

Hip Deformities

Contracture

Hip contractures commonly occur as a result of muscle imbalance (particularly in low lumbar-level patients); spasticity of hip musculature is commonly seen in patients with tethered cord, or the habitual posture of wheelchair patients with high-level lesions. Abduction and adduction contractures can lead to pelvic obliquity, asymmetric gait, and compensatory scoliosis. Adduction contracture is treated with an adductor myotomy if mild and with a subtrochanteric valgus osteotomy if necessary to correct pelvic obliquity. Abduction contracture is usually mild and will correct with the Ober-Yount procedure with its release of the tensor fascia latae. Postoperatively, a hip splint and early mobilization are used.

Flexion contracture can cause anterior pelvic tilt that is associated with decreased walking velocity and increased demand on the upper extremities. Treatment of flexion contracture varies with the child's neurologic level. For a patient with a high-level lesion, contracture up to 30 to 40 degrees can be tolerated if it does not interfere with bracing or walking. Surgical treatment consists of a radical release often including the anterior hip capsule. For a low lumbar-level patient contracture up to 20 degrees can significantly affect walking and bracing. Surgical treatment must retain hip flexor power and therefore some muscles that are released must be reattached more distally. Splinting and early mobilization are used postoperatively to maintain results.

Dislocation

The incidence of hip dislocation varies with the level of involvement. Nearly half of children with myelomeningocele experience hip instability in the first 10 years of life (Table 19-2).

Muscle imbalance between the hip flexors and extensors and between the abductors and adductors accounts for hip instability. Many studies have found that the presence of hip dislocation does not affect ambulation, bracing requirements, seating, or progression of scoliosis, or

TABLE 19-2 INCIDENCE OF HIP DISLOCATION BY LEVEL

Level	Incidence of Hip Dislocation
Thoracic	28%
L1-L2	30%
L3	36%
L4	22%
L5	7%
Sacral	1%

lead to hip pain. Given the high incidence of complications with hip relocation procedures in myelomeningocele patients, including redislocation, stiffness, seating difficulty, cost, infection, and decreased ambulatory function, some recommend against such procedures. Treatment can be recommended based on the functional classification shown in Table 19-1.

- For patients in group 1, hip stability has little clinical effect.
  - Treatment is limited to release of contractures and realignment osteotomies to facilitate proper sitting, perineal care, and brace fitting.
  - There is little evidence to support hip relocation in this group.
- Group 2 patients have a high incidence of unstable hip.
  - Maintaining a level pelvis and flexible hips is more important than reduction.
- Group 3 patients place a high demand on their hips and therefore concentric reduction is very important.
  - Hip dislocation is uncommon in this group.
  - Some recommend aggressive treatment to achieve and maintain reduction including hip and pelvic osteotomies.

For excessively stiff hips, proximal femoral resection with interposition arthroplasty is recommended but rarely necessary. Femoral head resection alone is not effective.

Knee Deformities

Flexion Contracture

One study found that all babies with myelomeningocele had a 10-degree knee flexion contracture at birth. In many children this corrects with growth. Factors that lead to knee flexion contracture include the following:

- The typical position when supine of hip abduction, flexion, and external rotation, knee flexion, and ankle equinus
- Gradual contracture of the hamstrings, biceps, and posterior knee capsule
- Spasticity of the hamstrings due to tethered cord
- Paralysis of the gastrocsoleus, gluteus medius, and gluteus maximus

In children with high-level lesions knee flexion contracture can be prevented with early splinting.

A crouched gait has a high-energy cost. Knee flexion greater than 40 degrees increases energy costs. External tibial torsion can also lead to a crouched gait and higher energy costs. This is addressed in the section on rotational deformities. One study suggests that knee flexion on the examination table is doubled with weightbearing. Therefore, knee flexion contracture of greater than 20 degrees requires surgical correction. This can be achieved in a variety of ways. For children with high-level lesions a radical flexor release can be performed. A knee flexor lengthening is recommended for children with low lumbar- and sacral-level lesions. Supracondylar extension osteotomy of the femur is rarely indicated but is used in patients who have not had success with a radical release. Anterior stapling of the physis can be done in a growing child to achieve gradual correction of the flexion deformity.

Extension Contracture

Extension contracture is much less common than flexion contracture. This usually occurs bilaterally and is associated with hip dislocation, external rotation hip deformities, valgus knees, and equinovarus feet. Treatment options include serial casting to achieve 90 degrees flexion or surgical treatment to lengthen the quadriceps mechanism.

Rotational Deformities

External Tibial Torsion

External tibial torsion, internal hip rotation, and excessive pelvic rotation and contribute to gait problems, particularly increased valgus knee stress. External tibial torsion of greater than 20 degrees has been shown to contribute to crouch gait and an increased valgus stress at the knee. Rotational correction of the tibia can decrease valgus stress and improve crouch gait. Because of the high rate of complications, osteotomy is recommended just above the distal tibial physis with a separate incision for the fibular osteotomy. Internal hip rotation can be corrected with an intertrochanteric external rotation osteotomy when necessary. Excessive pelvic rotation can be decreased only by the use of crutches.

Internal Tibial Torsion

Internal tibial torsion is usually present from birth and is often associated with talipes equinovarus, or clubfeet. Before age 5, correction can be attempted with AFOs and twister cables. After age 5, external rotation tibial osteotomies are usually necessary. Gait studies have revealed that internal tibial torsion does not significantly increase stress at the knee. Any dynamic deformities, such as a spastic anterior tibial tendon, must be recognized at the time of surgery.

Hip Rotation

Excessive internal and external hip rotation can occur with spina bifida. Initial treatment is with twister cables, but proximal femoral osteotomies may become necessary when the child gets older.

Foot and Ankle Deformities

Some 80% to 90% of children with myelomeningocele have deformities of the foot. Some of these are present at birth, such as talipes equinovarus or vertical talus, and others are developmental due to muscle imbalance, such as calcaneal and calcaneal–valgus deformity.

The final treatment goal for children with spina bifida is a plantigrade, supple, braceable foot. Surgical treatment is often necessary and two main principles should be followed:

1. Muscle balance should be achieved through tendon excisions, which are more reliable than tendon transfer or lengthening.
2. Arthrodesis should be avoided whenever possible.

Correction should be achieved through osteotomies to preserve joint motion. A mobile, flat foot is easier to brace than a rigid foot. Joint fusion can lead to arthritic changes in neighboring joints and to soft tissue ulceration. Untreated muscle imbalance can lead to bony changes and should be addressed in a timely manner.

Clubfoot

Approximately 30% of children with myelomeningocele have clubfoot. In spina bifida, the clubfoot deformity is far more rigid than the idiopathic clubfoot. The foot often has a supination deformity caused by the unopposed action of the anterior tibialis, rotational malalignment of the calcaneus, talus and calcanealcuboid joints, talonavicular subluxation, a cavus component, and severe internal tibial torsion. Casting is rarely completely successful but should be attempted because improvement in the soft tissue can be seen. Surgical correction is recommended around age 10 to 12 months.

Surgical treatment involves a radical posterior medial–lateral release:

- All tendons are excised rather than lengthened.
- The anterior tibialis is excised to correct the supination deformity.
- The subtalar joint, including the interosseous ligament, is completely released.
- The calcaneocuboid joint is released circumferentially and a plantar release is performed.
- Kirchner wires are used to correct and hold the correction of the talonavicular and subtalar joints.
- Correction of the rotational malalignment of the talus and calcaneus is very important.
- Postoperatively, a long leg splint is used with the foot in mild equinus to decrease tension at the suture line.
- A long leg cast is worn for an additional 6 weeks.
- Kirchner wires are removed at the time of final cast removal and an AFO is recommended for day and nighttime use.

Results are better in children with low lumbar- and sacral-level lesions; poor results have only been reported in 11%. On the contrary, poor results have been reported in 50% of children with thoracic- and high lumbar-level lesions. The most common residual deformity is adduction of the forefoot, which is secondary to growth imbalance between the medial and lateral columns. When bracing is unsuccessful, osteotomies can be done around the midfoot to correct this problem. This should be delayed until there is ossification of the medial cuneiform, which occurs at age 4 or 5 years. The best treatment for failed clubfoot surgery is a talectomy. Extensive scar tissue surrounding the neurovascular bundle makes revision very difficult.

Equinus Deformity

Equinus deformity occurs more frequently in children with high lumbar- and thoracic-level myelomeningocele.

- Bracing is recommended to prevent progression of deformity.
- When surgery becomes necessary, Achilles tendon excision may be all that is needed.
- For more severe deformity, release of the posterior tibiotalar and talocalcaneal joints, including the calcaneofibular ligament, is needed.
- Postoperatively, a child is treated in a short leg cast for 6 weeks followed by AFOs for day and nighttime use.

Vertical Talus

At birth, approximately 10% of children with myelomeningocele will have vertical talus deformity. The talus is positioned vertically, the calcaneus is in equinus and valgus, the navicular is dislocated dorsally and laterally on the talus, and the cuboid is often dorsally subluxated in relation to the calcaneus. These deformities are typically congenital but muscle imbalance can contribute to the deformity. Serial casting can help stretch soft tissues, but complete posteromedial–lateral release is almost always required at age 10 to 12 months.

Calcaneus and Calcaneovalgus Deformities

Calcaneus deformity occurs in 30% of children with myelomeningocele and is due to imbalance of the active dorsiflexors and weak plantarflexors of the ankle. The deformity is typical in a child with an L5-S1 level. Calcaneovalgus is caused by an imbalance between the invertors and the evertors. When the deformity is present at birth, it is most often flexible, but if rigid, it can be corrected with serial casting. More often this is a developmental deformity. Tendon excision of the ankle dorsiflexors, peroneus brevis, and peroneus longus can often achieve a braceable, supple, plantigrade foot. In one study, 18% of patients had recurrent deformity with this treatment and required either repeat tendon excision or correction of equinus deformity. In older children, bony correction of the calcaneus, along with soft tissue releases, is required to allow bracing and prevent pressure sores.

Ankle Valgus and Hindfoot Valgus

Valgus deformity of the ankle is commonly seen in children with L4-L5 level spina bifida. This can lead to problems with pressure sores and difficulty with brace fitting. Additionally, these children often have a calcaneus foot, due to absence of gastrocnemius–soleus strength, and external tibial torsion. The calcaneovalgus position of the foot can also be associated with an abnormally short fibula that promotes further valgus tilt of the talus in the ankle mortise.

Surgical treatment of ankle valgus is indicated when there are problems with orthotic fitting. Achilles tenodesis to the fibula has been described but is no longer recommended.

- Hemiepiphysiodesis of the medial malleolus is done for mild deformities with a single screw in the malleolus.
  - The screw is removed within 2 years after its insertion in order to cause only temporary growth arrest.
- For more severe deformities a supramalleolar varus internal rotation osteotomy is indicated.
- If valgus of the hindfoot is also present, a medial sliding osteotomy of the calcaneus may also be required.

Supination and Forefoot Adduction Deformities

Supination deformity, which is often associated with adduction deformity of the forefoot, is caused by the unopposed action of the tibialis anterior when the peroneus brevis and longus are paralyzed. This occurs in children with an L5-S1 level.

- For supple deformity, tenotomy of the anterior tibial tendon is recommended.
- For patients who are able to walk without an orthosis, the anterior tibial tendon can be transferred to the lateral cuneiform but split transfer is not recommended.
- When the deformity is fixed, tendon transfer or tenotomy, along with a plantar closing wedge of the medial cuneiform is performed to plantarflex the first ray and realign the forefoot.
- If the supination deformity is more severe, a midtarsal osteotomy is done.

The most common residual deformity is forefoot adduction. This is often secondary to growth imbalance between the medial and lateral columns.

- Surgical correction is achieved with medial opening and lateral closing wedge osteotomies with an abductor hallicus and plantar fascia release.

Varus and Cavovarus Deformities

A cavovarus deformity is seen primarily in patients with sacral-level lesions. Cavus is the primary deformity, and the varus is caused by the cavus.

- The Coleman block test is used to determine the rigidity of the deformity.
- For a supple deformity, a plantar release can be performed without hindfoot surgery.
- For a rigid deformity, plantar release, midtarsal or first metatarsal osteotomy, and calcaneal osteotomy are often required.
- Postoperatively, a short leg cast is worn for 6 weeks followed by day and nighttime bracing.

PEARLS

- A supple, plantigrade, braceable foot is the final goal of treatment.
- Early recognition and treatment of muscle imbalance can prevent bony deformity.
- Tendon excision is preferable to tendon transfer.
- Osteotomies to preserve joint motion are preferable to arthrodesis.
- Postoperatively, day and nighttime braces are used to prevent recurrence.

SUGGESTED READING

Beaty JH, Canale ST. Orthopaedic aspects of myelomeningocele. J Bone Joint Surg (Am) 1990;72:626–630.

Brinker MR, Rosenfield SR, Feiwell E, et al. Myelomeningocele at the sacral level: long-term outcomes in adults. J Bone Joint Surg (Am) 1994;76:1293–1300.

Dias L. Myelomeningocele and intraspinal lipoma. Orthopaedic Knowledge Update: Pediatrics 2, 2001.

Fraser RK, Hoffman EB, Sparks LT, et al. The unstable hip and mid-lumbar myelomeningocele. J Bone Joint Surg (Br) 1992;74:143–146.

Litner SA, Lindseth RE. Kyphotic deformity in patients who have a myelomeningocele: operative treatment and long-term follow-up. J Bone Joint Surg Am 1994;76:1301–1307.

Mazur JM, Shurtleff D, Menelaus M, et al. Orthopaedic management of high-level spina bifida: early walking compared with early use of a wheelchair. J Bone Joint Surg (Am) 1989;71:56–61.

Rodrigues RC, Dias LS. Calcaneus deformity in spina bifida: results of anterolateral release. J Pediatr Orthop 1992;12:461–464.

Tosi LL, Slater JE, Shaer C, et al. Latex allergy in spina bifida patients: prevalence and surgical implications. J Pediatr Orthop 1993;13:709–712.

Ward WT, Wenger DR, Roach JW. Surgical correction of myelomeningocele scoliosis: a critical appraisal of various spinal instrumentation systems. J Pediatr Orthop 1989; 9:262–268.

Williams JJ, Graham GP, Dunne KB, et al. Late knee problems in myelomeningocele. J Pediatr Orthop 1993;13:701–703.

NEUROMUSCULAR DISORDERS

20.1 MUSCULAR DYSTROPHY

DAVID EMERY ■ BENJAMIN A. ALMAN

The muscular dystrophies are a group of disorders characterized by weakness of muscle. The pattern and severity are variable and depend on the type of dystrophy.

PATHOGENESIS

Etiology

Muscular dystrophies are due to mutations in specific genes, the protein products of which play important roles in muscle function (Table 20.1-1). The first dystrophy in which a mutation was identified is Duchenne muscular dystrophy (DMD), the most common type. This disorder is inherited in an X-linked recessive manner and is caused by a mutation in a gene located at Xp21, encoding the *dystrophin* protein. Becker muscular dystrophy is due to a defect in the same gene, but has a milder phenotype (the clinical course tends to be less severe).

Epidemiology

Muscular dystrophy is the most common of the neuromuscular disorders, and the most common form of muscular dystrophy is DMD, with an incidence among boys of 1 in 3,500 and a prevalence of 60 per million. The others are less common:

- Congenital muscular dystrophy: 25 per million
- Becker muscular dystrophy: 16 per million
- Limb girdle muscular dystrophy: 8 per million
- Fascioscapulohumeral muscular dystrophy: 8 per million.

Pathophysiology

The dystrophin protein has a variety of cellular effects, but has a predominant role maintaining muscle membrane stability. Skeletal and cardiac muscle are lacking the protein dystrophin in DMD. Lack of dystrophin leads to membrane damage during contraction, activating the inflammatory cascade, resulting in muscle cell death, subsequent fibrosis, and loss of function. The damaged muscle is replaced by fat and fibrous tissue. The role in other cell types, such as in the central nervous system, seems to be related to its cell signaling function, and this may be responsible for findings such as a relatively low IQ in some affected boys.

Classification

The muscular dystrophies are classified according to pattern of muscle involvement and mode of inheritance.

- Sex-linked:
  - DMD
  - Becker
  - Emery-Dreyfus (mostly)
- Autosomal dominant:
  - Fascioscapulohumeral
  - Distal
  - Ocular
  - Oculopharyngeal
  - Myotonic dystrophy
- Autosomal recessive:
  - Limb girdle
  - Infantile fascioscapulohumeral
  - Congenital muscular dystrophy

TABLE 20.1-1 TYPES OF MUSCULAR DYSTROPHY WITH PROTEIN AFFECTED AND GENE DEFECT

Dystrophy	Inheritance	Gene and Protein Defect	Gene Locus
Duchenne	X-linked recessive	Dystrophin	Xp21
Becker	X-linked recessive	Dystrophin	Xp21
Emery-Dreyfus	Mostly X-linked recessive	Emerin	Xq28
Congenital	Autosomal recessive	Laminin Fukutin Others	6q; 12q; 9q
Limb girdle	Autosomal dominant (1a–f) Autosomal recessive (2a–i)	Myotilin Calpain-3 Others	Various
Myotonic dystrophy	Autosomal dominant	Dystrophia myotonica Protein kinase	19q
Oculopharyngeal dystrophy	Autosomal dominant	Poly(A) binding Protein 2	14q
Fascioscapulohumeral dystrophy	Autosomal dominant		4q

DUCHENNE MUSCULAR DYSTROPHY

Diagnosis

Many cases of DMD are not diagnosed until the boy is 2 years of age or older. It is not uncommon for an orthopaedic surgeon to be the first medical professional to entertain this potential diagnosis.

History

- Pregnancy, including lack of *in utero* movement
- Birth history (e.g., floppy baby)
- Developmental delays, especially milestones (e.g., slow to sit, walk, talk)
- Specific current symptoms:
  - ☐ Toe-walking: often benign, but always check creatine phosphokinase level to exclude DMD
  - ☐ Clumsiness
  - ☐ Inability to keep up with other children
  - ☐ Easily fatigued
  - ☐ Waddling
  - ☐ Abnormal gait
- Other systems: cardiac problems, ocular, seizures, skin
- Family history

Physical Examination

- Look:
  - ☐ General appearance and morphology
  - ☐ Posture: sitting and standing
  - ☐ Winging of scapula (fascioscapulohumeral dystrophy)
  - ☐ Excessive lumbar lordosis (to compensate for pelvic girdle muscle weakness)
  - ☐ Muscle wasting
  - ☐ Pseudohypertrophy of calves
  - ☐ Scoliosis (often the first sign of neuromuscular disease)
  - ☐ Gait—waddling (differential diagnosis: developmental dysplasia of the hip)
  - ☐ Skin—facial expression, skin markings
- Feel:
  - ☐ Muscle quality, tone
  - ☐ Contractures:
    - ☐ Hip abduction, fixed flexion (later)
    - ☐ Ankle equinus
- Move:
  - ☐ Gross and fine motor skills
  - ☐ Joint range of movement
  - ☐ Pattern of motor weakness (proximal/distal/generalized)
- Specific signs:
  - ☐ Gower: weak pelvic girdle muscles—child climbs up legs from sitting on the floor.
  - ☐ Meryon: weak shoulder girdle—child slips through when lifted by encircling arms

Clinical Manifestations and Natural History

- Transmission of DMD is sex-linked, therefore only boys are affected (though women with the mutated gene are carriers and may show subtle clinical findings).
- Usually normal during early infancy with normal milestones.
- Start to develop waddling gait at age 4.
- Proximal lower limb muscles first to be affected; therefore, difficulty ascending stairs.
- Toe-walking may be presenting complaint: need to exclude DMD in all boys with toe-walking due to tightness of Achilles tendon.
- "Clumsy": frequent falls.

- Pseudohypertrophy of muscles, especially calf, due to replacement of muscle by fat and fibrous tissue.
- Muscle feels rubbery and is larger than would be expected.
- Weakness of hip extensors leads to compensatory lumbar lordosis to maintain upright posture.
- Weakness of upper limbs develops later.
- Distal muscles are the last to be affected.
- Ability to walk is lost between 12 and 14 years of age.
- Fixed contractures develop quickly after loss of ambulation.
- Progressive scoliosis.
- Sphincter control and ability to eat maintained.
- Pulmonary function deteriorates after age 13.
- Intercostal muscles weaken and cardiomyopathy develops.
- Death occurs from respiratory failure or cardiac failure in late teens or early 20s.

This is the natural history of untreated DMD. With appropriate supportive therapy (including part-time use of a respirator) boys may survive up to their fourth decade. Recent work has suggested that use of the steroid deflazacort may significantly slow progression of the disease, particularly in terms of the pulmonary function and scoliosis, thus allowing patients to remain active and to live longer.

Investigations

Diagnosis of DMD is made mostly on the history and physical examination and a raised creatine phosphokinase.

- Blood:
  - Creatine phosphokinase is significantly raised to 20 to 300 times normal (i.e., a minimally raised level is unlikely to represent muscular dystrophy)
  - Aspartate aminotransferase (AST) is mildly elevated.

Essentially, once a possible diagnosis of muscular dystrophy has been made, and particularly if the creatine phosphokinase level is high, referral to a pediatric neurologist for further investigation is the appropriate next step. He or she will most likely involve a clinical geneticist to help with further diagnosis and genetic counseling.

- DNA testing:
  - The diagnosis can be confirmed using DNA testing from white blood cells in many cases.

Subsequent investigations may include one or more of the following:

- Radiologic:
  - Generally not helpful.
  - May show osteopenia, enlarged heart in cardiomegaly.
- Neurophysiologic:
  - Electromyelography should show a myopathic rather than a neuropathic picture.
    - Invasive and painful; use in children only if necessary.
- Cardiac:
  - Electrocardiography may show conduction defects or arrhythmias.
  - Echocardiography may show cardiomyopathy.
- Respiratory:
  - Pulmonary function tests show reduced functional vital capacity (FVC). This is particularly relevant in planning timing of scoliosis surgery (discussed later in the chapter).
- Muscle biopsy:
  - Histopathology
  - Monoclonal antibody staining
  - Electrophoresis (Western blot)

Muscle biopsy is required only in difficult-to-diagnose cases. If performed, the biopsy should be taken from a muscle that is not yet significantly weakened (since involved muscle will be replaced with fibrous tissue, making the histologic interpretation difficult).

Treatment

Treatment of all severe neuromuscular conditions is best undertaken in a multidisciplinary framework, with the input from pediatricians, neurologists, pulmonologists, physiotherapists, occupational therapists, and orthotists.

- Pediatrician:
  - To coordinate the care and treat medical complications (cardiac and respiratory).
- Physiotherapist:
  - To prolong muscle strength and prevent contractures.
  - Also to help with functional testing to assess progression of the disease.
- Occupational therapist:
  - To help maintain independence within the home as long as possible.
- Orthotist:
  - To provide ankle–foot orthoses (AFOs) or knee–ankle–foot orthoses (KAFOs) to assist with ambulation and possibly slow the onset of contracture formation.
  - Orthoses can also be helpful in allowing the patient to transfer to a wheelchair after loss of ambulation occurs.

The orthotist and occupational therapist together are vital in the provision of an appropriately molded custom wheelchair to help with comfortable upright sitting and therefore mobility after ambulation is lost.

Surgical Treatment

Orthopaedic surgery should be performed to improve function or to decrease pain. In some cases, surgery can help maintain ambulation, and when the patient becomes nonambulatory, surgery may help to allow comfortable sitting and wheelchair use.

Fractures. Fractures of the lower extremity can occur after ambulation is lost due to disuse of osteopenia. Management is generally with reduction and cast fixation although internal fixation is occasionally warranted.

Contracture Releases. Some centers recommend contracture release in ambulatory patients to extend ambulation. These take the form of Achilles tendon lengthening, gastrocnemius recession (Vulpius), or tibialis posterior transfer for equinovarus foot deformity; the Yount procedure (iliotibial band and tensor fascia lata release) for knee contracture; and anterior hip release/tensor fascia lata release for hip flexion and abduction contracture. No definitive evidence is available to support this; patients tend to become wheelchair dependent soon after, and there is a risk of decreasing the time the patient has walking prior to loss of ambulation by placing him in a cast.

Although this management remains controversial, we do not recommend routine release of lower limb contractures in ambulatory boys with DMD.

The release of contractures might be necessary to allow comfortable wheelchair placement, but there is no evidence to support the routine release of contractures in asymptomatic patients.

Upper extremity contractures, although common, do not tend to interfere with function and surgical release is very rarely required.

Scoliosis. Almost all (more than 90%) of boys with DMD experience a progressive scoliosis that is unresponsive to brace therapy. Surgery is indicated early when the Cobb angle reaches 30 degrees or possibly even less, so that the patients have sufficient residual pulmonary function to allow safe spinal surgery. FVC below 30% is associated with a very poor outcome in terms of postoperative recovery, and the FVC should ideally be above 45%. Early operation also allows for stabilization before significant deformity has occurred, making the surgery less complex.

Scoliosis in DMD is treated with posterior instrumentation and grafting with allograft, stabilizing from high thoracic to the sacrum. Select cases may be managed with fusion to L5, rather than the sacrum, although there is a risk of progressive pelvic obliquity, especially in cases where the apex of the curve is in the lumbar spine. For this reason, we recommend instrumentation and fusion to the sacrum.

OTHER SEX-LINKED MUSCULAR DYSTROPHIES

Becker Muscular Dystrophy

- Similar to DMD but less severe, with onset after age 7
- Progresses more slowly; orthotics may be of benefit
- Treatment otherwise as for DMD
- Life expectancy greater than with DMD; some patients survive into later adulthood

Emery-Dreyfuss Muscular Dystrophy

- Characterized by early contractures (ankle equinus, elbow flexion, neck extension, tightness of lumbar paravertebrals), slow, progressive weakness in a humeroperoneal distribution (upper limb proximal, lower limb distal), and subsequent cardiomyopathy with conduction defects
- Conduction defects often asymptomatic; high incidence of sudden death due to arrhythmias
  - Early pacemaker fitting recommended
- Scoliosis may be a feature but tends not to progress
- Creatine phosphokinase elevation mild to moderate
- Treatment by physiotherapy, with surgical heel cord release occasionally indicated

AUTOSOMAL DOMINANT MUSCULAR DYSTROPHIES

Fascioscapulohumeral Muscular Dystrophy

- Characterized by weakness of facial and shoulder girdle muscles
- Usually presents in later childhood or early adulthood
- Progression often slow or stop–start
- Heart and central nervous system are normal
- Life expectancy is normal
- Orthopaedic problems:
  - Loss of forward flexion and abduction
  - Winging of the scapula
- Surgical intervention:
  - Posterior scapulocostal fusion (Jakab and Gledhill) to stabilize the scapula and restore mechanical advantage to the deltoid and rotator cuff muscles

Distal (Gower/Welander) Muscular Dystrophy

- Rare
- Late onset (after 45 years of age)
- Starts in the intrinsic muscles of the hands
- May involve the calf muscles

Ocular Muscular Dystrophy

- Rare
- Starts during the adolescent years, with diplopia
- May eventually involve the proximal upper extremities and pelvis
- Myopathy is of a mitochondrial origin.

Oculopharyngeal Muscular Dystrophy

- Largely a disease of French Canadians
- Onset in the third decade, with dysarthria, dysphagia, and ptosis

Myotonia

- Group of disorders characterized by the inability of skeletal muscle to relax after a strong contraction
- Three forms:
  - Myotonic dystrophy (Steinert disease):
    - Comprises myotonia with progressive muscle weakness, heart defects, frontal baldness, gonadal atrophy, and dementia.
    - Onset is usually in late adolescence.

- The protein abnormality has been identified as a mutation in the dystrophia myotinician protein kinase gene on chromosome 19. The defect results in an amplified trinucleotide repeat in the 3′ untranslated region of the gene. The phenotypic severity of the disorder is directly related to the number of repeats an individual has. Normal is 5 to 30 copies; mildly affected individuals have 50 to 80 copies; and in severe cases, there may be more than 2,000 copies. Amplification tends to increase with generation and transmission. Extreme amplification is not transmitted along the male line, however, which is why the most severe congenital form of the disorder (see below) is almost always passed from mother to child.
- Congenital myotonic dystrophy:
  - Relatively common, with variable expression that tends to increase with the generations.
  - Although autosomal dominant, it tends to be passed on by the mother. The mother often has a *forme fruste* of the disorder, and shaking her hand may give you an early indication of what to expect in the examination of the child.
  - Sufferers have a long, narrow face, are hypotonic, and often have difficulty feeding.
  - 40% have severe involvement or die in infancy; 60% may be affected later.
  - Patients may suffer from severe clubfoot. They are often resistant to nonoperative treatment, and later develop teratologic hip dysplasia and scoliosis.
- Congenital myotonia:
  - Presents later (after age 10) although present at birth
  - Early myotonia decreases with repetitive movement
  - Variable clinical expression
  - May present as low back pain or decreased physical ability
  - No associated systemic abnormalities, no significant orthopaedic features; life span is normal

AUTOSOMAL RECESSIVE MUSCULAR DYSTROPHIES

Limb Girdle Muscular Dystrophy

- Relatively common
- Clinically and genetically heterogeneous (15 forms at last count)
- May be relatively benign, with a similar presentation to Becker, but with a normal dystrophin, or with a scapulohumeral form
- Onset tends to be later in childhood, with a more benign prognosis (survival to around age 40).
- Treatment tends to be as for DMD, but scoliosis less of a feature due to later onset

Infantile Fascioscapulohumeral Muscular Dystrophy

- More severe than the autosomal dominant form
- Earlier in onset with a more rapid clinical course, and loss of ambulation by the second decade
- Facial diplegia is noted in infancy with loss of hearing by age 5
- Weak glutei, resulting in a severe lumbar lordosis (pathognomic for this disorder)
- Weakness of shoulder girdle muscles so severe that stabilization is of little value

Congenital Muscular Dystrophy

- A variety of disorders are considered in this category.
- They present at birth, often with a floppy baby.
- Several forms are recognized, with a spectrum of severity.
- Joint stiffness and contractures may be a feature.
- Some types (e.g., Fukuyama) are rapidly progressive and may be fatal in the first decade, but most cases are not and survival into adulthood is common.
- Orthopaedic problems:
  - Hip dysplasia and dislocation—treat as for idiopathic disease, but beware of recurrence.
  - Clubfoot—treat vigorously.
  - Scoliosis—try bracing, but surgical stabilization is likely to be required.

SUGGESTED READING

Alman BA, Kim HK. Pelvic obliquity after fusion of the spine in Duchenne muscular dystrophy. J Bone Joint Surg (Br) 1999;81: 821–824.

Bach JR, McKeon J. Orthopedic surgery and rehabilitation for the prolongation of brace-free ambulation of patients with Duchenne's muscular dystrophy. Am J Phys Med Rehabil 1991;70:323–330.

Biggar W, Gigras M, Fehlings DL, et al. Deflazacort treatment of Duchenne muscular dystrophy. J Pediatr 2001;138:45–50.

Emery AEH. The muscular dystrophies. Lancet 2002;359:687–695.

Shapiro F, Specht L. Current concepts review: the diagnosis and orthopaedic treatment of inherited muscular diseases of childhood. J Bone Joint Surg (Am) 1993;75:439–454.

Vignos PJ, Wagner PT, Kartlinchak B, et al. Evaluation of a program for long-term treatment of Duchenne muscular dystrophy. J Bone Joint Surg (Am) 1996;78:1844–1852.

20.2 ARTHROGRYPOSIS MULTIPLEX CONGENITA NEUROLOGICA

LORIN M. BROWN

Arthrogryposis multiplex congenita neurologica (AMCN) is a symptom complex that consists of contractures of the upper and lower limbs and spine. These contractures may be in flexion or extension at any of the involved joints. The pattern of the deformity is related to the innervation levels of the involved musculature. There are many forms of arthrogryposis that cause contractures and contractions of the same anatomic areas of the extremities and spine. These are similar in clinical appearance to AMCN but in histologic, etiologic, or neurologic involvement are essentially very different entities.

PATHOGENESIS

Etiology

Though it is not a classically hereditable disease, recently the gene loci for several forms of AMCN have been mapped to the q region of chromosome 5. The heredity pattern appears to be recessive and incomplete penetrance. Distal arthrogryposis is autosomal dominant or, rarely, X-linked, and maps to the p regions of chromosome 9, 11, or the X chromosome. AMCN has not been shown to be infectious or to develop after birth. It is possible however, that some forms are acquired *in utero* through the fetal circulation carrying viral or bacterial organisms that specifically destroy the anterior horn cells of the spinal cord of the fetus. (This is the same pathophysiology that causes poliomyelitis.) It is also possible that there is an embryologic defect responsible for the malformation of the anterior horn cells. The final common pathway leads to the destruction of the motor neural innervation of muscles.

Pathophysiology

The paralytic pattern of AMCN has been shown to be directly correlated with the segmental innervation of the involved muscles. The lengths of the anterior horn cell columns show distinct correlation patterns when compared to the ratio of partial paralysis to paralysis in children with AMCN (Table 20.2-1). These patterns correlate well with the specific levels of neurosegmental innervations (Figs. 20.2-1 and 20.2-2). The shorter the length of the anterior horn cell column that innervates a motor nerve, the more likely deformities involving those muscles is to occur in the child with AMCN. Also, the length of the anterior horn cell column inversely correlates with the severity of the contractures. This is because a destructive lesion or agenesis of the anterior horn cells is more likely

TABLE 20.2-1 SUSCEPTIBILITY TO PARALYSIS OF MUSCLES OF THE LOWER EXTREMITIES COMPARED WITH LENGTH OF ANTERIOR HORN CELL COLUMN

Muscle	Anterior Horn Cell Column Length (mm)	Ratio of Paresis to Paralysis
Peronieal	10	0.18
Tibialis anterior	8	0.31
Tibialis posterior	8	0.33
Extensor hallucis longus	9	0.66
Extensor digitorum longus	10	0.66
Triceps surae	14	1.5
Hip abductors	16	1.5
Inner hamstrings	20	1.75
Gluteus maximus	17	2.0
Biceps femoris	14	4.5
Intrinsics	15	6.0

Adapted from Brown LM, Robson MJ, Sharrard WJW. The pathophysiology of arthrogryposis multiplex congenita neurologica. J Bone Joint Surg (Br) 1980;62B:291–296.

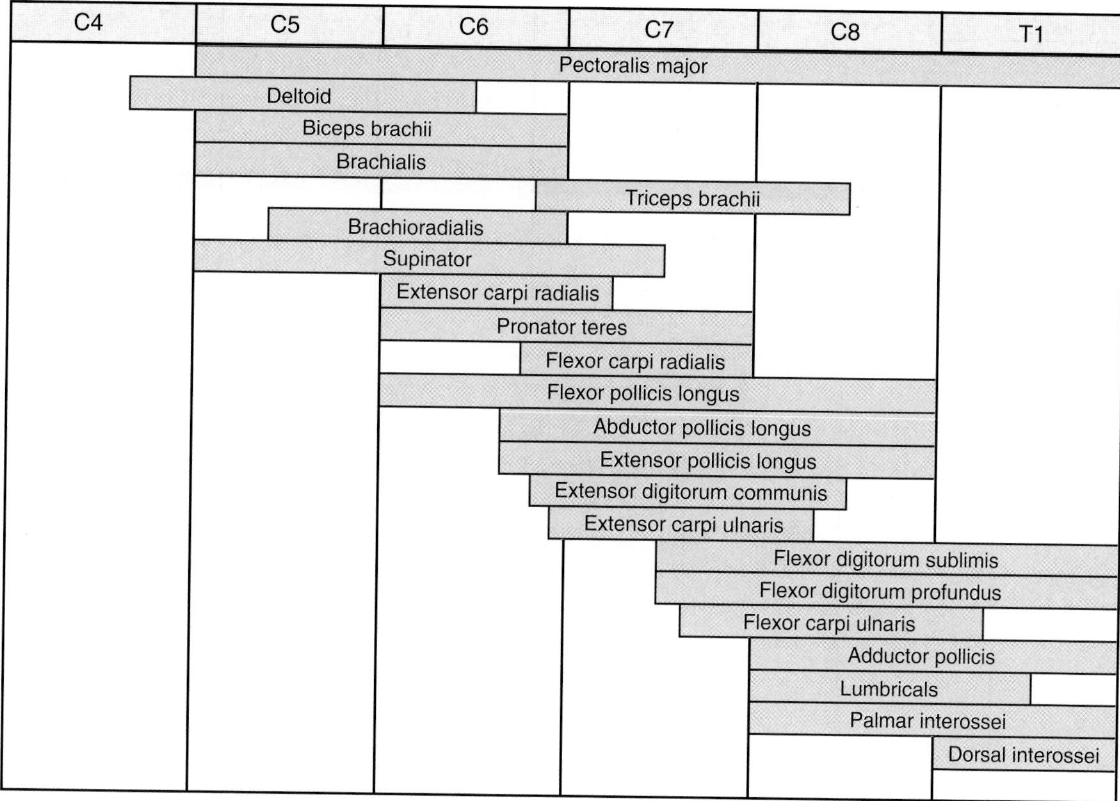

Figure 20.2-1 Segmental innervation of upper limb muscles. (From Brown LM, Robson MJ, Sharrard WJW. The pathophysiology of arthrogryposis multiplex congenita neurologica. J Bone Joint Surg (Br) 1980;62:291–296.)

to be able to affect a greater percentage of the cells when the column is shorter and has fewer cells. Therefore, a typical example would be the common fixed extension contracture of the knees. This is attributed to the short anterior horn cell column of the hamstrings at the level of L5-S1, which is more likely to be absent or largely destroyed than the longer anterior horn cell column of the quadriceps at the level of L2-L4.

Classification

Within AMCN, there are eight defined types of deformities. The most common deformities are type I in the upper extremities and type III in the lower extremities. See Table 20.2-2 for the classification of AMCN and Figures 20.2-3 and 20.2-4 for case examples.

DIAGNOSIS

The diagnosis is usually made on physical examination and evaluation of the deformed individual. Using physical diagnosis and keeping the types of deformity in mind, one can make an accurate diagnosis and assessment usually without the need for many other tests.

- Genetic consultation will usually exclude most known syndromes.
- Electromyelogram and nerve conduction velocities may be of some help in evaluating the patient's levels of innervation.
- If the correct levels and areas of muscle biopsy are performed, the muscles on the active motor side of the deformed joint should show normal fibers while the muscles not functioning on the opposite side of the deformed joint will show the pathologic features of denervation.
  - An example would be normal-appearing quadriceps muscles in a knee in fixed extension while the hamstrings have fatty replacement and fibrosis as well as other signs of denervation.
  - The muscle belly of the quadriceps may only deform extremely proximally in the anterior leg if the paralysis is severe.
  - Biopsy of the quadriceps more distally would show fibrosis as well.

Differential Diagnosis

It is important to accurately diagnose which type of arthrogryposis or arthrogrypotic-like syndrome a patient has. Certain syndromes (Box 20.2-1) may mimic some of the features of true AMCN but have other known causes and known sequelae that require different treatment. The term *amyoplasia* in the literature is probably synonymous with

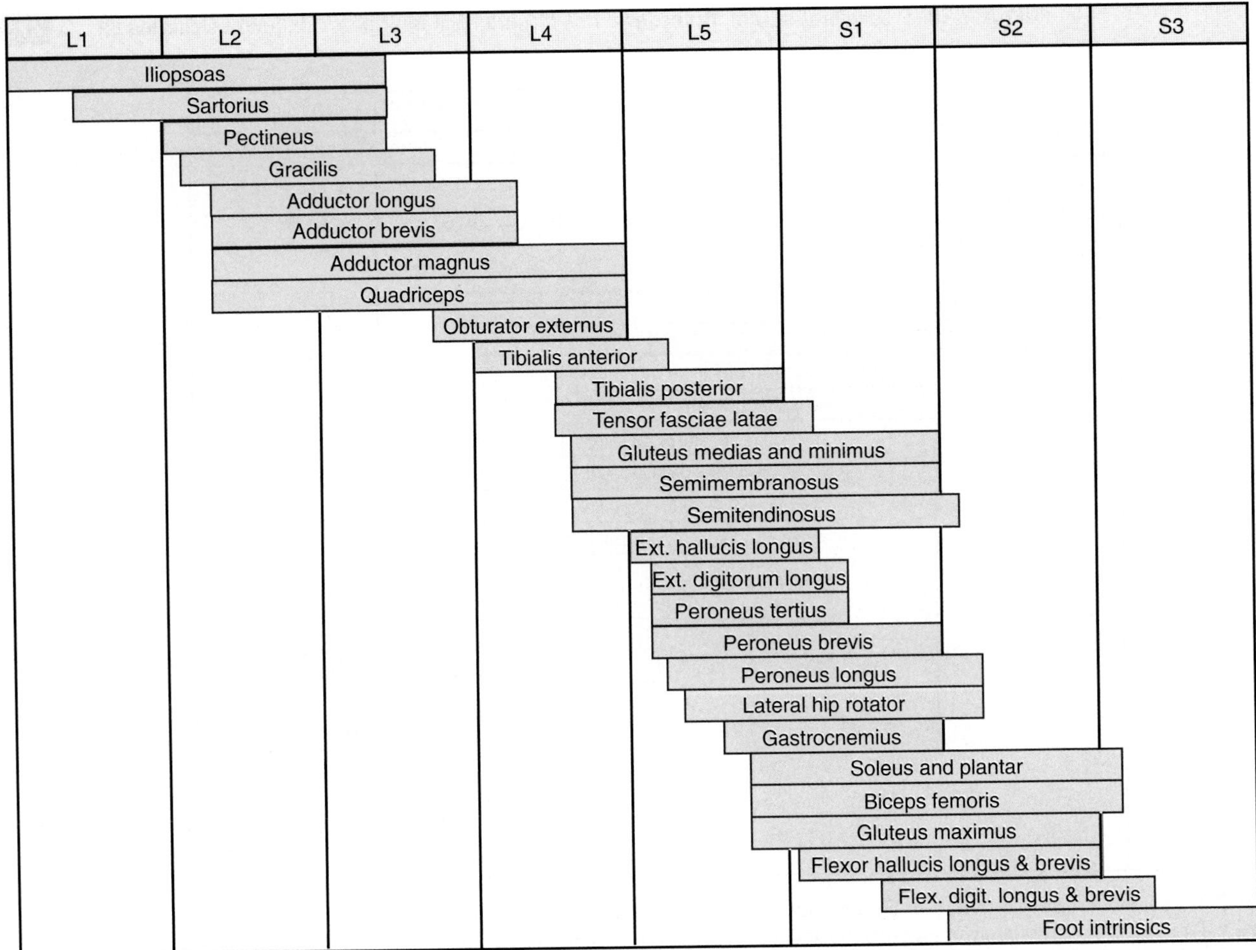

Figure 20.2-2 Segmental innervation of lower limb muscles. (From Brown LM, Robson MJ, Sharrard WJW. The pathophysiology of arthrogryposis multiplex congenita neurologica. J Bone Joint Surg (Br) 1980;62:291–296.)

TABLE 20.2-2 DEFORMITIES FOUND IN ARTHROGRYPOSIS MULTIPLEX CONGENITA NEUROLOGICA

Classification	Pattern of Deformity	Level	No. of Limbs Affected
Upper limb			
Type I	Adduction or medial rotation of the shoulder, extension of the elbow, pronation of the forearm, flexion and ulnar deviation of the wrist. In addition, 2 had weak intrinsic muscles of the hand, indicating T1 involvement.	C5, C6	13
Type II	Adduction or medial rotation of the shoulder, flexion deformity of the elbow, flexion and ulnar deviation of the wrist. In addition, 2 had weak intrinsic muscles of the hand, indicating T1 involvement.	Partial C5, C6, partial C7	3
Lower limb			
Type III	Flexion and adduction of the hip (with dislocation in 5 limbs), extension of the knee, equinovarus of the foot. In addition, 2 had weak intrinsic muscles, indicating S3 involvement.	L4, L5, S1	11
Type IV	Flexion of the knee, equinovarus of the foot	L3, L4, partial L5	1
Type V	Flexion and abduction of the hip, flexion of the knee, equinovarus of the foot	L3, L4, patchy S1-S2	2
Type VI	Flexion of the hip, extension of the knee with valgus, equinus of the foot	L4-L5	2
Type VII	Equinus of the foot	L4	2
Type VIII	Equinovarus of the foot, weak intrinsic muscles of the foot	L4, patchy L5, S3	1

Adapted from Brown LM, Robson MJ, Sharrard WJW. The pathophysiology of arthrogryposis multiplex congenita neurologica. J Bone Joint Surg (Br) 1980;62:291–296.

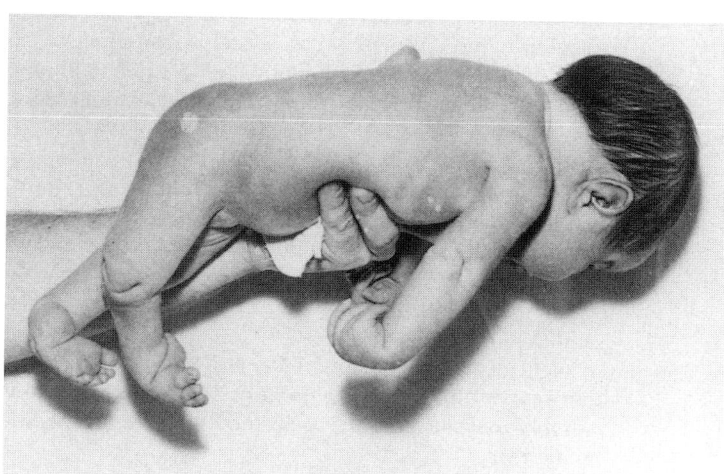
A

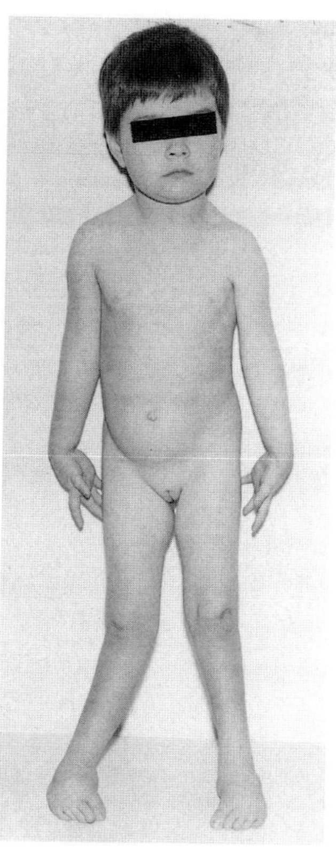
B

Figure 20.2-3 Neurogenic arthrogryposis. (**A**) Patient at birth exhibiting type I (upper limb) and type III (lower limb) deformities. There is adduction of the shoulders, extension of the elbows, pronation of the forearms, flexion of the wrists, flexion and adduction deformity of the hips, extension of the knees, equinovarus deformities of the feet, and dimples over elbows and knees. (**B**) Same patient at 4 years of age. (From Brown LM, Robson MJ, Sharrard WJW. The pathophysiology of arthrogryposis multiplex congenita neurologica. J Bone Joint Surg (Br) 1980;62:291–296.)

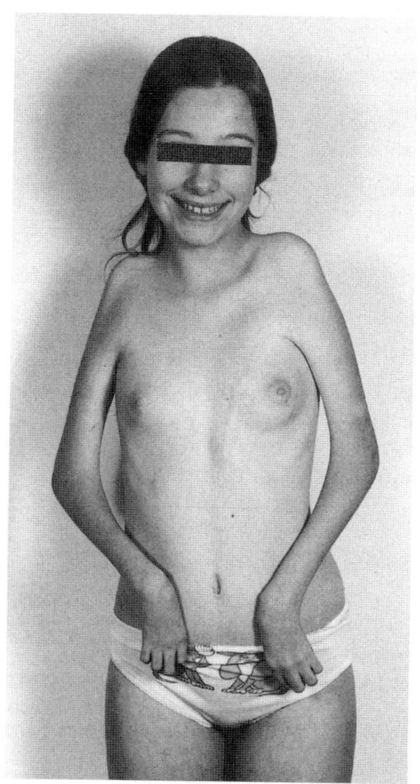

Figure 20.2-4 Type II deformity. There is adduction and medial rotation of the shoulders, flexion deformity of the elbows, flexion and ulnar deviation of the wrists, and weak intrinsic muscles of the hands in a teenage girl with only upper body involvement. Deformity of the chest is secondary to a right-sided pectoralis muscle transfer. (From Brown LM, Robson MJ, Sharrard WJW. The pathophysiology of arthrogryposis multiplex congenita neurologica. J Bone Joint Surg (Br) 1980;62:291–296.)

BOX 20.2-1 CONDITIONS AND SYNDROMES TO EXCLUDE FROM THE DIAGNOSIS OF ARTHROGRYPOSIS MULTIPLEX CONGENITA NEUROLOGICA

Skeletal dysplasias
Spinal dysraphism
Sacral agenesis
Laxity syndromes
Intrauterine postural malformations
Cerebral palsy
Birth palsy
Spina bifida
Schwartz syndrome
Moebius syndrome
Steinert myotonic dystrophy syndrome
Freeman-Sheldon syndrome
Zellweger syndrome
Mietens syndrome
Poland syndrome
Turner syndrome

Adapted from Brown LM, Robson MJ, Sharrard WJW. The pathophysiology of arthrogryposis multiplex congenita neurologica. J Bone Joint Surg (Br) 1980;62:291–296.

AMCN, if the levels of involvement in these published patients are consistent with the known types of deformities (Table 20.2-2).

TREATMENT

Overall treatment goals for children with AMCN are mobility, self-care, and lower extremity alignment which is optimal for standing and walking. If the patient is first seen at birth, when the paralysis is present but not complete, there is considerable joint range of motion that can be gained and maintained with frequent passive range of motion therapy by the parent and physical therapist. If the degree of paralysis is severe, and the joint has not moved with fetal motion since the limb developed, less motion can be gained.

Lower Extremity

- The initial goal is anatomic reduction of any dislocated or malpositioned joints.
- The entire situation of the individual child first needs to be taken into account.
  - For example, if both hips cannot be reduced, it is detrimental to reduce only one hip. All joints involved need to be treated simultaneously.
- If it is possible to loosen a contraction by passive stretch, then later osteotomies will require a less severe angular correction and, therefore, result in less juxtaarticular deformity.
- The longer a functional position can be maintained by therapy and bracing, the longer an osteotomy can be delayed at the major joints.
- Bracing and splinting will most likely be necessary through the child's lifetime.

Foot

- Foot deformities of AMCN are either a clubfoot (equinovarus and adductus deformity) or rarely vertical talus (valgus deformity).
- Goal of treatment is plantigrade feet for standing.
- Almost all severe vertical tali and clubfeet not attributed to other known conditions may in fact be arthrogryposis limited to these peripheral locations.
- Serial casting should be started at birth and manipulated more often than an idiopathic clubfoot deformity.
- After the maximum correction is obtained by stretch casting, it is maintained by physical therapy and removable splints.
- Open reconstruction is performed between 6 and 12 months of age.
- A high recurrence of some deformity through the growing years of life is expected, and other osteotomies and surgery may need to be performed to maintain plantigrade feet.
  - Soft tissue releases, medial open-wedge first cuneiform with lateral cuboid closing-wedge autograft osteotomies, midtarsal dorsal wedge osteotomies, metatarsal osteotomies, and potentially, triple arthrodesis for salvage.
- If the child has an untreated or extreme deformity that is resistant to the standard treatment procedures for the clubfeet or vertical tali feet, partial or complete talectomy is the treatment of choice.

Knee

- Either extension contracture or flexion contracture may be present.
- Flexion contractures initially can be somewhat corrected by serial casting or physical therapy of the knees to extension.
  - Care should be taken to not displace the physes during the manipulations or to cause laxity to the collateral ligament.
- After maximum correction is obtained by passive stretching, surgically lengthening the distal hamstrings and soft tissue may be of help.
- If the knees are not at less than 30 degrees from full extension at this point, supracondylar extension osteotomies are needed to get the legs straight enough to brace for standing.
- Extension contractures are also treatable by serial flexion casting.
- If this does not correct the problem by allowing knee flexion, a quadricepsplasty can be performed.
- Care must be taken to not lose the initial posture ability as well (i.e., to not overlengthen the quads to get flexion of the knee and therefore lose the opposing extension posture).

Hip

- Teratologic dysplasia of the hips is a frequent finding in AMCN.
- About 65% of patients manifest some degree of hip dysplasia.
- If initially there is a unilateral dislocated or subluxed hip, it should be reduced and splinted.
- If the hip is rigidly dislocated, then aggressive traction and therapy may allow it to reduce eventually.
- Surgical muscle releases of hip contractures may aid in the reductions and will help in later ambulation.
- Doing these as a first stage may shorten the time of the initial closed reduction attempts.
- If the hip fails to reduce, then an early, rather than late, open reduction of the hip with femoral shortening or acetabular reconstruction (as one would do for any developmental hip dysplasia) is performed.
- Less postoperative immobilization than usual is advisable (to reduce incidence of further contracture) and surgical intervention may allow this.
- If the child presents later in life, it is imperative to try to correct a unilateral dislocation.
- Bilateral dislocated hips in the older child should be left dislocated, and femoral osteotomies and soft tissue releases performed to correct the alignment if necessary.

Upper Extremity

- Correction of upper extremity deformities are usually performed after 3 years of age.
- Only functional reconstruction is done to the upper extremities.

Shoulders

- Fixed severe deformity only will require an osteotomy.
- Most deformities are acceptable and functional.

Elbows

- If there is a fixed extension deformity, serial casting at birth may improve the position.
- If function is not acceptable, osteotomies and muscle releases are then performed.
- Flexion can be obtained by triceps lengthening, and if not sufficient, supracondylar osteotomy is performed to obtain enough flexion so that the child can care for the head and neck area as well as performing self-feeding.
- Extension can be obtained by biceps tendon release. If not sufficient, then a supracondylar osteotomy to extension may be performed unilaterally to allow for lower body care.
- Children with upper extremity arthrogryposis develop many trick maneuvers to allow limb positioning for functional use.
- If needed to allow active flexion of one elbow, the pectoralis major may be transferred (Fig. 20.2-4).
  - This should not be done bilaterally because of the need for one arm to extend to allow for lower body care and to allow for the use of a cane for walking.
  - There must be 90 degrees of passive flexion before a pectoralis major transfer is undertaken.

Spine

- If the child has severe scoliosis or a spinal deformity, fusions should be performed as would be for any patient with neuromuscular disease.
- In an adolescent with a curve under 40 degrees, a plastic thoracolumbosacral brace works well.
- Congenital scoliosis secondary to malformed vertebrae most likely is not AMCN.

SUGGESTED READING

Brown LM, Robson MJ, Sharrard WJW. The pathophysiology of arthrogryposis multiplex congenita neurologica. J Bone Joint Surg (Br) 1980;62:291–296.

Canale ST, Beaty JH. Operative pediatric orthopaedics. St Louis: Mosby-Year Book, 1991:731–733.

Hau JG, Reed SD, Dricoll EP. Part I: Amyoplasia, a common, sporadic condition with congenital contractures. Am J Med Genet 1983;15: 571–590.

Hoppenfeld S. Orthopedic neurology. Philadelphia: JB Lippincott Co, 1977.

Jones KL. Smith's recognizable patterns of human malformation, 5th ed. Vol 2. Philadelphia: WB Saunders, 1997:687–690.

Sarwark JF, MacEwen GD, Scott CI Jr. Scoliosis in amyoplasia congenita. Orthop Trans 1986;10:19.

Sharrard WJW. Paediatric orthopaedics and fractures, 2nd ed. Oxford, UK: Blackwell Scientific, 1979.

Stahli LT, Chew DE, Elliott JS, et al. Management of hip dislocations in children with arthrogryposis. J Pediatr Orthop 1987;7:681–685.

20.3 NEUROFIBROMATOSIS

ERIC SHIRLEY ■ ARABELLA I. LEET

Neurofibromatosis is a genetic disorder characterized by an abnormal proliferation of cells from the neural crest. Clinical manifestations involve the skin, nervous tissue, bones, and soft tissues. There are two types of neurofibromatosis, NF-1 (peripheral) and NF-2 (central). NF-1, also referred to as von Recklinghausen disease, is more common and has orthopaedic manifestations, whereas NF-2 does not. NF-1 is characterized by café-au-lait macules, intertriginous freckles, neurofibromas, Lisch nodules, optic gliomas, bony dysplasias, and learning disabilities.

PATHOGENESIS

Etiology

The inheritance of NF-1 is autosomal dominant, though 50% of cases are due to spontaneous mutations. Penetrance is close to 100%. The gene for NF-1 has been localized to chromosome 17 at band q11.2. The protein product of this gene loci is neurofibromin. Neurofibromin acts as a tumor suppressor by down-regulating a protein (Ras) that enhances cell growth and proliferation. A point mutation or deletion of this gene results in diminished function of neurofibromin.

Epidemiology

NF-1 is the most common human single-gene disorder. The disease affects approximately 1 in 4,000 persons, and at least 1 million people throughout the world. NF-1 is seen in all racial and ethnic groups and affects the sexes equally.

Pathophysiology

The pathophysiology of NF-1 is relatively unclear. The diminished function of neurofibromin as a tumor suppressor may be related to the occurrence of certain tumors in neurofibromatosis. It is unclear how the gene mutation results in other disease manifestations. Spinal deformities may be due to osteomalacia, localized neurofibroma-related erosion and infiltration into bone, endocrine disturbances, or mesodermal dysplasia.

Classification

NF-1 is more common than NF-2 and has cutaneous, neurologic, skeletal, and neoplastic manifestations. These manifestations include café-au-lait macules, intertriginous freckles, neurofibromas, Lisch nodules, optic gliomas, bony dysplasias, and learning disabilities.

NF-2 has autosomal dominant inheritance as well, but affects roughly 1 in 40,000 persons. The mutation occurs on chromosome 22. NF-2 is characterized by schwannomas of cranial nerve VIII, meningiomas, and ependymomas.

DIAGNOSIS

In 1987, the National Institutes of Health Consensus Development Conference on Neurofibromatosis-1 concluded that the diagnosis can be established when two of seven criteria are met (Box 20.3-1). The criteria may be problematic for diagnosis in infants since 46% of patients with spontaneous mutations and 30% of all patients have met only one criterion by the age of 1 year. Ninety-seven percent of patients meet two or more criteria by age 8. Diagnostic testing may include x-rays, computed tomography (CT)/magnetic resonance imaging (MRI), electroencephalogram, visual evoked responses, skin lesion biopsies, slit lamp exams, and developmental/neuropsychiatric testing. Prenatal testing is available but requires chorionic villus sampling, a more complicated procedure than amniocentesis.

A diagnosis of NF-2 can be made when bilateral acoustic neuromas are present. The diagnosis can also be made when a first-degree relative has NF-2 and the patient has either a unilateral cranial nerve VIII palsy or has two of following present: neurofibroma, meningioma, glioma, schwannoma, or juvenile posterior subcapsular lenticular opacity.

BOX 20.3-1 NATIONAL INSTITUTES OF HEALTH GUIDELINES FOR DIAGNOSIS (1987)

Criteria for the diagnosis of neurofibromatosis-1 met if at least two of the following are present:

- Six or more café-au-lait macules, size >5 mm in prepubertal patients or >15 mm in postpubertal patients
- Two or more neurofibromas or one plexiform neurofibroma
- Freckling in axillary or inguinal region
- Presence of optic glioma
- Two or more Lisch nodules (iris hamartomas)
- Distinctive osseous lesion (i.e., sphenoid dysplasia, thinning of long bone cortex, pseudarthrosis)
- First-degree relative with neurofibromatosis-1 by above criteria

HISTORY AND PHYSICAL EXAMINATION

The patient history should be broad in order to cover the manifestations of NF-1. Patients and parents should be asked about skin lesions, pain, cognitive or psychomotor problems, progressive neurologic deficits, constipation, growth problems (precocious puberty or hypogonadism), orthopaedic problems, and hypertension. The family history should include first-degree relatives, grandparents, great aunts, and great uncles. The physical examination should include a blood pressure measurement, a thorough skin exam, ophthalmic exam, musculoskeletal exam, and neurologic exam; pubertal status should be assessed. Particular portions of the exam may be specific to specialty or clinic.

Clinical Features

NF-1 can affect many organ systems, and it is difficult to predict which signs will manifest in which patients with the disease. See Table 20.3-1 for the clinical manifestations of NF-1.

Café-au-Lait Macules

- Hyperpigmented tan macules with smooth well-defined borders.
- Lesions are present at birth or develop during infancy and are seen in 99% of cases by age 1.
- Lesions are found in skin areas not exposed to sun.

Neurofibromas

- Four types are recognized: cutaneous, subcutaneous, nodular plexiform, and diffuse plexiform.
- Cutaneous neurofibromas are mixed cell tumors rich in Schwann cells, but also contain fibroblasts, endothelial cells, and glandular elements. They have no malignant potential.
- Subcutaneous neurofibromas can be painful and tender to palpation.
- Nodular and plexiform neurofibromas can also be painful and have the potential to dedifferentiate into malignant neurofibrosarcomas.
- Nodular plexiform neurofibromas may involve dorsal nerve roots.
- Diffuse plexiform neurofibromas may invade muscle, bone, or viscera.
- Lesions are seen in 48% of patients by age 10 and in 84% of patients by age 20.
- The lesions increase during pregnancy and puberty.

Elephantiasis

- Large soft tissue masses with rough, raised villous skin.
- Underlying bone is typically dysplastic.

Verrucous Hyperplasia

- Skin overgrowth with thickening.
- Skin integrity can be compromised by superficial infection or by weeping in skin folds causing maceration.

Axillary and Inguinal Freckles

- Found in 90% of patients by age 7.

Lisch Nodules

- Asymptomatic iris hamartomas.
- The nodules, specific for NF-1, are seen in 90% of NF-1 patients more than 6 years old.

Optic Glioma

- Most common tumor in children with NF-1
- Only occur in 1% of patients by age 1 year and in 4% of patients by age 3 years
- Small percentage can cause exophthalmus and visual impairment

Spinal Deformities

- 10% to 60% of patients with NF-1 have scoliosis.
- Deformity of the spine may be associated with intraspinal abnormalities.
- Of all children and adolescents with scoliosis, 2% to 3% of cases are due to NF-1.
- Dystrophic and nondystrophic changes occur in vertebral bodies.
- Nondystrophic changes include wedging, angulation, and rotation.
- See Box 20.3-2 for dystrophic changes in the spine.

TABLE 20.3-1 CLINICAL FEATURES OF NEUROFIBROMATOSIS

Category	Manifestation
Cutaneous	Café-au-lait macules, neurofibromas, elephantiasis, verrucous hyperplasia, axillary and inguinal freckles
Ophthalmic	Lisch nodules, optic gliomas
Spine	Scoliosis, kyphoscoliosis, lordoscoliosis, dumbbell lesions, dural ectasia, meningoceles, plexiform venous channels
Orthopaedic	Congenital tibial dysplasia, bone growth disorders, short stature, sphenoid dysplasia, skull/facial deformities
Tumors	Neurofibrosarcoma, leukemia, rhabdomyosarcoma, Wilms tumor, parathyroid adenoma, pheochromocytoma, medullary thyroid carcinoma, central nervous system lesions, mediastinal tumors
Other	Vascular stenosis, cognitive deficits

BOX 20.3-2 DYSTROPHIC CHANGES IN SPINAL DEFORMITIES

- Scalloping of vertebral bodies
- Severe rotation of the apical vertebrae
- Vertebral wedging
- Widening of the spinal canal
- Enlargement of neural foramina
- Widened interpediculate distance
- Defective pedicles
- Presence of a paravertebral soft tissue mass
- Spindling of transverse process or ribs
- Penciling of ribs

- Pseudoarthrosis is more common after spinal fusion for dystrophic and nondystrophic curves.
  - Risk of pseudarthrosis further increases with kyphotic curves.
  - Neurofibromas are often found at pseudarthrosis sites.

Nondystrophic Scoliosis

- Curve characteristics are similar to idiopathic scoliosis, but a higher percentage have progression of deformity and postoperative pseudarthrosis.
- Deformations have ability to modulate (transform by acquiring dystrophic features). The curves are more likely to modulate if they manifest before 7 years of age.
- Likelihood of progression increases when a curve acquires either three penciled ribs or a combination of three dystrophic features.

Dystrophic Scoliosis

- Curves are characterized by short curves (four to six segments), dystrophic changes, and the tendency to progress to severe curves.
- Risk factors of early progression include:
  - Early age of onset
  - High Cobb angle at presentation
  - Kyphosis more than 50 degrees, apex in middle to lower thoracic area
  - Penciling of one or more ribs on concave or both sides
  - Penciling of four or more ribs, rotation more than 11 degrees at apex
  - Severely notched anterior vertebral body
- Natural history demonstrates high rate of progression.

Kyphoscoliosis

- Defined as kyphosis more than 50 degrees with associated scoliosis
- Associated with neurologic injuries
- Further increased risk of pseudarthrosis after surgery

Lordoscoliosis

- Curves with sagittal plane curvature less than normal curvature
- Associated with mitral valve prolapse and decreased pulmonary function
- Also associated with dystrophic deformities and dural ectasia

Dural Ectasia

- Expands spinal canal at the expense of bony and ligamentous elements.
- Results of expansion can lead to destabilization of vertebrae, spontaneous dislocation, and penetration of the spinal canal by the ribs.

Intrathoracic Meningocele

- Protrusion of meninges through intervertebral foramen or a bony defect in vertebrae
- Typically asymptomatic

Plexiform Venous Channels

- May surround spine and impede operative approach in patients with NF-1

Cervical Spine Abnormalities

- Abnormalities present with head and neck mass, torticollis, or dysphagia.
- Most common abnormality is asymptomatic kyphosis.
- More frequently associated with dysplastic changes
- 44% of NF-1 patients with scoliosis and 9% without scoliosis have cervical spine abnormalities.
- Anteroposterior and lateral cervical spine x-rays should be obtained prior to performing traction or general anesthesia in patients with NF-1.

Spondylolisthesis

- Cases due to NF-1 have occurred, but incidence lower than that in general population
- Typically due to dural ectasia with meningoceles or neurofibroma with involvement of lumbosacral nerve root

Paraplegia

- Etiology must be acutely defined.
- Typically due to neoplasm in the older patient. In younger patients, the paraplegia is more often due to spinal deformity, instability, dural ectasia, or rib penetration into the spinal canal.
- Kyphosis contributes to neurologic changes more than scoliosis.
- Intraspinal lesion, extradural dumbbell neurofibroma, and intradural extramedullary neurofibroma should be included in the differential diagnosis.

Dumbbell Lesions

- Dumbbell appearance results when a neurofibroma is constricted as it exits the foramina.
- Can be intraspinal or extraspinal

Vertebral Column Dislocation

- Rare in NF-1.
- Can occur with little clinical or radiographic warning
- Diagnosis should be considered in NF-1 patients with unexplained neck and back pain.

Congenital Tibial Dysplasia

- Preferred term over congenital pseudoarthrosis

- Anterolateral bowing of the tibia can occur with or without pseudoarthrosis.
- Seen in 1% to 2% of NF-1 cases, compared with 1 per 140,000 in the general population.
- Typically involves the middle or lower third of the tibia or fibula
- Often diagnosed in infancy, and fracture typically occurs before age 2.5 years.
- Occurs spontaneously or after fracture
- See Table 20.3-2 for radiographic types.
- Extremely difficult to resolve, as fracture and re-fracture are common
- Pseudoarthrosis also occurs in ulna, radius, humerus, femur, clavicle.

Bone Growth Disorders

- Segmental hypertrophy is most common in the extremities but may also occur in the skull, mandible, and pelvis.
- The cystic lesions that are often seen consist of nonspecific fibrous tissue.
- Periosteal dysplasia results in a loose attachment to bone and predisposes to subperiosteal hematoma.
- Limb length discrepancy

Other Musculoskeletal Manifestations

- Short stature
- Relative macrocephaly
- Sphenoid dysplasia, bony defects in skull
- Postaxial and preaxial polydactyly
- Protrusio acetabuli

Vascular Stenosis

- Can involve any organ system.
- Most commonly occurs in the renovascular system with resultant hypertension

Tumors Associated with NF-1

- Neurofibrosarcoma: presents as a symptom complex of unexplained pain, neurofibroma enlargement, focal neurologic deficit
- Leukemia
- Rhabdomyosarcoma of the urogenital tract
- Wilms tumor
- Parathyroid adenoma
- Sipple syndrome: triad of neurofibromas, bilateral pheochromocytomas, medullary thyroid carcinoma

Cognitive Deficits

- 50% of patients have learning disorders.
- Unidentified bright objects (seen as high signal-intensity lesions on a T2-weighted MRI) may correlate with the cognitive deficits.

Radiographic Features

Routine posteroanterior and lateral cervical, thoracolumbar, and sacral spine x-rays should be taken because of the potential for occult deformities in each location. Each film should be examined for abnormal lordosis, kyphosis, and dystrophic changes. A CT/MRI should be obtained preoperatively to rule out the presence of an intraspinal lesion. Other radiographs are acquired as dictated by signs and symptoms.

Differential Diagnosis

The differential diagnosis for NF-1 includes other disorders of pigmentation:

- McCune-Albright syndrome
- Watson syndrome
- Bannayan-Riley-Ruvalcaba syndrome
- Epidermal nevus syndrome
- Proteus syndrome
- Multiple lentigines syndrome
- Multiple café-au-lait lesions

TREATMENT

Patients require multidisciplinary care coordinated by a primary care physician or neurofibromatosis specialty clinic. Treatment involves both management of known symptoms of disease and prompt detection of new manifestations.

TABLE 20.3-2 FOUR RADIOGRAPHIC TYPES OF PSEUDARTHROSIS OF THE TIBIA

Type	Description
I	Anterolateral bow with dense medullary canal Usually followed up without bracing, may never have a fracture Best prognosis
II	Anterolateral bowing with increased medullary canal and a tubulation defect Should be protected at time of diagnosis and prepared for surgery
III	Anterolateral bow with a cystic lesion Should have early bone grafting because of tendency for early fracture
IV	Anterolateral bow with fracture, cyst, or frank pseudarthrosis Worst prognosis

Adapted from Crawford AH Jr, Bagamery N. Osseous manifestations of neurofibromatosis in childhood. J Pediatr Orthop 1986;6:2–88.

Routine Follow-Up

- Arrange for serial eye exams.
- Perform neurologic exams for signs of neural tumors.
- Inquire about milestone delays, learning disabilities, speech impairment, school performance problems, retardation.
- Check for scoliosis/kyphosis, pseudarthrosis, signs of tumors
- Educate about risk of progression during puberty, pregnancy.
- Evaluate first-degree relatives.

Problem Management

Neurofibromas

- Ketotifen can be prescribed for pruritus
- Surgical excision or carbon dioxide laser excision as needed

Nondystrophic Scoliosis

- Observe curves less than 20 degrees. Follow radiographs for signs of modulation and progression.
- Brace curves 20 to 35 degrees.
- Curves more than 35 degrees require posterior fusion with segmental instrumentation.
- Curves more than 60 degrees require anterior release with bone graft as well as posterior fusion and instrumentation.

Dystrophic Scoliosis

- Curves less than 20 degrees should be reevaluated every 6 months.
- Bracing has not been effective for dystrophic scoliosis and aggressive early surgery is recommended.
- For curves 20 to 40 degrees, posterior spinal fusion and segmental instrumentation should be considered. Posterior spinal fusion is only appropriate in selected patients with curves involving at least five segments and kyphosis less than 50 degrees. A CT should be obtained 6 months postoperatively for signs of pseudarthrosis.
- Curves more than 40 degrees require anterior and posterior fusion.
- Consider postoperative bracing.

Kyphoscoliosis

- The treatment of kyphosis less than 50 degrees depends upon the degree of the scoliosis.
- Anterior and posterior spinal fusion should be performed for a kyphosis of more than 50 degrees. A strong anterior strut graft such as the fibula is recommended.
- Curves more than 70 degrees may require bracing even after surgical intervention.
- A laminectomy alone for cord compression in kyphoscoliosis is contraindicated.

Lordoscoliosis

- These curves require fusion and instrumentation well above the lordosis because of the possible development of a junctional kyphosis at the cervicothoracic junction.

Spondylolisthesis

- Requires posterior spinal fusion and a postoperative hyperextension cast

Cervical Spine Abnormalities

- Posterior spinal fusion should be performed for cervical spine deformities with instability.

Congenital Tibial Dysplasia

- Multiple treatment options are available:
  - ☐ Ankle–foot orthoses (AFOs) should be started prior to ambulation. Orthotics should be maintained until maturity.
  - ☐ Autogenous bone graft with intramedullary rod fixation from proximal tibia to calcaneus
  - ☐ Vascularized autogenous graft, such as contralateral fibula, iliac crest, rib
  - ☐ Resection of nonunion followed by distraction osteogenesis using the Ilizarov method
- A Boyd or Syme amputation should be considered after three unsuccessful surgeries or when limb length discrepancy or foot and ankle deformity compromises function. These amputations allow the weightbearing surface of the foot to be maintained.
- Treatment of pseudarthrosis of fibula, ulna, os pubis, clavicle similar to tibia.

Bone Growth Disorders

- Empirical and individualized treatment is necessary, usually a combination of epiphysiodesis, debulking, and neurofibroma resection.

SUGGESTED READING

Bernauer T, Mirowski G, Caldemeyer K. Neurofibromatosis type 1. Part II. Non-head and neck findings. J Am Acad Dermatol 2001; 44:1027–1029.

Crawford AH. Neurofibromatosis. In: Weinstein SL, ed. The pediatric spine: principles and practice. Philadelphia: Lippincott Williams & Wilkins, 2001:471–490.

Crawford AH, Bagamery N. Osseous manifestations of neurofibromatosis in childhood. J Pediatr Orthop 1986;6:72–88.

Crawford AH, Schorry EK. Neurofibromatosis in children: the role of the orthopaedist. J Am Acad Orthop Surg 1999;7:217–230.

Debella K, Szudek J, Friedman JH. Use of the National Institutes of Health criteria for diagnosis of neurofibromatosis 1 in children. Pediatrics 2000;105:608–614.

Eichenfield L, Levy M, Paller A, et al. Guidelines for care of neurofibromatosis type 1. J Am Acad Dermatol 1997;37:625–630.

Kim HW, Weinstein SL. The management of scoliosis in neurofibromatosis. Spine 1997;23:2770–2776.

20.4 HAMARTOMATOUS DISORDERS

ROBERT P. HUANG ■ GEORGE H. THOMPSON

Hamartomas are congenital anomalies secondary to developmental disturbances that result in excessive focal overgrowth of mature tissues. This excessive overgrowth can be responsible for a variety of dysmorphic features affecting the musculoskeletal system, such as hemihypertrophy and macrodactyly, as well as other orthopaedic manifestations. In general, hamartomatous disorders occur as rare sporadic events. The true incidence and prevalence of these disorders are unknown. There does not appear to be specific predilection for race or sex or inheritance pattern. Germ line cells are not affected.

A number of hamartomatous disorders can affect the musculoskeletal system. The differential diagnosis of these disorders is presented in Box 20.4-1. Neurofibromatosis (Chapter 23) and Maffucci (Chapter 23) syndrome are presented in other chapters. This chapter focuses on congenital hemihypertrophy, macrodactyly, Proteus syndrome, and Klippel-Trenaunay syndrome.

CONGENITAL HEMIHYPERTROPHY

PATHOGENESIS

Etiology and Epidemiology

Congenital hemihypertrophy is broadly classified into nonsyndromic and syndromic disorders (Box 20.4-2). The former is the most common type. The etiology of nonsyndromic hemihypertrophy is unknown. Although numerous hypotheses have been proposed, including abnormalities in vascular or lymphatic flow, chromosomal mutations, localized endocrine or paracrine malregulation, and defects in embryologic development, there is insufficient evidence to lend credence to any proposed hypotheses of hemihypertrophy. In addition, epidemiologic studies have not clearly differentiated nonsyndromic from syndromic hemihypertrophy; thus, true incidence of nonsyndromic hemihypertrophy is unknown. Prevalence is estimated to be 1 per 50,000 individuals.

Classification

See Box 20.4-2 for the classification of congenital hemihypertrophy.

DIAGNOSIS

Hemihypertrophy is defined as asymmetry between the right and left sides of the body with 5% or greater difference in limb length or circumference (Fig. 20.4-1). Hemihypertrophy is easily diagnosed when severe discrepancies are clinically apparent; however, when discrepancies are mild, the distinction between hemihypertrophy and hemihypotrophy becomes difficult. Diagnosis of hemitrophy is made by comparison of measured limb lengths with expected lengths in relation to normal body proportions. Trunk height can be used to determine the patient's trunk height percentile, which can subsequently be used to determine the patient's expected limb lengths.

BOX 20.4-1 DIFFERENTIAL DIAGNOSIS OF HAMARTOMATOUS DISORDERS

- Idiopathic hemihypertrophy/hemihyperplasia
- Idiopathic macrodactyly
- Proteus syndrome
- Klippel-Trenaunay syndrome
- Parkes-Weber syndrome
- Maffucci syndrome
- Neurofibromatosis, type 1
- Epidermal nevus syndrome
- Bannayan-Riley-Ruvalcaba syndrome
- Hemihyperplasia/lipomatosis syndrome
- Familial lipomatosis
- Symmetric lipomatosis
- Encephalocraniocutaneous lipomatosis

BOX 20.4-2 CLASSIFICATION OF HEMIHYPERTROPHY

Acquired
Congenital
- Nonsyndromic
  - Total organ involvement
  - Limited
    - Classic (ipsilateral upper and lower limbs)
    - Segmental (single limb)
    - Facial
    - Crossed (contralateral upper and lower limbs)
- Syndromic

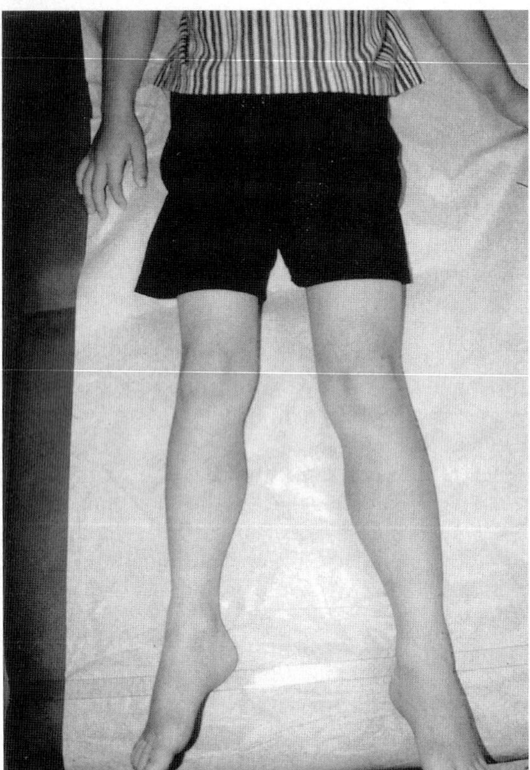

Figure 20.4-1 Eight-year-old boy with congenital hemihypertrophy involving the right side of the body. Observe the discrepancy in length and circumference of the left lower extremity.

Clinical Features

- Hemihypertrophy is rarely apparent at birth but clinically manifests during subsequent growth.
- Anatomic structures, including the eye, ear, tongue, thorax, abdomen, head on one side of the body, enlarge asymmetrically.
- The skin may be thicker and there may be more hair on the affected side.
- Ipsilateral internal organs are also increased in size.
- In contrast to syndromic hemihypertrophy, where the growth is irregular and unpredictable, the growth pattern in nonsyndromic hemihypertrophy is regular and proportionate with growth of the patient.
  - This allows for improved prediction of eventual lower extremity length discrepancy and appropriate timing of interventions.
  - Lower extremity length discrepancy rarely exceeds 5 cm by skeletal maturity.
- Nonsyndromic hemihypertrophy is not associated with cutaneous or vascular lesions.
- The presence of vascular or cutaneous anomalies, in the setting of hemihypertrophy, indicates a generalized overgrowth syndrome.
- Patients with nonsyndromic hemihypertrophy typically have normal mental capabilities.
- Hemihypertrophy can be clinically differentiated from hemihypotrophy/hemiatrophy, which may be characterized by the presence of mental retardation, muscle hypotrophy/atrophy, focal neurologic abnormalities, or joint abnormalities.
- Genitourinary abnormalities are commonly associated with nonsyndromic hemihypertrophy, including inguinal hernia, renal cysts, cryptorchidism, sponge kidney, and horseshoe kidney.
- Other associated orthopaedic findings include scoliosis, macrodactyly, syndactyly, lobster-claw hand, developmental dysplasia of the hip, and clubfoot.

Patients with nonsyndromic hemihypertrophy are at increased risk of malignancy, such as Wilms tumor, adrenal carcinoma, pheochromocytoma, hepatoblastoma, and leiomyosarcoma. Periodic abdominal ultrasound screening remains controversial because the benefits of early detection are unproved, and extraabdominal tumors remain undetectable by abdominal ultrasound. Despite these issues, current recommendations include abdominal ultrasound every 3 months until 7 years of age followed by physical examination every 6 months until skeletal maturity.

TREATMENT

Orthopaedic treatment may be indicated for lower extremity length discrepancy (Chapter 8).

MACRODACTYLY

PATHOGENESIS

Etiology

The etiology of idiopathic macrodactyly is unknown. Hypotheses include genetic mutations, neuroinduction, and localized endocrine or paracrine malregulation. None of these hypotheses have been adequately proven, although the frequent enlargement of digits in the sensory distribution of a major peripheral nerve provides abundant circumstantial evidence to the hypothesis of neuroinduction. In all cases of true idiopathic macrodactyly, hypertrophy of the digital nerves and median or ulnar nerve coincide with hypertrophy of the digits within the distribution of innervation.

Epidemiology

There is no evidence of any inheritance pattern for macrodactyly, although, there appears to be a slightly greater male predominance with a 3:2 male-to-female ratio. Some 90% to 95% of cases are unilateral with multiple adjacent digit involvement. Macrodactyly is equally likely to occur in the hands as in the feet. The second ray is the most commonly involved followed by third, first, fourth, and fifth in decreasing frequency of occurrence.

Pathophysiology

All tissues are enlarged in macrodactyly; however, fibrous bands and adipose tissue consistently infiltrate muscles and nerves. There is tumorlike proliferation of adipose tissue resembling that of adult adipose tissue. In addition, digital nerves, median, or ulnar nerves in the distal third of the forearm are prominent resulting from fibrolipomatous proliferation of endoneurium, perineural, and epineural tissues. There is diffuse periosteal fibromatosis resulting from proliferation of fibroblastic tissue underlying the periosteum with increased osteoblastic and osteoclastic activity that may account for phalangeal and metacarpal overgrowth.

Classification

The classifications of macrodactyly are presented in Boxes 20.4-3 and 20.4-4.

DIAGNOSIS

Macrodactyly is characterized by increased size of a single digit or several adjacent digits of the hand or foot with variable enlargement of the involved hand or foot proximal to the digits. True macrodactyly must be differentiated from pseudomacrodactyly where there is isolated enlargement of soft tissue without enlargement of bone. Pseudomacrodactyly can occur secondary to hemangiomas, congenital arteriovenous fistulas, or congenital constriction band syndrome.

Clinical Manifestations

- True macrodactyly presents without any evidence of cutaneous manifestations.
- There is maximal enlargement of the digit distally, which tapers proximally.
- Because the areas of enlargement lie in a particular regional peripheral nerve distribution, it is also known as nerve territory-oriented macrodactyly.
- The median nerve distribution is most commonly involved.
- Enlargement of the nerve extends well proximal to the macrodactyly, often beginning at the distal third of the forearm with gradual enlargement toward the tip of the involved digits.
    - Enlarged median and ulnar nerves are susceptible to compressive neuropathy.
    - Carpal tunnel syndrome is a common finding in adults with macrodactyly.
- The palmar or plantar surface is disproportionately hypertrophied in relation to the dorsal surface, resulting in hyperextension deformities of the metatarsophalangeal/metacarpophalangeal and interphalangeal joints.
    - The increased palmar or plantar soft tissue bulk results in limitation of flexion with ensuing joint stiffness.
    - Clinodactyly of the involved digit is common when half the digit is involved.
- In mild cases, enlargement is isolated to the digits; however, in severe cases, metatarsal/metacarpal bones are affected with hypertrophy of the interosseous muscles and widening of the affected hand or foot.
- The static form of macrodactyly is often present at birth.
    - The involved digits are 50% larger in length and width of normal digits and continue to enlarge proportionately to the rate of growth.
    - Patients can retain reasonable function if the condition is localized to one or two digits, and thus tend to present in adolescence for treatment.
- The progressive form is typically normal or nearly normal at birth, with unremitting and disproportionate digital overgrowth by 2 to 3 years of age.
- In both forms, longitudinal overgrowth continues until physeal closure or arrest, but transverse growth and soft tissue overgrowth may continue even after skeletal maturity.
- Documentation of hand and digit size with anteroposterior hand radiographs is essential to determine the growth pattern and differentiate the static and progressive forms of macrodactyly.
- Macrodactyly is associated with syndactyly in 10% of cases and can also be associated with polydactyly and cryptorchidism.

BOX 20.4-3 GENERAL CLASSIFICATION OF MACRODACTYLY

True macrodactyly
- Idiopathic macrodactyly
    - Static
    - Progressive
- Syndromic macrodactyly

Pseudomacrodactyly

BOX 20.4-4 FLATT'S CLASSIFICATION OF MACRODACTYLY

Gigantism and lipofibromatosis
- Static
- Progressive

Gigantism and neurofibromatosis
Gigantism and digital hyperostosis
Gigantism and hemihypertrophy

TREATMENT

Surgical treatment of macrodactyly depends on the age, location, type, and severity. Primary consideration in management of macrodactyly in the hand is function. Significant increases in girth and length of digits in the hand are tolerable if there is only minor functional impairment. On the other hand, the goals of treatment in the foot are for proper shoe fitting and painless weightbearing. This is more difficult to achieve since a small increase in width of the foot will prevent adequate shoe accommodation.

- Treatment options include nerve excision and grafting, soft tissue debulking, physeal arrest and hemiepiphysiodesis, osteotomies, digital shortening, amputation, ray resection, or a combination of procedures.
- Mild to moderate macrodactyly can usually be managed by epiphysiodesis of the involved bones and staged soft tissue debulking in children less than 6 to 8 years of age or digital shortening and staged debulking in older children and adolescents.
- This strategy is ineffective in the foot because it does not adequately address girth that may be more properly addressed with ray resection.
- Ray resection is not an option when the first ray is involved because of its unique role in balance and weightbearing.
- More extensive involvement of the foot may require a midfoot or Syme amputation.

The plethora of procedures signifies the difficulty in adequately addressing the challenges of macrodactyly. Patients and parents must be informed of the complexities involved and the potential number of surgeries required as good cosmetic result will be difficult to achieve and functional result decreases with each successive surgery.

KLIPPEL-TRENAUNAY SYNDROME

PATHOGENESIS

Etiology

Klippel-Trenaunay syndrome results from combined capillary, lymphatic, and venous malformations in the extremities without involvement of the arterial system. The increased capillary and lymphatic flow is thought to cause secondary hypertrophic effects on the extremities. Primary mesodermal abnormality may also be present because macrodactyly has been found to occur in the "uninvolved" limb. Somatic mutation for a factor critical to vasculogenesis during embryonic development is thought to be the causative factor; however, the underlying molecular basis of Klippel-Trenaunay syndrome has not been clearly elucidated.

Epidemiology

Klippel-Trenaunay syndrome affects the lower limbs in 95% of patients and the upper limbs in 5% of patients with 15% of patients having combined upper and lower limb involvement. Only 10% of patients will have discrepancies of more than 3 cm by skeletal maturity.

Pathophysiology

Klippel-Trenaunay syndrome occurs as a congenital mesodermal abnormality resulting in the malformation of combined capillary, venous, and lymphatic channels. The vascular channels in these combined capillary, venous, and lymphatic malformations are lined by a single layer of endothelial cells in distinction from hemangiomas and other vascular tumors that are characterized by endothelial hyperplasia. Venous fibromuscular dysplasia with a hypertrophied, irregular, or absent medial layer results in dilation of the superficial venous system. Deep venous system is absent in 14% of patients.

DIAGNOSIS

Clinical diagnosis of Klippel-Trenaunay syndrome is made by the presence of a distinctive clinical triad:

1. Combined vascular malformations of the capillary, venous, and lymphatic types
2. Varicosities in unusual distributions in infancy or childhood
3. Limb (bony and soft tissue) hypertrophy.

Distinction must be made between the slow-flow venous malformations characteristic of Klippel-Trenaunay syndrome and the fast-flow arteriovenous malformations of Parkes-Weber syndrome, in which lymphatic malformations are absent.

- Clinical diagnosis of Klippel-Trenaunay syndrome needs to be confirmed by magnetic resonance imaging (MRI) with gadolinium to distinguish between lymphatic, venous, and arterial malformations.
- The characteristic lateral venous anomaly and any deep venous abnormalities should be documented by MRI or venography.
- The combination of capillary malformation and hemihypertrophy is insufficient to make the diagnosis.

Clinical Manifestations

- Klippel-Trenaunay syndrome is commonly characterized by the classic lateral varicosities (vein of Servelle) in the lower extremity beginning as a venous plexus from the dorsolateral aspect of the foot, extending in a superolateral fashion with variable termination proximally.
- Full leg distribution of varicosities with drainage into gluteal veins is found in 33% of patients.
- Characteristic lymphatic vesicles and venous flares originating from the lateral varicosities appear on the surface as cutaneous capillary malformations.
- The lymphatic, venous, capillary malformations most commonly occur in the extremities, but have been

observed to occur in the head, neck, buttocks, chest, trunk, abdomen, bladder, and oral cavity.

- Abnormalities of the deep venous systems such as agenesis, atresia, hypoplasia, valvular incompetence, or aneurysmal dilatation are common.
- Other clinical manifestations include complications secondary to distal venous hypertension and congestion depending on the regional anatomy affected:
  - Lymphedema, chronic venous ulceration, gangrene, thromboembolism, thrombophlebitis, hematochezia, hematuria, vaginal bleeding, esophageal varices, chronic consumptive coagulopathy secondary to localized intravascular coagulation, and rapidly progressive limb/trunk overgrowth
- In contrast to Proteus syndrome, the overgrowth observed in Klippel-Trenaunay syndrome is present and severe at birth, although ultimate limb length discrepancy is not as pronounced as that found in Proteus syndrome and typically does not exceed 5 cm by skeletal maturity.

Disproportionate macrodactyly can occur and is not always ipsilateral to the vascular malformations (Fig. 20.4-2).

TREATMENT

Because patients with Klippel-Trenaunay syndrome tend to present with less severe hemihypertrophy and limb length discrepancy, the orthopaedic intervention tends to be more successful in patients with Klippel-Trenaunay syndrome. Treatment is generally supportive until the symptoms become intolerable or functional impairment becomes severe. There is recent evidence to suggest that early surgical treatment of the vascular malformation in Klippel-Trenaunay syndrome may prevent long sequelae of distal venous hypertension including hemihypertrophy; surgical treatment of vascular malformations however remains controversial.

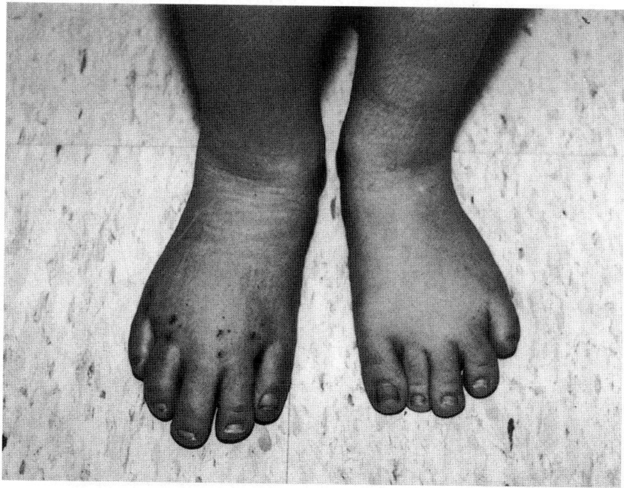

Figure 20.4-2 Postoperative photograph of a 7-year-old girl with Klippel-Trenaunay syndrome. She has disproportionate macrodactyly primarily of her right second, third, and forth toes and, to a lesser extent, the left third and fourth toes. The involved toes on the right foot have been treated with a percutaneous epiphysiodesis of the metatarsals and proximal phalanges to allow for progression shortening with subsequent growth.

PROTEUS SYNDROME

PATHOGENESIS

Etiology

Proteus syndrome is hypothesized to result from postzygotic somatic mutations in multiple cell lineages that occur only in the mosaic state. This mosaicism accounts for the variability of presenting clinical features. The hypothesized somatic mutations in Proteus syndrome are presumed to be lethal in the nonmosaic state such that there is no risk of recurrence or inheritance. There is recent evidence to suggest a somatic mutation in the PTEN tumor suppressor gene as the principal cause of many overgrowth syndromes including Proteus syndrome and Proteus-like syndromes.

Pathophysiology

Proteus syndrome occurs as patchy dysplasia across all three germ layers. There is irregular overgrowth of multiple tissues and cell lines resulting in highly variable phenotypic manifestations. Proteus syndrome is mainly characterized by connective tissue nevi, epidermal nevi, and hyperostoses. Commonly, there is excessive growth of mature tissues including epidermis, connective tissue, endothelium, adipose tissue, and bone. Overgrowth of tissues is progressive but plateaus after the adolescent growth spurt.

DIAGNOSIS

Diagnosis of Proteus syndrome is based on specific clinical manifestations; however, general syndromic criteria must be met regardless of the presence of multiple specific criteria. The diagnosis of Proteus syndrome must include the following:

- Mosaic pattern of distribution of tissue overgrowth
- Evidence of the progressive nature of the disease
- Lack of any mode of inheritance or transmission.

In addition, specific criteria within any one of three categories must be met for diagnosis (Box 20.4-5).

BOX 20.4-5 SPECIFIC CRITERIA FOR PROTEUS SYNDROME

Either A or two from B or three from C in addition to general criteria (mandatory)

A. Connective tissue nevus

B. 1. Epidermal nevus
  2. Disproportionate overgrowth
    a. Gigantism of limbs
      i. Hemihypertrophy (arms/legs)
      ii. Macrodactyly (hands/feet/digits)
    b. Skull hyperostosis
    c. External auditory meatus hyperostosis
    d. Megalospondylodysplasia
    e. Viceromegaly (spleen/thymus)
  3. Specific tumors before end of second decade
    a. Bilateral ovarian cystadenomas
    b. Parotid monomorphic adenoma

C. 1. Dysregulation of adipose tissue
    a. Lipomas
    b. Regional absence of fat
  2. Vascular malformations
    a. Capillary malformations
    b. Venous malformations
    c. Lymphatic malformations
  3. Facial phenotype
    a. Dolichocephaly
    b. Long facies
    c. Minor downslanting of palpebral fissures and/or minor ptosis
    d. Low nasal bridge
    e. Wide or anteverted nares
    f. Open mouth at rest

Clinical Manifestations

The presence of connective tissue nevi with fulfillment of the general criteria is pathognomonic for Proteus syndrome.

- Connective tissue nevi result from dense overgrowth of the underlying collagen resulting in the appearance of “cerebriform or gyriform” lesions.
- These connective tissue nevi most commonly occur in the plantar and palmar surfaces.
- Epidermal nevi, vascular malformations, and lipomas are also common findings in patients with Proteus syndrome.

The most common orthopaedic manifestations of Proteus syndrome are macrodactyly and hemihypertrophy.

- Macrodactyly may occur in any combination of digits in the hand, feet, or both and is not always ipsilateral with hemihypertrophy (Fig. 20.4-3).
- It is usually minor or absent at birth but rapidly progresses in the first few years of life.
- The degree of macrodactyly usually results in severe cosmetic and functional impairment.
- Growth of the affected digits typically decreases to a more proportionate rate in late childhood and plateaus at skeletal maturity.

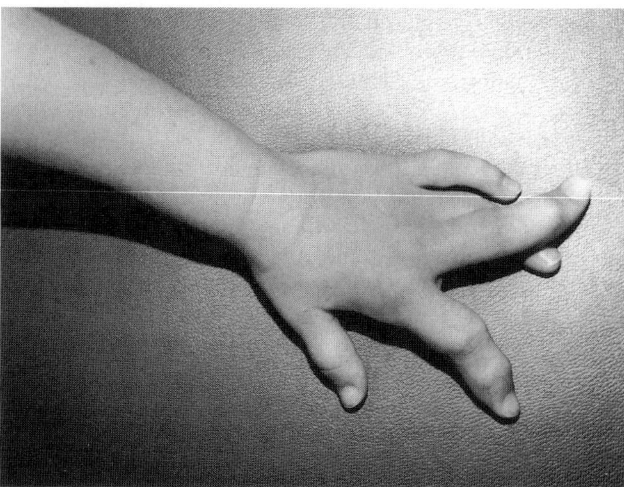

Figure 20.4-3 Severe macrodactyly of the index and long fingers of the left hand in a 5-year-old girl with Proteus syndrome. The fingers are essentially nonfunctional and were amputated. She also has ovarian abnormalities, macrodactyly of several toes, and other fibrous lesions of bone.

- Hemihypertrophy can be partial, complete, or crossed (Fig. 20.4-4).
- Hemihypertrophy of the upper extremity usually does not result in severe functional impairment; however, involvement of the lower extremity can result in severe limb length discrepancy.

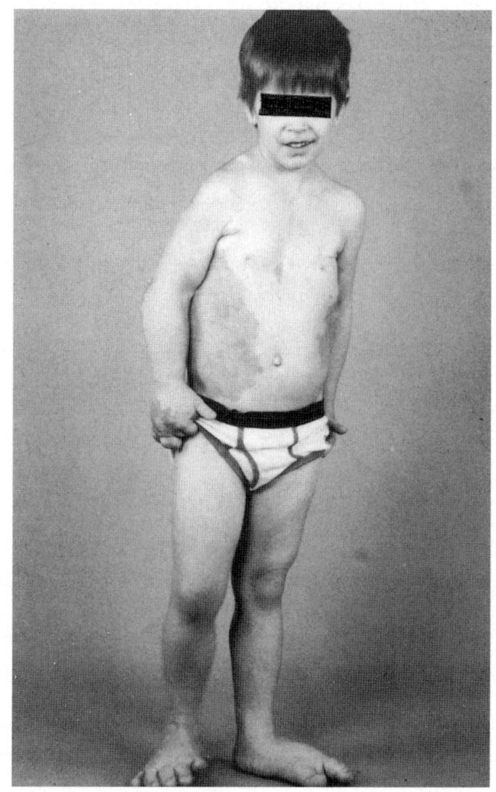

Figure 20.4-4 Four-year-old boy with Proteus syndrome. An extensive vascular malformation involves the right chest and abdomen, his right hand and both feet are enlarged, and there is hemihypertrophy of the right lower extremity.

BOX 20.4-6 OTHER ORTHOPAEDIC MANIFESTATIONS OF PROTEUS SYNDROME

- Spinal deformity (scoliosis, kyphoscoliosis, megalospondylodysplasia, gazelle neck)
- Angular limb deformities (coxa valga/vara, knee and ankle valgus/varus)
- Developmental dysplasia of the hip
- Exostosis of hands, feet, or skull
- Syndactyly, polydactyly, clinodactyly
- Joint contractures/ligamentous laxity
- Talipes equinovarus
- Calcaneovalgus

- In combination with macrodactyly of the foot and hemihypertrophy of the pelvis, leg length discrepancy in excess of 10 cm can be expected.

Other orthopaedic manifestations of Proteus syndrome are presented in Box 20.4-6.

TREATMENT

Because of the variable clinical manifestations affecting variable organ systems, patients with Proteus syndrome are often cared for by multiple subspecialists. In general, management for Proteus syndrome is individualized and directed toward each specific manifestation. Hemihypertrophy and macrodactyly are the most common reasons for orthopaedic consultation, however, there is dissociated or delayed skeletal age making growth prediction unreliable and treatment difficult.

Although orthopaedic intervention has been mostly successful for limb or digit length equalization, soft tissue bulk and digital and pedal girth continue to be problems. Surgical options include soft tissue debulking, epiphysiodesis, ray resection, and amputation. Many patients with Proteus syndrome with severe disproportionate overgrowth and multiple recurrences will go on to multiple amputations at increasingly more proximal levels.

SUGGESTED READING

Ballock RT, Wiesner GL, Myers MT, et al. Hemihypertrophy: concepts and controversies. J Bone Joint Surg (Am) 1997;79:1731–1738.

Baraldini V, Coletti M, Cipolat L, et al. Early surgical management of Klippel-Trenaunay syndrome in childhood can prevent long-term haemodynamic effects of distal venous hypertension. J Pediatr Surg 2002;37:232–235.

Biesecker LG, Happle R, Mulliken JB, et al. Proteus syndrome: diagnostic criteria, differential diagnosis, and patient evaluation. Am J Med Genet 1999;84:389–395.

Chang CH, Kumar SJ, Riddle EC, et al. Macrodactyly of the foot. J Bone Joint Surg (Am) 2002;84:1189–1194.

Cohen MM. Klippel-Trenaunay syndrome. Am J Med Genet 2000; 93: 171–175.

Demetriades D, Hager J, Nikolaides N, et al. Proteus syndrome: musculoskeletal manifestations and management: a report of two cases. J Pediatr Orthop 1992; 12:106–113.

Leung AK, Fong JH, Leong AG. Hemihypertrophy. J R Soc Health 2002;122:24–27.

Mackenzie WG, Gabos PG. Localized disorders of bone and soft tissue. In: Morrissey RT, Weinstein ST, eds. Lovell and Winter's pediatric orthopaedics, 5th ed. Philadelphia: Lippincott Williams & Wilkins, 2001:343–355.

Noel AA, Gloviczki P, Cherry KJ, et al. Surgical treatment of venous malformations in Klippel-Trenaunay syndrome. J Vasc Surg 2000; 32:840–847.

Ogino T. Macrodactyly. In: Buck-Gramcko D, ed. Congenital malformations of the hand and forearm. London: Churchill Livingstone, 1998:183–197.

Özturk H, Karnak I, Sakarya MT, et al. Proteus syndrome: clinical and surgical aspects. Ann Genet 2000;43:137–142.

Samuel M, Spitz L. Klippel-Trenaunay syndrome: clinical features, complications and management in children. Br J Surg 1995;82: 757–761.

Stricker S. Musculoskeletal manifestations of Proteus syndrome: report of two cases with literature review. J Pediatr Orthop 1992; 12:667–674.

Waite KA, Eng C. Protean PTEN: form and function. Am J Hum Genet 2002;70:829–844.

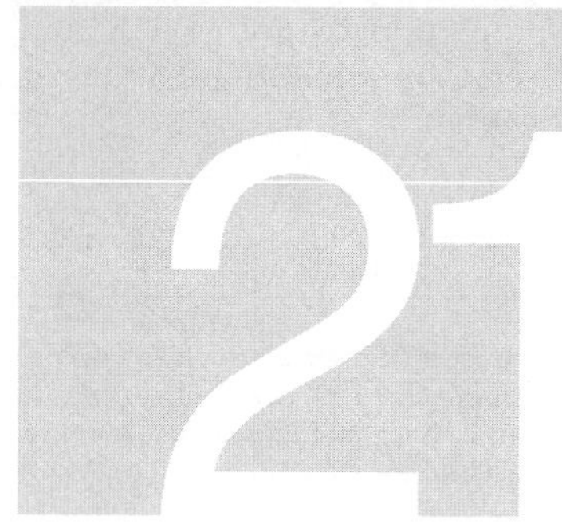

JUVENILE RHEUMATOID ARTHRITIS

KOSMAS J. KAYES
SUZANNE BOWYER
THOMAS F. KLING, JR.

Juvenile rheumatoid arthritis (JRA) is one of the most common rheumatic disorders of childhood. Although the term JRA is often used to refer to one disease, there are three variants with related host responses, which may have the same or different etiologies. All types are characterized by the insidious onset of idiopathic (nontraumatic) arthritis, often in the lower extremity, due to an immunoinflammatory process which may be activated by external antigens in children with a specific, although as yet undefined, genetic predisposition. Early diagnosis of JRA is facilitated by recognition of the three major variants, including oligoarthritis, polyarthritis, and systemic-onset arthritis. Each type is defined by a distinct constellation of clinical signs and symptoms, which present during the first 6 months of disease. Interestingly, JRA and adult rheumatoid arthritis rarely occur in the same family.

PATHOGENESIS

Classification

Table 21-1 describes a classification of JRA based on the types of onset.

Etiology

JRA is an autoimmune disease. The pathologic characteristics of chronic synovitis and T-cell abnormalities suggest a cell-mediated pathogenesis. In addition, multiple autoantibodies, complement activation, and immune complexes, suggest humoral abnormalities. It is also clear that JRA is associated with a complex genetic predisposition. Specific genetic traits occur in children with oligoarticular and pol-

TABLE 21-1 CHARACTERISTICS OF JUVENILE RHEUMATOID ARTHRITIS BY ONSET TYPE

Characteristic	Oligoarthritis (Pauciarticular)	Polyarthritis	Systemic Onset
Number of involved joints	≤4	≥5	Variable
Frequency of cases	60%	30%	10%
Age at onset	Early childhood Peak at 1–2 yr	Childhood Peak at 1–3 yr	Throughout childhood
Female to male ratio	5:1	3:1	1:1
Occurrence of uveitis	20%	5%	Rare
Systemic manifestations	None except uveitis	Moderate involvement	Always involved
Seropositivity			
ANA	75%–85% in girls with uveitis	40%–50%	10%
Rheumatoid factor	Rare	10%—increases with age	Rare
Prognosis	Excellent except for eyes	Fair	50% Excellent 50% Poor

ANA, antinuclear antibody.
Adapted from Cassidy JT, Petty RE. Juvenile rheumatoid arthritis. In: Textbook of pediatric rheumatology. Philadelphia: WB Saunders, 2001:218–321.

yarticular onset. Interaction of multiple genes is likely, given the non-Mendelian inheritance pattern displayed in the various types of JRA. Many of the identified genes are on the histocompatibility complex of chromosome 6. Elevated levels of pre-inflammatory (TH- 1) cytokines characterize all types of JRA. High levels of circulating tumor necrosis factor (TNF) are found in all types. Children with systemic-onset JRA have unusually high levels of interleukin-6 (IL-6). The correlation of IL-6 levels with disease manifestations of systemic JRA have fueled suspicion that cytokine plays a role in the pathogenesis of this condition.

Epidemiology

The incidence of JRA varies in the literature from 2 to 20 per 100,000 of the susceptible population per year. The incidence varies from country to country, and between different ethnic groups. Some authors have identified seasonal variations in incidence. JRA has been described in all races and geographic areas although its prevalence varies throughout the world. Data from North America indicate that children with African and Chinese ancestry have a lower incidence of JRA than Caucasian children. In addition, oligoarthritis is the least common type of arthritis observed in Africa.

The onset of JRA before 6 months of age is rare, although the age of onset is typically quite young, with a peak incidence occurring between 1 and 3 years. This peak age distribution is most evident in girls with oligoarthritis and less so in those with polyarthritis. Systemic onset has no increased frequency at any age.

Twice as many girls as boys develop JRA. Girls with oligoarthritis outnumber boys by 3:1. In patients with uveitis, the ratio of girls to boys is higher at 5 or 6:1. Girls with polyarthritis outnumber boys in a ratio of 2.8:1. Systemic-onset JRA occurs with equal frequency in girls and boys although there is a seasonal variation in frequency. These differences in sex ratios suggest that the disease expression is modified by sex chromosome factors.

Pathophysiology

The final pathway in all forms of JRA is arthritis associated with abnormalities of the immune system. Synovial proliferation and increased fluid production cause reduced joint activity that results in decreased range of motion and strength, as well as potential for development of flexion contractures. Ultimately, cartilage erosion and bony destruction occur as the result of a long-standing, active, or uncontrolled inflammatory process with persistent pannus formation.

DIAGNOSIS

The diagnosis of JRA is clinical and based on knowledge of each onset type and a high index of suspicion. No laboratory tests are pathognomonic for JRA. However, the laboratory does provide support for the diagnosis of JRA by providing evidence of inflammation in an appropriate clinical setting for each onset type.

TABLE 21-2 LABORATORY FINDINGS IN JUVENILE RHEUMATOID ARTHRITIS BY ONSET TYPE

Laboratory Test	Oligoarthritis	Polyarthritis	Systemic Onset
Elevated ESR	+	++	+++
Elevated CRP	+	++	+++
Anemia	No	+	+++
Leukocytosis	No	+	+++
Thrombocytosis	No	+	+++
ANA	++	+	No
Rheumatoid factor	No	+	No
Increased hepatic enzymes	No	+	++

ANA, antinuclear antibody; CRP, C-reactive protein; ESR, erythrocyte sedimentation rate.
Adapted from Cassidy JT, Petty RE. Juvenile rheumatoid arthritis. In: Textbook of pediatric rheumatology. Philadelphia: WB Saunders, 2001:218–321.

Useful laboratory tests vary by onset type and are presented in Table 21-2. It is appropriate to order complete blood count with differential, erythrocyte sedimentation rate, and antinuclear antibody (ANA) testing when considering the diagnosis of JRA. Interestingly, rheumatoid factors (RFs) are unusual in normal children under the age of 7 years and are seldom helpful in the diagnosis at onset of disease. Thus, as a diagnostic aid, RF is of little value. However, children with a high titer of RF likely represent a subgroup of those with polyarthritis who have a later age of onset, are older, and typically have a poor functional outcome.

Clinical Features

The common clinical manifestations of JRA are specific to the onset type, the duration, pattern, and number of joints involved and the presence of associated organ disease. These features are summarized in Tables 21-3 and 21-4.

The arthritis in JRA is usually insidious in onset and is associated with a gait abnormality or limb movement abnormality that is not described as painful. Morning stiffness and gelling after inactivity of the involved joint are common. Stiffness is infrequently mentioned by the child but frequently reported by parents as morning slowness or stiffness. Fatigue is rare in oligoarthritis but is common in children with polyarthritis and systemic onset, especially at onset. It may be expressed as a lack of energy, increased sleep requirement, or increased irritability. Children with oligoarticular onset are not ill while those with systemic onset appear quite ill. Those with polyarthritis may appear ill at onset when a large number of joints are involved.

The affected joint is swollen and warm but usually not erythematous, tender, or painful with gentle movement. If the disease has been present for several weeks, then there is usually mild to moderate muscle atrophy and a mild joint

TABLE 21-3 CLINICAL FINDINGS IN JUVENILE RHEUMATOID ARTHRITIS BY ONSET TYPE

Finding	Oligoarthritis	Polyarthritis	Systemic Onset
Number of joints involved (during 1st 6 mo)	≤4	≥5	Variable
Distribution of joint involvement	Lower extremity Large joints	Lower and upper extremities Large and small joints	Variable
Frequency of involved joints	Knees, ankles, elbows Hips almost always spared	Knees, wrists, elbows, ankle	Variable
Pattern of joint involvement	Usually unilateral Knee most common	Tends to be symmetric	Systemic symptoms often proceed arthritis by weeks or months
Small joints of hands and feet	No	IP joint of thumb; 2nd and 3rd MCP and PIP	May be involved
Cervical spine	Rare	Frequent	Frequent
Temporomandibular joints		Often develops later	
Systemic illness	No	Mildly	Pronounced

Adapted from Cassidy JT, Petty RE. Juvenile rheumatoid arthritis. In: Textbook of pediatric rheumatology. Philadelphia: WB Saunders, 2001:218–321.
IP, interphalangeal; MCP, metacarpal phalangeal; PIP, proximal interphalangeal.

flexion contracture. These changes can best be observed when the joint involvement is asymmetric.

Abnormalities of growth and development are frequently associated with JRA. Linear growth is retarded during periods of active systemic disease. Localized growth disturbance results from accelerated development of ossification centers of long bones or premature fusion of the physis. During active disease the growth and development of the epiphysis is accelerated related to the hyperemia of inflammation. When this occurs in the knee of a young child, it may result in overgrowth of the involved leg, which can be a long-term problem.

Radiographic Features

Plain films of the affected joint are the best investigation in most situations. Early radiographic changes reflect inflammation and include periarticular soft tissue swelling, and sometimes widening of the joint space secondary to synovial hypertrophy. Juxtaarticular localized osteoporosis, growth arrest lines, and advanced epiphyseal ossification center development are often seen within weeks of the onset of disease. These findings are most obvious when the disease is asymmetric. Overtubulation often accompanies linear overgrowth of long bones. Periosteal new bone for-

TABLE 21-4 FREQUENCY OF EXTRAARTICULAR JUVENILE RHEUMATOID ARTHRITIS FINDINGS BY ONSET TYPE

Finding	Oligoarthritis	Polyarthritis	Systemic Onset
Fever	No	30%	100%
Rheumatoid rash	No	2%	95%
Hepatosplenomegaly	No	10%	85%
Lymphadenopathy	No	5%	70%
Pericarditis	No	5%	35%
Pleuritis	No	1%	20%
Rheumatoid nodules	No	10%	5%
Uveitis	20%	5%	1%

Adapted from Cassidy JT, Petty RE. Juvenile rheumatoid arthritis. In: Textbook of pediatric rheumatology. Philadelphia: WB Saunders, 2001:218–321.

mation and metaphyseal rarefaction are found in some children with polyarticular- and systemic-onset disease.

Later radiographic changes include joint space narrowing, marginal joint erosion, joint subluxation, ankylosis, and aseptic necrosis of the femoral head and dome of the talus in those with severe polyarticular- and systemic-onset disease. These late changes are unusual in oligoarticular disease.

Radionuclide scans show early evidence of joint inflammation with increased uptake on both sides of the joint with increased uptake on the early blood flow phase. Unfortunately, they cannot differentiate JRA from septic arthritis or other causes of joint arthritis.

Differential Diagnosis

The differential diagnosis is different for each onset type. In monoarthritis of recent onset (within 72 hours), the diagnosis must include septic arthritis, trauma, and hemolytic disease, including hemophilia, leukemia, and malignancy. If a joint is acutely erythematous and painful, especially with movement, in a febrile child, then septic arthritis is most likely the cause. Immediate joint aspiration is always indicated to rule out septic arthritis.

Juvenile Rheumatoid Arthritis

- The most common cause of chronic arthritis, particularly in girls younger than 6 years of age.
- Psoriatic arthritis and Lyme disease may also present in a similar fashion.
- Rare causes of monoarthritis include juvenile ankylosing spondylitis, villonodular synovitis, and seronegative spondyloarthropathy.

Polyarticular-Onset JRA

- Differential diagnosis is different from oligoarthritis.
- Septic polyarthritis is rare, although *Neisseria gonorrhoeae* may have an early polyarticular phase.
- Lyme disease may be polyarticular, but can be differentiated from JRA by its intermittent pattern of activity and preceding cutaneous, neuralgic, and cardiac findings.

Systemic Lupus Erythematosus

- Can present as polyarthritis in a preadolescent or adolescent girl and mimic JRA.
- Difficult to distinguish the two without serologic studies and the later onset of the characteristic clinical features of systemic lupus erythematosus (SLE) including butterfly rash, alopecia, nephritis, central nervous system disease, Raynaud phenomenon, leukopenia, and hemolytic anemia.
- Presence of an active urinary sediment or Raynaud phenomenon strongly suggests the diagnosis of SLE.

Juvenile Ankylosing Spondylitis

- Should be considered in a boy older than 10 years with a family history of ankylosing spondylitis who develops lower extremity arthritis.
- The HLA–B-27 antigen is present in 92% of these children.
- Firm diagnosis of juvenile ankylosing spondylitis depends on the characteristic x-ray findings in the sacroiliac joint, which is observed later in the disease.

Systemic-Onset JRA

- Can be difficult to diagnose early in its course in a child with a high-spiking fever and evidence of systemic infection but no arthritis.
- Arthritis may not be present initially in this onset type.
- The differential diagnosis is that of fever of unknown origin and includes sepsis, malignancy, inflammatory bowel disease, polyarteritis nodosa, SLE, and juvenile dermatomyositis.
- Infectious mononucleosis and other viral illnesses may have transient arthritis.
- Documenting a rheumatoid rash and the presence of arthritis helps to make the diagnosis of JRA.
- Laboratory tests are of little value in systemic-onset JRA, which is often a diagnosis of exclusion when the associated features are observed in the ensuing weeks or months.

TREATMENT

JRA cannot yet be cured, but spontaneous remission eventually occurs in many children and, in the interim, disease control can be achieved in many with vigorous treatment. Most children with chronic arthritis require a combined regimen of pharmacologic, physical, and psychosocial treatment. The goals of treatment are as follows:

- Preserve range of motion and muscle strength.
- Restore function.
- Prevent deformity.
- Control pain if present.
- Diagnose and manage associated manifestations, particularly uveitis.
- Facilitate normal growth and psychological development.

Since it is not usually possible at outset to predict which child will recover and which will have unremitting disease, it is therefore prudent to initiate vigorous treatment in all children.

- All children should be referred to an ophthalmologist for slit-lamp examination to look for uveitis, which can be present at onset and is often asymptomatic.
  - Most children develop uveitis within 5 to 7 years of onset, making regular ophthalmologic exams mandatory.
  - Slit-lamp exams should be done every 3 months for the first 2 years in children in the high-risk group (early age of onset, oligoarthritis, female sex, ANA-positive) and every 4 to 6 months thereafter for at least 7 years.
  - The exam can be done every 4 to 6 months in children with polyarthritis.

- Inflammatory arthritis should initially be treated with nonsteroidal antiinflammatory drugs (NSAIDs).
  - Naproxen is effective in managing joint inflammation in a dose of 15 to 20 mg per kg per day given with food twice daily.
  - Available in a b.i.d. liquid.
  - Tolmetin in a dose of 25 to 30 mg per kg per day given in three divided doses with food is also effective, although it causes slightly more frequent gastric irritation.
  - Clinical response to NSAIDs is variable and relatively unpredictable.
  - Approximately 65% of children respond within 4 weeks of onset of treatment.
- Analgesia with acetaminophen given two to three times a day is useful to control pain and fever in systemically ill children.
  - Acetaminophen should not be used long term with NSAIDs, since it may contribute to interstitial nephritis.
- If NSAIDs are not effective in controlling the inflammatory arthritis after 1 to 2 months, second-line drugs such as methotrexate, sulfasalazine, or lefluramide can be used.
  - Glucocorticoid drugs are indicated in children with uncontrolled or life-threatening systemic disease, in the treatment of chronic uveitis, and as an intraarticular agent.
  - Chronic oral glucocorticoid therapy is to be avoided if at all possible.
- Physical therapy should be initiated early if there is any muscle atrophy or joint contracture.
  - Atrophy of the extensor muscles begins early and active exercise must be instituted to maintain strength and prevent contracture.
  - During periods of active inflammation, warming the joint with a hot bath in the morning and heat before physical therapy can reduce joint pain and stiffness.
  - Passive stretching is usually necessary to regain lost extension.
  - For resistant contractures, particularly of the wrist, elbows, or knees, serial casts or splints may be beneficial.
  - The maintenance of normal range of motion often requires long-term gentle stretching and the use of resting splints.
  - During periods of remission, an active exercise program to maintain range of motion and strength is recommended.
  - This exercise program also helps to alert parents of recurrent arthritis if atrophy or contracture intervenes.
  - It is usually not necessary to limit play since children determine their own level of activity and normal play is vital to the psychosocial development of the child.
  - Sports that place excessive stress on affected joints, particularly in the lower extremities of older children, should be avoided.
  - Physical therapy is critical to the total management program and should be a regular component of follow-up in children with JRA.
- Biologic medications became commercially available in November 1998 and have greatly benefited children with JRA.
  - Given by injection (etanercept) or intravenously (infliximab), these medications lead to remission in most of the children treated.
  - Etanercept (Enbrel) is given by subcutaneous injections twice a week.
    - In a study of children with JRA who were started on etanercept, approximately 70% responded favorably.
    - These patients had all failed treatment with methotrexate.
  - Infliximab (Remicade) is given intravenously on a monthly basis.
  - Newer biologics like anti–IL-1 (Anakinra) and anti–IL-6 should be available for children within the next few years.
    - The major side effect of this class of medication is decreased resistance to infection, especially infections such as tuberculosis and endemic fungi (histoplasmosis, coccidiomycosis).
- It is unclear whether these medications need to be discontinued prior to orthopaedic procedures such as total hip arthroplasty.
- Depot glucocorticoid can be very beneficial when injected into joints that have not responded to NSAIDs or as an aid to physical therapy of inflamed contracted joints.
  - Triamcinolone hexacetonide is the drug of choice in a dose of 20 to 40 mg for large joints.
  - Aseptic technique is necessary to prevent infection, and anesthesia or conscious sedation is often helpful.
  - Almost all patients respond favorably in 2 to 4 days and the effect lasts for 6 months in 60% of patients and for 1 year in almost 45%.
  - Side effects are uncommon.
  - Subcutaneous atrophy at the injection site can be avoided or minimized by careful prevention of leakage around the needle tract.
- Orthopaedic surgery to equalize leg lengths, relieve long-standing joint contractures, and joint replacement of the hip and knee are beneficial in older children with disability.
  - Synovectomy does not alter the long-term arthritis of JRA, although it can be beneficial to relieve mechanical blocks to joint motion secondary to chronic synovial hypertrophy.
  - Preservation of muscle strength in anticipation of surgery requires rehabilitation over many years and greatly improves the results of surgery.
  - Total joint replacement can be successful only if muscle strength and range of motion have been preserved through the years.

Course of Disease and Outcome

The course of JRA is unpredictable at the outset of disease since the arthritis is typically remitting and relapsing over a period of time. As a group, it is estimated that 70% to 85% of children have a good prognosis for recovery from their arthritis without serious disability. Some 10% to 17% of children with JRA have moderate to severe functional disabilities in adulthood. Children who have many involved joints or unremitting arthritis over a long period of time have a poor prognosis. As expected, there are differences in the course and prognosis for each onset type. However, even with group statistics, it is not possible to predict the outcome in any individual child.

Oligoarticular-Onset JRA

- Course is variable.
- Most children go into remission, although flares of arthritis may occur years later.
- A few have persistent arthritis, which can lead to cartilage erosion.
- Children with oligoarthritis fare best from the standpoint of joint disease and worst from the risk of uveitis.
- Because of the limited extent of joint involvement, serious functional disability is uncommon.
- Correct responce to intraarticular glucocorticoid injection.

Polyarticular-Onset JRA

- The prognosis is not nearly as good as in oligoarticular-onset disease due to the greater number of involved joints.
- Factors that correlate with an unsatisfactory course:
  - ☐ Older age at onset
  - ☐ Long duration of unremitting inflammatory activity
  - ☐ Early involvement of the small joints of the hands and feet
  - ☐ Rapid appearance of erosions
  - ☐ Positive RF
- Largest number of involved joints, often 20 or more
- Long-term disability is related to the extent of articular involvement.
- Limited range of motion often develops early, and remission is unlikely if the arthritis persists longer than 7 years.
- Hip disease occurs in 50% of sufferers and is almost always accompanied by persistent inflammation, which leads to abnormal development and distortion of the femoral head.
- Involvement of the small joints of the hands and feet is characteristically associated with polyarthritis and with a more guarded outlook.

Systemic-Onset JRA

- Acute manifestations vary in duration from weeks to months.
- About half the children eventually recover almost completely, usually after a pattern of oligoarticular disease for a variable period of time.
- The rest of affected children continue to show progressive involvement of more and more joints, which results in moderate to severe disability.
- Eventual outcome depends more on the number of involved joints and on the persistence of inflammatory activity in the joints than on the nature of the systemic disease.

SUGGESTED READING

Cassidy JT, Petty RE. Juvenile rheumatoid arthritis. In: Textbook of pediatric rheumatology. Philadelphia: WB Saunders, 2001:218–321.

DeBenedetti F, Martini A. Is systemic JRA an IL-6–mediated disease? J Rheumatol 1998;25:203–207.

Glass DN, Giannini EH. JRA as a complex genetic trait. Arthritis Rheumatism 1999;42:2261– 2268.

Lovell DI, Giannini EH, Brewer EJ. Time course of response to nonsteroidal anti-inflammatory drugs in JRA. Arthritis Rheuma 1984; 27:1433–1437.

Lovell DJ, Giannini EH, Reiff A, et al. Etanercept in children with polyarticular JRA. N Engl J Med 2000;16:763–769.

Petty RE, Southwood TR, Baum J, et al. Revision of the proposed classification criteria for juvenile idiopathic arthritis. Durban 1977. J Rheumatol 1998;25:1991.

Schaller JG. Juvenile rheumatoid arthritis. Pediatr Rev 1997;18: 337–349.

EQUIPMENT

CLIFFORD L. CRAIG
NICOLE PARENT
MARK D. CLARY
ROBERT N. HENSINGER

WHEELCHAIRS

A wheelchair is a type of mobility system. The following questions need to be considered when writing the prescription for a child who will need to use a wheelchair:

- How long will the child be in the chair each day?
- Will this be the child's primary means of mobility?
- Are there any fixed deformities of the trunk or lower extremities?
- Does the child have head and trunk control?
- What are the child's activities?
- What are the environmental requirements?

Writing the Prescription

Assistance of a knowledgeable physical or occupational therapist is essential. Include diagnosis, duration of need, and justification for type of chair, and each component or accessory. Table 22-1 details the many variables of wheelchairs.

- Type: frame and weight
- Back
  - ☐ Height: need to support mid-back
  - ☐ Fixed/reclining
- Components and accessories
  - ☐ Foot rests
  - ☐ Seat/cushion: abduction wedge; air, gel, or foam
  - ☐ Trochanter pads/hip guides
  - ☐ Scoliosis pads
- Control straps
  - ☐ Seat belt
  - ☐ "H" straps: kyphosis
  - ☐ Pelvic belt: controls sacral sitting
- Tray

ASSISTIVE DEVICES

Assistive devices enlarge the base of support in stance and swing phase of gait, enhance balance, and decrease the weightbearing load.

Types

- Crutches
  - ☐ Axillary
  - ☐ Forearm (Lofstrand/Canadian)
  - ☐ Platform
- Canes
  - ☐ C-handle
  - ☐ Four-pronged base
  - ☐ Hemiwalker
- Walkers
  - ☐ Standard
  - ☐ Folding: portable
  - ☐ Reciprocating: articulated, each arm can move independently
  - ☐ Rolling: wheeled—front, back, both
  - ☐ Platform: forearm support
  - ☐ Posterior: positioned behind the patient; promotes erect posture (sometimes called a Kaye walker)

PROSTHETICS

Prescribing a prosthesis for a child is particularly challenging given the dynamics of growth, activity level, and variable motor coordination.

Principles

- Provide components appropriate to the child's age and level of gross and fine motor function.
- Function should be a priority over cosmesis.
- Initial lower limb prosthesis fitted when starting to pull to stand (7 to 9 months)
- Initial upper limb prosthesis fitted when starting two-handed activities (6 to 9 months)

Prescription Considerations

- Suspension: belt versus socket
- Activity level: influences suspension, structural strength needed
- Structure
  - ☐ Endoskeletal: modular components with a soft cover

TABLE 22-1 WHEELCHAIR VARIABLES

Variable	Choices	Description
Weight	Ultralight	22 lb
	Lightweight	30 lb
	Standard	40 lb
Frame	Folding	More portable
	Rigid	Lighter
Components		
Wheels	Mag	Solid plastic
	Spoke	
Tires	Pneumatic	Air-filled
	Solid	
Hand rims	One-arm drive	For hemiplegics—where the user grips to propel the wheels
	Quad projections	Rubber extensions for improved leverage
Wheel locks	Standard	
	Brake extensions	Positioned at front of seat for ease of access
Back frame	Reclining	Changes orientation by seat to back and knee angles
	Tilt-in-space	Changes orientation of seat and redistributes pressure but maintains angle at hips, knees, and ankles
Head rest/collars	Support based on head and neck control	
	Hensinger collar	Circumferential collar
Arm rests	Standard	
	Tubular swing-away	
Foot rests	Rigid	Built into frame
	Swing-away	Can be moved to facilitate transfers
	Elevating	
Foot plates	Single or two piece	
	Heel and toe loops	Help center foot on footrest

- Exoskeletal: wood or polyurethane covered by plastic laminate; more durable

Lower Extremity Prostheses

Developmental Staging

- Birth to 6 months: usually not fitted
- 7 to 14 months
  - Foot: foam filling in shoe
  - Solid tube connecting foot to socket
  - Hip joint for sitting if needed
  - Omit knee joint
- 15 to 36 months
  - Consider articulated knee
  - Tube extension for growth
- 37 to 72 months: add solid ankle cushion heel (SACH) foot or articulated knee
- 7 to 12 years
  - Consider hydraulic polycentric knee
  - Depends on height and weight and muscle control
- 12 years to adulthood: transition to adult prosthesis

Amputation-Level Considerations

- Hip disarticulation
  - Socket
    - Extends to waist
    - Enclose contralateral side for suspension
    - Single-axis hip joint
    - Endoskeletal structure
    - Knee locked initially
- Transfemoral
  - Socket
    - Ischial containment variations
    - Adducts femur and locks ischial tuberosity
- Suspension
    - Silesian belt initially
    - Silicone socket at 2 to 3 years
    - Suction socket at maturity
- Transtibial
  - Socket
    - Patellar tendon bearing (PTB)
    - Supracondylar suprapatellar (SCSP)
    - Supracondylar (SC): patella-free
  - Suspension
    - SC cuff
    - Silicone suspension liners
- Ankle disarticulation (Symes)
  - Socket: extends to patellar tendon
    - Obturator (medial opening) design
    - Silicone bladder prosthesis
- Partial foot
  - Lange silicone partial foot prosthesis
    - Cosmetic foot shell
    - Silicone-laminated socket
    - Posterior zipper
- Prosthetic feet
  - SACH
    - No articulations
    - Motion depends on compression of material in foot
  - Single axis: allows passive sagittal motion

- Multiaxis: allows sagittal and coronal motion
- Dynamic response
  - Energy storing
  - Spring mechanism in heel
  - Preferred for feet more than 12 cm in length

Upper Extremity Prostheses

Control Systems

- Body powered
  - Shoulder movement activates terminal device
  - Grip strength from rubber bands
  - Bulky harness
  - Terminal device: hand or hook
- Externally powered
  - Switch or myoelectric control
  - No harness
  - Muscle in limb controls terminal device
  - Heavy; difficult to use in children under 2 years
  - Grip strength built into system
  - Terminal device: hand only

Terminal Devices

- Hands and hooks
  - Body or external power
  - Voluntary open and closing

Congenital Below-Elbow Amputation

- Most common congenital upper extremity deficiency
- Most ideal for prosthetic fitting
  - Initial fit at 6 to 15 months: passive hand
  - 15 to 18 months reaching begins: start body- or external-powered prostheses.

ORTHOTICS

The goal of an orthosis is to control motion, correct or accommodate deformity, and compensate weakness. Table 22-2 lists the acronyms that refer to orthoses, Table 22-3 describes joint motion control options, and Box 22-1 high-

TABLE 22-2 ACRONYMS USED: ORTHOTIC AND PROSTHETIC PRESCRIPTIONS

Acronym	Stands for	Notes
Orthoses		
Lower limb		
FO	Foot orthosis	
AFO	Ankle-foot orthosis	Solid, articulated, PLS, conventional (metal); custom molded or prefabricated
KAFO	Knee-ankle-foot orthosis	Single or double upright
HKAFO	Hip-knee-ankle-foot orthosis	May be bilateral or unilateral
RGO	Reciprocating gait orthosis	Type of HKAFO; allows hip flexion in swing, stability in stance
SMO	Supramalleolar orthosis	Controls subtalar motion, allows limited plantarflexion and dorsiflexion
UCBL	University of California, Berkeley, Laboratory orthosis	Orthosis was designed there; addresses flexible hindfoot deformity
SAAJ	Single-action adjustable joint	One channel only
DAAJ	Double-action adjustable joint	Two channels for control of dorsiflexion and plantarflexion (assist and stops)
Upper limb		
HO	Hand orthosis	Does not extend or control wrist
WHO	Wrist-hand orthosis	May or may not have thumb spica
EO	Elbow orthosis	May be protective or stretching
EWHO	Elbow-wrist-hand orthosis	Extends over wrist in addition to elbow
SEWHO	Shoulder-elbow-wrist-hand orthosis	
Spine		
CO	Cervical orthosis	Cervical collar
CTO	Cervicothoracic orthosis	Minerva or Somi
SOMI	Sternal occipital mandibular immobilizer	Type of CTO
LSO	Lumbosacral orthosis	Addresses injuries L1-L5
TLSO	Thoracolumbosacral orthosis	Addresses injuries T4-L5
CTLSO	Cervicothoracolumbosacral orthosis	Cervical extension for injuries above T4 in addition to other thoracic or lumbar injury
Prostheses		
Sockets		
PTB	Patellar tendon bearing	
SC	Supracondylar	
SCSP	Supracondylar suprapatellar	
Other		
SACH	Solid ankle cushion heel	Used for prosthetic feet
OTS	Off the shelf	Not custom molded

TABLE 22-3 JOINT MOTION CONTROL OPTIONS

Type	Description
Free	No restriction in plane of motion, with medial and lateral stability
Assisted	Spring added to increase range and velocity
Resisted	Spring added to decrease range and velocity
Stop	Blocks all motion or limits to a specific range
Lock	Mechanism to block motion when engaged

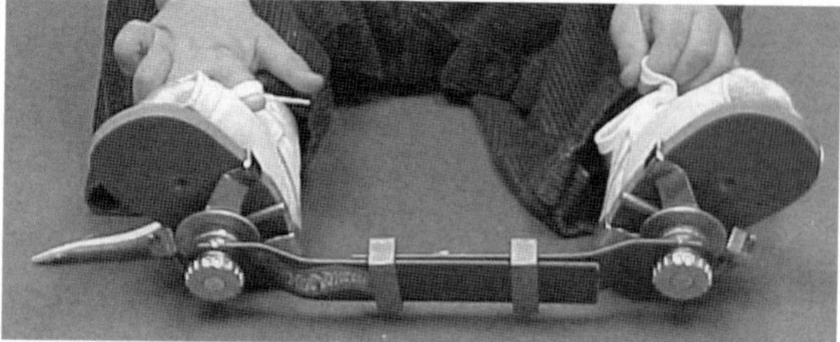

Figure 22-1 Denis Browne bar (attached to reverse-last shoes)

lights the elements that must be included in a prescription for an orthosis.

Lower Extremity Orthoses

Shoes

- Postoperative shoes
  - ☐ Hard sole (wooden)
  - ☐ Velcro closure
  - ☐ Open toe
- Extra-depth shoes
  - ☐ ⅓-inch longer, ½-inch wider than standard size shoe
  - ☐ Removable inner sole to accommodate orthosis
- Custom-molded shoes
  - ☐ Made from cast of foot
  - ☐ Accommodates severe rigid deformity
- Corrective shoes
  - ☐ Reverse last open-toe prewalker shoes—forefoot abducted
  - ☐ Reverse last closed-toe shoes (ambulatory)—forefoot abducted
  - ☐ Straight last open-toe prewalker shoes—forefoot neutral
  - ☐ Straight last closed-toe shoes (ambulatory)—forefoot neutral
- Shoe modifications
  - ☐ Heel
    - ☐ Thomas heel: additional medial support to control pronation
    - ☐ Medial wedge: controls midfoot and hindfoot pronation
    - ☐ Lateral wedge: controls midfoot and hindfoot supination
  - ☐ Sole
    - ☐ Medial sole wedge: controls forefoot eversion
    - ☐ Lateral sole wedge: controls forefoot inversion
    - ☐ Metatarsal bar: decreases pressure on metatarsal heads
- Denis Browne bar (foot abduction bar) (Fig. 22-1)
  - ☐ Attaches to reverse last or straight last shoes
  - ☐ Positions feet in adjustable amounts of external rotation
  - ☐ Able to set separate amounts of external rotation for unilateral applications
  - ☐ Width of bar should equal width of child's shoulders

BOX 22-1 ESSENTIAL ELEMENTS OF AN ORTHOTIC PRESCRIPTION

- Date
- Institution or office or origination
- Patient's name, age, gender, address, telephone number
- Diagnosis: status post is not sufficient; condition for which the surgery was done is also required
- Description of the orthosis and orthotic goal
- Acronym for orthosis and description of the motion control of each joint
- If shoes to be attached to or fit over the orthosis, include modifications
- Justification for orthosis (letter of medical necessity)
- Inclusion of office note may be sufficient

Foot Orthosis

- Accommodative
  - ☐ Soft materials
  - ☐ Custom molded or off-the-shelf (OTS)
- Semi-rigid
  - ☐ Multidensity layered materials
  - ☐ Custom molded or OTS
- Corrective
  - ☐ Rigid materials
  - ☐ Used for flexible deformities
  - ☐ Custom molded or OTS

Additional foot orthosis prescription criteria are based on individual control requirements.

- Medial wedge: controls pronation and heel valgus
- Lateral wedge: controls supination and heel varus
- Longitudinal arch support: controls pronation and heel valgus
- Metatarsal pad: pressure relieves metatarsal head, placed proximal to metatarsal heads

University of California, Berkeley, Laboratory (UCBL) Orthosis (Fig. 22-2)

- Plastic molded insert named for origin of development (UCBL)
- Controls flexible hindfoot deformity
- Accommodates rigid deformity and prevents progression of deformity
- Extended medial wall to control forefoot adduction
- Extended lateral wall to control forefoot abduction

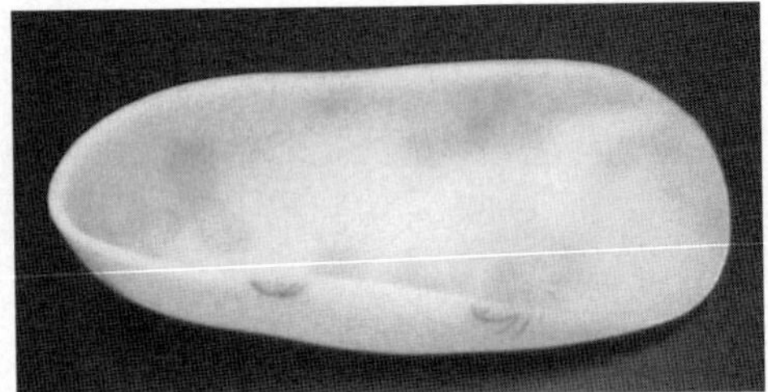

Figure 22-2 University of California, Berkeley, Laboratory (UCBL) orthosis.

Lace-Up Ankle Orthosis

- Canvas orthosis with lace-up anterior support and medial and lateral corrective straps to control inversion, eversion, or both
- Fits in athletic shoe

Ankle Stirrup

- Restricts inversion and eversion (coronal plane motion)
- Allows free dorsiflexion and plantarflexion (sagittal plane motion)
- Fits in athletic shoe

Cast Boot

- Prefabricated ankle immobilizer
- Immobilizes ankle but allows knee flexion
- Smallest size: accommodates 6-inch foot length

Supramalleolar Orthosis (SMO) (Fig. 22-3)

- Molded or prefabricated plastic orthosis that extends above malleoli
- Allows limited plantarflexion and dorsiflexion, restricts inversion and eversion
- Controls pronation and supination, forefoot motion

Ankle–Foot Orthosis (AFO)

- AFOs can be custom molded or fit from prefabricated design components.
- Solid ankle (Fig. 22-4): restricts sagittal and coronal plane motion

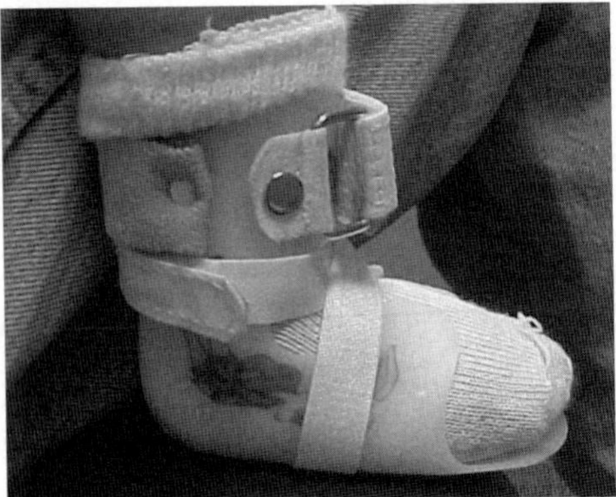

Figure 22-3 Supramalleolar orthosis.

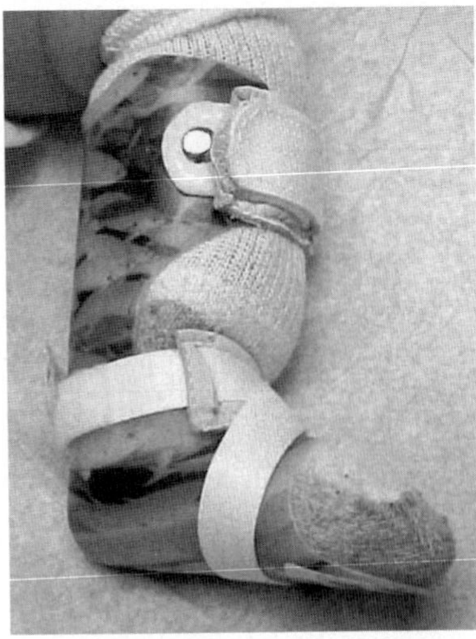

Figure 22-4 Solid ankle–foot orthosis.

- Articulated ankle
  - Provides controlled motion at the ankle
  - Limited or assisted motion (plantarflexion and dorsiflexion)
  - Dorsiflexion stop: check strap or pin in anterior channel of metal joint
  - Plantarflexion stop: plastic stop or pin in posterior channel of metal joint
  - Dorsiflexion assist: assist joint or spring in metal joint
  - Plantarflexion assist: assist joint or spring in metal joint
  - Free motion: free dorsiflexion and plantarflexion with restricted subtalar motion
- Dorsiflexion assist
  - Nonarticulated
    - Posterior leaf spring design
    - Plastic trimmed posterior to malleoli
    - Low-profile design
    - Restricts plantarflexion and allows limited dorsiflexion
  - Articulated (Fig. 22-5)
    - Jointed with dorsiflexion spring assist
    - Limits inversion and eversion
    - Resists plantarflexion but allows range of motion
    - Allows free assisted dorsiflexion

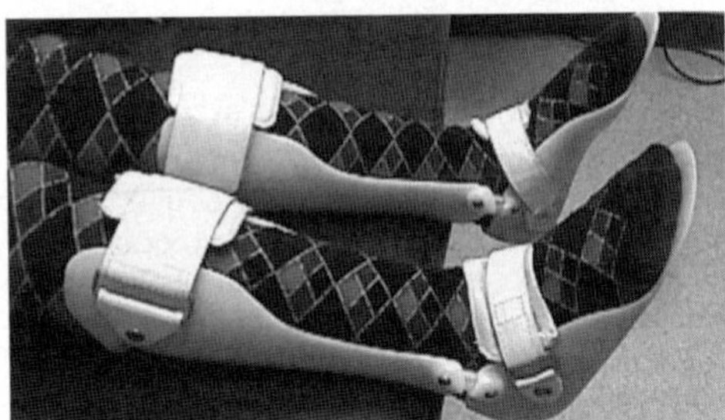

Figure 22-5 Articulated ankle–foot orthosis.

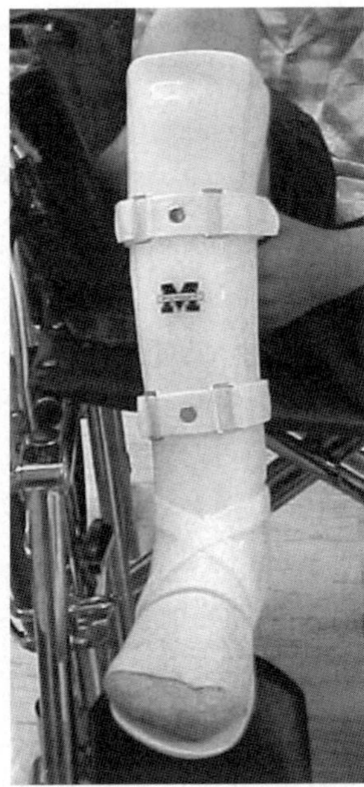

Figure 22-6 Patellar tendon-bearing orthosis.

- Patellar tendon bearing (Fig. 22-6)
  - □ Modifications done to positive cast to lessen weight on lower extremity
  - □ May include solid or articulated ankle
- Conventional metal (Fig. 22-7)
  - □ Can be rigidly attached to shoe with metal stirrup
  - □ Can be fit inside shoe with plastic insert attached to metal stirrup
  - □ Double upright: increased stability and rigidity, heavier person, more adjustability
  - □ Single upright: smaller lever arm (shorter leg), less rigidity
  - □ Single-action adjustable joint (SAAJ): dorsiflexion assist or stop
  - □ Double-action adjustable joint (DAAJ): dorsiflexion and plantarflexion assist and stop

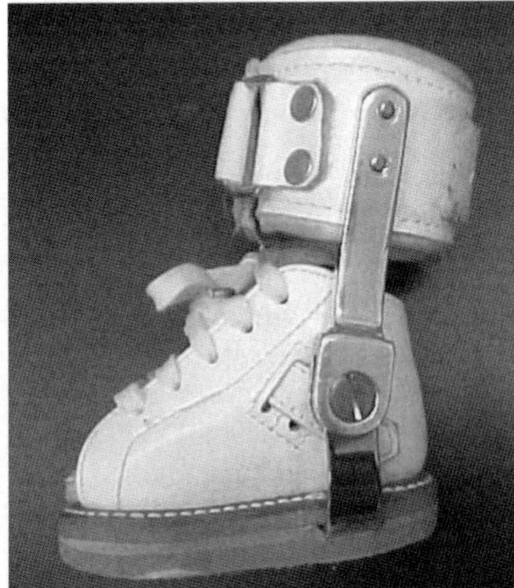

Figure 22-7 Conventional metal ankle–foot orthosis.

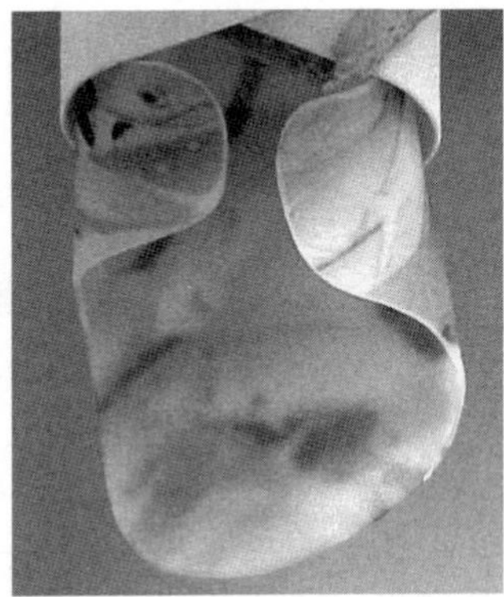

Figure 22-8 Extended lateral wall–forefoot abduction control.

Additional AFO prescription criteria based on individual control requirements:

- Extended medial wall to control forefoot adduction
- Extended lateral wall to control forefoot abduction (Fig. 22-8)
- Toe sulcus length footplate to allow metatarsal phalangeal (MTP) extension
- Full-length footplate to protect toes and allow for growth
- Tone-reducing footplate to apply contact and stimulation to decrease hypertonicity or spasticity
- Total contact: includes anterior shell (clamshell design)
- Sustentacular tali or longitudinal arch pads to control pronation
- Eversion and inversion control straps
- Lateral flanges to control supination and inversion
- Medial flanges to control pronation and eversion

Knee–Ankle–Foot Orthosis (KAFO)

KAFOs can be custom molded or assembled from prefabricated components based on a series of measurements. Support is provided to the knee, ankle, and foot. Parameters for control needed at each joint must be provided on the prescription.

- Foot control options
  - □ Full-length footplate
  - □ Sulcus-length footplate
  - □ Tone-reducing footplate
  - □ See additional foot orthosis prescription criteria based on individual control requirements (described earlier).
- Ankle control options
  - □ Solid ankle
  - □ Articulated ankle
    - □ Dorsiflexion or plantarflexion assist
    - □ Dorsiflexion or plantarflexion stop
    - □ Free motion
  - □ Conventional metal
  - □ See additional AFO prescription criteria based on individual control requirements (described earlier)
- Knee control options
  - □ Drop lock
    - □ Engaged locks in full extension
    - □ Disengaged allows free flexion

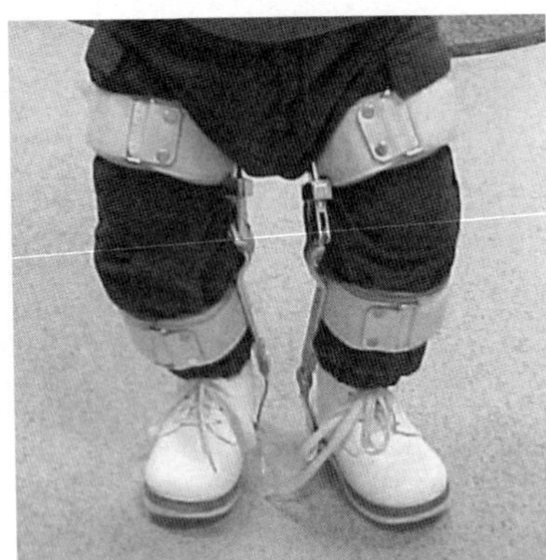

Figure 22-9 Single metal upright ankle–foot orthosis.

- □ Adjustable extension
  - □ Allows knee to lock in position other than full extension
  - □ Combined with drop lock will allow full flexion when lock disengaged
- □ Posterior offset: allows extension movement to prevent knee flexion (buckling) without need for manual drop lock
- □ Bail lock
  - □ Locks in full extension
  - □ Releases into flexion with lever located behind the knee
- □ Static progressive
  - □ Allows incremental increases in range of motion
  - □ No motion, locks at position set, used for stretching or contracture management
- □ Single upright (Fig. 22-9) or double upright (Fig. 22-10)

Hip–Knee–Ankle–Foot Orthosis (HKAFO) (Fig. 22-11)

HKAFOs provide motion control to the hip, knee, ankle, and foot. They are generally custom molded but can be assembled from measurements using prefabricated components. Parameters for control required or range of motion to be limited/allowed must be specified on the completed prescription for each joint included. They may be unilateral or bilateral.

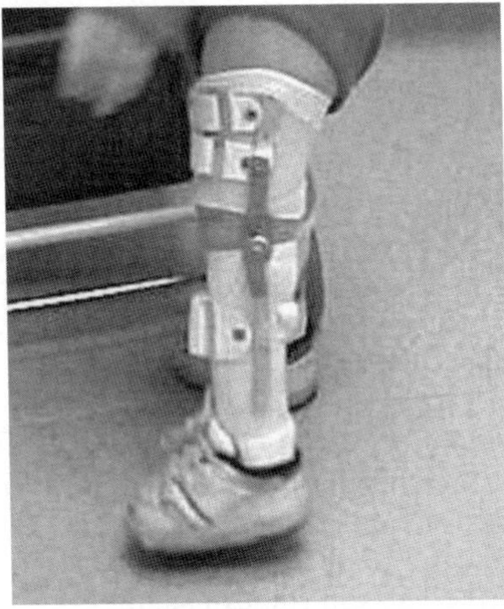

Figure 22-10 Double metal upright knee–ankle–foot orthosis.

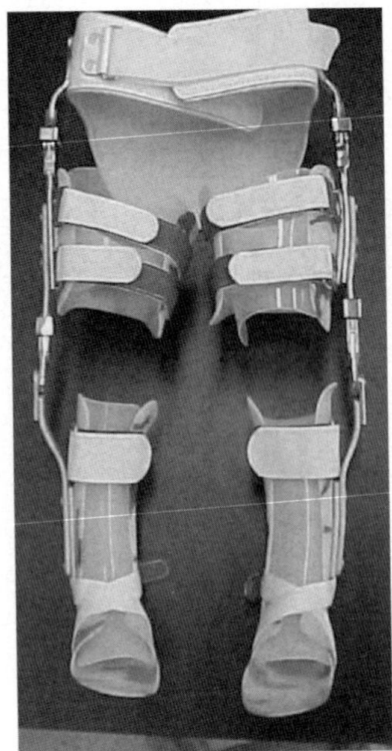

Figure 22-11 Hip–knee–ankle–foot orthosis.

- For foot, ankle, and knee options, see previous section on knee–ankle–foot orthosis.
- Hip control options
  - □ Drop locks
    - □ Lock in full extension
    - □ Free flexion when unlocked
  - □ Adjustable extension
    - □ Lock in set amount of flexion or extension
    - □ Used with drop lock generally
  - □ External and internal rotation control: twister cable from knee to hip joint or offset in metal upright
  - □ Abduction and adduction control: allows range of motion between set parameters or locked at abducted position
  - □ Hip control provided with pelvic band (molded or prefabricated) or extended thoracic support (molded or prefabricated) for additional trunk control

Standing Frame (Parapodium) (Fig. 22-12)

- Adds component of thoracic stability to HKAFO
- Can be used with or without HKAFO system
- Some models flex at knee, allow swivel walking (limited mobility)

Twister Cables

- Reverse-wound cables attached to pelvic band to provide external or internal rotation assist.
- Can be attached to HKAFO or AFO system
- Can be used unilaterally or bilaterally

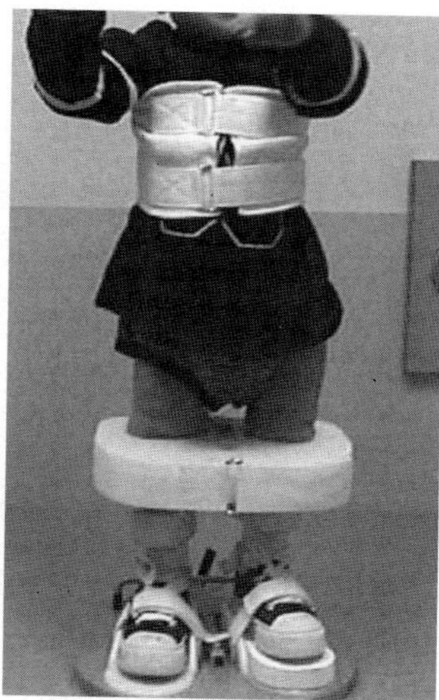

Figure 22-12 Standing frame (parapodium).

Upper Extremity Orthoses

Wrist–Hand Orthosis (WHO)

- Custom molded (Fig. 22-13)
  - ☐ May include anterior shell for total contact
  - ☐ Impact protection for postfracture healing
  - ☐ Allows metacarpal phalangeal (MP) flexion to 90 degrees, should not extend past palmar crease
  - ☐ Allows elbow flexion, should end distal to bicipital crease
  - ☐ May include thumb spica
- Prefabricated
  - ☐ Elastic or neoprene
  - ☐ Aluminum palmar or dorsal support (aluminum stay)
  - ☐ Limited motion control and impact protection
  - ☐ May include thumb spica

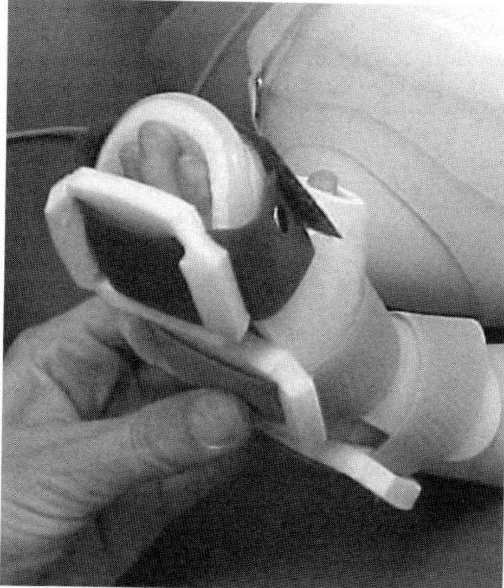

Figure 22-13 Molded wrist–hand orthosis.

Neoprene Wrist–Hand Orthosis, Neoprene Hand Orthosis

- Ventilated neoprene material
- Measured or used prefabricated
- Used to maintain wrist in extension or thumb abducted

Elbow Orthosis (EO) and Elbow–Wrist–Hand Orthosis (EWHO) (Fig. 22-14)

- Provides varus and valgus control at elbow
- Usually custom molded
- Provides total contact, free or limited range of motion at elbow
- Sarmiento design for fracture management of distal humeral fractures

Shoulder–Elbow (Sarmiento) Orthosis

- Fracture management of proximal-third humeral fracture
- Includes thoracic stability strap to decrease rotation of orthosis
- Trimmed distally to allow elbow flexion

Midshaft Humeral (Sarmiento) Orthosis

- Midshaft humeral fractures: total contact design
- Can be custom molded or prefabricated (smaller patients custom molded)

Shoulder Abduction Orthosis

- Controls and limits shoulder motion: abduction and adduction, flexion and extension, internal and external rotation
- Generally custom molded for small children
- Prefabricated options for adolescent or larger children

Sling

- Immobilizes arm in shoulder adduction and internal rotation, with elbow flexed
- Pediatric sizes available with smaller envelopes to free fingers

Sling and Swathe (Shoulder Immobilizer Sling)

- Sling combined with rotation-control thoracic strap
- Further immobilizes the shoulder and prevents abduction and flexion

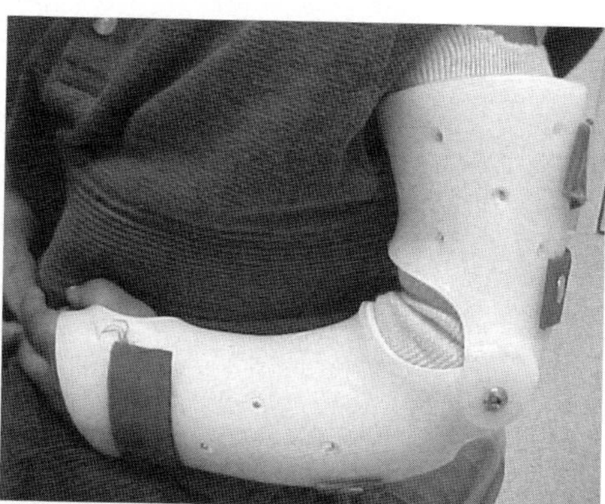

Figure 22-14 Elbow–wrist–hand orthosis.

Figure-of-Eight (Clavicle Strap)

- Prevents scapular protraction and encourages scapular retraction
- Postural correction, clavicle fracture management
- Can be added to spinal orthosis for kyphosis correction

Spinal Orthoses

Cervical Orthosis (CO)

- Soft collar
  - Support for cervical muscle spasms or minor ligamentous injuries
  - Serves simply as kinesthetic reminder, provides soft tissue warmth
- Hard collar
  - Limits sagittal motion better than the soft collar
  - Support for muscle spasms and atlantoaxial rotary subluxation
  - Many types: Philadelphia, Aspen (Fig. 22-15), Miami J

Cervicothoracic Orthosis (CTO)

- Increases stability of cervical orthosis alone by extending inferiorly over thoracic region
- Addresses C1 fractures without subluxation, stable hangman fracture, and flexion injuries of C3-C5
- Minerva
  - Plastic with removable liner
  - Good flexion control
- SOMI: sternal occipital mandibular immobilizer
  - Can be easily applied in a supine position
  - Good flexion control, limited extension control
- Halo (Fig. 22-16)
  - Addresses unstable cervical injuries
  - Most rigid control through skeletal fixation
  - Excellent flexion, extension, and rotation control

Lumbosacral Orthosis (LSO)

- Addresses acute or chronic low back pain, acute low back and leg pain, sacroiliac disorders
- Support from L1 to L5
- Provides varying degrees of abdominal support, motion control, and pain relief
- Nonoperative and operative types
  - Corset or elastic wraparound styles sized (OTS)
  - Rigid plastic LSO (custom molded)

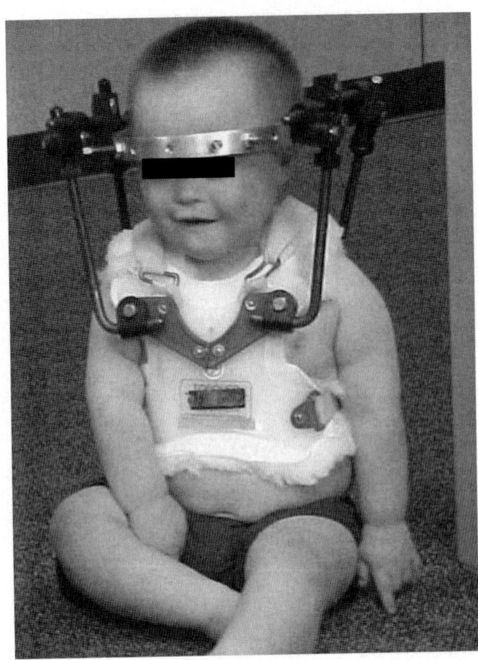

Figure 22-16 Halo.

Thoracolumbosacral Orthosis (TLSO)

Addresses fractures (e.g., anterior compression, burst), congenital malformation, neurologic disease with muscle paralysis, spondylolisthesis, disc herniation, stenosis

- Hyperextension TLSO (Jewett, CASH): addresses anterior compression fracture and prevents flexion
- Knight-Taylor TLSO
  - Fabricated from measurements only
  - Applicable for obese patients
  - Easily accommodates weight fluctuations
  - Provides good ventilation
- Custom-molded TLSO
  - Provides intimate fit and maximum control of flexion, extension, lateral flexion, and rotation
  - Can be molded in desired position (Fig. 22-17)
- TLSO with thigh extension: used to control motion at L5-S1 level

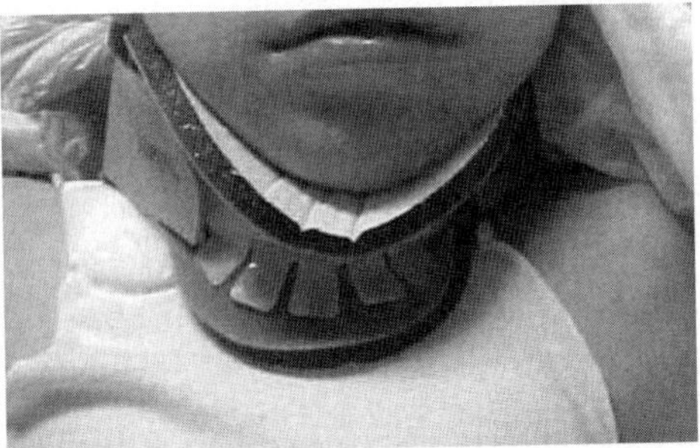

Figure 22-15 Aspen cervical collar.

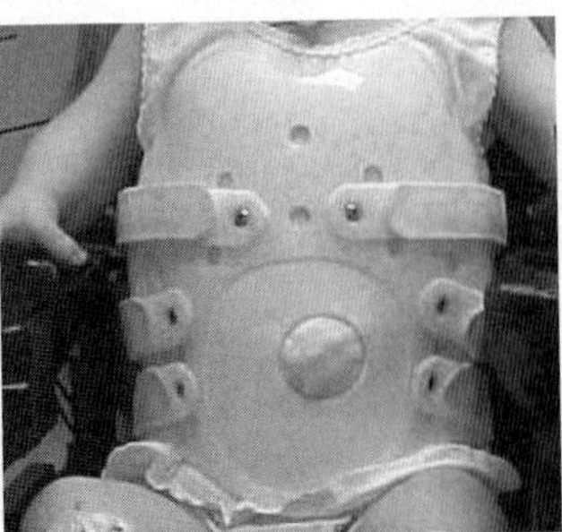

Figure 22-17 Molded thoracolumbosacral orthosis.

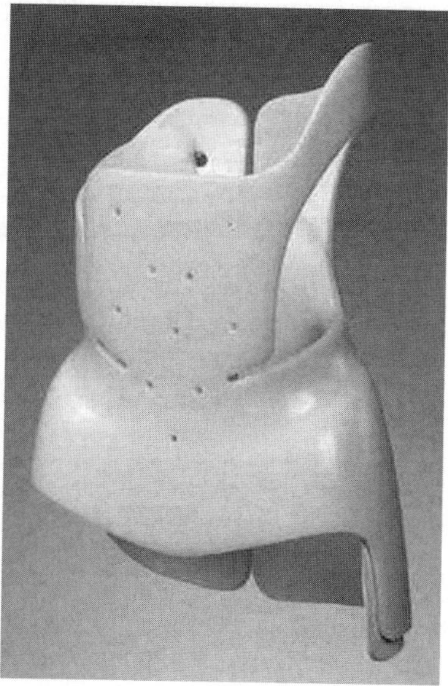

Figure 22-18 Scoliosis—thoracolumbosacral orthosis.

- Scoliosis—TLSO
  - ☐ Used to manage idiopathic (not neuromuscular) scoliotic curves from 25 to 40 degrees
  - ☐ Uses specific trim lines to a module with interior pads to apply counteractive forces
  - ☐ Boston brace: worn up to 23 hours a day (Fig. 22-18)
  - ☐ Charleston bending brace (overcorrection): molded in bent position to reverse scoliotic curve; nighttime use only
  - ☐ Wilmington, Lyon, Milwaukee: used to address higher thoracic curves

Cervicothoracolumbosacral Orthosis (CTLSO)

- Cervical extension added to TLSO to address multiple spinal injuries
- Halo, Minerva, or SOMI extension may be added to TLSO depending on stability needed
- Milwaukee CTLSO
  - ☐ Addresses kyphosis or high scoliotic curves
  - ☐ Very low compliance because of metal extensions in cervical region

SUGGESTED READING

Birch JG, Carter PR, Cummings DB, et al. Limb deficiencies. In: Herring JA, ed. Tachdjian's pediatric orthopaedics, 3rd ed. Philadelphia: WB Saunders, 2002:1745–1810.

Bowker JH, Michael JW, eds. Atlas of limb prosthetics: surgical, prosthetic, and rehabilitation principles, 2nd ed. St. Louis: Mosby-Year Book, 1992.

Goldberg B, Hsu JD, eds. Atlas of orthoses and assistive devices, 3rd ed. St. Louis: Mosby-Year Book, 1997.

Herring JA, Birch JG, eds. The child with a limb deficiency. Rosemont, IL: American Academy of Orthopaedic Surgeons, 1998.

Morrissey RT, Giavedoni B, Coulter-O'Berry C. The limb-deficient child. In: Morrissy RT, Weinstein SL, eds. Pediatric orthopaedics, 5th ed. Philadelphia: Lippincott Williams & Wilkins, 2001: 1217–1272.

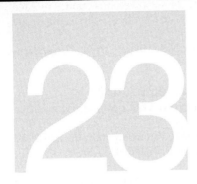

TUMORS

BULENT EROL
JOHN P. DORMANS
LISA STATES
BRUCE PAWEL

BACKGROUND

Pediatric musculoskeletal tumors (MSKTs) are uncommon; although when they occur, they usually are benign. Early detection of a malignant MSKT may not only make the difference between life and death, but also may allow for successful limb salvage surgery rather than amputation of the limb. The primary bone and soft tissue tumors of childhood can be classified based on their tissue origin (Table 23-1). This chapter is not intended as an exhaustive survey of childhood musculoskeletal neoplasm. It will cover general principles of MSKT diagnosis and treatment, and some of the more common individual entities.

A thorough evaluation of the history of the patient and physical examination are the basis for determining the correct diagnosis and therapy. That type of tumors seen in children with an MSKT are presented in Box 23-1. The age of the patient is important in establishing a differential diagnosis, because certain tumors tend to occur in certain age groups (Table 23-2).

Imaging Studies

- Plain radiographs give the most detailed information about skeletal lesions.
  - ☐ Orthogonal views showing the entire lesion are necessary.
  - ☐ 30% to 40% of a bone must be destroyed before lytic changes can be seen in plain radiographs.
  - ☐ It is often difficult to see soft tissue tumors and soft tissue extension from bony neoplasms with plain radiographs.

TABLE 23-1 CLASSIFICATION OF PEDIATRIC MUSCULOSKELETAL TUMORS BASED ON TISSUE OF ORIGIN

Origin	Tumor
Bone tumors	
Bone origin	Osteoid osteoma, osteoblastoma, osteosarcoma
Cartilaginous origin	Osteochondroma, chondroblastoma, chondromyxoid fibroma, enchondroma, periosteal chondroma
Fibrous origin	Nonossifying fibroma, fibrous dysplasia, osteofibrous dysplasia, desmoplastic fibroma
Miscellaneous	Unicameral bone cyst, aneurysmal bone cyst, giant cell tumor Langerhans cell histiocytosis, Ewing sarcoma; musculoskeletal manifestations of leukemia, bone lymphomas
Metastatic tumors	Neuroblastoma, retinoblastoma, hepatoblastoma
Soft tissue tumors	
Vascular tumors	Hemangioma, vascular malformations
Nerve origin	Neurolemmoma, neurofibroma, malignant peripheral nerve sheath tumor
Fibrous origin	Fibromatosis, fibrosarcoma
Muscular origin	Rhabdomyosarcoma
Miscellaneous	Synovial sarcoma, primitive neuroectodermal tumors, ganglion and synovial cyst

BOX 23-1 CLINICAL PRESENTATIONS OF PEDIATRIC MUSCULOSKELETAL TUMORS[a]

Pain
- Duration
- Localization
- Severity
- Character
- Relief and how obtained

Mass
- Duration
- Size
- Consistency
- Mobility

Pathologic fracture spectrum from microfractures to displaced fractures
- Prior symptoms and signs
- Mechanism of fracture
- Characteristics of fracture

Incidental radiographic findings
- Prior symptoms and signs
- Why radiograph obtained

[a]For soft tissue masses, small (<5 cm), superficial, soft, and moveable lesions are usually (but not always) benign. Large (>5 cm), deep, firm, fixed, tender masses raise the index of suspicion for malignancy.

- Magnetic resonance imaging (MRI) best demonstrates the soft tissue anatomy and intramedullary extension of the tumor.
- MRI remains the modality of choice for staging, for evaluating response to preoperative chemotherapy, and for long-term follow-up of most bone and soft tissue sarcomas.
- Computed tomography (CT) can demonstrate bone destruction and mineralization and is particularly helpful for bone tumors involving axial skeleton.
- A total body radionuclide bone scan will evaluate the biologic activity of the primary bone lesion and search for other lesions within the skeletal system.

Features of Bony Lesions

- Location (Box 23-2)
  - □ Epiphyseal, metaphyseal, or diaphyseal
  - □ Central or eccentric
- Destruction of bone (Fig. 23-1)
  - □ Geographic: typical of slow-growing, benign lesions
  - □ Moth-eaten (multiple, small, often clustered lytic areas) and permeative (ill-defined, very small oval radiolucencies or lucent streaks) typical of rapidly growing, infiltrating tumors
- Replacement of bone
- Response of bone
  - □ "Walled off" by cortex: static lesion
  - □ Destroyed cortex and soft tissue mass: aggressive lesion
- Periosteal reaction (Fig. 23-2)
  - □ Continuous: benign
  - □ Interrupted: malignant
  - □ Sunburst ("hair-on-end")
  - □ Lamellated (onion-skin).
  - □ Reactive cuff (Codman triangle)

Staging of lesions that appear to be malignant is required prior to biopsy. Box 23-3 outlines staging recom-

TABLE 23-2 PEAK AGE OF COMMON PEDIATRIC MUSCULOSKELETAL TUMORS[a]

Age (yr)	Benign	Malignant
0–5	Langerhans cell histiocytosis Osteomyelitis	Metastatic tumors Leukemia Ewing sarcoma[b] Fibrosarcoma
5–10	Unicameral bone cyst Aneurysmal bone cyst Nonossifying fibroma Fibrous dysplasia Osteomyelitis Osteoid osteoma Langerhans cell histiocytosis	Osteosarcoma Rhabdomyosarcoma Ewing sarcoma
10–20	Fibrous dysplasia Osteoid osteoma Fibroma Aneurysmal bone cyst Chondroblastoma Osteofibrous dysplasia	Osteosarcoma Ewing sarcoma Rhabdomyosarcoma Synovial cell sarcoma Chondrosarcoma

[a]Musculoskeletal tumors are more common in boys than girls.
[b]Ewing sarcoma is prevalent in Caucasians and rare in African Americans.

BOX 23-2 COMMON LOCATIONS OF PEDIATRIC BONE TUMORS

Epiphysis
- Chondroblastoma
- Brodie abscess of the epiphyses
- Giant cell tumor
- Fibrous dysplasia

Metaphysis
- Any tumor

Diaphysis (FAHEL)
- Fibrous dysplasia
- Osteofibrous dysplasia/adamantanoma
- Langerhans cell histiocytosis
- Ewing sarcoma
- Leukemia, lymphoma
- *Occasional diaphyseal:*
  - Osteoid osteoma
  - Unicameral bone cyst

Multiple
- Leukemia (metastasis)
- Multiple hereditary exostoses
- Langerhans cell histiocytosis
- Polyostotic fibrous dysplasia
- Enchondromatosis

Pelvis
- Ewing sarcoma
- Osteosarcoma
- Osteochondroma
- Metastasis
- Fibrous dysplasia

Anterior elements of spine
- Langerhans cell histiocytosis
- Leukemia
- Metastatic
- Giant cell tumor

Posterior elements of spine
- Aneurysmal bone cyst
- Osteoblastoma
- Osteoid osteoma
- Metastasis

Rib
- Fibrous dysplasia
- Langerhans cell histiocytosis
- Ewing sarcoma
- Metastasis

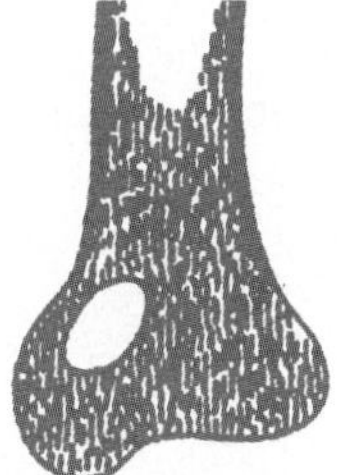

IA: Geographic destruction well-defined with sclerosis in margin

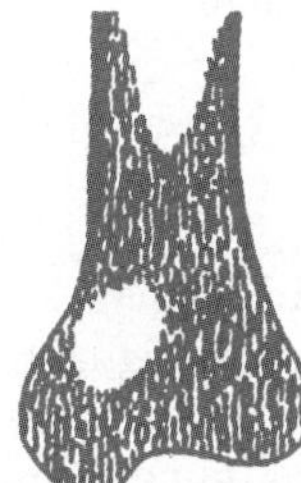

IB: Geographic destruction well-defined but no sclerosis in margin

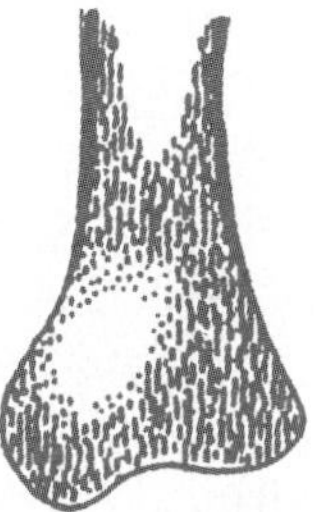

IC: Geographic destruction with ill-defined margin

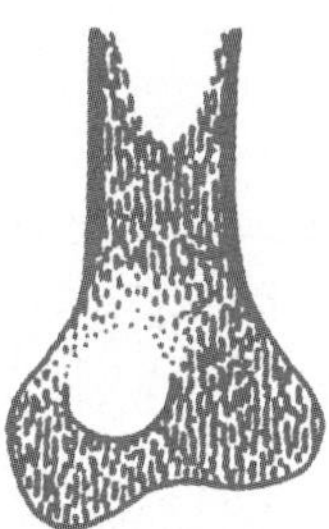

Changing IA margin (destruction of rind)

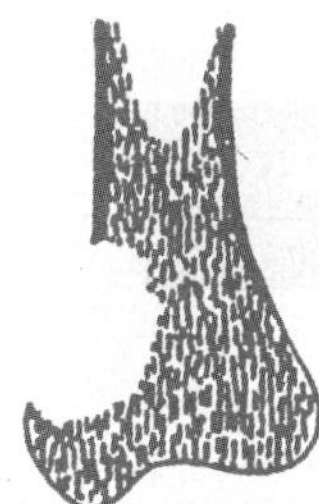

Changing IB margin (cortical breakout)

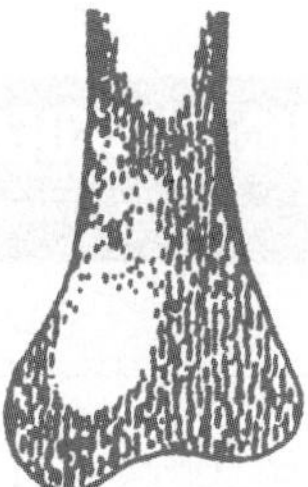

Changing IB margin (transition to II)

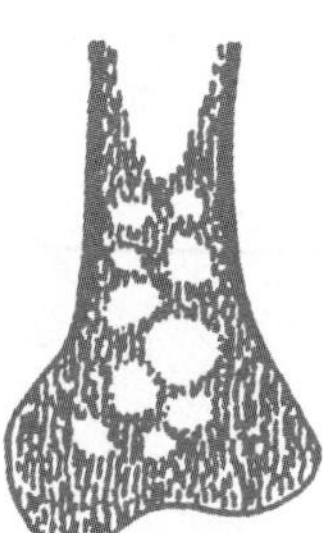

Cancellous

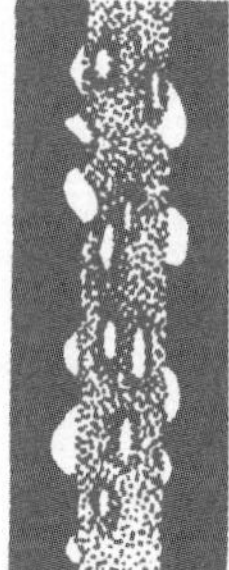

Cortical

II: Motheaten

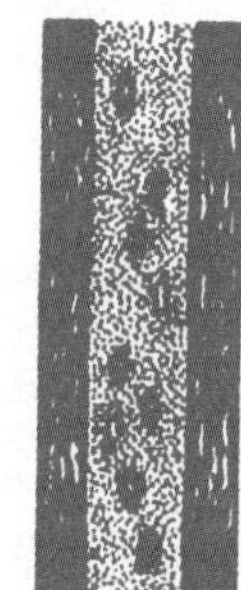

III: Permeated

Figure 23-1 Different patterns of bone destruction. (Adapted from Madewell JE, Ragsdale BD, Sweet DE. Radiologic and pathologic analysis of solitary bone lesions. Part I. internal margins. Radiol Clin North Am 1981;19:715–748.)

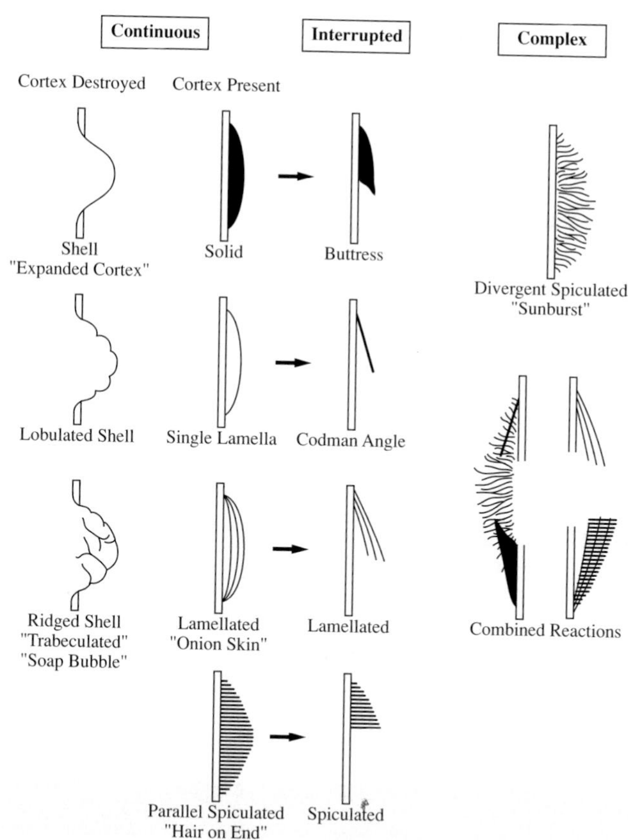

Figure 23-2 Different patterns of periosteal reaction. (Adapted from Ragsdale BD, Madewell JE, Sweet DE. Radiologic and pathologic analysis of solitary bone lesions. Part II. periosteal reaction. Radiol Clin North Am 1981;19:749–783.)

BOX 23-4 BASIC PRINCIPLES OF AN INCISIONAL BIOPSY

- Longitudinal incisions should be used in the extremities.
- Smallest incision compatible with obtaining an adequate tumor specimen should be used.
- The most direct route from the skin to the tumor should be taken; to prevent tumor spreading, the biopsy should go through muscle rather than through intermuscular planes and should avoid exposure of neurovascular bundle or joint.
- Intraoperative frozen section should be done to confirm the adequacy of the specimen.
- Meticulous hemostasis should be obtained for the prevention of tumor spread by hematoma.
- Drains should be placed close and in line with the incision.

mendations. Biopsy should be the last step in the evaluation of a patient with a bone or soft tissue sarcoma and should be performed following completion of the radiographic staging and preoperative consultation with the oncologist, radiologist, pathologist, and surgeon. After staging studies are completed, a differential diagnosis can be formulated. Box 23-4 summarizes the basic principles that should be followed in performing an incisional biopsy.

A precise definition and classification of surgical margins are useful for evaluation, planning, and treatment in the care of MSKTs. There is usually a capsule (or pseudocapsule) surrounding soft tissue tumors or a rim of reactive bone around bone tumors. Within the reactive zone is a variable amount of microscopic tumor extension and beyond the reactive zone is normal tissue. High-grade tumors may have neither a capsule nor reactive rim of bone. Four types of surgical margins of resection have been

BOX 23-3 TREATMENT PRINCIPLES FOR OSTEOSARCOMA AND EWING SARCOMA

Staging of primary lesion and search for other lesions
- Magnetic resonance imaging of the primary site including the joint above and below
- Total body radionuclide bone scan; to search for bone metastases and skip lesions
- Computed tomography of the chest; to search for lung metastases

Pediatric oncology consultation

Incisional biopsy
- Intraoperative frozen section
- Bone marrow aspiration/biopsy for Ewing sarcoma
- Broviac placement for chemotherapy

Preoperative neoadjuvant chemotherapy (usually multiagent chemotherapy)

Repeat magnetic resonance imaging after chemotherapy and prior to definitive surgery
- Radiographic evaluation of the tumor response to chemotherapy (change in size of tumor, change in amount of tumor edema, involvement of neurovascular structures)
- Surgical planning

Surgery; excision of the tumor with wide surgical margins
- Limb-salvage surgery; resection of the tumor with wide surgical margins and reconstruction; currently possible in most patients with extremity sarcoma
- Amputation

Histologic examination of resection specimen
- Histologic evaluation of the tumor response to chemotherapy (>90% tumor necrosis demonstrates good response)
- Verification of wide surgical margins

Continued chemotherapy (adjuvant chemotherapy) after local control surgery
- Usually same protocol with neoadjuvant chemotherapy if tumor response to chemotherapy is good

Radiation
- Usage limited to lesions that cannot be resected, or that have recurred
- Keep dose <60 Gy to prevent a secondary sarcoma

Follow-up
- Every 3 months first year, then 6- to 12-month intervals

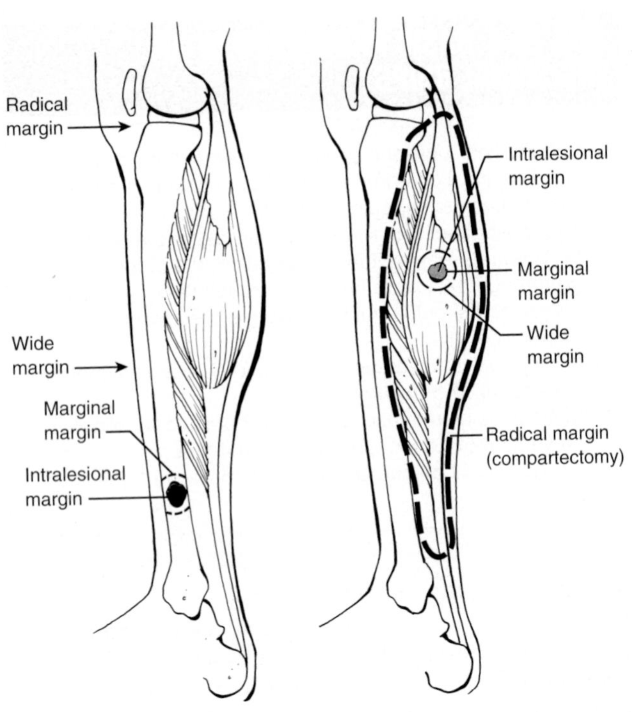

Figure 23-3 Surgical margins for bone (**left**) and soft tissue (**right**) lesions. Intralesional margin; within the lesion, marginal margin; through the reactive zone of the lesion, wide margin; beyond the reactive zone through normal tissue within compartment, radical margin; normal tissue extracompartmental. (Adapted from Himelstein BP, Dormans JP. Malignant bone tumors of childhood. Pediatr Clin North Am 1996;43:967–984.)

TABLE 23-3 SURGICAL MARGINS

Surgical Margins	Limb Salvage	Amputation	Histology
Intralesional	Curettage, piecemeal resection within lesion	Through tumor	Tumor at margin
Marginal	Marginal excision through reactive tissue	Along reactive tissue	Reactive tissue with or without satellites
Wide	Wide excision through normal surrounding tissue	Through normal tissue in compartment	Normal tissue with or without skip lesions
Radical	Radical resection with entire compartment	Extracompartmental amputation or disarticulation	Normal tissue

defined: intralesional (or intracapsular), marginal, wide, and radical (Fig. 23-3 and Table 23-3).

BONE TUMORS

Osteoid Osteoma

- Nidus of osteoid tissue is surrounded by dense reactive bone (Fig. 23-4).
- 10% of benign bone tumors.
- The femur is the single most common site of involvement.
- More than half are found in either the femur or the tibia.
- Pain is typically worse at night.
- Relieved by salicylates and nonsteroidal antiinflammatory drugs (NSAIDs).
- The posterior elements of the spine may also be involved.

Radiographic and Histologic Features

See Table 23-4.

Natural History and Treatment

- Burns out with time (years)
- Standard treatment is complete removal of the nidus by open surgical or CT-guided percutaneous techniques.

Osteoblastoma

- "Giant osteoid osteoma" (Fig. 23-5)
- Less than 1% of primary bone tumors
- Predilection for the posterior elements of the spine
- Gradually increasing pain
- Not totally relieved with salicylates or NSAIDs

Radiographic and Histologic Features

See Table 23-4.

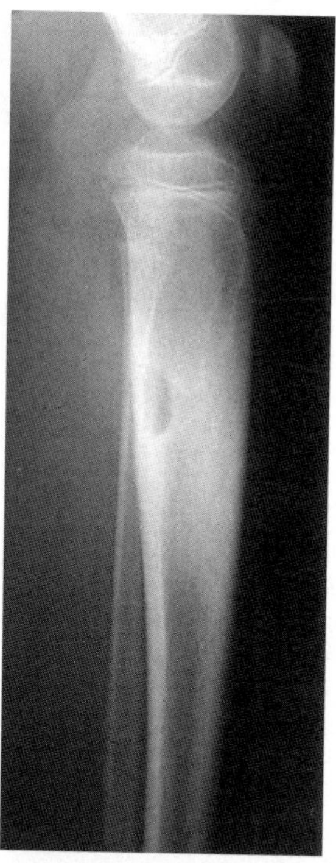

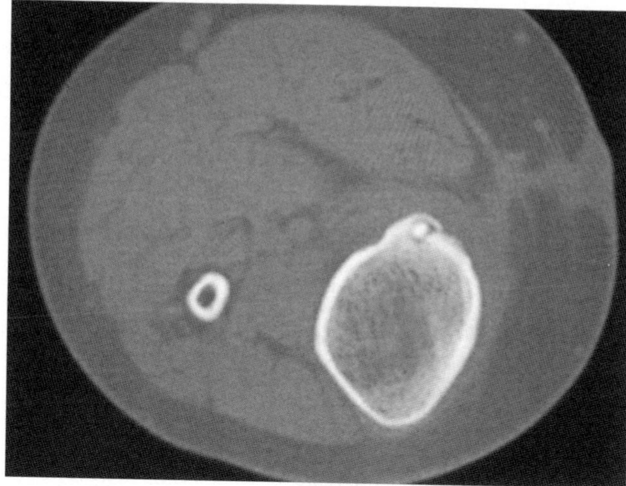

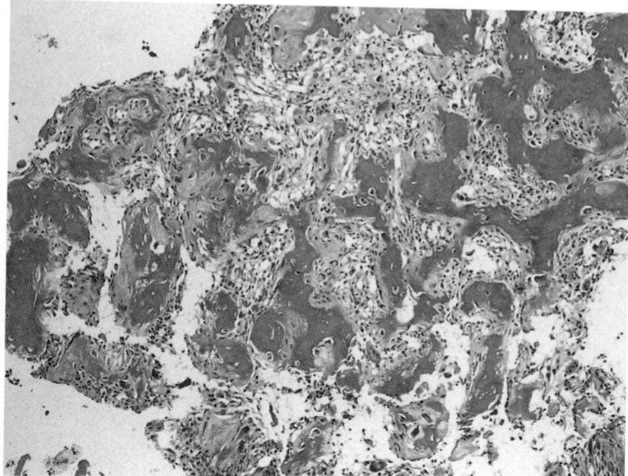

Figure 23-4 Osteoid osteoma. (A) Lateral radiograph of the proximal leg shows a well-circumscribed lytic lesion in the posterior cortex of the proximal tibia. There is significant cortical thickening surrounding the lesion. The cortical thickening has caused widening of the tibia. (B) Axial computed tomography image demonstrates the cortical location of the lesion. There is a dense, central nidus surrounded by a lucent rim. Note the extensive cortical thickening. (C) Photomicrograph of the lesion shows a nidus composed of irregular woven bone trabeculae within a background fibroblastic stroma rich in blood vessels.

Natural History and Treatment

- Excised surgically by extended intralesional curettage or *en bloc* excision

Osteosarcoma

- Most common malignant primary bone tumor of childhood
- Classified by whether it is primary (occurring with no evidence of a preexisting lesion or prior treatment of the bone, such as radiation therapy) or secondary, and by the site of origin, either within the bone (intramedullary) or on the surface (juxtacortical)
- More than 95% of osteosarcomas involving children and young adults are primary.
- Osteosarcomas generally have complex karyotypic abnormalities without chromosomal translocations. Several nonrandom deletions have been identified, however. The two most obvious gene deletions in osteosarcomas are located on chromosome 13 and 17, which are the chromosomes containing tumor suppressor genes—retinoblastoma (*RB1*) and *p53* genes, respectively.

High-Grade Intramedullary Osteosarcoma (Conventional Osteosarcoma)

- 85% of all forms of osteosarcoma
- Occurs at the metaphyseal ends of the long bones, which have the greatest growth potential
- 50% are located in the distal femur or proximal tibia.

TABLE 23-4 TYPICAL RADIOGRAPHIC AND HISTOLOGIC FEATURES OF OSTEOID OSTEOMA AND OSTEOBLASTOMA

Features	Osteoid Osteoma	Osteoblastoma
Histologic		
Gross (macroscopic)	Round or oval, reddish brown, most ~ 1 cm diameter	Similar, but larger than osteoid osteoma (most 2–6 cm)
Histologic (microscopic)	Distinct demarcation between nidus and surrounding reactive bone Interlacing network of immature bone and bony trabeculae, with focal areas of osteoblastic and osteoclastic activity	Demarcation is not significant Interlacing woven bone lined by osteoblasts within a fibrovascular stroma
Radiographic		
Plain radiography	Long bone; metaphysis or diaphysis Spine; posterior elements Small (~ 1 cm), round-elliptical, lucent, intracortical (mostly) lesion surrounded by extensive reactive sclerotic bone	Spine; posterior elements Long bone; metaphysis or diaphysis 2–6 cm, round-elliptical lytic lesion surrounded by moderate reactive sclerotic bone
Computed tomography	Thin (1–2 mm) sections; provides exact localization of the nidus	

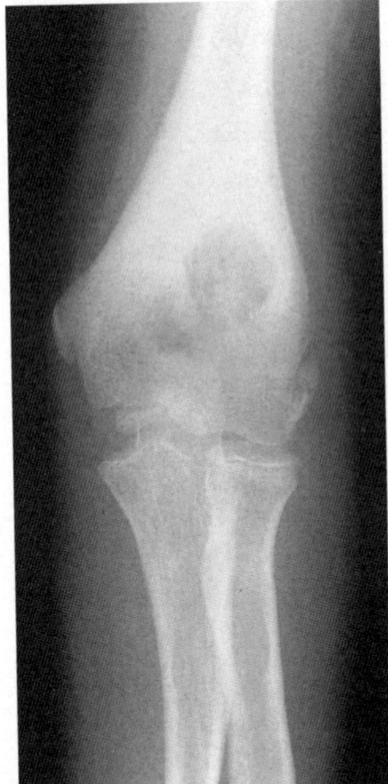
A

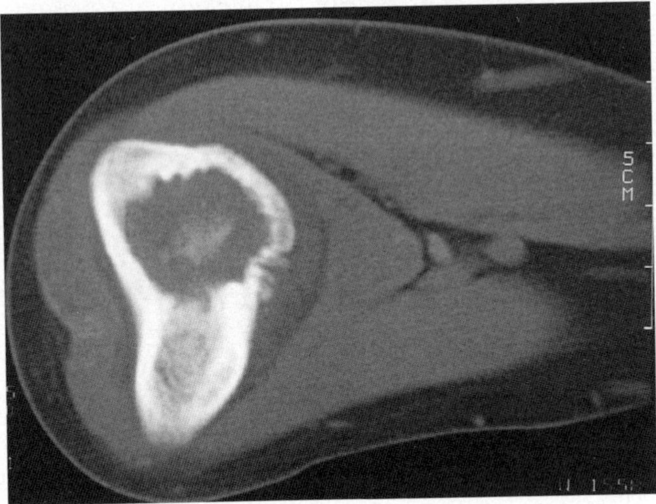

B

Figure 23-5 Osteoblastoma. (**A**) On anteroposterior radiograph of the elbow, a well-circumscribed lytic lesion with sclerotic borders is seen in the metaphysis of the distal humerus. Note the significant cortical thickening. The location is unusual but the features are classic for osteoblastoma. (**B**) Axial computed tomography image shows the typical central nidus of bone formation within the lytic lesion. Note the diffuse, reactive cortical thickening.

- The proximal humerus, proximal femur, and pelvis are the next most common sites.
- Pain and swelling are the most common presenting symptoms.
- Approximately 15% of patients with high-grade intermedullary osteosarcoma present with clinically evident metastases, most commonly in the lungs, but also in other bone locations and brain.
- Metastases at diagnosis indicate poor prognosis.

Radiographic Features

- Plain radiographs: metaphyseal lesion involving the medullary canal with mixed lytic (radiolucent) and blastic (radiodense) activity
- Sunburst periosteal reaction with a Codman triangle (Fig. 23-6A)
- Soft tissue mass which may contain sclerotic foci (tumor bone formation) is also a common finding
- Bone scan shows increased uptake in the area of the tumor.
- MRI is the method of choice for evaluating the tumor and its relationship to adjacent structures.

Histologic Features

- Several histologic subtypes, all with the same prognosis, and characterized by the formation of osteoid tissue or new bone by the neoplastic cells
- Osteoblastic subtype is the most common (50%).
- Highly pleomorphic spindle-shaped and polyhedral tumor cells (see Fig. 23-6C).
- Nuclear hyperchromasia, abundant mitotic activity, and atypical mitotic figures.

A
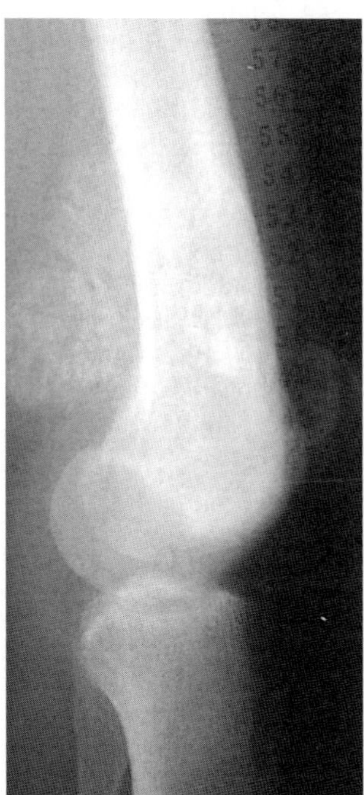
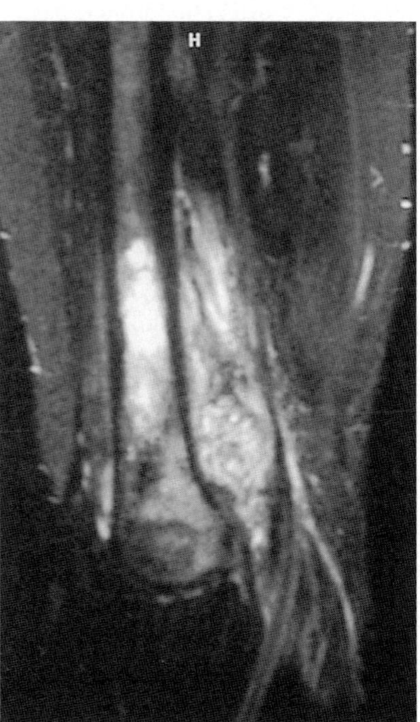

B

C
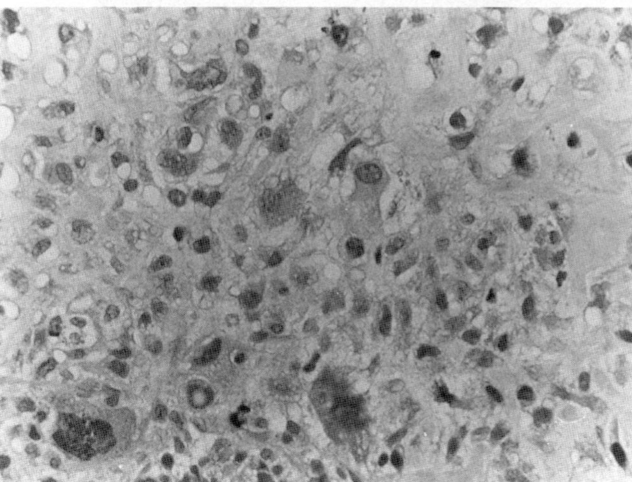

Figure 23-6 High-grade intramedullary osteosarcoma (conventional osteosarcoma). (**A**) Lateral radiograph of the knee shows a lacy, spiculated mass of new bone formation in the metaphysis of the distal femur. Irregular, patchy sclerosis is seen in the metaphysis and epiphysis. (**B**) On sagittal T2-weighted image a heterogenous mass is seen in the marrow of the metaphysis and epiphysis with extension into the soft tissues posterior to the femur. (**C**) Photomicrograph (high-power magnification) of the lesion reveals a cellular neoplasm with scattered pleomorphic and bizarre nuclei. Focal osteoid production is evident.

Treatment

- Combination of chemotherapy and surgical resection of the tumor.
- Current standard protocols consist of preoperative multiagent neoadjuvant chemotherapy, followed by surgical resection, and subsequent additional chemotherapy (adjuvant chemotherapy) (Box 23-3).
- Osteosarcoma responds poorly to radiation therapy.
- Neoadjuvant chemotherapy is to treat micrometastatic disease, to cause necrosis of the primary tumor and to decrease the primary tumor size in order to facilitate limb salvage procedures.
- Following surgical resection, adjuvant chemotherapy is continued to eliminate any micrometastases still present.
- A good response to chemotherapy, usually defined as greater than 90% necrosis of the tumor (detected in the resection specimen), is associated with higher survival rates than a lesser response.
- Surgery is the mainstay of local control of osteosarcoma.
  - □ Excision of the tumor with wide surgical margins, which can be achieved through limb salvage or amputation, is the goal of the surgery.
  - □ Currently, limb salvage is possible in most patients with an extremity osteosarcoma.
  - □ Limb salvage reconstruction includes techniques such as endoprosthetic reconstruction, allograft reconstruction, or rotationplasty reconstruction.
  - □ In some locations, such as the fibula and clavicle, no bony reconstruction is necessary.
- The indications for an amputation are inability to achieve wide surgical margins, a grossly displaced pathologic fracture, a tumor that enlarges during preoperative chemotherapy, and neurovascular bundle involvement that cannot be appropriately addressed with reconstructive techniques.

Surface or Juxtacortical Osteosarcoma

The term *juxtacortical* is a general designation for a group of osteosarcomas that arise on the surface of a bone. Three subtypes are recognized; parosteal, periosteal, and high-grade. The great majority of juxtacortical osteosarcomas are low-grade tumors (parosteal osteosarcoma), although there are moderately (periosteal osteosarcoma) and highly malignant (high-grade surface osteosarcoma) variants.

Treatment

- Low-grade juxtacortical osteosarcomas (parosteal and periosteal) should be treated with wide excision.
  - □ Although the metastatic potential of these low-grade surface lesions is much lower than conventional osteosarcoma, these are locally aggressive malignant tumors and inadequate resection will result in recurrence.
  - □ Repeated local recurrence also may result in progression of the tumor to a more aggressive, high-grade lesion.
- High-grade surface osteosarcomas require aggressive treatment similar to that of conventional osteosarcoma.

TUMORS OF CARTILAGINOUS ORIGIN

Osteochondroma

- Most common skeletal tumor
- 20% to 50% of benign bone tumors and 10% to 15% of all bone tumors
- Involves the metaphysis of long bones, particularly around the knee (40% of lesions) and the proximal humerus
- A firm mass, usually of long duration, adjacent to a joint
- Pain may result due to irritation of overlying soft tissues by the lesion.

Radiographic Features

- Plain radiographs show a bony projection composed of a cortex continuous with that of the underlying bone and a spongiosa, similarly continuous.
- The lesions consist of a cartilaginous cap with a broad (sessile osteochondroma) or narrow (pedunculated osteochondroma) base (Figs. 23-7 and 23-8).
- CT can demonstrate the continuity of cancellous portions of the lesion and the host bone and the thickness of the noncalcified cap (it is usually less than 3 mm).
- CT may be useful in differentiating atypical osteochondromas from malignant lesions.

Natural History and Treatment

- Malignant transformation of osteochondroma to chondrosarcoma occurs in less than 1% of solitary lesions.
- In a skeletally mature patient, a growing lesion with a thick cartilaginous cap in an axial location (i.e., pelvis, scapula) is highly suggestive of this complication.

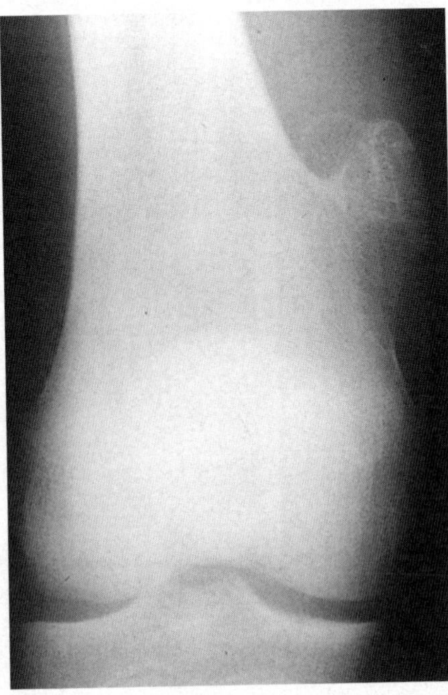

Figure 23-7 Osteochondroma. A patient with a pedunculated osteochondroma. Note the narrow pedicle.

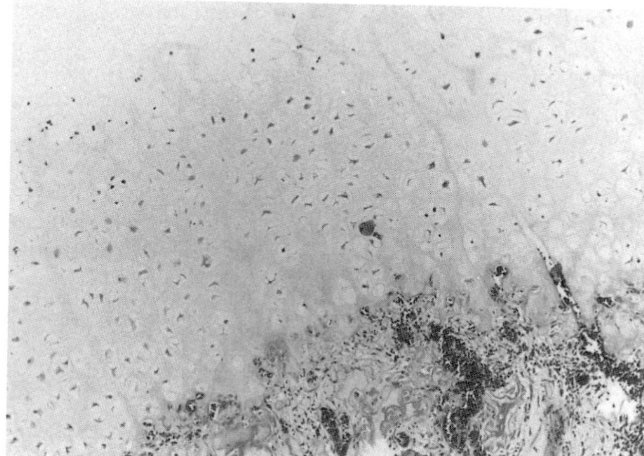

Figure 23-8 Photomicrograph of osteochondroma, demonstrating a thick cartilaginous cap overlying cancellous bone.

- Asymptomatic osteochondromas do not require any treatment.
- For osteochondromas that cause pain or neurovascular compromise (i.e., lesions in the popliteal fossa) or are cosmetically unappealing, surgical excision is indicated.
  - A potential complication of surgery is injury to an adjacent physis, which may lead to deformity, if the lesion is in close proximity to the growth plate.
- The incidence of local recurrence after surgical excision is very low (less than 2%). The entire cartilaginous cap should be removed to prevent recurrence.

Hereditary Multiple Exostosis

- Autosomal dominant disorder with a variable penetrance
- Associated with tumor-suppressor genes, termed *exostosin* (EXT) genes
- After the age of 30, patients with this disorder have an increased risk of developing a secondary chondrosarcoma.
- Excision of one or more exostoses often is necessary.

Chondroblastoma

- 1% of all benign bone tumors
- Occurs primarily in the epiphysis of the growing skeleton
- The most common sites are the proximal humerus, proximal and distal femur, and proximal tibia.
- Pain, swelling, and limited motion are usually localized to the adjacent joint.

Radiographic Features

- Plain radiographs show a well-marginated, radiolucent lesion, usually with a sclerotic rim of bone (Fig. 23-9A). The lesion may have small foci or calcifications.
- Bone scan shows increased uptake.
- Chest radiography or CT should be performed, because chondroblastoma is one of the benign tumors that can have lung metastasis.

Histologic Features

- Small cuboidal cells (chondroblasts) closely packed together to give the appearance of a cobblestone street (see Fig. 23-9B). There are areas with varying amounts of amorphous matrix that often contains streaks of calcification ("chicken-wire" calcification), and there are numerous multinucleated giant cells.

Natural History and Treatment

- Chondroblastoma is a benign, but locally aggressive lesion (Box 23-5).

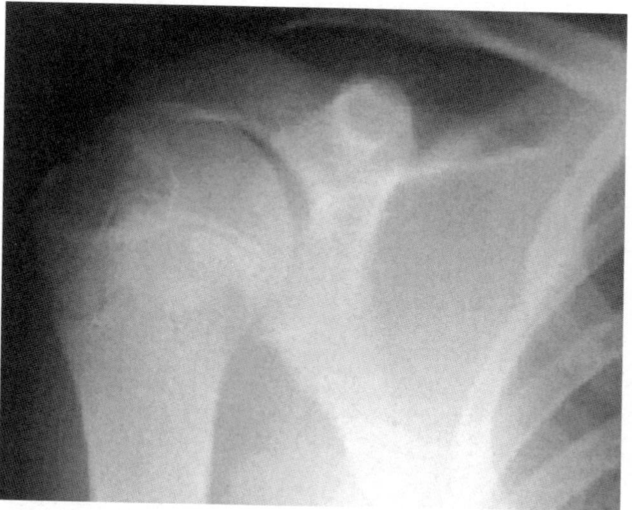

A

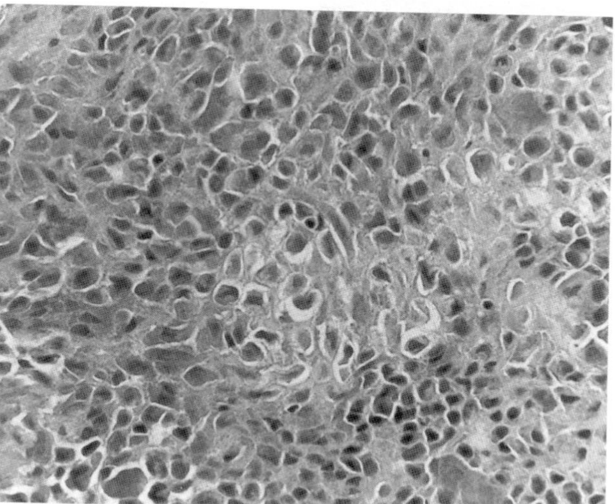

B

Figure 23-9 Chondroblastoma. (**A**) Anteroposterior radiograph of the shoulder shows a well-circumscribed, lytic lesion in the lateral epiphysis of the humerus. The lesion does not cross the physis. (**B**) Photomicrograph of the lesion demonstrates tumor cells that are uniform, closely packed and polyhedral, and are focally enveloped by a lace-like, lightly calcified chondroid matrix.

BOX 23-5 BENIGN BUT LOCALLY AGGRESSIVE BONE TUMORS

- Osteoblastoma
- Chondroblastoma
- Osteofibrous dysplasia
- Aneurysmal bone cyst
- Giant cell tumor
- Chondromyxoid fibroma

- Most patients are close to skeletal maturity and damage to the growth plate is not a major concern. However, the lesions may progress and invade the joint.
- Chondroblastomas should be treated when detected.
- Intralesional extended curettage is the initial treatment of choice.
- Recurrence rates of approximately 10% have been reported after intralesional excision.
- The majority of recurrences are adequately addressed with a second curettage. Rarely, recurrent lesions require *en bloc* excision.
- In rare cases of severe bone destruction or recurrence, wide resection and segmental reconstruction sometimes is indicated.

Enchondroma

- Benign tumor of mature hyaline cartilage
- 10% of benign bone tumors
- Usually present as solitary lesions
- Short tubular bones of the hand and foot are common sites.
- Most present with a pathologic fracture through the lesion, or as an incidental finding on a radiograph taken for another reason.

Radiographic Features

- Plain radiographs show a sharply circumscribed radiolucent lesion located centrally in the medullary canal (Fig. 23-10A).

Histologic Features

- Grossly, enchondromas are lobular lesions with a bluish color.
- Histologically, lobules of hyaline cartilage with varying cellularity are seen and are recognized by their blue matrix (see Fig. 23-10B). The chondrocytes are located in rounded spaces called lacunae.

Natural History and Treatment

- Malignant transformation of enchondromas occurs infrequently (less than 1%), and is rare before skeletal maturity.
- Patients experiencing pain in a previously asymptomatic lesion without evidence of a pathologic fracture should be evaluated for this possibility.
- Asymptomatic solitary enchondromas do not require any treatment other than a periodic follow-up evaluation.
- Symptomatic or large lesions in the short tubular bones of the hand without a pathologic fracture can be managed with curettage and bone grafting.
- If a pathologic fracture occurs through an enchondroma, the fracture should be allowed to heal prior to curettage and bone grafting.
- Recurrence after curettage and bone grafting is rare.

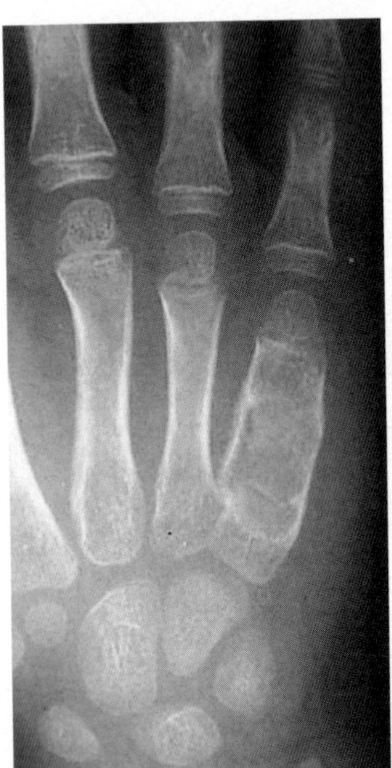
A

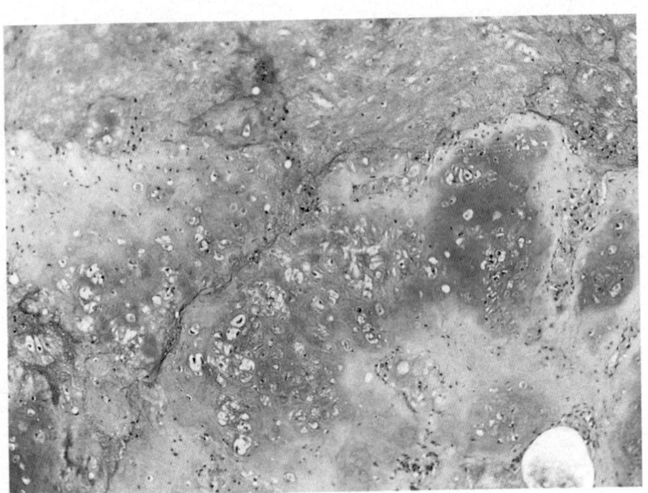
B

Figure 23-10 Enchondroma. (**A**) Anteroposterior radiograph of the ulnar three digits of the hand shows an expansile, lytic lesion involving the diaphysis of the fifth metacarpal with extension into the distal metaphysis. There is saucerization (scalloping) of the inner cortex. (**B**) Photomicrograph demonstrates a lobular lesion composed of mature cartilaginous tissue.

- Incisional biopsy usually is contraindicated.
  - Pathologists may have difficulty distinguishing an active enchondroma (most pediatric patients have active lesions) from a low-grade chondrosarcoma.
  - An incisional biopsy alters the histologic and radiographic status of the lesion and may make subsequent evaluation difficult.

Multiple Enchondromatosis

- Also known as *Ollier disease*, it is an inherited condition with widespread enchondromas.
- It is much less common than solitary enchondroma.
- Patients with Ollier disease have an increased risk of developing secondary chondrosarcoma later in life.
- Multiple enchondromatosis with vascular anomalies of soft tissues is known as *Maffucci syndrome* (see "Vascular Tumors" later in the chapter). Patients with this disorder have an even greater risk of developing malignant cartilage tumors than patients with Ollier disease; importantly, they also have a greater risk of developing carcinoma of an internal organ.

TUMORS OF FIBROUS ORIGIN

Nonossifying Fibroma

- *Nonossifying fibroma* (NOF), *fibrous cortical defect*, *metaphyseal fibrous defect*, and *fibroma* all refer to the same histopathologic process in bone.
- Fibrous cortical defects are small asymptomatic lesions that occur in 30% of the population during the first and second decades of life.
- NOF refers to a lesion that enlarges and encroaches on the medullary bone.
- Benign proliferation of fibroblast-like mesenchymal tissue that is more likely a hamartomatous process than a true neoplasm
- Most common in the long bones, especially the distal femur and the tibia
- Asymptomatic lesion that is often found only when a radiograph is taken for another reason or when the patient has a pathologic fracture

Radiographic Features

- Plain radiographs show an eccentric, metaphyseal lesion, involving the medullary canal, with a loculated appearance and a radiodense rim (Fig. 23-11A).
- NOFs range in size from 0.5 to 7 cm, with their long axes aligned with the long axis of the affected bone.

Histologic Features

- Histologically, NOF consists of benign, spindle, fibroblastic cells arranged in a storiform pattern (see Fig. 23-11B).
- Multinucleated giant cells are common, and foam cells containing lipid often can be seen.
- Hemosiderin within the spindle cells and multinucleated giant cells are usual.
- Typically, the lesion does not contain bone.

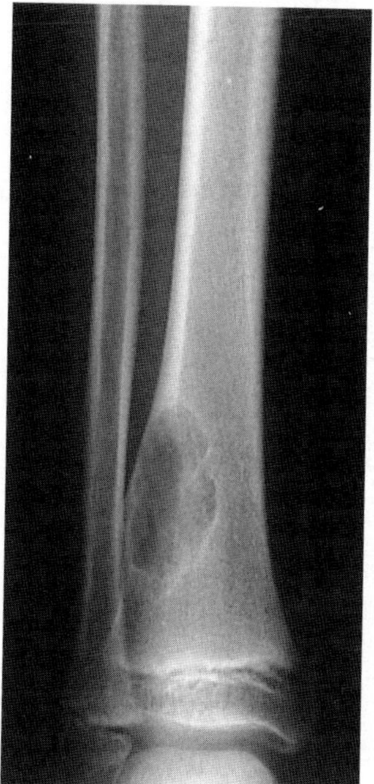

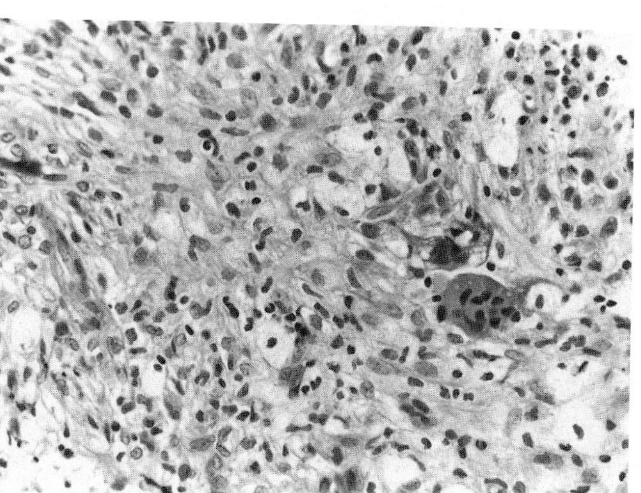

Figure 23-11 Nonossifying fibroma. (A) Anteroposterior and lateral radiographs of the distal tibia show a cortically based, lytic lesion with well-defined margins. Note the typical scalloped appearance. Involvement greater than 50% of the diameter of the bone puts this lesion at risk for pathologic fracture. (B) Photomicrograph (high power magnification) of the lesion demonstrates foamy histiocytic cells and giant cells discerned within the fibroinflammatory spindle cell stroma.

Natural History and Treatment

- Fibrous cortical defects need no treatment, they heal spontaneously.
- NOFs less than 50% of the diameter of the bone and that are asymptomatic and can be observed.
- NOFs occupying more than 50% of the diameter of the bone, have an increased risk of developing pathologic fractures, and should be considered for curettage and bone grafting.
- Patients who present with pathologic fractures can usually be managed nonoperatively.

Fibrous Dysplasia

- A nonneoplastic condition of aberrant bone development.
- Produces a variety of complaints and physical findings.
- 85% of cases are a single skeletal lesion (monostotic fibrous dysplasia).
- 15% have numerous lesions (polyostotic fibrous dysplasia).
- The most common locations for monostotic fibrous dysplasia are ribs, proximal femur, tibia, and the base of the skull.
- The patient with monostotic fibrous dysplasia usually presents without significant symptoms, and the lesion is usually discovered incidentally on radiographs obtained for other reasons.
- Occasionally, a child presents with a pathologic fracture or angular deformity (Fig. 23-12A).

Radiographic Features

- Fibrous dysplasia is a medullary process usually involving the full width of the bone.
- Plain radiographs show a radiolucent lesion with slight expansion and thinning of the cortex, and partial loss of trabecular pattern in the cancellous bone, which gives the characteristic ground-glass appearance (see Fig. 23-12A).
  - Cystic areas can also be seen within the abnormal bone.
  - There may be an angular deformity or bowing in the bone, especially when the lesion is large.
  - The lesions are usually diaphyseal, and the differential diagnosis may include other common diaphyseal lesions of bone.
- On the bone scan, uptake within the lesion is usually intense.

Histologic Features

- Histologically, fibrous dysplasia (both the monostotic and polyostotic variants) is composed of trabeculae of immature, woven bone within a background stroma of collagen-rich tissue (see Fig. 23-12B).
- The osteoid and bone appear to arise in a haphazard fashion from the fibrous stroma.
- The trabeculae often obtain a variety of shapes (C's and O's) and are sometimes referred to as alphabet soup or Chinese letters.

Treatment

- Monostotic fibrous dysplasia usually does not require any treatment other than observation.
- Surgical treatment may be required for lesions that are very large or enlarging, in a high-stress location (i.e., proximal femur), or have become symptomatic.
- Intralesional extended curettage is performed for eradication of the lesion; curettage often results in healing with dysplastic, mechanically deficient bone, similar to the pattern of fracture healing in fibrous dysplasia.
- Therefore, the goals of surgical treatment, when indicated, are clearly different from other benign active or aggressive lesions.

A
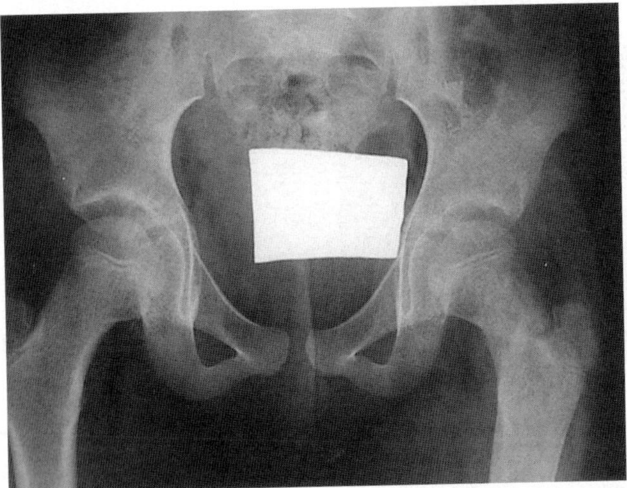

B
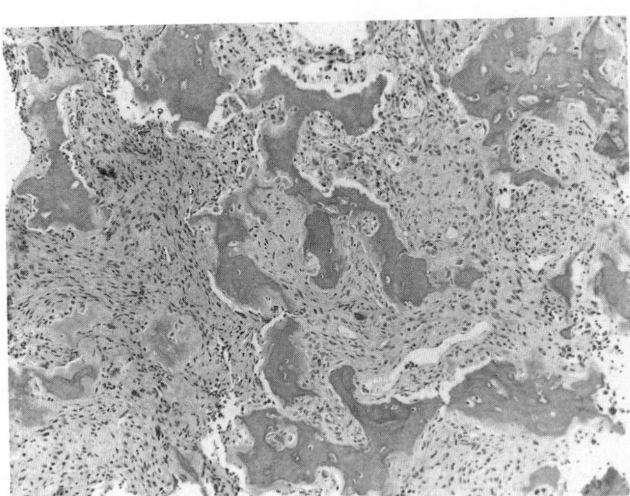

Figure 23-12 Fibrous dysplasia. (**A**) Anteroposterior radiograph of the pelvis shows subtle ground-glass density of the left femoral neck and proximal diaphysis. The cortex blends imperceptibly with the medullary canal. A pathologic fracture is seen at the base of the femoral neck. (**B**) Photomicrograph of the lesion demonstrates irregular woven bone trabeculae (so-called Chinese letters) in a background of bland fibroblastic stroma. Note absence of osteoblastic rimming.

- Rather than resect the lesional tissue, the goals are to stabilize the bone, prevent or correct deformity, and relieve pain.
- Prophylactic internal fixation may be required depending on the size and location of the lesion.

Albright Syndrome

- Polyostotic fibrous dysplasia may occur as a part of a condition known as *McCune-Albright syndrome* which is characterized by a classic triad of polyostotic fibrous dysplasia, café-au-lait skin lesions, and precocious puberty.
- Activating missense mutations of the guanine nucleotide-binding protein gene (*GNAS*), encoding the α-subunit of the stimulatory G protein, have been identified in patients with this syndrome.

MISCELLANEOUS LESIONS

Unicameral Bone Cyst (Simple Bone Cyst)

- Tumor-like cystic lesion of unknown cause, attributed to a local disturbance of bone growth
- Arises on the metaphyseal side of the growth plate and is displaced from the physis with skeletal growth
- The most common locations are the proximal humerus and femur, accounting for 90% of lesions, followed by calcaneus
- Commonly are asymptomatic, and often come to attention only after pathologic fracture has occurred

Radiographic and Histologic Features

See Table 23-5 and Figure 23-13A.

Natural History and Treatment

- Tend to enlarge with skeletal growth
- Enters a latent phase after skeletal maturity, ceases growing, is resorbed, and is replaced by normal bone
- Some unicameral bone cysts remain small and do not present a significant risk of a pathologic fracture. Observation and activity restriction may be all that is necessary for these lesions.
- In most cases, a pathologic fracture should be treated nonoperatively until it heals.
- Healing of the fracture usually does not result in healing of the bone cyst (less than 10% of cysts heal with pathologic fracture).
- Surgical treatment options include curettage and bone grafting, and fluoroscopically guided percutaneous corticosteroid injection, which are both associated with high persistence and recurrence rates, and some morbidity.
- Newer techniques include injection with autologous bone marrow or demineralized bone matrix, and percutaneous intramedullary decompression, curettage, and grafting using bone graft substitutes (calcium sulfate pellets) (see Fig. 23-13B and C).
  - The short-term results of these techniques are very promising, with high healing and low complication and recurrence rates.

Aneurysmal Bone Cyst (ABC)

- Vascular lesions consisting of widely dilated vascular channels that are not lined by identifiable endothelium.
- 1% to 2% of all benign bone lesions.
- Etiology is not known.
- Occur in association with other benign (i.e., giant cell tumor, chondroblastoma, osteoblastoma) and malignant

TABLE 23-5 TYPICAL RADIOGRAPHIC AND HISTOLOGIC FEATURES OF ANEURYSMAL AND UNICAMERAL BONE CYSTS

Features	Aneurysmal Bone Cyst	Unicameral Bone Cyst
Histologic		
Gross (macroscopic)	Blood-filled sponge with thin periosteal membrane	Cystic cavity usually filled with yellowish fluid
Histologic (microscopic)	Cavernous blood-filled spaces lacking endothelial cell lining Fibrous septa forming the walls contain woven bone trabeculae, giant cells, and hemosiderin-laden macrophages	A cyst lining consisting of a single layer of mesothelial cells with underlying connective tissue or bone
Radiographic		
Plain radiographs	Metaphysis of long bones Eccentric or involve entire width of bone Expansile, lytic lesion circumscribed with a thinned, but intact bony cortex Internal septations within the lesion	Metaphysis of long bones Centrally located Well-circumscribed, lucent lesion with sclerotic margins
Magnetic resonance imaging	Internal septations and multiple fluid–fluid levels Marked bony expansion	Fluid–fluid levels, only if hemorrhage has occurred Minimal bony expansion

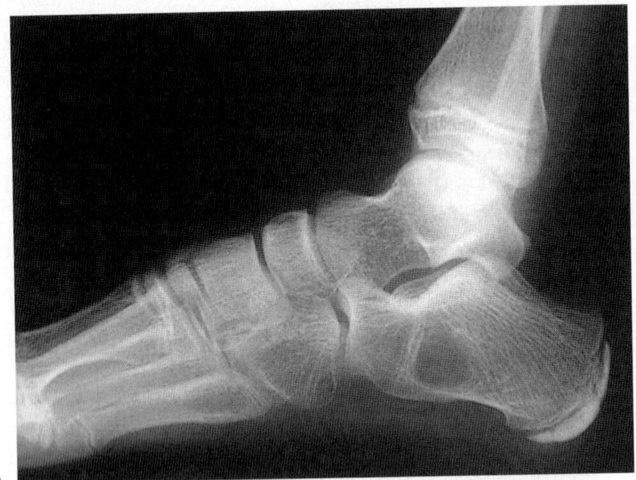

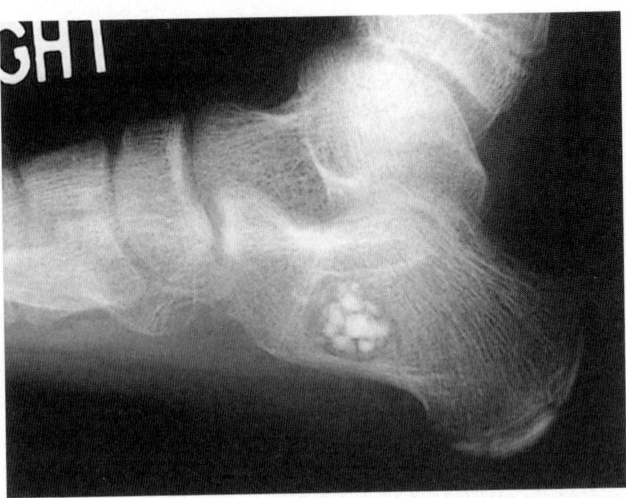

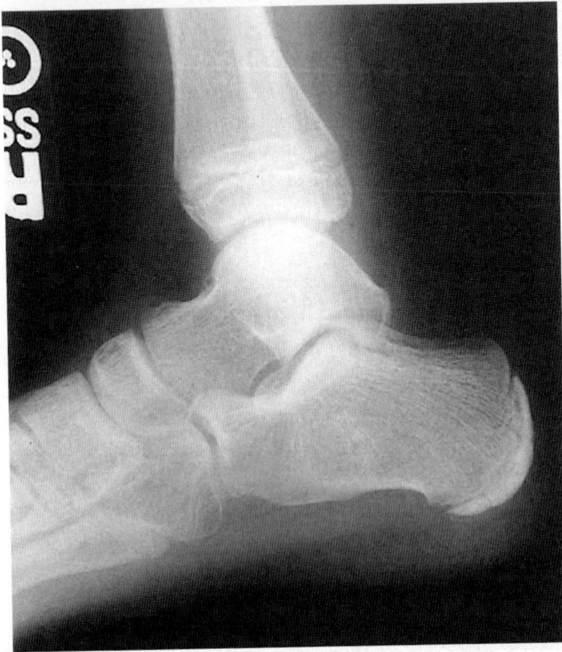

Figure 23-13 Unicameral bone cyst. (**A**) Lateral radiograph of the foot depicts a lytic lesion in calcaneus with well-defined margins. (**B**) This lesion was treated by percutaneous intramedullary decompression, biopsy, curettage, and grafting with calcium sulfate pellets. (**C**) Postoperative 1-year follow-up radiograph shows complete healing of the lesion.

(i.e., osteosarcoma) processes as "secondary ABCs" in up to 30% of cases.

- More than 50% of ABCs arise in large tubular bones, and almost 30% occur in the spine.
- Mild, dull pain; only rarely is there a clinically apparent pathologic fracture.

Radiographic and Histologic Features

See Table 23-5 and Figure 23-14.

Natural History and Treatment

- ABCs are benign by histology, but can be locally aggressive (Box 23-5).
- They should undergo biopsy to establish the diagnosis, and then be treated surgically.
- The usual treatment for ABCs is extended curettage and bone grafting.
- ABCs in expendable bones, such as fibula, ribs, distal ulna, metacarpal, and metatarsal bones, may be treated by *en bloc* resection.
  - ☐ Resection is also appropriate for recurrent aggressive lesions.
- An ABC of the spine can present a challenging problem.
  - ☐ The lesion usually involves the posterior elements, but can also invade into vertebral body.
  - ☐ Surgery is recommended for most patients as the initial means of treatment.
  - ☐ Radiotherapy is contraindicated.
- More recently, selective arterial embolization has been used in conjunction with surgery or as a curative procedure alone for some pelvic and spinal lesions.

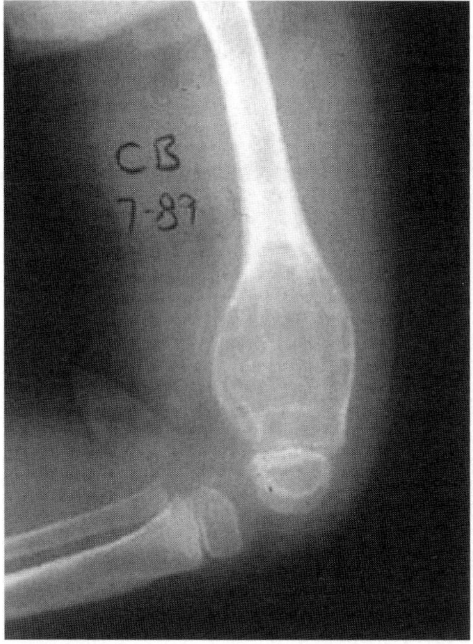

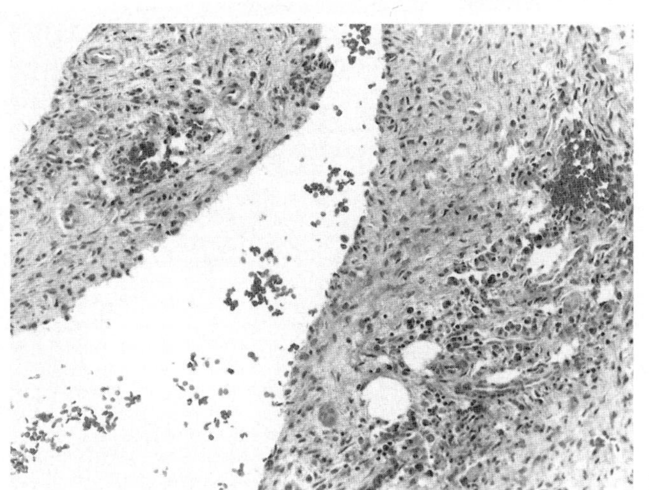

A B

Figure 23-14 Aneurysmal bone cyst. (A) Lateral radiograph of the knee shows a large lytic lesion expanding the distal femoral metaphysis. Note the trabeculated, nonossified matrix. (B) Photomicrograph of this lesion demonstrates salient features including scattered erythrocytes within the cyst cavity, lack of an endothelial lining, and an occasional giant cell in the underlying stroma.

Ewing Sarcoma

- Second most common primary malignant bone tumor in children
- Ewing sarcoma (EWS) is closely related to primitive neuroectodermal tumor (PNET); both these tumors are thought to arise from the neural crest and at least 90% have a characteristic chromosomal translocation [t(11:22)(q24:q12)], which leads to a novel fusion protein called EWS-FLI1 (Table 23-6).
- The femur is the most common site of origin, followed by the pelvis and humerus.
- Pain and local swelling are the most common presenting symptoms.
- EWS may present with fever and an elevated sedimentation rate and may mimic bacterial osteomyelitis.

TABLE 23-6 PEDIATRIC MUSCULOSKELETAL TUMORS WITH NONRANDOM/SPECIFIC TRANSLOCATIONS

Tumor	Translocation
Ewing sarcoma/primitive neuroectodermal tumors	t(11;22); t(21;22)
Alveolar rhabdomyosarcoma	t(2;13); t(1;13)
Synovial sarcoma	t(X;18)
Myxoid liposarcoma	t(12;16)

- Approximately 5% of patients with EWS present with pulmonary metastasis.

Radiographic Features

- Plain radiographs demonstrate diffuse destruction of bone, usually occurring in the diaphyseal regions of long bones or in flat bones of the axial skeleton (Fig. 23-15A).
  - The lesion usually is associated with a periosteal reaction (Fig. 23-2), which has an "onion-skin" or sunburst appearance, and a large soft tissue mass.
- On bone scan, EWS shows a very increased uptake; it may be multicentric.
- MRI is essential for definitive demonstration of extraosseous soft tissue mass, determining relationship of the tumor to surrounding structures, and determining medullary canal involvement, both of which are usually more extensive than what was expected from the plain radiographs (see Fig. 23-15B and C).

Histologic Features

- Histologically, EWS consists of small, uniform-sized cells characterized by an almost clear cytoplasm and nuclei that are round and slightly hyperchromatic (see Fig. 23-15D).
  - Necrotic areas usually are seen.
  - There are glycogen granules in the cytoplasm, and these produce the positive periodic acid–Schiff (PAS) stain on routine histology.
- Increasingly, genetic analysis is being done for EWS to identify the 11:22 translocation as a means of establishing the diagnosis.

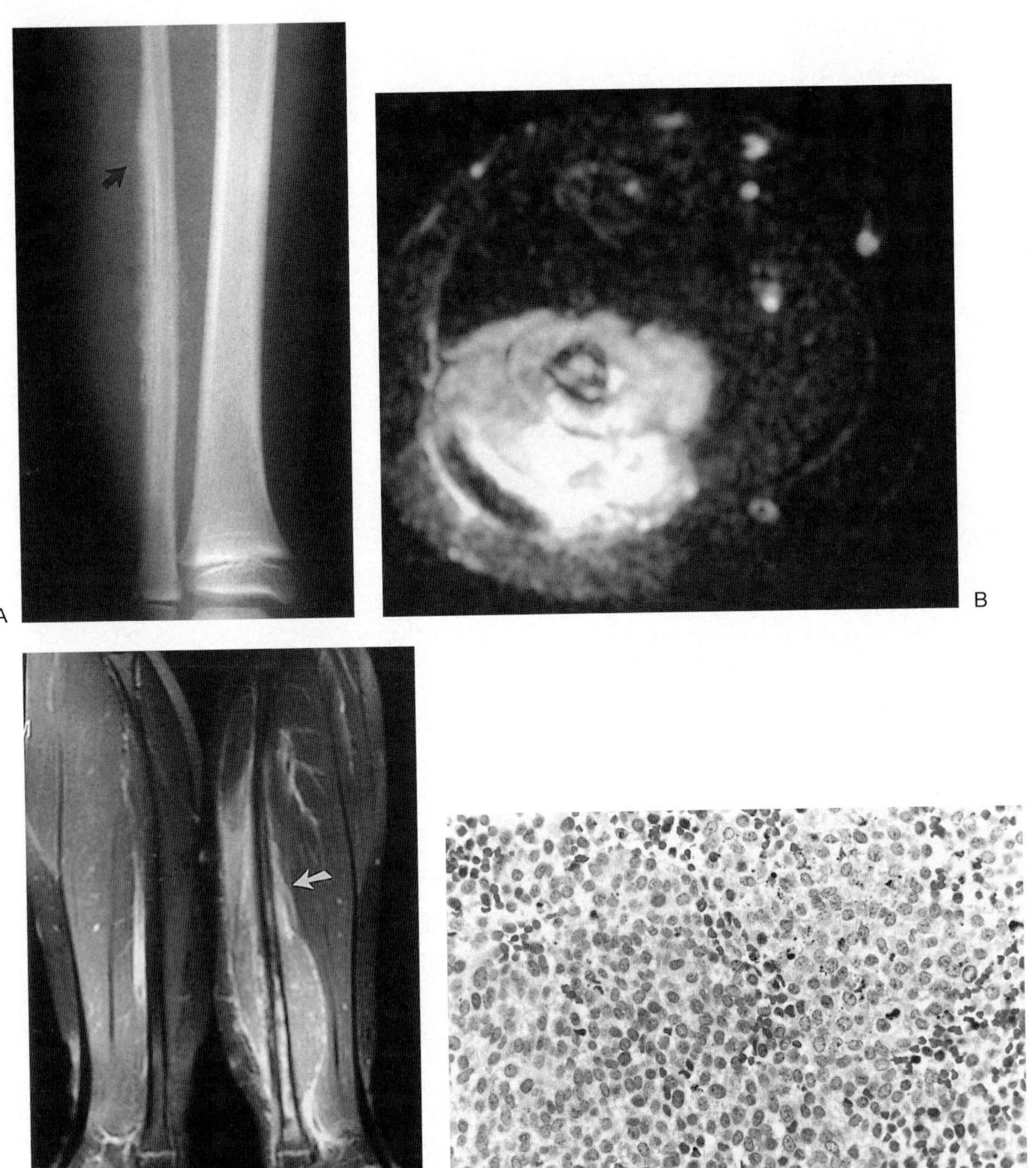

Figure 23-15 Ewing sarcoma. (**A**) Anteroposterior radiograph of the distal fibula reveals an irregular, hazy patterned, periosteal new bone formation with fine spiculations and a Codman triangle at the superior edge (*arrow*). This aggressive pattern of new bone formation is associated with enlargement of the soft tissues and obliteration of the fat planes due to a soft tissue mass. The underlying bone has a permeative pattern of bone destruction. (**B**) Axial T2-weighted magnetic resonance image shows abnormal, hyperintense signal in the marrow of the fibula. Patches of hypointense signal are scattered throughout the cortex as well. Spicules of new bone formation are well seen. A large, fairly homogeneous, soft tissue mass invades the lateral compartment. (**C**) Coronal T1-weighted, fat-saturated image with contrast enhancement shows (abnormally) enhancement extending from the distal metaphysis to the mid-fibula (*arrow*). An enhancing soft tissue mass encompasses the fibula and extends up into the proximal soft tissues above the marrow abnormality. (**D**) Photomicrograph of the lesion demonstrates primitive, small, and uniform malignant cells with inconspicuous cytoplasm. Darker staining cells are pyknotic.

Treatment

- Multiagent chemotherapy has made a significant difference in the prognosis for patients with EWS, improving the 5-year survival rate from 5% to 10% to over 70%.
- Current treatment principles of EWS are summarized in Box 23-3.
- Treatment of EWS is a combination of chemotherapy and either surgery or irradiation.

SOFT TISSUE TUMORS

VASCULAR TUMORS

Hemangiomas are true neoplastic lesions with endothelial hyperplasia. They are the most common benign soft tissue tumors of childhood, occurring in 4% to 10% of all children. They infrequently are present at birth but grow rapidly during the first 2 to 3 weeks of life. Hemangiomas may be located in the superficial or deep dermis, subcutaneous tissue, musculature, bone, or viscera. Head and neck are the most commonly involved sites.

The second category of vascular anomalies is *vascular malformations*, which are congenital lesions with normal endothelial turnover. They are subclassified by the predominant vessel found in the lesion (i.e., venous, arterial, capillary, lymphatic, mixed) and by the blood flow within the lesion (high vs. low flow). Vascular malformations are not seen as commonly as hemangiomas. Many of the common vascular malformations are present at birth, however some may manifest in adolescence or adulthood. The majority of these lesions involve the skin and subcutaneous tissue, but deep or extensive involvement of structures such as muscle, joint, bone, abdominal viscera, and central nervous system is not uncommon. The most commonly affected sites are head and neck.

MRI is an excellent imaging modality for confirming the nature of vascular anomalies and defining their relationship to adjacent structures (Fig. 23-16). Ultrasound or color Doppler may also be used.

Treatment

Hemangiomas

- In the absence of intervention, partial or complete involution of hemangiomas usually occurs, and correction of cosmetic defects typically follows.
- When intervention for a rapidly expanding hemangioma is necessary, the first line of treatment is intralesional or systemic corticosteroids.
- Occasionally, when surgical resection is indicated for larger, deeper lesions that threaten normal function, staged excisions may be considered.

Venous Malformations

- Compression stockings to prevent progressive venous dilation, pain, ulceration, and bleeding are the mainstay of treatment, and low-dose aspirin may also be used to minimize thrombophlebitis.

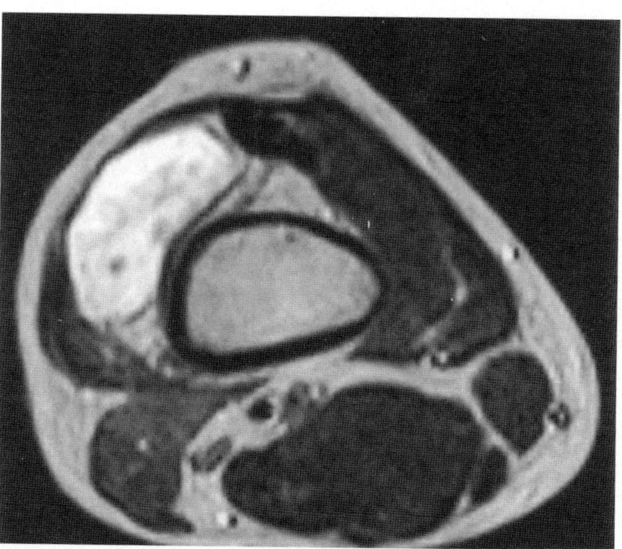

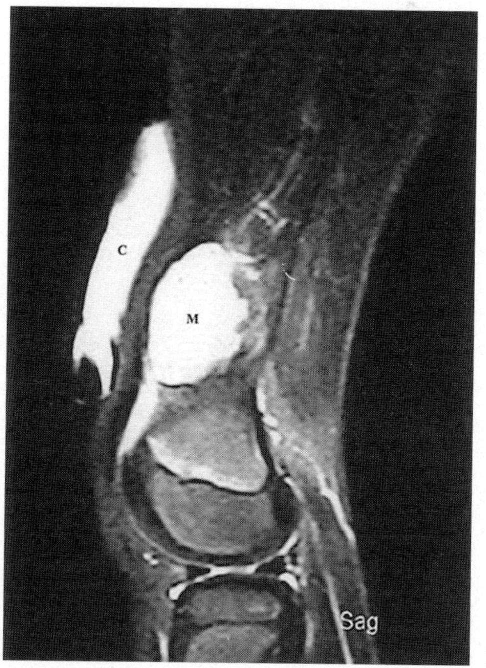

Figure 23-16 Vascular malformation: lymphangioma. (**A**) Axial T2-weighted magnetic resonance image of the distal thigh shows a high-signal intensity mass similar to fluid. No vessels or septations are seen within the mass. (**B**) On sagittal T2-weighted image, a vitamin E capsule (**C**) is used to mark the site of the palpable mass. Note the high signal of this fluid-filled mass (*M*). A small suprapatellar effusion, just inferior to the mass, has the same signal intensity.

- When the patient does not receive adequate benefit from compression stockings, laser surgery, sclerotherapy (i.e., 100% ethanol), or surgical resection are all widely accepted treatment methods.
- Surgical intervention may be required for deep venous malformations involving muscle or bone, which have led to pain, functional impairment or pathologic fracture.
- Epiphysiodesis may be performed in patients with extensive venous malformations that have resulted in skeletal overgrowth.

Arteriovenous Malformations

- AVMs can prove deceptively problematic and even dangerous to treat.
- Most experts agree that conservative treatment is preferred in the absence of significant symptoms.
- Deep AVMs may cause significant muscle or bone changes and will necessitate surgical debulking or epiphysiodesis.
- When surgery is required, angiographic studies followed by selective embolization is usually done 24 or 72 hours before resection.
- Embolization or ligation of feeding arteries without surgical resection is contraindicated because occlusion of the major feeding arteries usually results in rapid recruitment and dilation of previously microscopic collateral blood flow.

TUMORS OF NERVE ORIGIN

Neurolemmoma and neurofibroma are the most common benign tumors of peripheral nerves. Both arise from benign proliferation of periaxonal Schwann cells that embryologically arise from the neural crest.

Neurolemmomas, also known as *schwannomas*, can be seen in patients of all ages, but they are most often encountered in early adulthood. They have a predilection for the head, neck, and flexor surfaces of the extremities (i.e., peroneal, ulnar nerves). The patient usually presents with a painless, slow-growing, solitary mass in the subcutaneous tissue. Although they arise from the nerve sheath, nerve dysfunction is uncommon, and is seen only when the nerve is compressed between the tumor and an adjacent rigid structure. A positive Tinel sign with percussion over the mass is not uncommon. Neurolemmomas rarely are associated with neurofibromatosis.

Neurofibromas, like neurolemmomas, usually present during young adulthood. They may present as solitary lesions or as multiple lesions in association with neurofibromatosis, but the majority (90%) are solitary. Like neurolemmomas, they grow slowly as a painless mass in the skin, subcutaneous tissue, or the distribution of a peripheral nerve. Unlike neurolemmomas, they tend to be intimately associated with the nerve fibers (Fig. 23-17).

Natural History and Treatment

The risk of malignant transformation of neurolemmomas or solitary neurofibromas is exceedingly rare. In contrast, malignant transformation of neurofibromas in the face of neurofibromatosis is well documented; this risk has been reported in about 2% of cases. Therefore, patients and parents should be aware of the clinical symptoms leading to suspicion of malignant transformation, such as enlargement of a neurofibroma and pain. If sarcomatous degeneration occurs, the prognosis for long-term survival is poor. Neurofibrosarcomas can also rarely arise de novo.

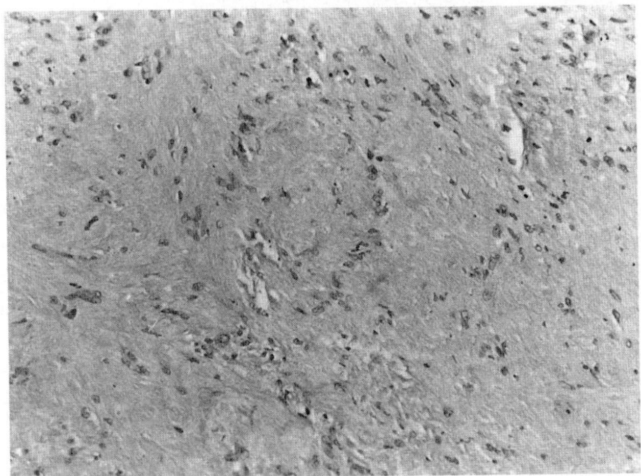

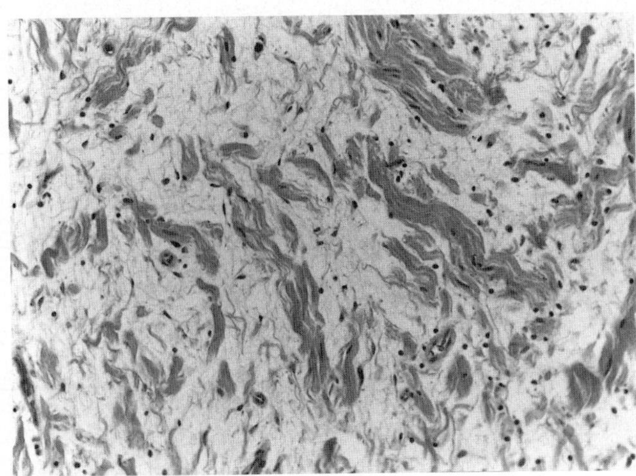

Figure 23-17 Histopathology of benign peripheral nerve sheath tumors. **A:** Neurolemmoma. This tumor demonstrates a classic palisading of Schwann cells (Verocay bodies) within a spindle-cell background. (**B**) Neurofibroma. The lesion is composed of fascicles of Schwann cells and fibroblasts within an edematous and mildly inflamed background stroma, imparting a histologic appearance that has been compared to shredded carrots.

Neurolemmoma

- Treatment of neurolemmomas consists of marginal surgical excision.
- Overlying nerve fibers can usually easily be mobilized and preserved as the lesion is marginally shelled out.
- Neurolemmoma usually does not recur following marginal excision.

Neurofibroma

- Marginal surgical excision is recommended for symptomatic solitary neurofibromas involving a peripheral nerve.
- Those arising from a major nerve can be resected, but they should be approached cautiously.

TUMORS OF MUSCULAR ORIGIN

Rhabdomyosarcoma

- Most common soft tissue tumor in children
- 5% of all pediatric cancers
- Arises from the same embryonal mesenchyme that is destined to give rise to striated skeletal muscle.
- Peak incidence is in the 1- to 5-year age group.
- There are four histologic patterns: embryonal, botryoid-type, alveolar, and pleomorphic.
  - □ Embryonal and alveolar types are common.
  - □ Embryonal tumors are most often found in the head and neck or the genitourinary tract.
  - □ Alveolar rhabdomyosarcomas are more commonly found in the extremities and trunk.
- Extremity lesions usually present as a painless mass, while paravertebral tumors may cause back pain.
- Characteristic chromosomal abnormalities have been identified in the alveolar rhabdomyosarcoma (Table 23-6).

Radiographic Features

- MRI shows a heterogeneous mass, indicating the presence of blood or necrosis.
- Tumor invasion and extent are variable (Fig. 23-18A and B).

A

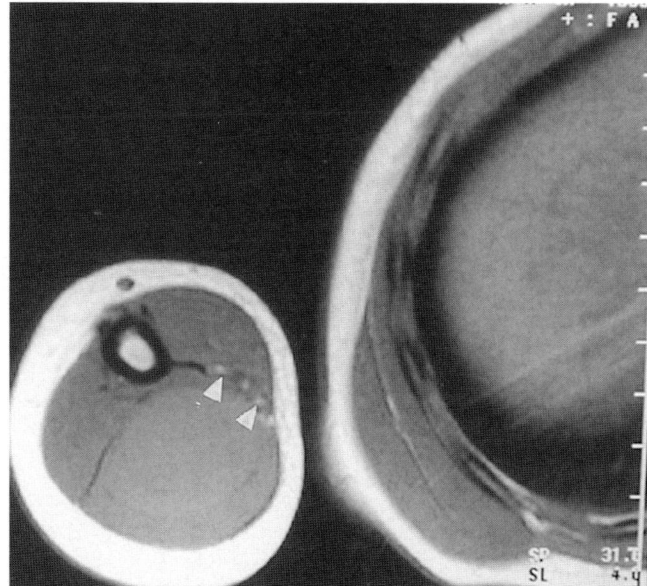

B

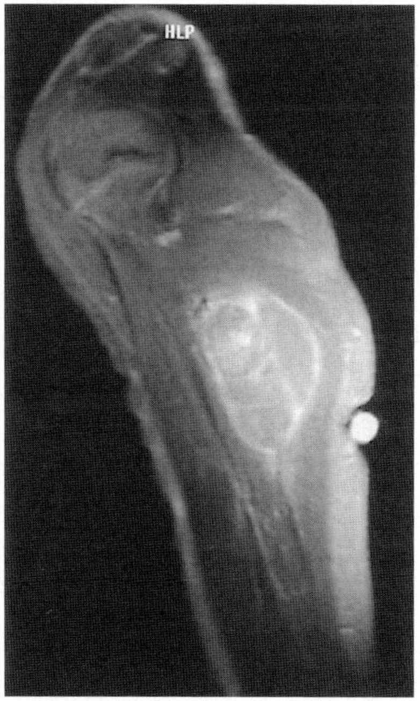

C

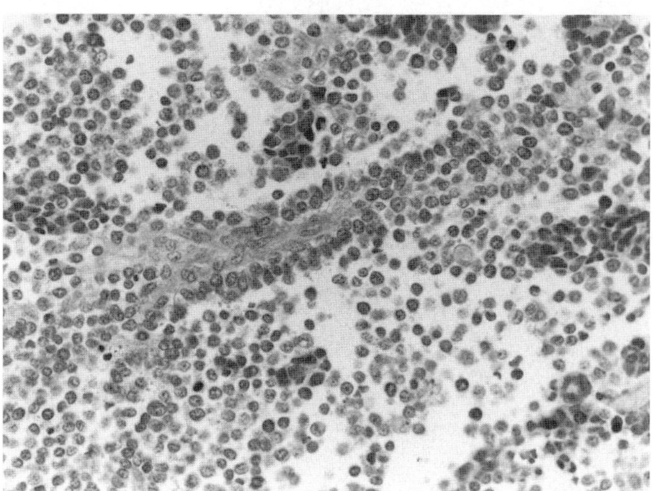

Figure 23-18 Alveolar rhabdomyosarcoma. (**A**) Axial T1-weighted magnetic resonance image through the humerus shows a slightly hyperintense mass replacing the triceps muscles of the arm. The neurovascular bundle (*arrowheads*) is contiguous with the anterior medial edge of the mass. (**B**) After contrast administration, there is heterogeneous enhancement of the mass. (**C**) Photomicrograph of the lesion demonstrates undifferentiated small blue cells lining fibrovascular septae with central discohesion, imparting an alveolar appearance.

- MRI provides important information about tumor extent which is necessary for treatment planning.

Histologic Features

- Embryonal rhabdomyosarcoma consists of poorly differentiated rhabdomyoblasts with a limited collagen matrix.
  - The rhabdomyoblasts are small, round-to-oval cells with dark-staining nuclei and limited amounts of eosinophilic cytoplasm (see Fig. 23-18C).
- Alveolar rhabdomyosarcoma is composed of poorly differentiated small, round-to-oval tumor cells that show central loss of cellular cohesion and formation of irregular alveolar spaces.
  - The individual cellular aggregates are separated and surrounded by irregularly shaped fibrous trabeculae.

Natural History and Treatment

- Prognostic variables for rhabdomyosarcomas include histologic subtype, size of the tumor, site of the tumor, and age of the patient.
- Alveolar subtype, larger tumors, extremity location, and patients older than 10 years of age are more often associated with a poorer prognosis.
  - Alveolar rhabdomyosarcoma, like the other subtypes, is treated with a combination of chemotherapy and surgery.
  - Irradiation can be used if total surgical resection cannot be achieved without excessive morbidity.
  - Total resection of the tumor with wide surgical margins is recommended, and preoperative chemotherapy often makes total resection of an extremity lesion possible.
- Lymph node biopsy should be considered if the patient has any suggestion of lymph node involvement.
- Postoperative irradiation may be used when the surgical margins are positive for tumor or there is poor necrosis of excised tumor from chemotherapy.
- The overall survival for a patient with extremity rhabdomyosarcoma is approximately 65%.

Acknowledgment

The authors thank Ms. Julia Lou for her research assistance during the writing of this chapter.

SUGGESTED READING

Coffin CM, Dehner LP, O'Shea PA. Pediatric soft tissue tumors: a clinical, pathological, and therapeutic approach. Baltimore: Williams & Wilkins, 1997.

Copley L, Dormans JP. Benign pediatric bone tumors. Pediatr Clin North Am 1996;43:949.

Dormans JP, Flynn J. Pathologic fractures associated with tumors and unique conditions of the musculoskeletal system. In: Rockwood and Wilkins fractures in children, 5th ed., Beatty JH and Kasser JR, eds., 2001, pp. 139–240.

Enneking WF. Musculoskeletal tumor surgery. New York: Churchill Livingstone, 1983.

Greenspan A, Remagen W. Differential diagnosis of tumors and tumor-like lesions of bones and joints. Philadelphia: Lippincott-Raven, 1998.

Himelstein BP, Dormans JP. Malignant bone tumors of childhood. Pediatr Clin North Am 1996;43:967.

Madewell JE, Ragsdale BD, Sweet DE. Radiologic and pathologic analysis of solitary bone lesions. Part I: internal margins. Radiol Clin North Am 1981;19:715.

Ragsdale BD, Madewell JE, Sweet DE. Radiologic and pathologic analysis of solitary bone lesions. Part II: periosteal reactions. Radiol Clin North Am 1981;19:749.

Simon MA, Biermann JS. Biopsy of bone and soft tissue lesions. J Bone Joint Surg (Am) 1993;75:616.

SPORTS MEDICINE

24.1 KNEE PAIN

LAWRENCE WELLS

Knee pain as the presenting symptom or complaint can come from a variety of sources. The approach to diagnosis, and to ultimately recommending a course of treatment, lies in four steps:

1. Have an appreciation of normal knee anatomy.
2. Obtain a thorough history, including onset and duration of symptoms, mechanism of injury, and precipitating causes of pain.
3. Perform a complete physical examination if necessary, taking into account surrounding areas (spine, hip, ankle) that may be sources of referred knee pain.
4. Order supplemental studies, such as radiographs, magnetic resonance imaging (MRI), bone scans, and special procedures (arthrocentesis, arthrometer testing, and examination under anesthesia) if they can aid in identifying the cause of knee pain.

The knee is a hinged joint with three major bony articulations surrounded by a complex array of ligaments and tendons (Figs. 24.1-1 to 24.1-3 and Table 24.1-1). The menisci are found between the medial and lateral femoral tibial articulations. They provide increased surface area to dispense weightbearing forces between the femur and tibia, as well as provide supplemental stability for the knee (Fig. 24.1-4).

There are several bursae, which are fluid-filled sacs that allow adjacent soft tissue envelopes to glide across one another about the knee. The most commonly involved in injury are the prepatellar bursa (Fig. 24.1-5), pes anserine bursa, and infrapatellar tendon fat pad. When inflamed, they present as tender, soft, boggy structures overlying the area of injury.

The knee also is surrounded by a complex array of neurovascular structures—the popliteal artery and vein and the tibial, common peroneal, and saphenous nerves.

Appreciating the anatomy of the knee helps one to conduct specific examinations of each area previously listed and identify areas of injury. Localizing the pain to a particular area is the key to making the correct diagnosis. If the pain cannot be localized on physical examination, one should consider a referred pain from another area, such as the hip, spine, or ankle (Fig. 24.1-6).

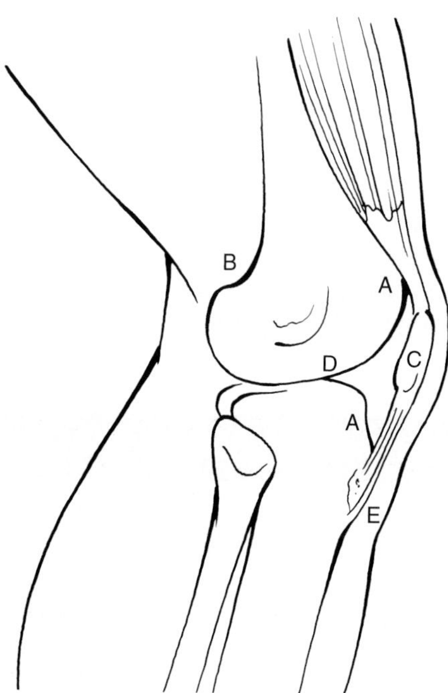

Figure 24.1-1 Surface anatomy of the knee. *A*; Suprapatellar and infrapatellar depressions. *B*; Adductor tubercle. *C*; Patella. *D*; Joint line. *E*; Tibial tubercle.

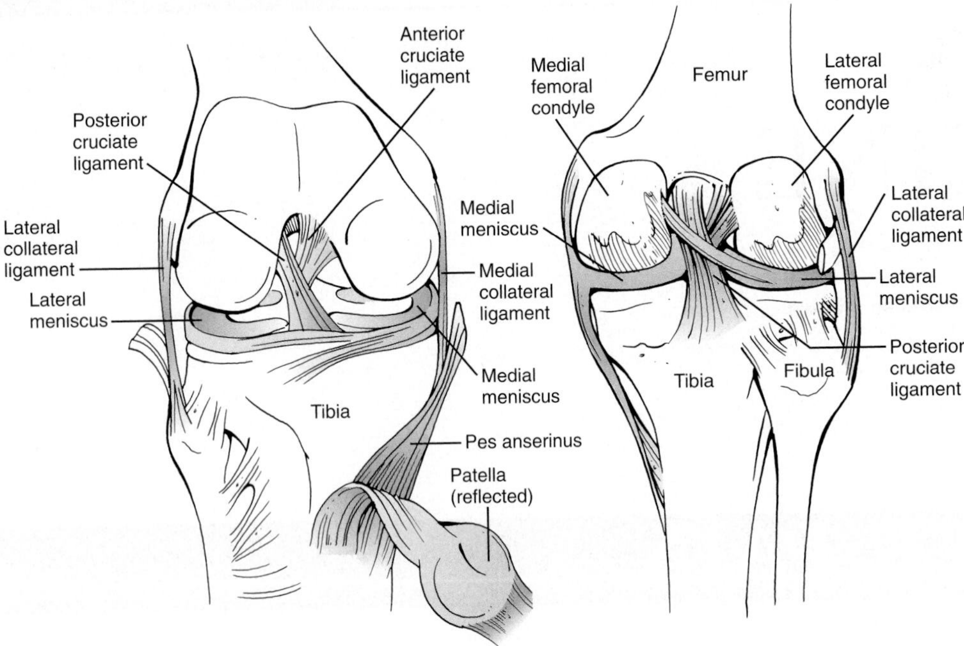

Figure 24.1-2 Normal knee anatomy.

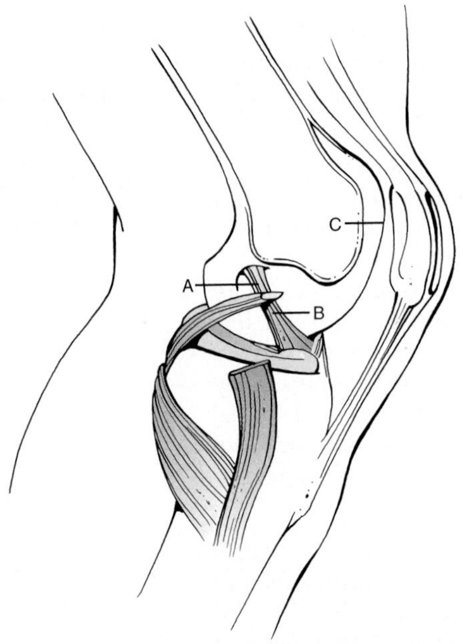

Figure 24.1-3 Ligaments of the knee. *A*; Posterior cruciate ligament. *B*; Anterior cruciate ligament. *C*; Patellofemoral articulation.

TABLE 24.1-1 KNEE LIGAMENT AND TENDON ANATOMY

Structure	Origin	Insertion
Anterior cruciate	Posterior lateral intercondylar notch	Medial tibial spine
Posterior cruciate	Anterior medial femoral notch	Proximal posterior tibia
Lateral collateral ligament	Lateral femoral condyle	Fibular head
Medial collateral ligament	Medial femoral epicondyle	Medial tibial shaft
Quadriceps tendon	Rectus femoris and 3 vastus muscles	Superior patella
Patella tendon	Inferior patella	Tibial tubercle
Pes anserine tendons	Gracilis, semitendinosis, and semimembranosus muscles	Medial tibial shaft superficial to medial collateral ligament
Lateral hamstring	Long and short biceps femoris muscle	Fibular head and proximal tibia
Iliotibial band	Tensor fascia lata	Gerdy tubercle

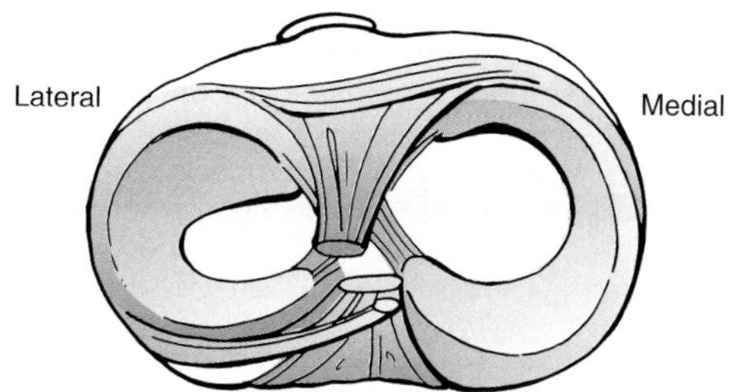

Figure 24.1-4 Axial view of knee menisci.

PATHOGENESIS

The most common causes of knee pain are from traumatic injuries—acute versus repetitive microtrauma accumulated over time. However, one needs to take a comprehensive approach in identifying the cause of pain. The anagram VINDICATER is a useful tool as one begins to formulate a differential diagnosis for knee pain (Box 24.1-1).

DIAGNOSIS

Patient History

The history can frequently provide many helpful clues to identify the cause of knee pain. Obtaining a complete history can be difficult in a young child. Therefore, in addition to the child, it is important to interview the caretakers who are familiar with the child and circumstances related to the child's symptoms (Tables 24.1-2 and 24.1-3).

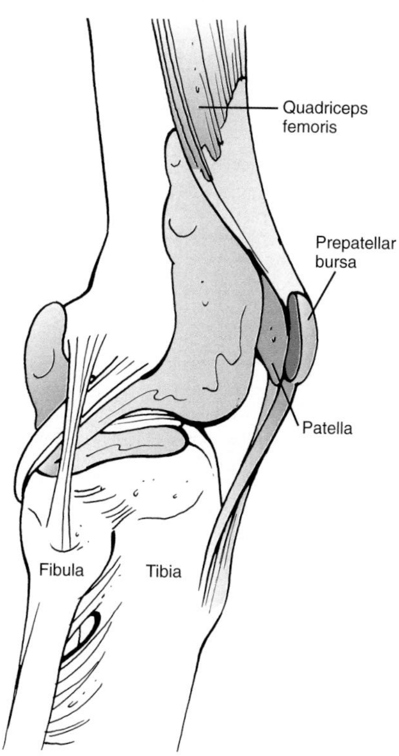

Figure 24.1-5 Prepatellar bursa.

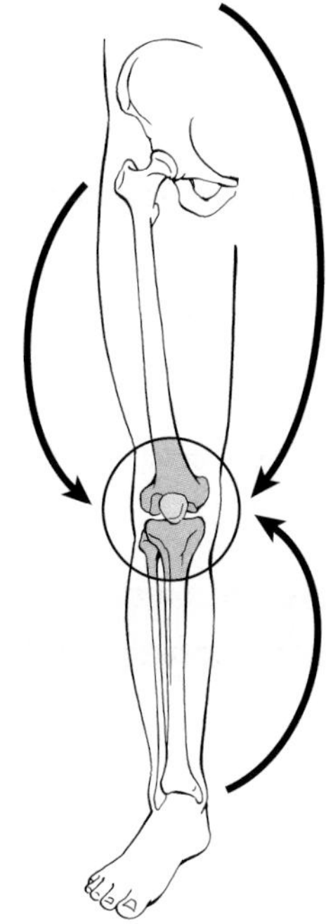

Figure 24.1-6 Sources of referred pain.

Physical Examination

- Begin with inspection of the knee alignment (Fig. 24.1-7), observation of the gait pattern, palpating pulses, and a neurologic exam (Table 24.1-4).
- Follow with evaluation of joint motion, tests for ligament stability, and direct palpation to identify specific areas of injury.
  - Localized tenderness is an important finding to identify the source of pain (Fig. 24.1-8).

BOX 24.1-1 DIFFERENTIAL DIAGNOSIS OF KNEE PAIN: "VINDICATER"

- Vascular
- Infectious
- Neoplastic
- Degenerative
- Inflammatory
- Congenital
- Arthritic
- Traumatic
- Endocrine
- Referred

TABLE 24.1-2 HISTORY OF KNEE INJURY

Question	Areas to Consider
Is the pain localized to a specific area? Ask patient to point to exact area.	Joint line, patella tendon, pes anserine bursa
Is there a sense of giving way or locking?	Meniscal tear, loose body, chronic muscle weakness
What is nature of pain? Activity-related, sharp, dull, burning, acute, or chronic?	Overuse syndrome, fracture, reflex sympathetic dystrophy
Is one awakened at night from pain? Is pain relieved by salicylates or nonsteroidal antiinflammatory medications?	Infection or tumor
Was a "pop" felt or heard preceding symptoms? Was patient able to continue activity?	Ligament injury
Did knee swell immediately?	Meniscal, ligament injury or fracture
Is the pain accentuated with going up or down stairs?	Patellofemoral joint irritation

TABLE 24.1-3 OUTCOMES ANALYSIS OF KNEE INJURY MECHANISM

Mechanism	Potential Outcomes
Twisting planted foot	Meniscal or ligament injury
Fall directly onto knee	Contusion extensor mechanism or PCL injury
Valgus or varus stress	MCL, MM or LCL, LM injury, respectively
Sense of "pop," immediate swelling, inability to continue activity participation	ACL or fracture
Sense of "giving way" or locking	Meniscal tear or patellofemoral injury
Constant or nighttime pain, relief with nonsteroidal antiinflammatory medications	Infection or tumor
Pain with use of stairs or prolonged sitting/squatting	Patellofemoral injury

ACL, anterior cruciate ligament; LCL, lateral collateral ligament; LM, lateral meniscus; MCL, medial collateral ligament; MM, medial meniscus; PCL, posterior cruciate ligament.

TABLE 24.1-4 PHYSICAL EXAMINATION FOR KNEE PAIN

Inspection	Varus/Valgus Alignment	Thigh and Calf Circumference	Foot Position	Swelling, Absence of Normal Parapatellar Concavities
Gait	Limp	Short leg	Kneeling	Jump—double/single leg
Joint motion	Extension: normal 0 degrees	Flexion: normal 145 degrees	Popliteal angle: normal <20 degrees	
Neurovascular examination	Popliteal, dorsalis pedis, posterior tibial artery	Tibial, common peroneal, and saphenous nerves	Skin color, warmth	

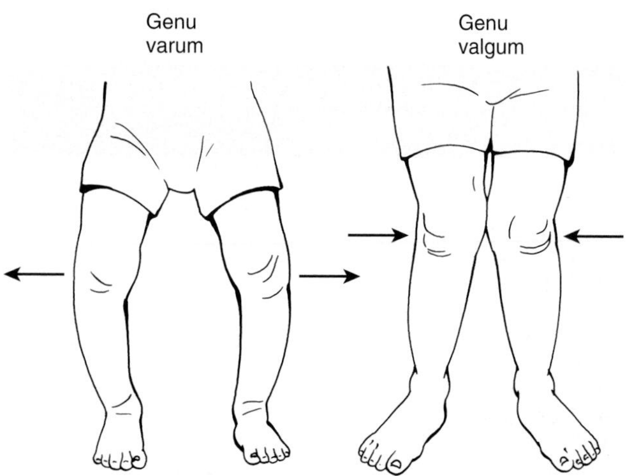

Figure 24.1-7 Knee alignment.

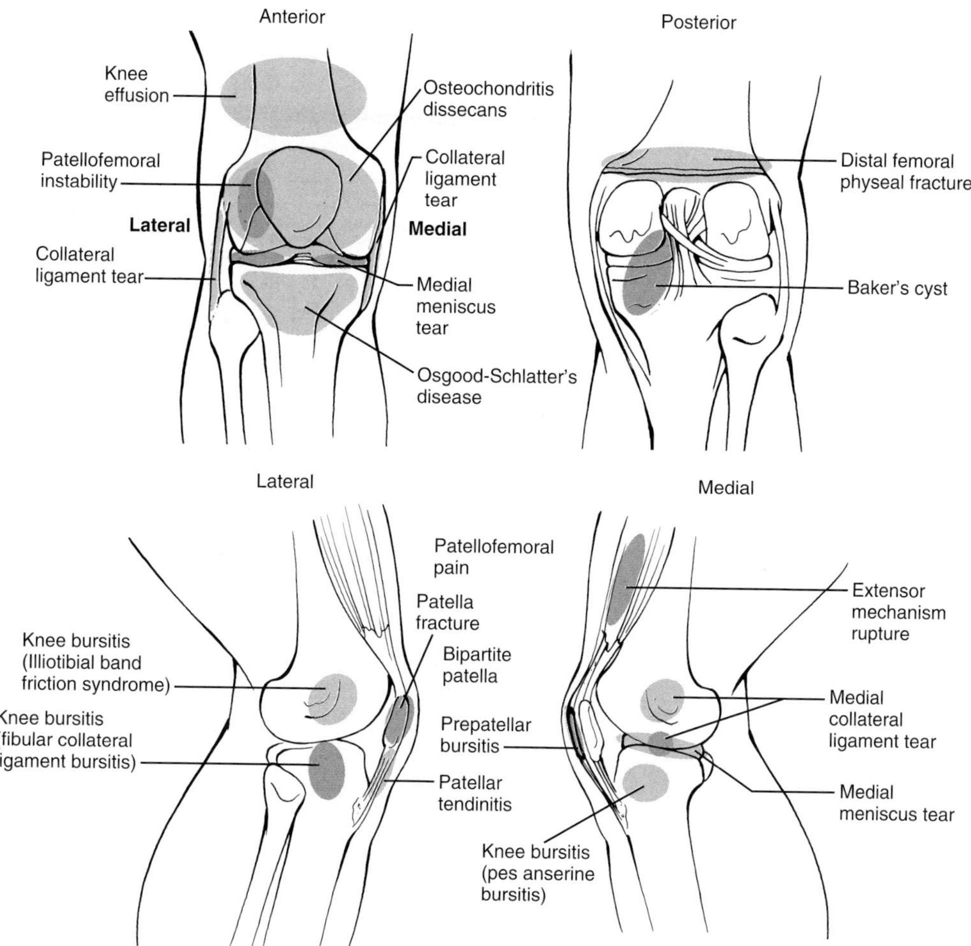

Figure 24.1-8 Potential causes of knee pain and their respective anatomic locations.

- Meniscal injuries often present with joint line tenderness extending from the midportion of the knee in the coronal plane posteriorly behind the femoral condyle.
- Tender crepitance along the joint line with flexion–rotation (McMurray test) or compression–rotation maneuvers (Appley test) suggest a meniscal tear.
- Severely displaced menisci often found in bucket-handle type tears can also limit full knee motion, especially extension.

- The patellofemoral joint is assessed with the patient lying supine and sitting with the knee bent at 90 degrees (Fig. 24.1-9).
  - Attempts at translating the patella medially and laterally can elicit a sense of apprehension or resistance from the patient in the case of patellar subluxation or dislocation (Fig. 24.1-10).
  - Painful crepitance and tenderness along medial or lateral parapatellar retinaculum are also signs of patellofemoral injury.
  - Malalignment is determined by measuring the Q angle, which is formed by the intersection of a line drawn along the long axis of the thigh and a line

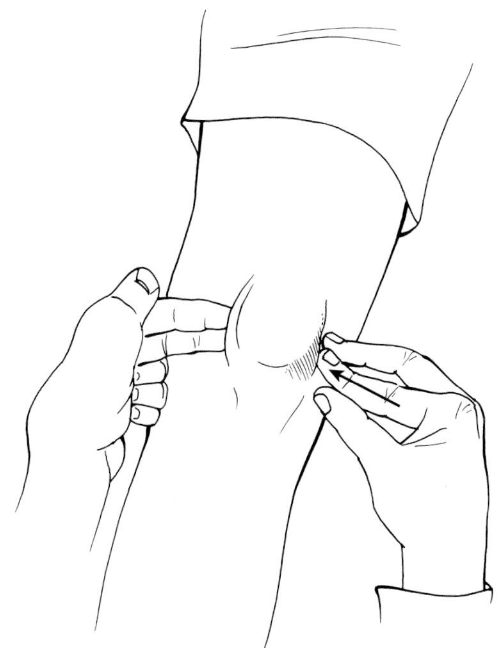

Figure 24.1-9 Supine evaluation of patellofemoral joint.

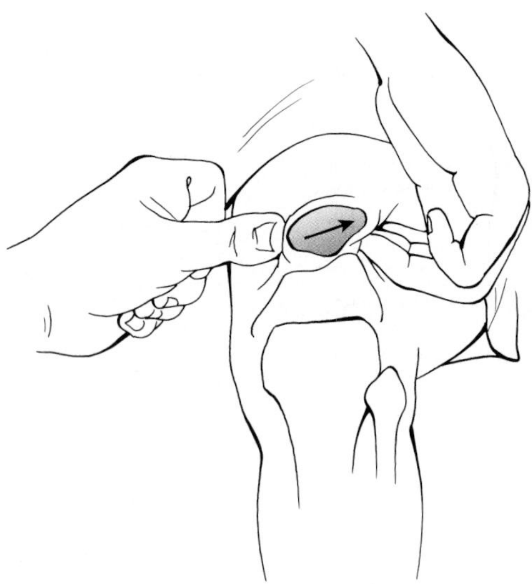

Figure 24.1-10 Lateral translation and palpation of lateral patellar facet.

drawn from the midpoint of the patella to the tibial tubercle.

- □ The normal value of the Q angle is 10 degrees in men and 15 degrees in women.
- □ Increased Q angles are thought to represent lateral tracking or misalignment of the patellofemoral joint.

□ Direct tenderness of the infrapatellar tendon can represent patellar tendonitis, commonly seen in repetitive jumping sports.

□ Sinding-Larsen-Johansson syndrome and Osgood-Schlatter disease are represented by tenderness over the inferior pole of the patella and tibial tubercle, respectively.

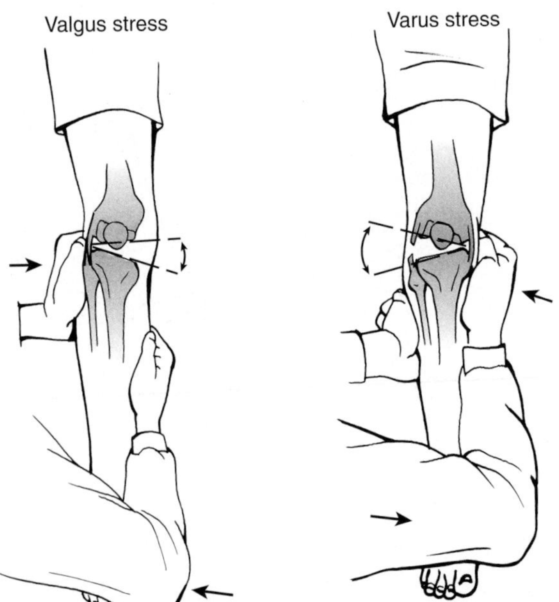

Figure 24.1-11 Testing collateral ligaments of the knee.

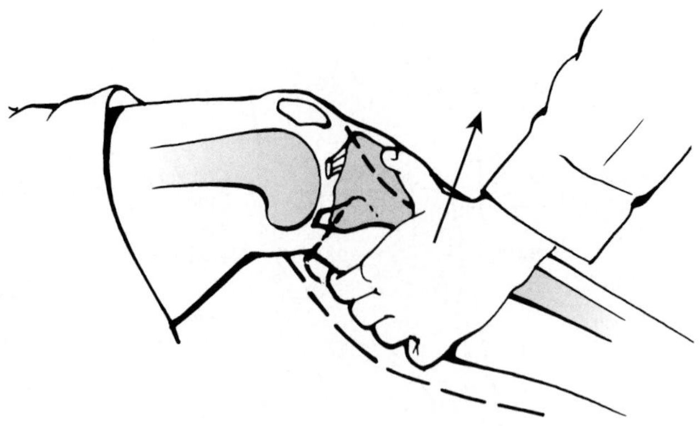

Figure 24.1-12 Lachman test for anterior cruciate ligament deficiency.

□ Tenderness over the lateral femoral epicondyle is often present with iliotibial band tendonitis, and tenderness over the pes anserine area can represent an inflamed bursa adjacent to medial hamstring insertions (Figs. 24.1-8B and 24.1-11 to 24.1-14; Table 24.1-5).

- The knee ligament exam is conducted with both the patient sitting and supine.
  - □ Lying supine often helps the patient to relax, thus avoiding inadvertent hamstring contraction that can compromise the examination results (Table 24.1-6).

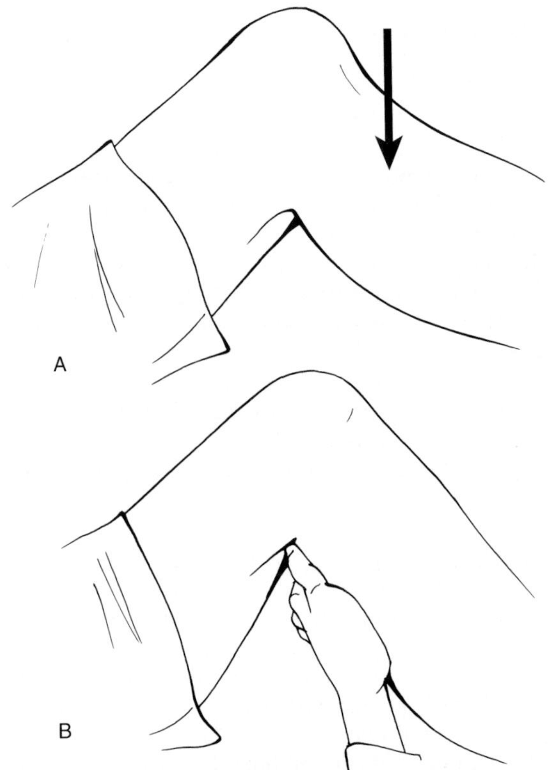

Figure 24.1-13 (A) Posterior sag sign, indicating posterior cruciate injury. (B) Absence of posterior sag, indicating normal posterior cruciate ligament.

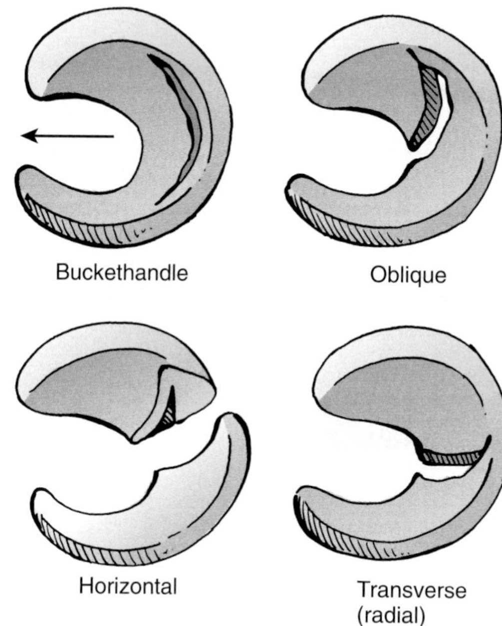

Figure 24.1-14 Meniscal injuries.

Radiographic Features

- Routine x-rays of the knee should be part of every "painful knee" evaluation.
  - A standard knee x-ray exam should include a weight-bearing posteroanterior (10 to 15 degrees flexed), lateral, Merchant or sunrise patella view, and an intercondylar notch view of the knee.
  - When the patient is unable to stand, an anteroposterior view of the knee should be obtained.
  - After a satisfactory film is obtained, systematic careful evaluation of the x-ray is performed.
  - Although seemingly evident, it is wise to confirm the name on the films with the name of the patient being examined.
  - Appropriate indicators of the side (right vs. left) being examined should also be noted (Table 24.1-7).
- When knee x-rays are normal, evaluate the spine, hip, and ankle regions to rule out sources of referred pain.
- Additional imaging studies such as MRI and bone scans can be useful in determining and localizing the extent of injury and in making treatment decisions, but they should not be used as primary screening studies.

TABLE 24.1-5 DIAGNOSIS OF KNEE PAIN[a]

Localized Tenderness	Diagnostic Considerations
Joint line	Meniscal injury
Patellofemoral	Patellar subluxation/prepatellar bursitis
Inferior patella	Sinding-Larsen-Johansson syndrome
Infrapatella tendon	Patellar tendonitis/anterior fat pad
Tibial tubercle	Osgood-Schlatter disease
Gerdy tubercle/lateral femoral epicondyle	Iliotibial band syndrome, lateral collateral ligament injury
Pes anserine	Pes anserine bursitis

[a]See also Figure 24.1-8.

TABLE 24.1-6 LIGAMENT EXAMINATION

Ligament	Test	Treatment	Outcome
MCL	Valgus stress at 30 degrees of flexion (Fig. 24.1-11)	Brace/early ROM	4–6 wk recovery
LCL	Varus stress at 30 degrees of flexion (Fig. 24.1-11)	Brace/early ROM	Same as MCL
ACL	Lachman, anterior drawer, pivot shift (Fig. 24.1-12)	Acute: ROM, hamstring strengthening, avoid sudden deceleration sports; ACL reconstruction after full ROM restored	Excellent with ACL reconstruction and post-op rehabilitation; return to sports 6–12 mo
PCL	Posterior drawer, posterior sagittal (Fig. 24.1-13), quad active test	Rehabilitate quads	Generally good for grade 1 and 2 injuries
PCL/PLC	Same as PCL plus reverse pivot shift and increased external rotation at 30 and 90 degrees of flexion	Surgical reconstruction within 2 wk of injury	Expect mild residual but improved laxity

ACL, anterior cruciate ligament; LCL, lateral collateral ligament; MCL, medial collateral ligament; PCL, posterior cruciate ligament; PLC, posterior lateral corner; ROM, range of motion.

TABLE 24.1-7 RADIOGRAPH EVALUATION GUIDELINES

Areas to Study	Significant Findings
Soft tissue contours	Effusion, soft tissue mass
Cortical margin	Erosions, lytic changes
Marrow contents	Lucency, blastic changes, calcification
Air–fluid levels	Open knee joint, penetrating trauma
Cortical discontinuity	Fracture

- Special procedures for diagnosing knee pain are given in Table 24.1-8.

Differential Diagnosis

- Vascular causes of knee pain are listed in Table 24.1-9.
- Infectious causes of knee pain are listed Table 24.1-10.
- As a whole, primary bone tumors around the knee are rare.
  - The most common and the most dangerous neoplastic lesions are listed in Table 24.1-11. Recognizing

TABLE 24.1-8 SPECIAL PROCEDURES

Procedure	Benefits
Arthrocentesis	Decreased symptoms, diagnostic information; acute hemarthrosis suggests meniscal or ACL injury
Stress radiographs[a]	Rule out underlying physeal injury
Arthrometer testing	Noninvasive tool for ACL/PCL laxity assessment
Examination under anesthesia	Preoperative injury confirmation, improved clinical examination

[a]Caution: avoid iatrogenic popliteal artery injury with overzealous stress.
ACL, anterior cruciate ligament; PCL, posterior cruciate ligament.

TABLE 24.1-9 VASCULAR CAUSES OF KNEE PAIN

Cause	History	Physical Examination	Treatment	Outcome
Sickle cell disease	Pain crisis, +HbSS electrophoresis	Joint effusion, pyoarthrosis	Arthrotomy, antibiotics	Arthritis, disability
Hemophilia	Male gender, factor VIII deficiency	Painful swollen joint	Factor replacement, RICE, joint motion, arthroscopic synovectomy	Good with attention to prevention, maintaining adequate factor level

HbSS, homozygosity for hemoglobin S; RICE, rest, ice, compression, elevation.

TABLE 24.1-10 INFECTIOUS CAUSES OF KNEE PAIN

Cause	History	Physical Examination	Laboratory Findings	Diagnostic Tests	Treatment	Outcome
Septic arthritis	Sexually active adolescent	Swollen, tender, limited motion	↑Synovial WBC, ↑ESR, CRP, +blood culture, bone scan	Aspiration, culture	Arthroscopic lavage, RICE, joint motion after acute symptoms resolved	Excellent if treated within a few days of onset; delayed treatment results in arthritis
Osteomyelitis	Low-grade fever, dull pain	Metaphyseal tenderness, limited motion	↑WBC, ESR	X-ray shows osteolytic changes; biopsy, culture routine, +AFB	Surgical débridement, antibiotics	Physeal injury; limb length inequality if extensive

AFB, acid-fast bacillus; CRP, C-reactive protein; ESR, erythrocyte sedimentation rate; RICE, rest, ice, compression, elevation; WBC, white blood cell count.

TABLE 24.1-11 NEOPLASTIC CAUSES OF KNEE PAIN

Cause	History	Physical Examination	Laboratory Findings	Radiographic Findings	Treatment	Outcome
Baker cyst	Painless mass popliteal fossa	Firm rubbery nodule, transilluminates light	None needed	Normal	Observation	Many resolve spontaneously
Meniscal cyst	Painful nodule at joint line	Lateral mass, aspiration yields yellow gelatinous fluid	Normal	Usually associated with meniscal tear on MRI	Aspiration and arthroscopic partial meniscectomy	Good; unlikely recurrence with treatment of meniscal tear
Osteogenic sarcoma	2nd decade, insidious pain day and night	Tender soft tissue mass	↑Alkaline phosphatase, ↑LDH	Lytic/blastic changes; may present as pathologic fracture	Chemotherapy, limb salvage, rotationplasty, or amputation	70% 5-yr survival without metastatic disease
Chondroblastoma	Ill-defined pain	Swelling; may have localized tenderness	Normal	Epiphyseal location	Excision and curettage	<25% recurrence
Osteochondroma	Painful snapping sensation, adolescent	Palpable nodule in metaphyseal area	Normal	Metaphyseal nodularity; may be multiple	Excise if enlarged or increased tenderness	Generally benign
Osteoid osteoma	2nd decade; boys/girls 2:1; dull achy pain increased at night; relief possible but not certain with NSAIDs	Occasionally area of point tenderness is found; thigh/calf atrophy	Normal	Radiolucent nidus surrounded by reactive bone; increased uptake on bone scan	NSAIDs provide temporary relief; excision for persistent symptoms; preoperative CT helpful for defining lesion	Excellent with complete excision
Myositis ossificans	Recurrent contusions, contact sports	Swelling commonly of the distal thigh; limited ROM	Normal	Organized zonal pattern of peripheral ossification	RICE, ROM; avoid contracture formation	Excellent, full recovery expected

CT, computed tomography; LDH, lactate dehydrogenase; MRI, magnetic resonance imaging; NSAIDs, nonsteroidal anti-inflammatory drugs; RICE, rest, ice, compression, elevation; ROM, range of motion.

them is vital to delivering appropriate treatment without delay.

- Degenerative conditions are typically not found in the pediatric age group.
- Primary inflammatory conditions of the knee are rare.
  - Generally, juvenile rheumatoid arthritis presents in the 2- to 6-year-old age group as a swollen knee and a limp.
  - Workup to rule out trauma, infection, and tumor are normal.
  - Treatment is primarily medical, and patients should be referred to a rheumatologist.
  - Outcomes are generally good with appropriate medical management.
  - Other considerations for inflammatory causes of knee pain include Lyme disease and lupus erythematosus.
  - Extensor mechanism disorders typically fall under the scope of overuse syndromes (Box 24.1-2), which are considered more fully in section 24.2.
- Congenital causes—conditions with generalized ligamentous laxity, such as Ehlers-Danlos syndrome, Down syndrome, and nail–patella syndrome—typically make children more prone to injury, particularly of the patellofemoral joint.

BOX 24.1-2 OVERUSE SYNDROMES

- Osgood-Schlatter disease
- Sinding-Larsen-Johansson syndrome
- Patellar tendonitis
- Adolescent anterior knee pain
- Symptomatic plica
- Iliotibial band syndrome

- □ Treatment protocols usually do not differ from those of children without congenital conditions.
- Traumatic causes of knee pain are listed in Table 24.1-12.
- In cases in which the physical examination is unremarkable, one needs to consider referred sources of knee pain, which are given in Box 24.1-3.

TREATMENT

In general, most sources of knee pain in children are from minor contusions, muscle strains, or tendonitis related to minor trauma or overactivity. Most are resolved with conservative measures, which include *r*est, application of *i*ce to reduce swelling, *c*ompressive wraps, temporary bracing or splinting, and *e*levation to prevent edema. This is known as the RICE program, which also includes activity modification or restriction until symptoms have resolved. Occasionally, a course of physical therapy is needed to aid in restoring joint range of motion and muscle strength.

Referral should be made when the patient is not responding to conservative measures, or if there is suspicion of infection, vascular injury, obvious deformity, or fracture.

TABLE 24.1-12 TRAUMATIC CAUSES OF KNEE PAIN

Cause	History/Mechanism	Physical Examination	Treatment	Outcome
Contusion	Fall, blunt trauma	Localized tenderness	RICE	Self-limited recovery
Patellar subluxation, dislocation, or malalignment	Blunt trauma Twisting injury	Parapatellar tenderness Apprehension ↑Q angle	RICE, ROM, quadriceps strengthening	Typically resolves with nonoperative treatment Proximal or distal realignment procedures for recurrent cases
Meniscal injuries (Fig. 24.1-14)	Twisting injury "Locked knee"	Effusion Joint line tenderness	RICE, ROM Arthroscopy for persistent mechanical symptoms	Prognosis good with preservation of as much meniscus as possible
Ligament injuries	Planted foot ± contact with sudden deceleration or valgus/varus stress	Point tenderness, instability on exam	RICE, restore ROM Ligament reconstruction for persistent instability or multiple ligament injuries	Prognosis generally good for isolated single ligament injuries; combined injuries have longer rehab. and more guarded chance of full recovery
Osteochondritis desiccans	Diffuse pain, limp in adolescents	Effusion, occasional point tenderness	RICE, activity modification, arthroscopy for persistent or mechanical symptoms	Prognosis age-dependent; spontaneous healing can occur in those <13 yr old
Bipartite patella	Adolescent, parapatellar pain Usually discovered after blunt injury	Tenderness corresponds to superior lateral defect in patella ossification (75%)	RICE, activity modification Surgical excision and reattachment of extensor mechanism for recalcitrant cases	Most respond to conservative treatment with resolution of symptoms
Knee dislocation	Older adolescent High-impact injury, obvious deformity	Obvious deformity, generalized tenderness, may have associated neurovascular injury	Correct deformity emergently, careful neurovascular exam and repair for sustained vascular injury. Ligament reconstruction 7–10 days after injury	Good for discovered and repaired vascular injuries. Residual instability (PCL) expected but minimal symptoms if repaired
Reflex sympathetic dystrophy	Disproportionate burning pain relative to injury	Marked tenderness to light touch, skin discoloration, atrophy, stiffness	Sympathetic block, TENS, physical therapy	Variable; advanced cases have poorer prognosis for recovery

LDH, lactate dehydrogenase; PCL, posterior cruciate ligament; RICE, rest, ice, compression, elevation; ROM, range of motion; TENS, transcutaneous electrical nerve stimulation.

BOX 24.1-3 REFERRED SOURCES OF KNEE PAIN

- *Lumbar spine:* herniated disc, spondylolisthesis
- *Hip:* slipped capital femoral epiphysis
- *Ankle:* osteoid osteoma, osteochondritis desiccans

Acknowledgment

I thank Kathrin Halpern for her assistance in the preparation of this manuscript.

SUGGESTED READING

Bruns DM, Maffuci N. Lower limb injuries in children in sports. Clin Sports Med 2000;19:4:637–662.

DeVellis JP, Andrish JT. Knee ligament injuries in the skeletally immature athlete. In: Orthopaedic knowledge update: sports medicine 2. Rosemont, IL: American Academy of Orthopaedic Surgeons, 1999:355–364.

Gebhardt MC, Hornicek FJ. Osteosarcoma. In: Orthopaedic knowledge update: musculoskeletal tumors. Rosemont, IL: American Academy of Orthopaedic Surgeons, 2002:175–186.

Gebhardt MC, Ready JE, Mankin HJ. Tumors about the knee in children. Clin Orthop 1990;255:86–110.

Iobst CA, Stanitski CL. Acute knee injuries. Clin Sports Med 2000; 19:621–635.

Smith A, Scoles PV. The knee. In: Pediatric orthopaedics in clinical practice, 2nd ed. Chicago: Yearbook Medical Publishers, 1988: 122–139.

Stanitski CL. Anterior knee pain syndromes in the adolescent. Instruct Course Lect 1994:211–220.

Stanitski CL. Knee disorders. In: Orthopaedic knowledge update: pediatrics. Rosemont, IL: American Academy of Orthopaedic Surgeons, 2002:191–201.

Stanitski CL, DeLee JC, Drez D. Pediatric and adolescent sports medicine. Vol 3. Philadelphia: WB Saunders, 1994.

Swenson TM, Harner CD. Knee ligament and meniscal injuries. Orthop Clin North Am 1995;26:529–545.

24.2 OVERUSE INJURIES

MICHAEL BUSCH ■ DAVID L. MARSHALL ■ KEITH H. MAY

An increasing number of young athletes are participating in organized sports programs. Sports programs and recreational, seasonal participation in a variety of sports are being replaced by year-round competition in a single sport or activity. This trend toward early specialization in a single activity has increased the number of sports-related injuries in young athletes. In addition, there has been a change in the pattern of injuries observed with the microtraumatic or overuse injury predominating over the acute, or macrotraumatic injury.

PATHOPHYSIOLOGY

Overuse injuries are defined as those that occur when repetitive submaximal stresses are applied to otherwise normal tissues. If there is adequate time for the tissue to repair itself, the tissue adapts to the demand and is able to undergo further loading without injury. Without adequate recovery, the normal reparative processes are overwhelmed; tissue failure (due to microtrauma) develops and stimulates the body's inflammatory response, leading to clinical injury.

Overuse injuries can occur in a variety of tissues such as bone, tendons, or growth cartilage (Box 24.2-1). Growth cartilage is found in three locations in the child: the physes, the epiphyseal surfaces, and the apophyses, all of which are susceptible to overuse injuries.

DIAGNOSIS

Patient History

As in any aspect of physical diagnosis, the history is important in diagnosing and treating overuse injuries. One must remember that the period of abusive training may have occurred weeks to months before the onset of clinical pain. Predisposing factors leading up to the onset of pain must be sought.

Predisposing factors for overuse injuries can be grouped into two broad categories: intrinsic factors and extrinsic factors (Box 24.2-2). Intrinsic factors such as limb alignment and resulting biomechanics are innate to the athlete. Extrinsic factors are determined by the athlete, and these include training regiments, shoes, and running surfaces.

OVERUSE SYNDROMES OF BONE

Stress injuries of bone can occur in any part of the bone. Much like repetitive bending of a paperclip, repetitive loading of virtually any element of the musculoskeletal system can lead to structural fatigue. Ideally, this leads to remodeling and strengthening that allows more activity as time

BOX 24.2-1 COMMON OVERUSE INJURY SITES BY LOCATION AND TISSUE TYPE

Metaphyseal/diaphyseal
- Stress fracture
- Spondylolysis

Epiphyseal
- Osteochondritis dissecans—capitellum

Physeal
- Little League shoulder
- Gymnast's wrist

Apophyses
- Osgood-Schlatter disease
- Sinding-Larsen-Johansson syndrome
- Sever disease
- Little League elbow
- Iselin disease

Periosteal
- Medial tibial stress syndrome

Tendon
- Achilles tendonitis
- Patellar tendonitis
- Rotator cuff tendonitis

BOX 24.2-2 PREDISPOSING FACTORS FOR OVERUSE INJURIES

Intrinsic Factors

Anatomic malalignment
- Pes planus
- Hyperpronation
- Tibial torsion
- Femoral anteversion
- Patellofemoral malalignment (Q angle)
- Leg length discrepancy

Growth-related factors
- During growth, lengthening of bone occurs more rapidly than surrounding muscle leaving the muscle–tendon unit tight
- Susceptibility of growth cartilage

Underlying disease states
- Scoliosis
- Arthritis
- Nutritional deficiency
- Excessive ligament laxity
- Previous injury

Extrinsic Factors

Training errors
- Sudden increase in intensity, frequency, or duration of an activity
- Addition of new program or sport
- Attendance at a specialty camp

Incorrect technique
- Pitching style

Improper equipment
- Wornout footwear (should be replaced every 250–400 miles)
- Grip size, string tension

Environmental factors
- Change in surface (wood, pavement, grass)
- Hill or bleacher training

goes on. If fatigue occurs faster than remodeling, the tissue fails resulting in clinical injury.

METAPHYSEAL/DIAPHYSEAL STRESS INJURIES

The simplest example of stress injury in bone is the stress fracture. Among youths, these most commonly occur with distance running. The athlete may experience gradual onset of symptoms and eventually be unable to run because of pain. Acute failure can occur through the weakened bone resulting in a complete fracture.

Pathogenesis

- Virtually any bone can be affected
- Most common metaphyseal and diaphyseal stress fractures in young athletes include the fibula, metatarsals, tibia, femur, and ulna.
- Stress fractures of the metatarsals (typically the second or third) and the distal fibula rarely have complications other than pain and disability.
- Fractures of the tibia, humerus, and forearm rarely displace but do represent potential risk for morbidity.

Epidemiology

- Most occur in later adolescence, ages 16 to 19.
- Boys and girl are equally affected.

Diagnosis

- Initially, only about 10% of radiographs are abnormal.
- Bone scan and magnetic resonance imaging (MRI) are much more sensitive.
- Bones scans result in radiation exposure, but are useful if the exact area of involvement is in question. Findings must be correlated to the clinical symptoms. As many as 50% of adolescents with stress fractures will show multiple areas of stress response on bone scans that do not correlate to areas of symptoms.
- MRI detects subtle marrow edema and early cortical failure.

Treatment

- Rest treats most diaphyseal and metaphyseal stress fractures.
- Crutches are often necessary. Occasionally, immobilization is needed.
- Healing time can range from 4 to 12 weeks.
- Alternative training, gradual resumption of sports, and monitoring for recurrent symptoms are necessary.
- Some stress fractures require surgery.
  - Stress fractures of the hip are rare but have the highest potential for morbidity. Femoral neck fractures can displace, disrupt the blood supply to the femoral head, and lead to avascular necrosis.
  - Stress fractures of the fifth metatarsal tend to be recurrent and are often best managed with an intramedullary screw.

SPONDYLOLYSIS

Pathogenesis

- Fracture through the pars interarticularis of the lumbar vertebrae.
- Commonly seen in athletes who are under the age of 20 and involved in a sport that requires repetitive extension of the lumbar spine, such as gymnastics, cheerleading, diving, football (linemen), and dance.
- The most common location is L5-S1, followed by L4-L5.

Diagnosis

- Pain with palpation is worse with single or dual leg hyperextension.
- Flexion usually is painless.
- Hamstrings frequently are tight.
- Anteroposterior, lateral, and oblique x-rays of the lumbar spine may be negative.
- Look for the fracture through the neck of the "Scotty dog" on the obliques.
- If clinical suspicion is high, and x-rays negative, consider computed tomography (CT), single-photon emission computed tomography (SPECT), or MRI.

Treatment

- Modify activities to avoid extension for 4 to 8 weeks.
- Consider rigid lumbar support bracing for 4 to 8 weeks.
- Physical therapy for truncal stabilization, and functional progression back to sport.
- Can resume activities without the brace 8 to 12 weeks from diagnosis.

APOPHYSEAL CONDITIONS

OSGOOD-SCHLATTER DISEASE

Pathogenesis

- A disorder of the proximal tibial apophysis that commonly affects young athletes, but may bother other active youngsters who are not involved in formal, organized sports.
- The tubercle of the proximal tibia is the insertion site of the patellar tendon.
- Because of the strength or the quadriceps, large tensile forces are transmitted through the patellar tendon insertion.
- The normal transition from the ossified and unossified tubercle into the tendon undergoes fatigue failure and a healing response ensues.

Epidemiology

- While activity plays a role, some individuals appear to be predisposed to this condition; 20% to 30% of youngsters will have siblings who have had the same problem.
- Typically, the child is between 10 to 15 years of age at the onset.
- Boys are more commonly affected than girls; however, female gymnasts seem to be particularly prone to this problem.
- Approximately 15% of teenage boys and 10% of teenage girls are affected.
- Incidence of bilaterality varies considerably.

Diagnosis

- Typically significant pain and prominence on the presenting side and some degree of findings on the contralateral side.
- Many patients have a prior history of heel pain compatible with Sever disease (calcaneal apophysitis).
- Pain is usually well localized to the prominent tibial tubercle.
- Pain is typically related to activities.
- There should be no signs or symptoms of intraarticular problems of the knee joint itself.
- The diagnosis can then be made clinically.
- A lateral radiograph of the knee can be helpful to confirm the diagnosis by showing irregularity of the tibial tubercle.
- The radiograph should also rule out any other osseous problems, such as tumor or infection.

Treatment

- In most, it simply runs its course with time, with symptoms lasting 1 to 4 years.
- In approximately 3% of patients a persistent ossicle forms, which can remain symptomatic and ultimately require surgical excision.
- Associated tuberosity fractures are so rare that there appears to be no sound evidence that activity restriction is required.
- Symptomatic measures include ice, nonsteroidal antiinflammatory drugs (NSAIDs), compressive sleeve or band, activity modifications as indicated by the symptoms, and hamstring stretching.
- Casts/rigid braces are rarely used, except for severe acute exacerbation.

SINDING-LARSEN-JOHANSSON SYNDROME

Pathogenesis

- Pathophysiology is similar to Osgood-Schlatter disease but the pain is located over the inferior pole of the patella.
- Typically patient is between 8 to 13 years of age at onset.
- Bilaterality varies considerably.

Diagnosis

- The pain is well localized over the inferior pole of the patella.
- The pain is related to activities.
- The diagnosis is clinical.
- Lateral radiograph may show irregular ossification over the distal patella.

Treatment

- Same as Osgood-Schlatter disease.

SEVER'S DISEASE (CALCANEAL APOPHYSITIS)

Pathogenesis

- Heel pain is a common complaint of the young adolescent.
- It is due to the very powerful but tight gastrocsoleus complex as it inserts on the back of the calcaneus.

Epidemiology

- Seen more often in boys age 9 to 13.
- More common in gymnastics, running, and sports in which cleats are worn (football, soccer).
- Bilateral in 50% of cases.

Diagnosis

- Pain localized to posterior aspect of calcaneus.
- Pain with medial and lateral pressure on the heel (squeeze test).
- Disease is associated with hyperpronation, femoral anteversion, tibial torsion.
- Those affected usually have tight plantarflexors and weak dorsiflexors.
- The diagnosis is made clinically. A lateral radiograph may show fragmentation and irregularity of the calcaneal apophysis, but this can be seen in asymptomatic heels.

Treatment

- The condition is self-limited so treatment is conservative and aimed at symptomatic relief: ice, NSAIDs, modification of activities, ¼-inch silicone or Sorbothane heel cups, orthotics to correct any mechanical problem, physical therapy, and home exercises to stretch the plantarflexors and strengthen the dorsiflexors.
- Casting for 2 to 3 weeks may be needed in extreme cases.

ISELIN'S DISEASE

Pathogenesis

- This is an uncommon traction apophysitis at the base of the fifth metatarsal at the insertion of the peroneus brevis.
- It occurs in skeletally immature athletes.

Diagnosis

- Pain is located on the lateral side of the foot and exacerbated by running, jumping, and cutting.
- Pain with resisted eversion.
- Radiographs may show a widened and prominent apophysis at the base of the fifth metatarsal.

Treatment

- Ice
- NSAIDS
- Activity modification to avoid pain.
- Physical therapy to stretch the ankle evertors and strengthen the invertors.

APOPHYSITIS OF THE MEDIAL EPICONDYLE

Pathogenesis

- Throwing produces a valgus moment at the elbow with compressive loads applied to the lateral side (radiocapitellar joint) and traction loads across the medial side.
- In the late teen years and above, repetitive traction injuries involve the medial collateral ligament itself, and can lead to rupture of the ligament.
- In the immature skeleton, the apophysis of the medial epicondyle can begin to fragment, which leads to a reparative process leading to pain and prominence.

Diagnosis

- Point tenderness over the medial epicondyle.
- Little or no loss of extension.
- Radiographs usually show some degree of irregularity or fragmentation of the apophysis.

Treatment

- Pain usually resolves with time and rest.
- Avulsion of the medial epicondyle can occur with forceful throwing, so restriction of rigorous throwing, such as pitching, is prudent.
    - ☐ Batting is usually not troublesome, and many can play an infield position while this resolves.
    - ☐ Return to pitching in less than 6 months often results in recurrence.

APOPHYSITIS OF THE PELVIS

Pathogenesis

- During periods of rapid growth, there is a strength–flexibility imbalance in the muscle tendon unit due to rapid growth of the bone relative to the muscle tendon.
- Several apophyses in the pelvis are susceptible to traction injuries (Table 24.2-1).
- These are most commonly seen in runners, sprinters, football players, and soccer players.

TABLE 24.2-1 APOPHYSES IN THE PELVIS

Apophysis	Muscle
Iliac crest	External obliques, gluteus medius, tensor fascia lata
Anterior superior iliac spine	Sartorius
Anterior inferior iliac spine	Rectus femoris
Ischial tuberosity	Hamstrings
Greater trochanter	Gluteus medius
Lesser trochanter	Iliopsoas

Treatment

- Ice
- NSAIDs
- Modification of activities to maintain cardiovascular endurance
- Stretching of the involved muscle–tendon unit once acute pain subsides
- Gradual return to activities usually by the direction of a physical therapist (usually after 2 to 4 weeks; 4 to 6 weeks if avulsion is present)

REPETITIVE PHYSEAL INJURIES

LITTLE LEAGUE SHOULDER

Pathogenesis

- Repetitive stress to the shoulder can lead to widening and resorption around the proximal humeral physis.
- This "physiolysis" has been termed "Little League shoulder" since it occurs primarily in Little League baseball players.
- While typically affecting pitchers, other rigorous throwers, such as catchers, can develop this as well.

Diagnosis

- Typically 12- to 15-year-old boys
- Shoulder pain related to overhead throwing
- Usually more painful in the deltoid region than the subacromial region
- Differential diagnosis: rotator cuff tendonitis and impending pathologic fracture from a simple bone cyst to the upper humerus
- Radiographic widening of the proximal humeral physis on the affected side confirms the diagnosis of Little League shoulder.
    - Need comparison with other shoulder.

Treatment

- Primarily involves rest
- Complications are uncommon, so if the symptoms are minimal, batting and playing infield positions are usually not painful.
- Resolution can take up to 6 months.
- Pitching is gradually resumed.
- Monitor for resumption of symptoms.

GYMNAST'S WRIST

Pathogenesis

- Gymnastic training often begins as early as age 4 or 5 and peaks in the early to mid-teens, during which the time spent in training may reach as high as 30 to 40 hours per week.
- Because many maneuvers in gymnastics involve weight-bearing on the dorsiflexed wrist, often with a rotational component, the wrist is a common site of overuse injury.
- The term *gymnast's wrist* is a catchall term often used to describe any of a wide variety of wrist injuries in gymnasts.
- The most common chronic injury seen is at the level of the distal radial physis.

Epidemiology

- 80% to 90% of affected athletes are female.
- Typically 12 to 14 years of age
- Symptoms are bilateral in approximately one-third of patients.
- Usually seen in gymnasts whose weekly training regimen exceeds 20 hours per week.
- Vault and floor exercise are the events most likely to cause symptoms.

Diagnosis

- Patients have pain with palpation over the distal radial physis.
- There is pain at extremes of dorsiflexion.
- This can be differentiated from dorsal impingement by the presence of pain on the volar and radial aspects of the physis.
- Radiographs may be normal (stage 1), and the diagnosis is made clinically.
- Radiographs may show widening of the distal radial physis, irregularity or cystic changes on the metaphyseal side of the growth plate, or breaking of the radial physis (stage 2).
- With late presentations, the radiographs may show positive ulnar variance due to premature closure of the radial physis.

Treatment

- Stage 1 (no radiographic changes)
    - Modified rest, which involves avoidance of axial compressive loads for a period of 2 to 4 weeks. During this time the athlete may continue to condition, maintain flexibility, and continue to train on the beam, practice aerial stunts, as well as footwork on the floor exercise.

- After the pain resolves, a gradual return to activity is allowed with close supervision.
- Stage 2 (radiographic changes with no ulnar variance)
  - Avoidance of axial compressive loads for 6 to 12 weeks. Casting may be appropriate for the noncompliant athlete.
  - To improve compliance, it is important to inform the gymnast that absolute rest will provide the best chance of returning to a competitive level.
- Stage 3 (positive ulnar variance)
  - Same as stage 2.
  - Consider MRI arthrography for triangular fibrocartilage complex (TFCC) tears. This should be suspected in any gymnast with wrist pain on the ulnar side.
  - Possible need for shortening osteotomy of the ulna.

Prevention

- Educate athletes and coaches on the importance of wearing variance braces with workouts.
- Recommend bi-annual routine wrist radiographs in all gymnasts training more than 16 hours per week.
- Encourage strength and flexibility training of the wrists year-round.
- Alternate compressive, axial-loading workouts (vault) with traction workouts (uneven bars).
- Early stage diagnosis: encourage gymnasts at all ages to have wrist pain evaluated.

EPIPHYSEAL OVERUSE CONDITIONS

Perhaps the best example of a repetitive stress injury of the epiphyses occurs at the capitellum—Panner disease and osteochondritis of the capitellum. In these conditions, a segment of epiphyseal bone becomes necrotic and can result in separation of the bone segment and overlying articular cartilage. While technically classified as an "osteochondrosis," these have features of repetitive stress-induced injuries, much like stress fractures.

PANNER'S DISEASE

- Panner described a lesion of a young boy's capitellum that he compared with Legg-Calvé-Perthes disease.
- In patients under 10 years of age who develop irregularity of the capitellum, the course is usually quite benign.
- An avascular segment of bone develops in the center of the capitellum, revascularizing in time.
- Loose bodies do not typically form.
- Sequelae are rare and treatment is simply rest.

OSTEOCHONDRITIS DISSECANS OF THE CAPITELLUM

Pathogenesis

- While the term *osteochondritis dissecans* implies that there is an inflammatory process present, histologic studies have in fact failed to confirm this.
- Appears to be a repetitive stress phenomenon
- Most commonly occurs in baseball pitchers.
- As the ball is accelerated during the pitching motion, a valgus moment is created at the elbow.
  - There is tension on the medial side of the elbow and compressive forces across the radial capitellar articulation.
- The capitellum has an end arterial blood supply, which may explain its susceptibility to develop avascular necrosis from chronic repetitive compression loads.

Diagnosis

- Side arm pitches, many curve ball techniques, and others can increase the compression loads across the lateral side of the elbow by bringing the ball further away from the midsagittal plane and accentuating the valgus moment.
- Typically patients complain of an aching pain in the lateral side of the elbow.
- Often they have flexion contractures.
- Displaced fragments can result in a loose body sensation, a locked elbow, or significant synovitis and pain.
- Plain radiographs typically show a sclerotic region or radiolucency. Tangential views may help.
- Occasionally, CT scan or MRI are indicated.

Treatment

- Osteochondritis of the capitellum can result in permanent arthrosis of the elbow joint.
- Prevention through education is key.
  - Junior baseball programs should have rules limiting how much youngsters can pitch, typically three innings per game, up to six innings per week.
- Occasionally, intact lesions heal with prolonged rest, but surgery is often necessary to remove unstable or displaced fragments.
- Compared with simple arthroscopic débridement, there is no proven benefit to grafting, or other procedures.

TENDINOSES

ROTATOR CUFF TENDONITIS

Pathogenesis

- Unlike in adults, tendon degeneration and rupture are rarely seen in youths.

- The rotator cuff is a convergence of the tendons of the subscapularis, supraspinatus, infraspinatus, and teres minor.
  - These extend from the scapula out over the humeral head.
  - Together, they stabilize the humeral head against the glenoid fossa and they prevent the humeral head from rubbing beneath the arch of the acromion.
  - The supraspinatus muscle is the most important of these.

Etiology

- Many factors contribute to rotator cuff tendonitis.
  - In young athletes, inherent laxity of the glenohumeral capsule is likely a significant factor.
  - Overhead throwing in baseball, swimming, serving motion in tennis, and gymnastics precipitate symptoms.
- Pain produces inhibition of the rotator cuff muscles, which precipitates impingement of the humeral head beneath the acromion.
  - With time, a well-established bursitis and tendonitis develop.

Diagnosis

- Typical complaints: pain with overhead activities, and sensation of the arm becoming heavy, tired or "dead."
- Thoroughly examine the neck and shoulder looking for restriction of motion, muscle atrophy, and focal tenderness.
  - There may be tenderness along the course of the biceps tendon, as well.
- The supraspinatus strength should be tested.
  - Glenohumeral laxity is common.
- Plain radiographs are useful to rule out other bony abnormalities.
- MRI can be diagnostic for rotator cuff tendonitis; however the diagnosis can usually be made clinically.
  - Partial and full thickness rotator cuff tears are rarely seen before 18 years of age.

Treatment

- The principles of treatment center on restoring strength and motion of the rotator cuff and scapular stabilizers.
- NSAIDs.
- Often overhead activities are curtailed while physical therapy is initiated. Rehabilitation of the entire scapular thoracic complex is key.
- As pain diminishes and strength returns, overhead sporting activities are initiated, with careful monitoring for evidence of recurrent impingement.
- In recalcitrant cases, a subacromial or intraarticular injection of steroids can hasten resolution of the inflammatory phase.
- Occasionally, surgical stabilization is necessary, though subacromial decompression is rarely indicated for youths.

SHIN PAIN

Shin pain is a common complaint in young athletes. Much like the term *headache*, the diagnosis of "shin splints" refers to a collection of maladies with the common feature being activity-induced pain in the midportion of the leg. Specific diagnoses include:

- Periostitis
- Chronic exertional compartment syndrome
- Stress fracture
- Muscle herniation
- Superficial nerve entrapment

Shin pain in youths should be evaluated for a specific diagnosis. Other considerations in the differential diagnosis include:

- Deep venous thrombosis
- Tumor
- Infection
- Popliteal artery entrapment

PERIOSTITIS

Pathogenesis

- This clinical entity is also termed *medial tibial stress syndrome* and *soleus syndrome*.
- The soleus muscle and its investing fascia originate in this area and are also implicated in causing the syndrome.
- Three-fourths of running athletes with shin pain have posteromedial tenderness, and half of them are bilateral.
- Boys and girls are equally affected.
- Predisposing factors include:
  - Muscle weakness
  - Running shoes with a lack of heel cushion, inadequate arch support
  - Hard training surfaces.
  - Training errors such as sudden increases in intensity or mileage
  - Abnormal lower limb biomechanics

Diagnosis

- Activity-related pain
- No associated numbness
- Recent increase in the intensity of sports participation, training, and competition schedule
- Recent change in regimen or shoes, and surface training conditions
- Pain and tenderness along the distal third of the posteromedial tibia—extending longitudinally along several centimeters, and not across to the anterior tibia
- Varus hindfoot alignment, excessive forefoot pronation, genu valgum, excessive femoral anteversion, and external tibial torsion
- No muscle herniation

- Negative Tinel test
- Normal radiographs
- If confirmation of the clinical diagnosis is needed, bone scan shows a longitudinal pattern of radionuclide concentration rather than a transverse pattern more typical of a stress fracture.

Treatment

- NSAIDs
- Ice
- Strengthening and stretching
- Ultrasound
- Foot orthoses
- Graduated running program
- Surgery rarely indicated

CHRONIC EXERTIONAL COMPARTMENT SYNDROME

Pathogenesis

- With repetitive exercise, the interstitial pressure within the osseofascial compartments of the leg can become elevated.
- When compartment pressures exceed capillary filling pressure, the muscle becomes ischemic and produces pain.
- This usually has an onset associated with activity and is relieved by rest.
- Unlike acute compartment syndromes resulting from trauma or arterial insufficiency, the pressure and blood flow to the muscles normalizes in chronic compartment syndromes and rarely result in tissue necrosis or residual disability.
- The anterior compartment is the most commonly involved, although any of the four compartments in the lower leg may be affected.

Diagnosis

- Typical complaints: aching pain, tightness, or a squeezing sensation brought on by and interfering with athletics
- Usually relieved promptly after exercise
- Some experience transient foot-drop with paresthesias across the dorsum of the foot if the anterior compartment is involved.
- Plantar paresthesias with chronic posterior compartment syndrome.
- Fascial defects with muscle herniation may be present over the anterior and lateral compartments.
- If clinically indicated or desired, dynamic measurement of compartment pressures during exercise can confirm the diagnosis.
  - In chronic compartment syndrome, resting pressures typically are not elevated.
  - With exercise, the pressures rise to 70 to 100 mm Hg, while normal compartments rise to less than 30 mm Hg
  - MRI done immediately after exercise may have a role as well.

Treatment

- Initial treatment includes activity modification, foot orthoses, physical therapy, and time.
- Recalcitrant cases may require a fasciotomy.
  - All involved compartments should be released.
  - This can be done through limited skin incisions rather than through the extensive releases suggested for adequate management of the acute traumatic compartment syndrome.
  - Care must be taken to protect the saphenous vein, saphenous nerve, and the superficial branch of the peroneal nerve.
- All compartments should be assessed because symptoms may not be adequate to identify all involved compartments.
- History of bilateral symptoms should be specifically sought.
  - After unilateral surgical release, patients frequently increase their activity levels, only to develop pain on the side that had been asymptomatic.
- Failures result from failing to appreciate multiple compartment involvement; from inadequate decompression, especially of the deep posterior compartments; and from excessive scar tissue response.

SUGGESTED READING

Busch MT. Sports medicine. In: Morrissey RT, Weinstein SL. Lovell & Winter's pediatric orthopaedics, 4th ed. Philadelphia: Lippincott Williams and Wilkins, 2001.

Combs JA. Hip and pelvis avulsion fractures in adolescents. Physician Sports Med 1994; 22:41–49.

Detmer DE. Chronic shin splints. Classification and management of medial tibial stress syndrome. Sports Med 1986;3:436–446.

Detmer DE, Sharpe K, Sufit RL, et al. Chronic compartment syndrome: diagnosis, management, and outcomes. Am J Sports Med 1985;13:162–170.

DiFiori J. Overuse injuries in children and adolescents. Physician Sports Med 1999; 27:75–84.

Kocher MS, Waters PM, Micheli LJ. Upper extremity injuries in the paediatric athlete. Sports Med 2000;30:117–135.

Kujala UM, Kvist M, Heinonen O. Osgood-Schlatter's disease in adolescent athletes. Am J Sports Med 1985;13:236–241.

Mandelbaum BR, Nativ A. Gymnastics. In: Reider B, ed. Sports medicine, the school age athlete, 2nd ed. Philadelphia: WB Saunders, 1996:459–462.

Outerbridge AR, Micheli LJ. Overuse injuries in the young athlete. Clin Sports Med 1995;14:503–516.

Schenck RC. Athletic training and sports medicine, 3rd ed. Rosemont, IL: American Academy of Orthopaedic Surgeons, 2000.

Walker RN, Green NE, Spindler KP. Stress fractures in skeletally immature patients. J Pediatr Orthop 1996;16:578–584.

Zetaruk M. The young gymnast. Clin Sports Med 2000;19:758–780.

ENDOCRINOLOGY

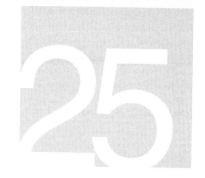

25.1 RICKETS

JAMES F. MOONEY III

The diagnosis of rickets includes a series of disease processes with a common pathologic mechanism. In each situation, a relative decrease in serum calcium, phosphorus, or a combination of each, causes abnormalities of normal physeal development and mineralization in the immature patient. While these abnormalities affect both the axial and appendicular skeleton, it is the effect on the extremities that becomes most clinically apparent, and is of most interest and concern to the pediatric orthopaedic surgeon. Similar perturbations of serum chemistries may be found in adults, as seen in association with renal disease, and with some malignancies, but the classic clinical appearance of rickets is found only in the skeletally immature.

PATHOGENESIS

Multiple underlying diagnoses present with similar clinical symptoms and signs. As such, there is no singular disease that can be termed *rickets*. *Classic (dietary) rickets* is secondary to dietary abnormalities and deficiency of vitamin D, which in turn lead to abnormalities in calcium uptake and metabolism. This is relatively infrequent in the Western world, but troubling reports have appeared recently of an increased incidence of dietary (vitamin D deficiency) rickets in children who are exclusively breast-fed.

Breast milk contains a minimal amount of either inactive or activated vitamin D. As such, infants who are exclusively breast-fed require vitamin D supplementation prior to the introduction of more advanced foods. This is particularly problematic in those infants with darker skin color, in whom melatonin competes with vitamin D for the ultraviolet (UV) radiation in the skin cells, thus increasing the amount of sun exposure required to activate an appropriate level of vitamin D. Premature infants, and those of families with particular religious considerations that require significant coverage of the head and face, particularly in females, may be at greater risk for rickets secondary to a lack of activated vitamin D.

This is also more of a problem in northern latitudes, especially in fall and winter months in which the opportunity for natural UV exposure is limited both by the cold and by clothing cover. Other groups that may develop similar findings include children with severe milk allergies who do not receive appropriate supplementation, and children made to follow a strict vegetarian diet, which may be low in vitamin D content. Overall, rickets secondary to deficiency of vitamin D is uncommon in modern Western society, but does occur, particularly in some cultures, and the pediatric orthopaedic surgeon must remain vigilant.

Other causes of rickets involve abnormalities of calcium, phosphate, or vitamin D metabolism. Many of these have an underlying genetic basis. The most common genetic abnormality is *hypophosphatemic rickets* which is usually transmitted in an X-linked dominant pattern, but may occur secondary to a spontaneous mutation. Females appear to be more commonly affected than males. Patients with this disorder possess a defect within the proximal and distal convoluted renal tubules, which inhibits appropriate resorption of phosphate, thereby leading to profound hypophosphatemia due to severe phosphate wasting in the urine. Such abnormal levels of serum phosphate inhibit normal mineralization and cause development of changes similar to those seen in classic rickets, despite normal calcium intake and uptake, and normal intake and ability to activate vitamin D. This type of rickets is often termed *vitamin D resistant*, as the levels and activity of vitamin D are generally normal, and further vitamin D supplementation without addressing the phosphate issue does not improve the clinical situation. Medical management of such patients requires significant oral supplementation with neutral phosphate to maintain appropriate serum levels in the face of persistent renal loss.

Various other genetic and metabolic conditions may cause clinical signs and symptoms consistent with rickets.

The most problematic of those remaining would be renal osteodystrophy in patients with chronic renal insufficiency. These patients will have the well established underlying problem of chronic renal disease, and the skeletal manifestations should be expected to varying degrees. The causes described previously make up most cases seen by pediatric orthopaedic surgeons, and certainly the most common causes of clinical findings for which the pediatric orthopaedic surgeon would be the primary diagnostician. More detailed descriptions of these less common entities are beyond the scope of this review, and one should consult standard pediatric and endocrinology texts for further information.

DIAGNOSIS

Physical Examination and History

Findings on physical examination of patients with possible rickets vary, but some consistencies do exist.

- Generally, patients are of short stature, but often heavier than children of similar chronologic age.
- Classically, their demeanor has been described as lethargic or irritable.
- Examination of the appendicular and axial portions of the skeleton, as well as the bones of the skull, provides reliable findings.
  - Frontal bossing, flattening of the skull due to changes of the growth regions about the cranial suture lines, and varying levels of dental disease.
  - Enlargement of the growth centers of the ribs (costal cartilages) has been described as "rachitic rosary" because it feels like a string of beads, and pectus carinatum can be seen occasionally.
- The patient may develop an increased thoracic kyphosis, termed "rachitic catback," but significant scoliosis associated with, or attributable to, rickets is uncommon.

Abnormalities of the appendicular skeleton are extremely common in patients with rickets, and are often the primary reason for pediatric orthopaedic evaluation.

- There is generalized shortening of all long bones, and the joints will appear bulbous and widened, especially in the face of severe, untreated disease.
- The humeri usually develop varus deformities, while the lower extremities may demonstrate either varus or valgus angulation.
- Commonly, the younger the patient, the more likely the lower extremities will present in varus, rather than valgus, and overall varus deformities of the lower extremities are much more common than valgus.
- In contrast, skeletal manifestations of chronic renal disease generally become apparent later in development, and the lower extremity deformities in these patients tend toward valgus.
- In addition to the structural abnormalities, children with rickets may present with significant ligamentous laxity, which will exacerbate the angular deformities, particularly in the lower extremities during weightbearing.

Radiographic Features

The radiographic evaluation of patients with suspected or known rickets relies exclusively on the use of standard radiographs. No special studies using computed tomography, magnetic resonance imaging, or bone scan are necessary.

- The histologic abnormalities resulting from the alterations in physeal development and maturation lead to standard radiographic changes directly adjacent to the growth plates.
- Plain radiographs demonstrate widening, irregularity, and cupping of the growth plates of all bones that undergo endochondral ossification (Fig. 25.1-1).

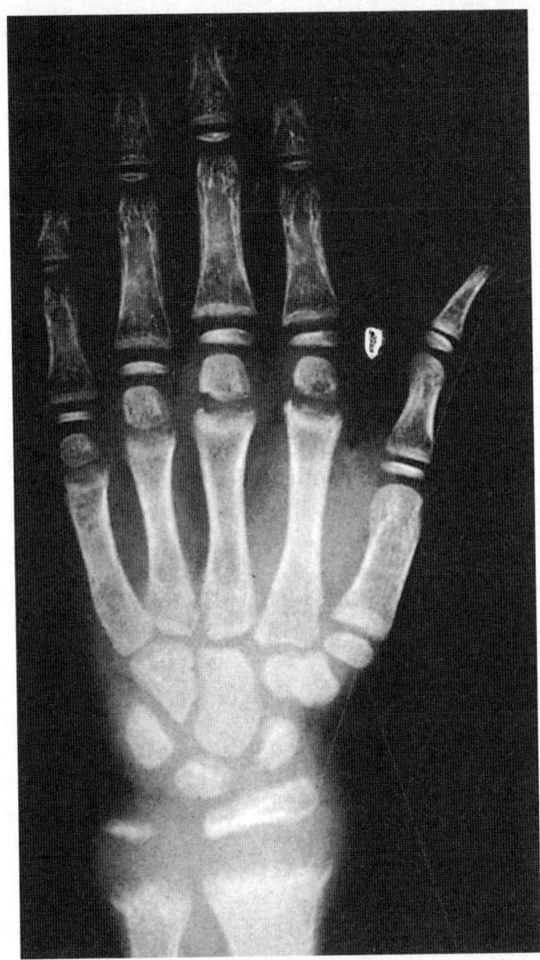

Figure 25.1-1 The changes in the epiphyseal plates of the wrist and hand are clearly seen in this radiography of an 8-year-old child with florid rickets. The distal radial and ulnar epiphyseal lines are markedly increased in axial height and show cupping; the zone of provisional calcification is absent. The changes in the slower-growing physes of the more distally placed bones are less marked, emphasizing the fact that rickets is a disease of the growing skeleton (in contrast to osteomalacia), and, if the physeal regions grow slowly, the findings are less prominent. (From Zaleske DJ. Metabolic and endocrine abnormalities. In: Morrissey RT, Weinstein SL, eds. Lovell and Winter's pediatric orthopaedics, 4th ed. Vol 1. Philadelphia: Lippincott Williams & Wilkins, 2001:189.)

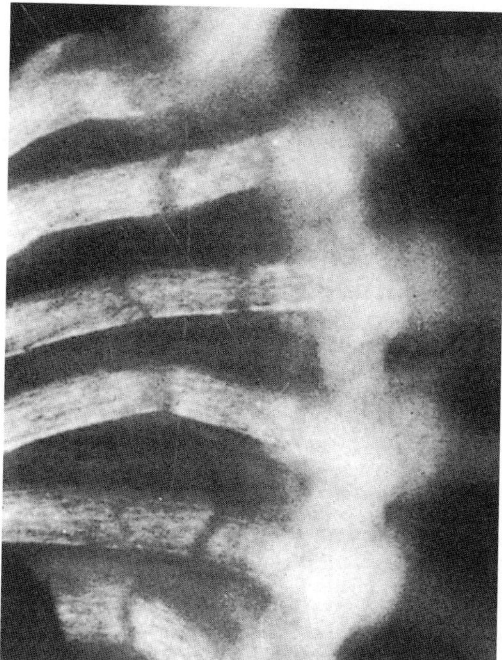

Figure 25.1-2 Looser lines seen in the rib cage of a child with florid rickets. These linear transverse radiolucent lines, which resemble incomplete fractures, are localized accumulations of osteoid of unknown cause. They are pathognomic for rickets and osteomalacia. (From Zaleske DJ. Metabolic and endocrine abnormalities. In: Morrissey RT, Weinstein SL, eds. Lovell and Winter's pediatric orthopaedics, 4th ed. Vol 1. Philadelphia: Lippincott Williams & Wilkins, 2001:190.)

- The zone of provisional calcification is much less distinct than that of an unaffected individual.
- As a result of these abnormalities, the metaphyses of the appendicular skeleton appear widened or flared, and angular deformities will occur over time and may be influenced by weightbearing.
- Similar changes may be seen in the long bones of those patients with a number of the metaphyseal dysplasias, most commonly those of the Schmid or McKusick type.
  - Assessment of serum chemistries may be necessary to differentiate patients with certain skeletal dysplasias from those with changes secondary to rickets.
- Radiographic abnormalities are also evident within the diaphyseal regions of the more tubular bones.
- Deposits of nonossified osteoid present as transverse radiolucent lines that may resemble fractures.
  - These areas are often referred to as Looser lines, or Milkman pseudofractures, and may be seen in up to 25% of patients with rickets (Fig. 25.1-2).
  - These lesions classically occur along the compressive sides of long bones, including the proximal femur, as well as the ribs, clavicle, and pelvis.
  - The etiology of Looser lines is unclear, but they may be the result of incomplete fractures through areas weakened by the generalized abnormality of bone maturation and development.

Laboratory Data

Serum blood chemistry evaluation is an essential part of the diagnosis of rickets, and is the basis of the differential diagnosis process, particularly since the radiographic findings are fairly consistent within multiple etiologies. Information regarding the differences in laboratory values between the various causes of rickets of interest to the pediatric orthopaedic surgeon is presented in Table 25.1-1.

TREATMENT

Management of rickets begins with determination of the exact cause of the bone changes, thereby allowing initiation of appropriate medical care. It cannot be stressed too highly that *medical therapy directed toward correction of the underlying biochemical abnormality must be the initial step.* Any surgical intervention in the face of untreated or active rickets is doomed to fail and presents significant risk to the patient. Because of this, coordination between health care professionals providing medical/endocrinologic care and those providing orthopaedic management is essential.

Once adequate medical intervention is established, and improvement is documented through biochemical data and radiographic evidence of stabilization or improvement of the growth plates, it is then appropriate to contemplate surgical management. Bracing of the lower extremities may be instituted during the period of attempted medical treatment; however, there is controversy in the literature

TABLE 25.1-1 SERUM LEVELS IN RICKETS

Type	Calcium	Phosphate	25(OH) Vitamin D	1,25(OH)$_2$ Vitamin D	Alkaline Phosphotase
Vitamin D deficiency	↓ or ↔	↓	↓	↓	↑
Calcium deficiency (rare)	↓	↔	↔	↔	↑
Phosphate deficiency	↔	↓	↓	↓ or ↔	↑
Malabsorption rickets	↓	↓	↓	↓ or ↔	↑
Vitamin D resistant (hypophosphatemic)	↔	↓	↔	↔	↑
Renal osteodystrophy	↓	↑	↓	↓	↑
Diminished vitamin D activation	↓	↓	↔	↓	↑

regarding benefit. Some very young patients with dietary (or vitamin D sensitive) rickets demonstrate spontaneous improvement of their limb deformities after the metabolic issues are stabilized and do not require any surgical or orthotic intervention.

- Surgical management of angular deformities associated with rickets involves realignment osteotomies, and such procedures are required most frequently for distal femoral and proximal tibial deformities.
  - Traditionally, corrections have been performed acutely within the metaphyseal regions of the involved bones, and have been stabilized with trans-fixing pins, compression plating, or casts.
  - Modern methods of angular correction using external fixation (monolateral or circular frames) have greatly enhanced the process through more precise correction and improved stability of fixation, thereby eliminating the need for additional cast immobilization.
  - Compartment syndromes, delayed unions and malunions, and superficial and deep infections are reported risks of realignment procedures, particularly of the tibia.
- Either acute or gradual correction may be obtained using external fixation techniques, and both allow greater patient mobility and activity in the postoperative period than those methods requiring supplemental cast treatment.
- Immobility is a particular problem in this patient population as it may cause significant shifts in serum calcium levels, exposing the patient to the inherent risks posed by such changes.
- Regardless of the type of procedure or fixation system, there is a significant risk of recurrence for any skeletally immature patient in whom medical or dietary management of the underlying process is not maintained.
- This is more of a problem for those patients with rickets secondary to genetic abnormalities of mineral absorption or excretion, or vitamin D metabolism.
- Because of heightened awareness and greater vigilance regarding appropriate intake and the need for adequate UV light exposure, dietary rickets rarely recurs.

SUGGESTED READING

Biser-Rohrbaugh A, Hadley-Miller N. Vitamin D deficiency in breast-fed toddlers. J Pediatr Orthop 2001;21:508–511.

Kanel JS, Price CT. Unilateral external fixation for corrective osteotomies in patients with hypophosphatemic rickets. J Pediatr Orthop 1995;15:232–235.

Lee DY, Choi IH, Lee, CK, et al. Acquired vitamin D-resistant rickets caused by aggressive osteoblastoma in the pelvis: a case report with ten years' follow-up and review of the literature. J Pediatr Orthop 1994;14:793–798.

Pinkowski JL, Weiner DS. Complications in proximal tibial osteotomies in children with presentation of technique. J Pediatr Orthop 1995;15:307–312.

Rohmiller MT, Tylkowski C, Kriss VM, et al. The effect of osteotomy on bowing and height in children with X-linked hypophosphatemia. J Pediatr Orthop 1999;19:114–118.

Rubinovitch M, Glorieux FH, Cruess RL, et al. Principles and results of lower limb osteotomies for patients with vitamin D-resistant hypophosphatemic rickets. Clin Orthop 1988;237:264–270.

Specker BC, Valanis B, Hertzber V. Sunshine exposure and serum 25-hydroxyvitamin D concentrations in exclusively breast-fed infants. J Pediatr 1985;107:372–376.

Verge CF, Lam A, Simpson JM, et al. Effects of therapy of x-linked hypophosphatemic rickets. N Engl J Med 1991;325:1843–1848.

Zaleske DJ. Metabolic and endocrine abnormalities. In: Morrissey RT, Weinstein SL, eds. Lovell and Winter's pediatric orthopaedics, 4th ed. Vol 1. Philadelphia: Lippincott Williams & Wilkins, 2001: 177–241.

25.2 RENAL OSTEODYSTROPHY

SUSAN A. SCHERL

Renal osteodystrophy is the name given to describe the constellation of pathologic bony entities that can occur in the patient with underlying renal disease.

PATHOPHYSIOLOGY

- Damage to the glomerular tubules of the kidney leads to phosphate retention and decreased production of the active form of vitamin D (1,25-dihydroxy vitamin D).
- This leads to the inability of the gut to absorb calcium.
- The resulting hypocalcemia leads to secondary hyperparathyroidism and bone resorption, in the body's attempt to maintain normal serum calcium levels.

There are four clinical entities of renal osteodystrophy:

- Rickets or osteomalacia—decreased mineralization of osteoid.
- Osteitis fibrosis cystica—severe lytic lesions of bone caused by increased levels of parathyroid hormone.
- Osteosclerosis—due to increased *numbers* of bony trabeculae, *not* increased mineralization of bone. This occurs in 20% of patients, and is most evident in the long bones and spine.
- Ectopic calcification—a by-product of the hypophosphatemia of renal patients. They are typically acidotic, which allows for increased serum solubility of calcium salts. However, if the level of serum calcium increases to

near normal, either spontaneously or secondary to diet or dialysis, calcium salts will precipitate out of the bloodstream into the corneas, conjunctivae, skin, arteriolar walls, and periarticular soft tissues.

DIAGNOSIS

Clinical Features

- Short stature
- Developmental delay
- Delay in appearance of secondary growth characteristics
- All of the clinical findings associated with any form of rickets
- Infections and pathologic fractures: frequently the side effects of treatment with either steroids or dialysis
- Bony tenderness
- Soft tissue itching and irritation: secondary to ectopic calcification
- Joint pain and decreased range of motion: secondary to ectopic calcification
- Gait disturbances
- Slipped epiphyses: due to severe hyperparathyroidism, which causes resorption of metaphyseal bone and leads to epiphyseal lysis
  - Most commonly proximal femur, but can be proximal humerus, distal femur, or distal tibia
  - Slipping of the distal radius and ulna occurs in older children; can lead to significant deformity

Radiographic Features

- Findings typical of rickets
- Lesions typical of osteitis fibrosis cystica:
  - "Salt and pepper" skull
  - Absence of the cortical outline of the distal centimeter of the clavicles
  - Subperiosteal resorption of the ulnae, phalangeal distal tufts, and medial proximal tibiae
- Brown tumors—large, lytic lesions with indistinct borders, often in the pelvis or long bones, characteristic of hyperparathyroidism

TREATMENT

- Usually multidisciplinary, involving a nephrologist and endocrinologist as well as an orthopaedist.
- Management of the underlying primary renal disorder, using steroids, dialysis, or renal transplantation.
- Control of calcium and phosphate levels using drug regimens.
- Parathyroidectomy is sometimes necessary to control hyperparathyroidism.
- Vitamin D must be used carefully to avoid the complication of ectopic calcification.
- Pinning of epiphyseal slips.
- Osteotomies for limb deformity are sometimes necessary.

SUGGESTED READING

Zaleske DJ. Metabolic and endocrine abnormalities. In: Morrissey RT, Weinstein SL, eds. Lovell and Winter's pediatric orthopaedics, 4th ed. Vol 1. Philadelphia: Lippincott Williams & Wilkins, 2001: 177–241.

HEMATOLOGY

26.1 HEMOPHILIC ARTHROPATHY

DANIEL W. GREEN ■ CEMIL YILDIZ

Hemophilia is a sex-linked genetic coagulation disorder that occurs primarily in males, resulting in clotting factors that are nonfunctional or absent. Intraarticular hemorrhages in patients with poorly controlled hemophilia can lead to progressive joint arthropathy. The natural history of the disorder has changed significantly over the past several decades, due to the development of factor replacement therapy, but considerable orthopaedic morbidity still occurs.

PATHOGENESIS

Epidemiology and Etiology

- The incidence of hemophilia is estimated to be 1 per 10,000 male births in the United States.
- Approximately 95% of cases are caused by a variable lack of factors VIII or IX.
- Hemophilia A (factor VIII deficiency) is the most common (about 80% of cases).
  - Several different mutations cause the disorder, which accounts for the variable clinical severity.
  - It is an X-linked recessive disorder that affects males.
  - Hemophilia A is the result of a new mutation in approximately 33% of patients.
- Hemophilia B (factor IX deficiency), also known as Christmas disease, is the next most common.
  - Clinically indistinguishable from hemophilia A.
  - Also transmitted as an X-linked disorder.
- The third most common inherited coagulation disorder is von Willebrand disease, caused by a variable lack not only of factor VIII coagulant activity but also of factor VIII–related activity responsible for adhesion of platelets to exposed vascular subendothelium.
  - This form is characterized by abnormal bleeding from mucosal surfaces, therefore major hemophilic arthropathy is relatively uncommon.

Pathophysiology

- The exact pathophysiology of hemophilic arthropathy remains controversial.
- Both the inflammatory cascade and iron deposition have been implicated in cartilage destruction.
- The degree of hemarthropathy does not always directly correlate with the number of joint bleeds.
- Hemarthrosis probably starts as a subsynovial, intramural hemorrhage that then ruptures into the joint cavity.
- Spontaneous hemorrhages without antecedent trauma commonly occur in patients with a severe deficiency.
- With repeated exposure to blood, the synovium of joint hypertrophies and becomes hypervascular, leading to a progressive cycle of synovitis and more bleeding.
- Histology of the hypertrophic synovium is characterized by villous formation, markedly increased vascularity, and chronic inflammatory cells.
- Hemosiderin deposits accumulate in the lining cells of the synovial villi, and the inflammatory cells congregate around the vessels and hemosiderin deposits.
- In summary, the result of repeated hemorrhage into a joint with chronic synovitis
- Proteolytic enzymes released by the inflamed synovium attack both cartilage and bone.

TABLE 26.1-1 GRADING OF SYNOVITIS AND ARTICULAR INVOLVEMENT IN HEMOPHILIC PATIENTS

Grade	Classificaiton	Description
I	Transitory synovitis	No bleeding sequelae, and no more than 3 episodes in 3 months. No evidence of chronic inflammation remains after treatment.
II	Permanent synovitis	Persistence of increased joint size/volume, synovial membrane thickening, and joint range limitation. Muscle atrophy cannot be detected in 1st week. However, vastus medialis is 1st muscle to become atrophic and quadriceps volume reduction becomes noticeable in 2nd week.
III	Chronic arthropathy	Grade II findings are present in grade III together with axial deformities and severe muscular atrophy. Joint changes are irreversible.
IV	Ankylosis	

Adapted from Battistella LR. Maintenance of musculoskeletal function in people with hemophilia. Haemophilia 1998;42:26–32.

- As the hypertrophied synovium continues to expand, and the articular cartilage erodes, the joint space narrows.
- Osteoporosis occurs from disuse, and the joint becomes immobile.
- Grading of articular involvement can be seen in Table 26.1-1.
- In children, chronic synovitis may also cause asymmetric physeal growth, or early physeal closure, leading to angular deformities or leg length discrepancies.

DIAGNOSIS

Clinical Features

- A history of similarly affected males on the maternal side of the family, or typical behavior
- A history of hemorrhage from major surface wounds and musculoskeletal sites.
- Hemophiliacs rarely experience bleeding during the first years of life in the absence of trauma or surgery.
  - Hemarthroses usually begin after the child starts to walk.
- The frequency and severity of bleeding episodes commonly increase as the child attends school and becomes more physically active and socially interactive.

TABLE 26.1-2 DIFFERENTIATING BLEEDING FROM SYNOVITIS

Bleeding	Synovitis
Acute onset	Slow onset
Painful	Minimal pain
Warm and tender	Warm and nontender
Marked limitation of motion	Good range of motion
Responds rapidly to factor replacement	Does not respond rapidly to factor replacement (responds to prednisone)

- Patients with severe hemophilia typically develop their initial joint pathology between the ages of 5 to 15 years.
- Abnormal bleeding may occur in any area of the body, but joints are the most frequent sites of repeated hemorrhage (Table 26.1-2).
- The weightbearing joints are the most common sites of hemophilic arthropathy, with the frequency of involvement being, in decreasing order, the knee, elbow, shoulder, ankle, wrist, and hip. The vertebral column is rarely involved.
- Clinical findings depend on the severity of hemorrhage and whether the hemarthrosis is acute, subacute, or chronic (Table 26.1-3).
- Other musculoskeletal problems in hemophilia include:
  - Pseudotumor (slowly progressive hemorrhage that increases in size within a confined space, causing pressure necrosis and erosion of the surrounding tissues)
  - Neuropraxias (femoral, peroneal, sciatic, median, and ulnar)
  - Ectopic ossifications
  - Fractures
  - Ischemic contractures or compartment syndrome
- After history and physical examination, laboratory tests should be ordered (Table 26.1-4). If these screening procedures suggest a bleeding tendency, factor assays must be carried out to establish not only the specific deficiency but also its degree.
- Most patients with hemophilia present to an orthopaedist with a known diagnosis. Clinical manifestations of hemophilia A and B are similar and depend on the blood levels of factor VIII or IX (Table 26.1-5).

Radiologic Features

Features of radiographs in knee hemarthrosis (Fig. 26.1-1):

- Distended capsule
- Synovitis
- Cartilage thinning
- Widening and erosion of intercondylar notch
- Enlargement of ossification centers (especially distal end of femur)

TABLE 26.1-3 CLINICAL STAGES OF HEMARTHROSIS

Stages of Hemarthrosis	Characteristic Findings	Response of Factor Replacement Therapy
Acute	Pain and swelling with distention of the joint capsule are the principal findings. Local tenderness and increased heat are present. The joint will assume the position of minimal discomfort, which is also the position of minimal intraarticular pressure (e.g., knee joint is held in flexion).	Rapid
Subacute	Develops after several episodes of bleeding into the joint. Pain is minimal. Joint motion is moderately restricted.	Slow
Chronic	Develops after 6 months of involvement. Progressive destruction of the joint takes place, with the end stage being a fibrotic, stiff, totally destroyed joint	No

TABLE 26.1-4 ROUTINE LABORATORY TESTS FOR PATIENTS WITH COAGULOPATHY

Tests	Objectives
Platelet count combined with inspection of the blood smear	
Ivy bleeding time	To assess platelet function, defective in hemophilia A and B
Plasma prothrombin time (PT)	To assess the extrinsic and common pathways of coagulation (I, II, V, VII, X)
Plasma partial thromboplastin time (PPT)	To assess the intrinsic and common pathways of coagulation (II, V, VIII, IX, X, XI, XII). Defective in hemophilia A and B

TABLE 26.1-5 CLINICAL MANIFESTATIONS OF HEMOPHILIA ACCORDING TO BLOOD LEVELS OF FACTORS VIII AND IX

Degree	Level of Hemostasis (% of Normal Blood Level)	Clinical Findings
Normal	>50	None
Mild	25–50	Excessive bleeding occurs only after major trauma or during surgery
Moderate	5–25	Severe and uncontrolled bleeding occurs only after minor injury or during an operative surgery
Moderately severe	1–5	Major hemorrhages occurring after minor injury or unrecognized mild trauma
Very severe	<1	Repeated spontaneous hemorrhages into joints and bleeding into deep soft tissues

- Widening of distal femoral epiphysis
- Squaring of inferior pole of patella
- Flattening of distal femoral condyles
- Hemophiliac pseudotumor
- Epiphyseal overgrowth with leg length discrepancy
- Osteopenia

The radiologic evaluation classification recommended by the orthopaedic advisory committee of the World Federation of Hemophilia is shown Table 26.1-6. It includes functional status. An additional radiographic classification useful for bony changes is shown in Table 26.1-7.

Evaluation of the clinical stage of hemophilic arthritis has improved with the use of ultrasound and magnetic resonance imaging (MRI), which can provide early, detailed information about the synovium, cartilage, and the joint spaces.

- Hemosiderin deposits can be seen on MRI (Fig. 26.1-2), as can subchondral and intraosseous cysts or hemorrhage (Figs. 26.1-3 and 26.1-4).

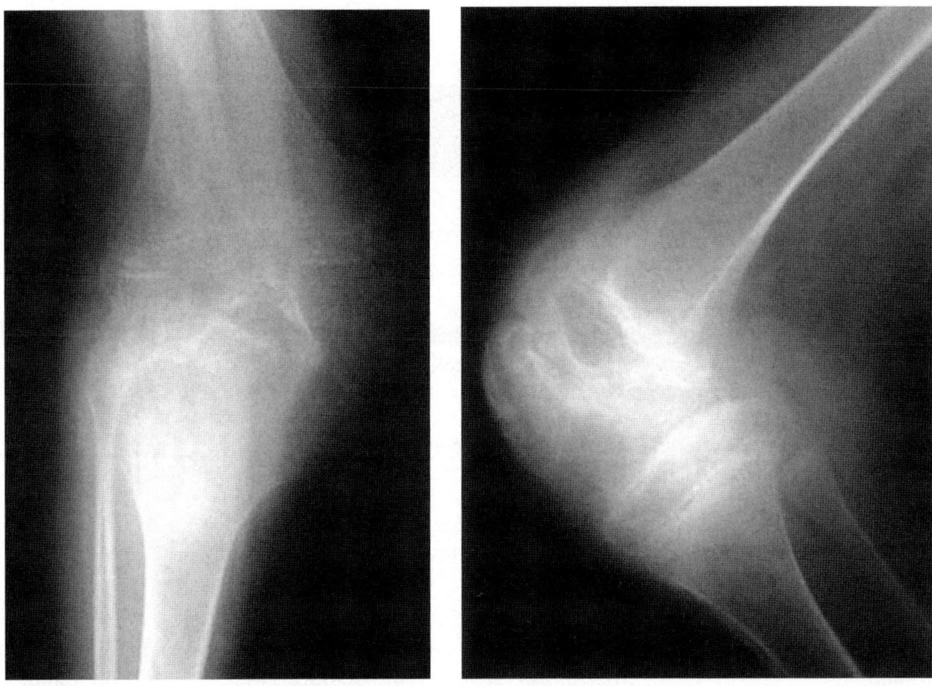

Figure 26.1-1 Anteroposterior (**A**) and lateral (**B**) knee plain radiographs of a 10-year-old boy with hemophilia: loss of joint cartilage space, marked enlargement of the epiphysis, and extensive joint destruction (stage V according to Arnold and Hilgartner radiographic classification).

TABLE 26.1-6 ROENTGENOGRAPHIC CLASSIFICATION OF HEMOPHILIC ARTHROPATHY

Radiologic Change	Score
Osteoporosis	
Absent	0
Present	1
Enlarged epiphysis	
Absent	0
Present	1
Irregular subchondral surface	
Absent	0
Present	1
Narrowing of joint space	
Absent	0
Present, joint space >1 mm	1
Present, joint space <1 mm	2
Subchondral cyst formation	
Absent	0
Present	1
Erosions at joint margins	0
Absent	1
1 cyst	2
>1 cyst	
Gross incongruence of articulating bone ends (angulation or displacement between articulating bone ends)	
Absent	0
Slight	1
Pronounced	2
Joint deformity	0
Absent	1
Slight	2
Pronounced	
Possible total	*0 to 13*

Adapted from Petterson H, Ahlberg A, Nilsson IM. A radiologic classification of hemophilic arthropathy. Clin Orthop 1980;149:153–156.

TABLE 26.1-7 RADIOGRAPHIC CLASSIFICATION OF HEMOPHILIC ARTHROPATHY

Stage	Description
0	Normal joint
I	No skeletal abnormalities; soft tissue swelling present
II	Osteoporosis and overgrowth of epiphysis; no erosions; no narrowing of cartilage space
III	Early subchondral bone cysts; squaring of the patella; intercondylar notch of distal femur or humerus widened; cartilage remains preserved
IV	Findings of stage III more advanced; cartilage space narrowed
V	Fibrous joint contracture; loss of joint cartilage space; marked enlargement of the epiphysis and substantial disorganization of the joint (extensive joint destruction)

Adapted from Arnold WD, Hilgartner MW. Hemophilic arthropathy. J Bone Joint Surg (Am) 1977;59:287–290.

- The limitation of MRI is that the cost may be prohibitive when serial exams are necessary.
- Ultrasound has been shown to be a sensitive and reproducible technique to assess synovial proliferation in a variety of joints.
- The activity of disease, in terms of acute synovitis, may further be assessed with power Doppler ultrasound.

TREATMENT

Treatment of hemophilia is generally overseen by a hematologist, with input from a variety of other medical professionals including orthopaedists, physical therapists, vocational therapists, nurses, dentists, social workers, psychiatrists, and genetic counselors. There are several factors that affect the choice of type of therapy (Table 26.1-8).

Medical Treatment

The most common approach to medical management in North America involves early intervention for bleeding episodes with increased factor given at the onset of discomfort and, if possible, even prior to the observation of joint swelling. This approach is often referred to as an on-demand treatment. It involves the use of home infusion of factor VIII without the need to be seen initially at a hospital or a clinic. Factor levels of 30 to 50 IU/dL are optimal in controlling an acute hemorrhage.

Prophylactic factor replacement (to maintain plasma factor levels greater than 1%) prevents hemophilic arthropathy better than on-demand therapy (Table 26.1-9).

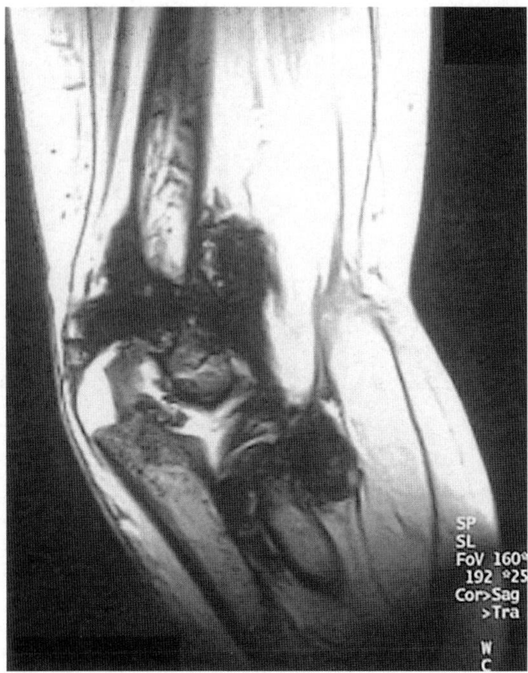

Figure 26.1-2 Right elbow magnetic resonance image of a 6-year-old boy with hemophilia. Synovial hypertrophy and large hemosiderin deposit are seen.

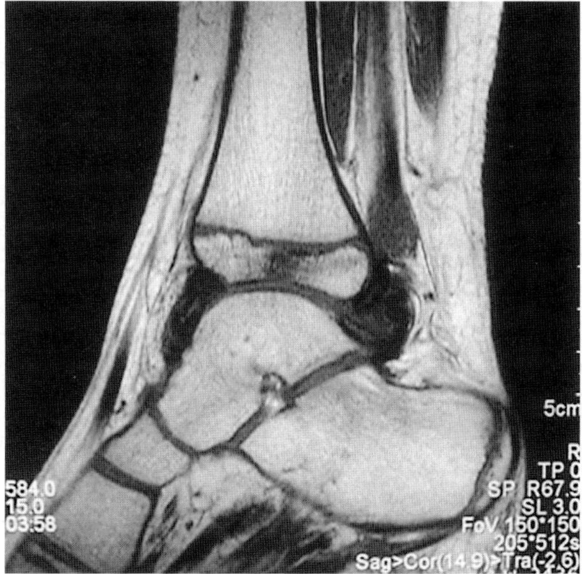

Figure 26.1-3 Left ankle sagittal magnetic resonance image of a 6-year-old boy with hemophilia. Subchondral bone cyst is seen.

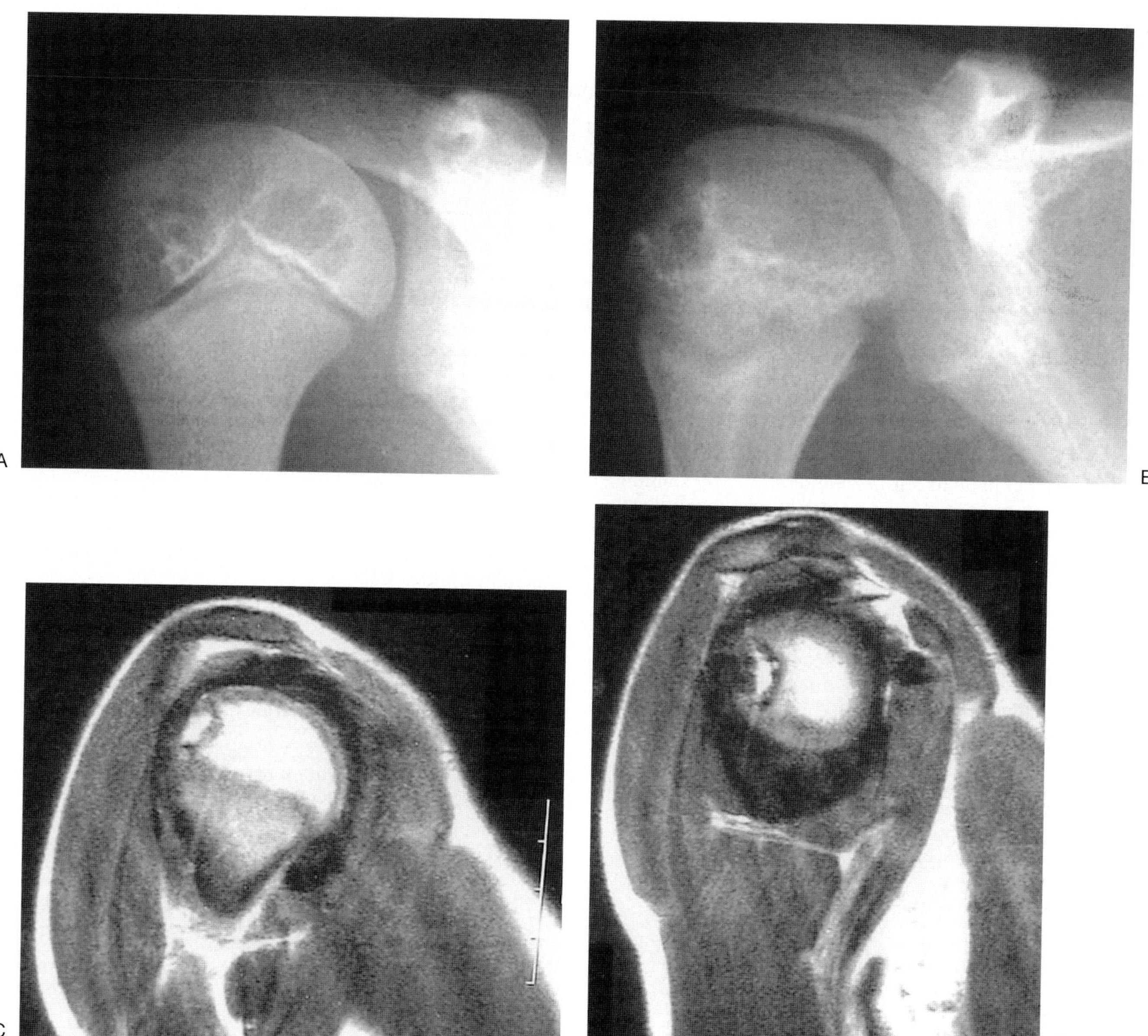

Figure 26.1-4 Eight-year-old boy with factor VIII deficiency. (**A and B**) Anteroposterior plain x-rays of the shoulder show cyst formation in the humeral head. (**C and D**) Coronal magnetic resonance images reveal marked synovial hyperplasia and hemosiderin deposits, called a *blooming* appearance.

TABLE 26.1-8 FACTORS THAT AFFECT THE CHOICE OF THERAPY FOR HEMOPHILIC ARTHROPATHY

Factor	Effects
Age	3–6 mo of conservative care is indicated at any age
Inhibitor status	Chemical synovectomy, which involves only an injection and not a surgical approach, is the procedure of choice
Associated medical factors	In cases in which HIV or hepatitis are advanced, radiosynovectomy is procedure of choice
Joint status	With advanced arthritis changes, results of synovectomy are less successful
Multiple joint involvement	Indication for chemical or radiation synovectomy because several joints can be treated at same time
Economic/geographic	Not all treatment modalities are available at hemophilia treatment centers throughout the world
Other	Expertise of treating physician

HIV, human immunodeficiency virus.

TABLE 26.1-9 PROPHYLACTIC TREATMENT OF HEMOPHILIC ARTHROPATHY

Model	Definition
Primary prophylaxis	Regular continuous treatment started before age of 2 yr or after first joint bleed
Secondary prophylaxis	A. Regular continuous (long-term) treatment, started at the age of >2 yr or after 2 or more joint bleeds B. Periodic (short-term) treatment, due to frequent bleeds

It has been useful in preventing the spontaneous bleeding typically seen in patients with severe disease. The amount of product necessary to achieve a nonbleeding state with few breakthrough bleeding episodes varies from patient to patient. The age of onset at which a patient may begin to experience hemarthrosis also varies, but is usually before the age of 4 years. Decreased hemophilic joint destruction and arthropathy have been demonstrated in patients who have started prophylaxis at 2 to 3 years of age. In certain situations, factor VIII levels should be increased for prophylaxis (Table 26.1-10).

Because of the risk of human immunodeficiency virus (HIV) transmission and hepatitis in human factor VIII replacement, recombinant products are preferred and are available for factors VII, VIII, and IX. The dosage required to replace a factor deficiency depends on the patient's weight and plasma volume. The hematologist makes the calculation and is in charge of administering the factor. The orthopaedic surgeon, however, should be aware of the fact that 20 to 30 minutes after administration of the antihemophilic factor, the plasma level will rise.

Pain Management

Analgesics such as aspirin, that are known to inhibit platelet aggregation and prolong the bleeding time, should be avoided in patients with hemophilia. Patients should be warned against the use of any medication containing an aspirin compound, guaiacolate, or antihistamine. Proxyphene, paracetamol, meperidine, codeine amitriptyline, or methadone may be used. Narcotic analgesics are used with care because in such a chronic disease, addiction can easily become a problem.

TABLE 26.1-10 SITUATIONS IN WHICH FACTOR VIII LEVELS SHOULD BE INCREASED

Situation	Percentage of Normal Level
Physical therapy	20
Treatment of hematoma	30
Acute hemarthrosis	>50
Soft tissue surgery	>50
Skeletal surgery	100 (preoperatively); >50 (postoperative 10 days)

Physical Therapy

Early physical therapy helps to prevent complications and yields the best results. Adequately prescribed and correctly supervised physiotherapy very rarely requires concurrent replacement therapy, except after surgery. Every patient generally requires individual exercise programs.

Orthosis

Any orthosis must be lightweight and should have a cushioned lining. Care should be taken to avoid muscle atrophy. There are four distinct functions for orthoses used in hemophiliac arthropathy:

1. Protection and stabilization of an unstable joint
2. Nocturnal use, in the immediate postoperative period or to complete casting
3. Prevention of some joint contractures, in particular flexion deformity
4. Braces, splints, and walking bandaging are useful to enhance joint stability without limiting movement.

Surgical Treatment

Surgical procedures useful in the management of hemophilic arthropathy are generally divided into two groups: procedures such as synovectomy that are done to control repetitive joint bleeding episodes and the more conventional orthopaedic procedures designed to correct or reconstruct joint deformities.

Surgery in hemophiliacs should be carried out with careful technique using tourniquet control when feasible and securely ligating all vessels insofar as possible. Cautery is a less satisfactory method of hemostasis in hemophiliacs. Before the wound is closed, the tourniquet must be released and bleeding surgically controlled. Appropriate perioperative factor replacement is imperative.

Aspiration

The need for routine joint aspiration has been debated. Some experts recommend aspiration only for an extremely tense hemarthrosis and avoid aspiration in ordinary cases, citing the risk of introducing infection, the discomfort to the patient, and the possibility that aspiration will incite more bleeding of the joint. Aspiration of the joint should be performed under strict aseptic conditions.

BOX 26.1-1 SYNOVECTOMY INDICATIONS IN HEMOPHILIC ARTHROPATHY

- Severe recurrent hemarthrosis (2 or 3 major bleeding episodes/mo)
- Hemarthrosis that does not respond to aggressive medical management maintained for ≥6 mo
- Failure to respond to orthopaedic nonsurgical treatment consisting of physical therapy and protection with crutches and orthoses
- Radiographic stage II or III hemophilic arthropathy

Synovectomy

The objective of synovectomy is to prevent progression of hemophilic arthropathy. The general consensus of opinion is that synovectomy relieves pain, decreases swelling, and diminishes the number of bleeding episodes per year (Box 26.1-1). Synovectomy is ineffective and contraindicated patients with radiographic stage IV or V hemophilic arthropathy.

Traditional open synovectomy is often complicated by loss of range of motion of the affected joint. Arthroscopic synovectomy is most useful when performed before severe degenerative changes have developed. Contraindication for arthroscopy of hemophilic patients is inhibitory antibodies to factor replacement. As complete a synovectomy as possible should be performed. After surgical synovectomy the knee should be immobilized in a Jones bandage for 3 days and active movement encouraged. Postoperative factor replacement supervised by a hematologist is required. Weidel has shown with a 10- to 15-year follow-up that the procedure was effective in stopping the bleeding episodes, and by maintaining the range of motion, joint deterioration continued to progress at a slower rate.

Radiosynovectomy consists of destruction of synovial tissue by intraarticular injection of a radioactive agent (yttrium-90, gold-198, phosphorus-32, and rhenium-186). It requires only one session, but has a higher cost (Box 26.1-2). A possible concern is that the damaging effects of the radioactivity are not strictly limited to the synovium but may also affect the articular chondrocytes. In addition, there is a theoretic concern of future oncogenesis (Fig. 26.1-5).

Chemical synovectomy has been performed with rifampicin, D-penicillamine, and osmic acid. Rifampicin is commonly used with successful results for chemical synovectomy in developing countries where there is a lack of radioactive materials. However, it is quite painful during injection and must be injected weekly, with the number of injections ranging from 5 (in ankles and elbows) to 10 (in knees). Osmic acid is another agent for using chemical synovectomy, but its results are no better than those of rifampicin.

BOX 26.1-2 POTENTIAL ADVANTAGES OF CHEMICAL OR RADIATION SYNOVECTOMY OVER SURGICAL SYNOVECTOMY IN HEMOPHILIC ARTHROPATHY

- A minimal requirement of antihemophilic factor
- Performance on an outpatient basis
- Concurrent treatment of several joints
- Low risk of hemorrhage in patients with inhibitors
- Administration of local anesthetic only, which is beneficial in patients who are not candidates for surgery because of systemic illness
- Low cost

Arthroplasty

The ultimate procedure for hemophilic arthropathy is total joint replacement. Disabling pain with advanced destruction of articular cartilage is the prime indication for surgery. It has been done routinely for knees, hips, and shoulders and sporadically for elbows and ankles. The problems of arthroplasty in hemophiliacs are considerable and include difficulties with lack of bone stock, deformities of the joint, muscle contractures, adhesions, and soft tissue contractures. The most common cause of failure is infection. It is difficult to salvage prostheses complicated by infection. However, the life expectancy of hemophilic patients is lower than that of the general population of patients treated with total knee arthroplasty, and the improvement in the quality of life after knee arthroplasty for hemophilic arthropathy may outweigh the risk of failure.

Total hip replacement is indicated in stage IV or stage V hemophiliac arthropathy when pain is persistent with severe disability not relieved by conservative measures. The most common problem is aseptic loosening of cemented components, probably because of microhemorrhages at the bone–cement surface. Studies suggest that arthroplasty, particularly of the hip and knee, can be a valuable option in the management of severe hemophilic arthropathy although complications are commonly described and the surgery is technically demanding.

Arthrodesis

Arthrodesis is a salvage procedure for hip and knee joints in which arthroplasty has failed or become infected. Arthrodesis of the ankle, subtalar, and midtarsal joints in the foot, elbow, or shoulder may be indicated when these joints are destroyed.

Fractures

Fractures usually heal in the normal time. Whenever possible, fractures are treated by closed reduction and immobilization in a cast. External fixators should be avoided. Open reduction and internal fixation are carried out when closed methods are not appropriate.

Hemophilic Pseudotumors

Symptomatic pseudotumors should be excised if they are accessible. Prior to surgical intervention, angiography, computed tomography, and nuclear MRI should be performed to provide accurate anatomic detail of adjacent vessels. Rarely, radiotherapy may be considered in surgically inaccessible sites.

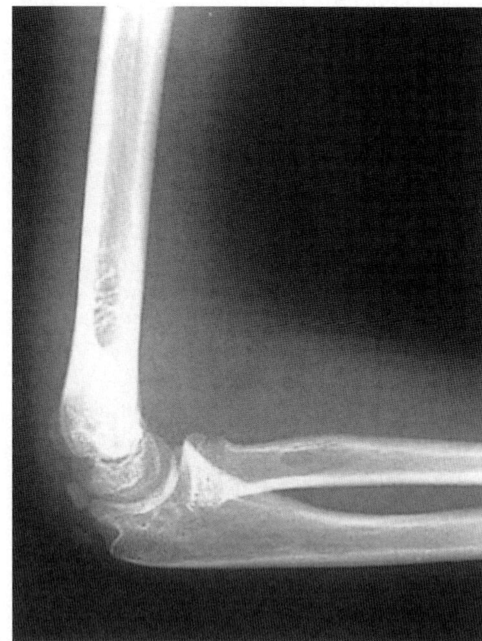
A

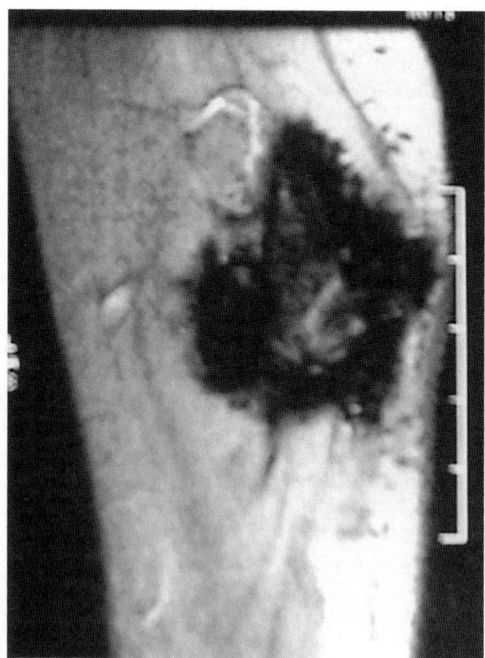
B

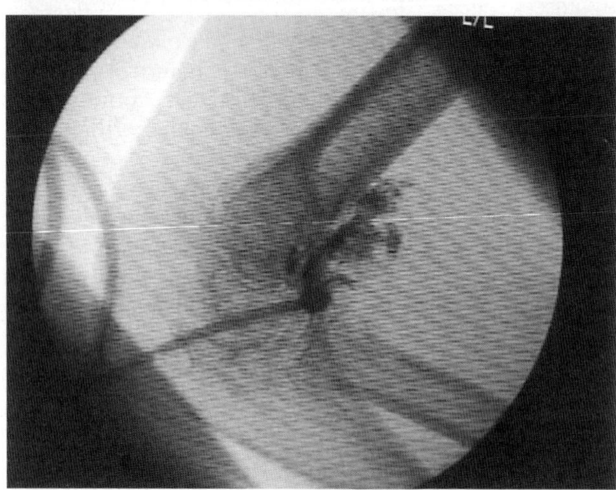
C

Figure 26.1-5 Right elbow lateral plain radiograph (**A**) and coronal magnetic resonance image (**B**) of an 8-year-old boy with hemophilia A and recurrent bleeding approximately eight times a year despite factor treatment. (**C**) Right elbow P-32 radioisotope synovectomy was performed.

Neuropraxia

Neuropraxia is treated by factor replacement therapy. Occasionally, decompression of the entrapped nerve may be required.

SUGGESTED READING

Arnold WD, Hilgartner MW. Hemophilic arthropathy. J Bone Joint Surg (Am) 1977;59:287–290.

Battistella LR. Maintenance of musculoskeletal function in people with hemophilia. Haemophilia 1998;4 2:26–32.

Beeton K, Rodriguez-Merchan EC, Altree J. Total joint arthroplasty in hemophilia. Haemophilia 2000;6:474–481.

Eickhoff HH, Koch W, Raderschadt G, et al. Arthroscopy for chronic hemophilic synovitis of the knee. Clin Orthop 1997;343:58–62.

Fernandez-Palazzi F, Rivas S, Viso R, et al. Synovectomy with rifampicine in hemophiliac haemarthrosis. Haemophilia 2000;6: 562–565.

Gilbert MS, Radomisli TE. Therapeutic options in the management of hemophilic synovitis. Clin Orthop 1997;343:88–92.

Greene WB, Wilson FC. The management of musculoskeletal problems in hemophilia. Part II (Pathophysiologic and roentgenographic changes in hemophilic arthropathy). AAOS Instr Course Lect 1983;32:217–233.

Hermann G, Gilbert MS, Abdelwahab IF. Hemophilia: evaluation of musculoskeletal involvement with CT, sonography, and MR imaging. AJR Am J Roentgenol 1992;158:119–123.

Hilgartner MW. Current treatment of hemophilic arthropathy. Curr Opin Pediatr 2002;14:46–49.

Norian JM, Ries MD, Karp S, et al. Total knee arthroplasty in hemophilic arthropathy. J Bone Joint Surg (Am) 2002;84:1138–1141.

Petterson H, Ahlberg A, Nilsson IM. A radiologic classification of hemophilic arthropathy. Clin Orthop 1980;149:153–156.

Rodriguez-Merchan EC, Wiedel JD. General principles and indications of synoviorthesis (medical synovectomy) in haemophilia. Haemophilia 2001;7(Suppl 2):6–10.

Saphiro F. Hematologic disorders. In: Pediatric orthopaedic deformities—basic science, diagnosis, and treatment. San Diego: Academic Press, 2001:909–933.

Siegel HJ, Luck JV Jr, Siegel ME, et al. Phosphate-32 colloid radiosynovectomy in hemophilia: outcome of 125 procedures. Clin Orthop 2001;392:409–417.

Wiedel JD. Arthroscopic synovectomy of the knee in hemophilia: 10- to 15-year follow-up. Clin Orthop 1996;328:46–53.

26.2 SICKLE CELL ANEMIA

SUSAN A. SCHERL

Sickle cell diseases are a group of hereditary hemoglobinopathies, which cause chronic hemolytic anemia, immunosuppression, and pain and organ damage secondary to vascular occlusion. Variants include sickle cell anemia (SCA), hemoglobin SC disease, and hemoglobin S β-thalassemia. SCA is the most common form, and can present with numerous musculoskeletal manifestations and complications. The diagnosis and management of the musculoskeletal problems associated with SCA can pose a considerable challenge to the orthopaedist.

PATHOGENESIS

Etiology

Sickle cell disorders occur as the result of an inherited genetic mutation that codes for the substitution of normal adult hemoglobin (HbA) with sickle hemoglobin (HbS), or less commonly, with another variety of abnormal hemoglobin. Normal HbA consists of two α-polypeptide chains and two β-polypeptide chains. In HbS, a mutation on chromosome 11 substitutes valine for glutamine in the sixth amino acid position of the β-globin chain. Children who are homozygous for the mutation have SCA; heterozygotes have sickle cell trait (SCT).

Epidemiology

About 8% of African Americans (approximately 2 million people) have SCT, and approximately 1 in 400 has SCA. In regions where malaria is endemic, the incidence of SCT can be as high as 40%, since heterozygotes have slightly increased resistance to malaria. Individuals of a variety of other ethnicities (Mediterranean, Asian, Hispanic, and Middle Eastern) may also inherit the trait or disease. The total number of persons in the United States with a clinically manifest variant of sickle cell disease is about 72,000.

Pathophysiology

Low oxygen tension causes hemoglobin S to polymerize, which changes it from a liquid to a gel. The orientation of the hemoglobin S molecules into longitudinal fibers, combined with their decreased plasticity due to increased viscosity, is what causes the characteristic sickling of the erythrocytes. The presence of other forms of hemoglobin mitigates the severity of the sickling. That is why heterozygotes, whom have a significant proportion of HbA, are clinically asymptomatic, except under conditions of severe hypoxia. Similarly, sickle cell disease does not clinically manifest itself in children under the age of 1 year, since fetal hemoglobin (HbF), which persists until that time, is protective. Even other abnormal hemoglobins, such as those with the thalassemia mutation, which decreases the amount of β-globulin produced, generally are less severely affected than HbSS homozygotes.

Other conditions that increase the rate of HbS polymerization include dehydration, increased temperature, and falling pH. Though sickling is reversible, repeated episodes cause cell membrane damage that leads to permanently sickled cells. These cells are hemolyzed intravascularly or in the spleen. The average life span of a red blood cell in a patient with SCA is only 10 to 30 days (120 days is normal). The relative inelasticity of the sickled cells (and even nonsickled cells with increased amounts of polymerized HbS) causes increased blood viscosity, and decreased blood flow rate; this contributes to occlusion and infarction of the microvasculature.

Classification

See Table 26.2-1 for the classification of Sickle cell disorders.

TABLE 26.2-1 CLASSIFICATION OF SICKLE CELL ANEMIA

Syndrome	Abbreviation	Hemoglobin (Hb) Make-Up	Clinical Manifestation
Sickle cell anemia	SCA	Homozygous: HbSS	Severe
Sickle cell trait	SCT	Heterozygous: HbSA	None
Sickle cell C	SCC	Heterozygous: HbSC	Milder than SCA
β^0-Thalassemia	$S\beta^0$	No HbA, HbS with ↓β-globin chains	Similar to SCA
β^+-Thalassemia	$S\beta^+$	Some HbA, HbS with ↓β-globin chains	Similar to SCC
Sickle cell D and E		Heterozygous: HbSD and HbSC	Similar to SCC

DIAGNOSIS

The gold standard diagnostic test for sickle cell disease is a hemoglobin electrophoresis. The different disease variants have characteristic electrophoresis patterns. A 5-minute solubility test, called a Sickledex, can be used in initial screening, or in an emergency setting, but if it is positive, an electrophoresis needs to be done to differentiate between a carrier and disease state. The Sickledex also has a relatively high false-negative rate.

Clinical Features

The common clinical manifestations seen in SCA are the result of vascular occlusion, hemorrhage, infarction, and ischemic necrosis secondary to increased blood viscosity caused by sickling. They can be summarized by use of the mnemonic *HBSS PAIN CRISIS* (problems for which an orthopaedist is frequently consulted are highlighted in italics):

H: hemolysis, *hand–foot syndrome (dactylitis)*
B: *bone marrow hyperplasia*
S: *stroke (thrombotic or hemorrhagic)*, subarachnoid bleeding
S: *skin ulcers* (usually leg)
P: *pain crises*, priapism, psychosocial problems
A: anemia, aplastic crisis, *avascular necrosis* (AVN; usually femoral head)
I: *infections* [central nervous system (CNS), pulmonary, genitourinary, *bone, joint*]
N: nocturia (urinary frequency)
C: cholelithiasis, cardiomegaly, congestive heart failure, chest syndrome
R: retinopathy, renal failure, renal concentration defects
I: *infarction* (*bone*, spleen, CNS, *muscle*, bowel, renal)
S: sequestration crisis (spleen, liver)
I: increased fetal loss in pregnancy
S: sepsis

Orthopaedic manifestations of SCA can be divided into two groups, based on cause (Box 26.2-1).

Dactylitis

- Affects short tubular bones of hands and feet
- Age 6 to 12 months (when HbF is replaced by HbS)
- Distal extremities become swollen, tender, and painful
- Triggered by cold weather
- Lasts 1 to 2 weeks
- Incidence: 45%
- Recurrence: 41%
- Rare after 6 years of age (when marrow activity in hands/feet ceases)

Pain Crises

- Age between 3 and 4 years
- Lasts 3 to 5 days
- Localized bone marrow or muscle infarction secondary to sequestration of sickled cells
- Commonly: humerus, tibia, femur
- Clinically: swelling, decreased range of motion, increased temperature

Osteomyelitis

- Clinically: fever, pain, swelling
- Polyostotic: 12% to 47%
- Erythrocyte sedimentation rate unreliable (usually low) secondary to sickled red blood cells
- *Staphylococcus aureus* and MRSA common, but patients also susceptible to encapsulated organisms secondary to decreased splenic function:
  - *Streptococcus pneumoniae*
  - *Haemophilus influenzae*
  - *Salmonella*
  - *Meningococcus*
  - *Klebsiella*
- Septic and reactive arthritis are less common than osteomyelitis but do occur
- Joint fluid in reactive arthritis will show less than 20,000 white blood cells/mm3
- Can lead to destruction of the physis, growth arrest, and limb deformity

Stroke

- Incidence: 8%
- May be hemorrhagic or infarct
- Greater than 50% recurrence rate, unless chronic lifetime transfusion therapy instituted
- May result in spastic hemiplegia requiring orthopaedic management

Pathologic Fractures

- May be secondary to bone marrow hyperplasia, osteomyelitis, or disuse osteopenia
- Attempt to minimize immobilization during treatment to prevent recurrence

Avascular Necrosis

- Femoral head most common, followed by humeral head
- Incidence: approximately 10%; bilateral: 54%
- Usually diagnosed on plain x-ray, but magnetic resonance imaging may be useful to show extent of head involvement

BOX 26.2-1 CAUSES OF ORTHOPAEDIC MANIFESTATIONS OF SICKLE CELL ANEMIA

Vascular Occlusion
- Dactylitis
- Avascular necrosis
- Osteomyelitis
- Septic arthritis
- Growth retardation
- Leg ulcers

Hemolysis
- Bone marrow hyperplasia
- Increased tendency to fracture

Radiographic Features

- Skull: thickened calvarium: 33% to 50%
- Long bones:

- □ Patchy osteosclerosis
- □ Cortical thinning
- □ Widened intramedullary canal
- □ Areas of infarction
- Spine: biconcave vertebrae

Differential Diagnosis

See Table 26.2-2 for the differential diagnosis of sickle cell disease and Table 26.2-3 for diagnosis based on bone and marrow scan results.

TREATMENT

Although most children with SCA are cared for primarily by a hematologist, the systemic nature of the illness and the clinical manifestations in various organ systems practically guarantee that most patients will also be treated by a variety of other subspecialists. The various acute crises and complications common to the disease often necessitate presentation in the emergency department as well. Treatment of patients with SCA can be thought of in three groups: preventive, problem management, and systemic.

Preventive

- Daily supplemental folate, to keep up with red blood cell production demand
- Periodic complete blood count check, to catch changes/problems early
- Use supplemental iron sparingly; iron overload can become a problem in older patients
- Maintain immunizations
- Encourage adequate oral hydration
- Encourage patients to seek early medical attention when ill
- Discourage smoking and alcohol intake
- Discourage excessive physical exertion
- Avoid extremes of temperature

Problem Management

Pain

- Nonsteroidal antiinflammatory drugs (NSAIDs) for chronic pain

Acute Pain Crisis

- Analgesia with NSAIDs/narcotics
- Hydration
- Bed rest
- Identify and correct underlying precipitators (especially infection)
- Administration of oxygen, and monitoring, if the patient has documented hypoxemia

Osteomyelitis

- Antibiotic coverage for *S. aureus* and *Salmonella*
- Surgical drainage for chronic osteomyelitis with sequestrum formation, or for patients who are systemically septic or not responding to antibiotic therapy

Septic Arthritis

- Arthrotomy and drainage, in conjunction with antibiotics

TABLE 26.2-2 DIFFERENTIAL DIAGNOSIS OF SICKLE CELL ANEMIA

Differentiation to be Made	Similarities	Diagnostic Strategy
Dactylitis vs. osteomyelitis	Pain, fever, ↑WBC count X-rays: lytic lesion, periosteal reaction	Bone scan unhelpful Perform aspiration of bone
Osteomyelitis vs. infarct	Pain, fever, swelling X-rays initially normal	Infarct much more common ESR unreliable Bone scan alone unhelpful Sequential bone marrow and bone scans may be helpful

ESR, erythrocyte sedimentation rate; WBC, white blood cell.

TABLE 26.2-3 DIAGNOSIS BASED ON SEQUENTIAL BONE MARROW AND BONE SCANS RESULTS

Results		
Bone Marrow Scan Uptake	Bone Scan Uptake	Diagnosis
Decreased	Increased	Acute infarct
Normal	Increased	Osteomyelitis
Normal	Normal	Neither
Decreased	Normal	Old infarct (usually asymptomatic)

TABLE 26.2-4 PROBLEM MANAGEMENT IN AVASCULAR NECROSIS

Extent	Treatment	Caveats
Lateral pillar intact	Conservative: Activity modification Physical therapy Protected weightbearing Bracing	May be ineffective Need to control the underlying sickling as much as possible
Whole head involvement		
Younger patient	Core decompression (early) Redirectional femoral or pelvic osteotomies (late)	Usually stopgap or salvage measures
Older patient	Total joint arthroplasty	↑ Rate of infection High intraoperative blood loss ↑ Rate of intraoperative femoral fracture Early aseptic loosening

Avascular Necrosis

See Table 26.2-4 for problem management in AVN.

Systemic

Oral Hydroxyurea

- Dose 1 to 35 mg/kg/day (see Table 26.2-5 for pros and cons)

Transfusion Therapy

- Simple transfusion to hemoglobin level of 10 g per dL now preferred over exchange transfusions for preoperative optimization.
- Use of antigen-matched blood and adequate hydration/oxygenation helps prevent complications during transfusion therapy and postoperatively.
- Acute transfusions are indicated for life-threatening complications of SCA such as stroke and aplastic anemia.
- Chronic transfusion therapy for life is indicated to prevent recurrent strokes.

TABLE 26.2-5 PROS AND CONS OF ORAL HYDROXYUREA THERAPY

Pros	Cons
↓ Pain crises	Can cause bone marrow suppression
↓ Hospital admissions	Long-term risks/benefits not known
↓ Need for transfusion by up to 50%	Not recommended for children

Central Nervous System Ischemia Screening

- By use of transcranial Doppler ultrasound or magnetic resonance imaging/magnetic resonance angiography
- 15% of patients have asymptomatic CNS ischemic injury
- Trials ongoing to establish role of transfusion therapy for *prevention* of CNS ischemic injury

SUGGESTED READING

Bennett OM, Namnyak SS. Bone and joint manifestations of sickle cell anaemia. J Bone Joint Surg (Br) 1990;72:494–499.

Bishop AR, Roberson JR, Eckman JR, et al. Total hip arthroplasty in patients who have sickle-cell hemoglobinopathy. J Bone Joint Surg (Am) 1988;70:853–855.

Diggs LW. Bone and joint lesions in sickle-cell disease. Clin Orthop 1967;52:119–143.

Ebong WW. Pathological fracture complicating long bone osteomyelitis in patients with sickle cell disease. J Pediatr Orthop 1986;6:177–181.

Engh CA, Hughes JL, Abrams RC, et al. Osteomyelitis in the patient with sickle-cell disease. J Bone Joint Surg (Am) 1971;53:1–15.

Hernigou P, Bachir D, Galacteros F. Avascular necrosis of the femoral head in sickle-cell disease: treatment of collapse by the injection of acrylic cement. J Bone Joint Surg (Br) 1993;75:875–880.

Robbins SL, Cotran RS, Kumar V. Sickle cell disease: pathologic basis of disease, 3rd ed. Philadelphia: WB Saunders, 1984:618–622.

Skaggs DL. Differentiation between bone infarction and acute osteomyelitis in children with sickle-cell disease with use of sequential radionuclide bone-marrow and bone scans. J Bone Joint Surg (Am) 2001;83:1810–1813.

Stevens MC, Padwick M, Serjeant GR. Observations on the natural history of dactylitis in homozygous sickle cell disease. Clin Pediatr 1981;20:311–317.

Walters MC, Patience M, Leisenring W, et al. Marrow transplantation for sickle cell disease: results of a multicenter collaborative investigation. N Engl J Med 1996;355:369–376.

SKELETAL DYSPLASIAS

MICHAEL CRAIG AIN
GEORGE S. NASEEF III

Skeletal dysplasias are a diverse group of disorders characterized by developmental abnormalities of the structure of bone and cartilage. They may be classified according to their specific deficiency (i.e., protein deficiency) or by the anatomic region they predominately affect (i.e., epiphysis, metaphysis, or spine). Skeletal dysplasias typically result in short stature, which is defined as height below the third percentile. Short stature may be proportionate, with symmetric decreases in both truncal and limb lengths. Disproportionate statures (dwarfing conditions) may be divided into shortened trunk, shortened limb, or shortened trunk and limb types. Short limb types may be subdivided by the region of limb involvement. Rhizomelic refers to shortening of the proximal portion of the limb; mesomelic, to the middle segment; and acromelic, to the distal segment. Over 300 skeletal dysplasias are now recognized, presenting myriad orthopaedic abnormalities. This chapter reviews six of the most common skeletal dysplasias, emphasizing orthopaedic evaluation and treatment.

ACHONDROPLASIA

PATHOGENESIS

- Most common type of short limb disproportionate dwarfism
- Incidence is estimated at 1 per 25,000 live births.
- Incidence correlates with greater paternal age.
- Achondroplasia is an autosomal dominant condition with 100% penetrance.
- It arises from a point mutation on the short arm of chromosome 4 at nucleotide 1138 of the fibroblast growth factor receptor 3 (FGFR3) gene (Table 27-1), resulting in a single amino acid change (glycine to arginine) in the transmembrane domain of the receptor.
- FGFR3 is expressed in the cartilaginous precursors of bone, where it is believed to decrease chondrocyte proliferation in the proliferative zone of the physis and to regulate growth by limiting endochondral ossification.
- 80% of new cases arise from a spontaneous mutation

DIAGNOSIS

PHYSICAL EXAMINATION AND HISTORY

Clinical Features (Table 27-2 and Fig. 27-1)

- Enlarged head with frontal bossing
- Midface hypoplasia
- Appearance of mandibular protrusion
- Flattened or depressed nasal bridge
- Normal trunk length
- Proximal limb shortening (rhizomelic)
- Mild elbow flexion contractures

TABLE 27-1 GENETIC DISORDERS OF DYSPLASIAS

Dysplasia	Defect
Achondroplasia	FGFR3
Pseudoachondroplasia	COMP (cartilage oligometric matrix protein)
Diastrophic dysplasia	Diastrophic dysplasia sulfate transporter gene (DTDST)
MED	
MED1	COMP
MED2	Alpha-2 polypeptide chain of type IX collagen
SED	Alpha-1 polypeptide chain of type II collagen
Mucopolysaccharidoses	Specific lysosomal enzyme deficiencies

MED, multiple epiphyseal dysplasia; SED, spondyloepiphyseal dysplasia.

TABLE 27-2 ORTHOPAEDIC MANIFESTATIONS OF DYSPLASIAS

Dysplasias	Atlantoaxial Instability	Spinal Stenosis	Lower Extremity Malalignment	Precocious Arthritis	Scoliosis/ Kyphosis
Achondroplasia	–	+	+	–	+
Pseudoachondroplasia	+	–	+	+	+
MED	–	–	+	+	–
SED	+	–	+	+	+
Diastrophic dysplasia	–	–	+	+	+
Morquio syndrome	+	–	+	+	+

- Trident hands with inability to approximate the long and ring fingers
- Genu varum (bow leg) is most common; genu valgum may occur
- Internal tibial torsion and ankle varus may be present

Children with achondroplasia are typically delayed in reaching motor milestones during the first few years of life.

- This is secondary to their enlarged head size, relative hypotonia, joint laxity, and the presence of foramen magnum stenosis.
- The timeframe of motor milestones in achondroplasia is:
  - Head control at 4 months
  - Sitting up at 10 months
  - Standing and ambulation begin between 17 and 20 months

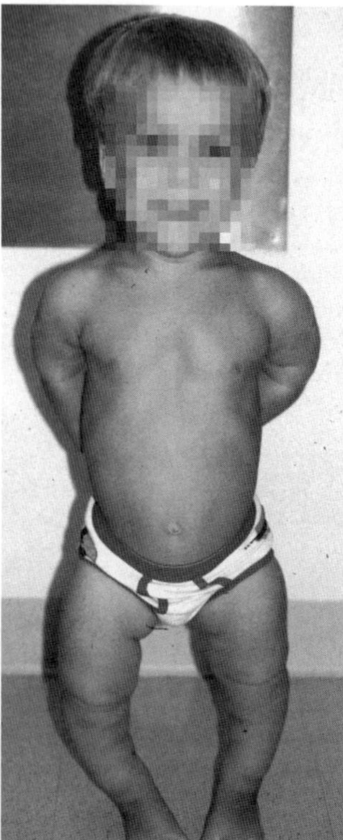

Figure 27-1 Typical clinical appearance in achondroplasia.

The foramen magnum is narrowed in achondroplasia.

- This occasionally causes cervical cord compression at either the posterior portion of the foramen or at the atlas.
- Cord compression is best visualized using magnetic resonance imaging (MRI).
- Symptoms of cord compression include respiratory difficulties (apnea), hypotonia, hyperreflexia, and clonus.

Radiographic Features

The lumbar spine of achondroplasts has unique anatomic findings:

- The interpedicular distance consistently decreases from upper to lower lumbar levels (best seen on posteroanterior radiograph of lumbar spine), which is opposite to what is found in unaffected individuals.
- The pedicles are approximately 30% to 40% thicker than unaffected individuals.
- These findings contribute to an overall decrease in the area of the lumbar spinal canal [best seen on computed tomography (CT) scan].

TREATMENT

GENU VARUM

- Present in 40% of patients with achondroplasia, but clinically significant in only 25%.
- Fibular overgrowth has been suggested as the source of this deformity.
- Several operations based on this assumption, including proximal fibular epiphysiodesis, have been reported, but no long-term satisfactory results have been published.
- Indications for operative intervention include pain, progressive deformity, and presence of a fibular thrust (lateral subluxation of the knee joint) while ambulating.
- Surgical options:
  - Proximal tibial osteotomy with fibular osteotomy with or without fibular epiphysiodesis
  - Distal femoral osteotomy
  - Supramalleolar osteotomy

THORACOLUMBAR KYPHOSIS (FIG. 27-2)

- Centered between T10 and L4.
- Most pronounced when the child begins to sit up.

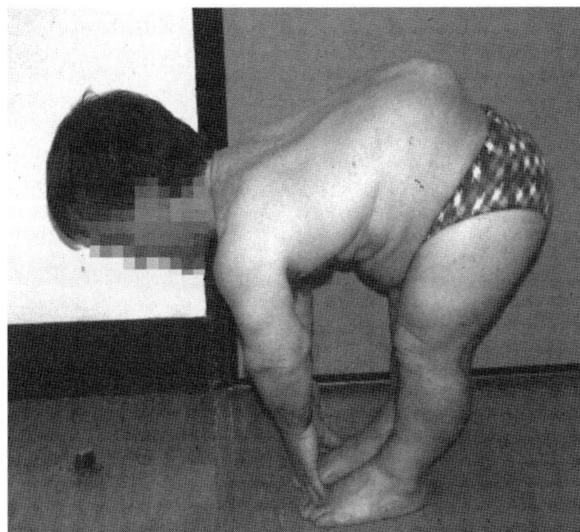

Figure 27-2 Achondroplasia with thoracolumbar kyphosis.

- 90% spontaneously regress when the child begins to ambulate.
- Small, wedge-shaped, slightly recessed apical vertebrae predict persistent deformity.
- Kyphosis beyond the age of 3 years should be treated with extension bracing.
- Anterior and posterior spinal fusion may be considered for significant kyphosis (greater than 50 degrees) beyond the age of 5 years.

RESPIRATORY DEPRESSION

- May contribute to cases of sudden infant death
- Central or obstructive in nature
- Treatment based its source and the severity of symptoms
- Severe central apnea treated with foramen magnum decompression
- Milder symptoms usually resolve with normal growth.

LUMBAR STENOSIS

- During the second or third decade of life, degenerative changes of the intervertebral discs further compromise the lumbar canal leading to development of lumbar stenosis.
- Patients with achondroplasia will typically present with complaints of lower back pain, leg pain, and progressive weakening of the extremities.
- Symptoms are decreased with squatting or bending over, which reduces lumbar lordosis.
- CT scan myelogram through cisternal puncture or MRI is useful to visualize the areas of stenosis (Fig. 27-3).
- Surgical treatment includes a wide multilevel laminectomy with care to preserve the facet joints.
- If thoracolumbar kyphosis is present, posterolateral fusion with instrumentation is recommended.

LIMB LENGTHENING

- Controversial within the Little People community
- Femur, tibia, and humerus are most often lengthened.

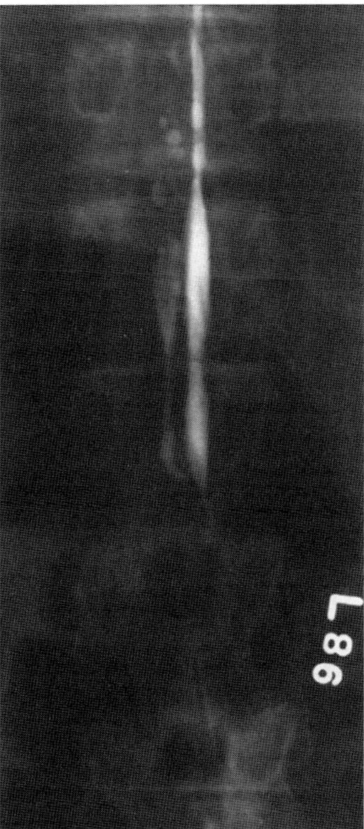

Figure 27-3 Myelogram showing lumbar spine stenosis.

- Multiple techniques described; most involve osteotomy and distracting ex-fix
- Limb lengthening of 40% to 50%
- Complications include infections, hardware failures, nerve injuries, osteomyelitis, soft tissue deformities, bone or joint deformities, high fracture rate, and progression of spinal stenosis.
- Requires up to 3 years to obtain desired results
- Decision best made by the well-informed and mature patient and not by the parents

PSEUDOACHONDROPLASIA

PATHOGENESIS

- Second most common short limb dwarfism
- Incidence is estimated to be 4 per million live births.
- Autosomal dominant condition
- Most cases are secondary to a spontaneous mutation.
- Arises from a mutation occurring on chromosome 19, affecting the gene coding for cartilage oligometric matrix protein (COMP)
  - COMP is a large extracellular matrix protein normally found surrounding chondrocytes in developing bone.
  - Several studies have shown intracellular accumulation of abnormal COMP in the rough endoplasmic reticulum of affected chondrocytes but the specific

mechanisms of this genetic disorder have yet to be elucidated.

DIAGNOSIS

PHYSICAL EXAMINATION AND HISTORY

Clinical Features (Table 27-2)

- Normal faces, head sizes, and stature at birth
- Rhizomelic shortening recognized around the age of 2 or 3 years
- Thoracolumbar kyphosis, scoliosis, or lumbar lordosis.
- Windswept knees, genu valgum, or genu varum are common.
- Shortening of the digits of the hands and feet
- Pes planus and marked ligamentous laxity
- Patients with hypoplasia or aplasia of the odontoid must be monitored for the development of atlantoaxial instability.
- Myelopathic symptoms, including increasing fatigability and hyperreflexia, are cause for further studies.

Radiographic Features

- Flattened vertebrae (platyspondyly) with anterior wedging
- Odontoid hypoplasia in 50%, warranting flexion–extension radiographs of the cervical spine
- Delayed epiphyseal ossification and flaring of the metaphysis
- Articular deformities in weightbearing joints (precocious osteoarthritis)

TREATMENT

ATLANTOAXIAL INSTABILITY

- Indication for posterior cervical fusion: atlantoaxial translation greater than 5 mm on flexion–extension radiographs in conjunction with progressive myelopathic symptoms or translation greater than 8 mm are the absolute numbers

SPINAL DEFORMITIES

- Kyphosis and scoliosis are usually flexible and compensatory to pelvic obliquity arising from lower extremity malalignment and hip flexion contractures.
- Bracing can be used to prevent lesser curves (25 to 45 degrees) from progressing.
- Curves greater than 50 degrees typically require posterior spinal fusion.
- Younger patients and those with greater kyphotic deformities often require anterior and posterior spinal arthrodesis.

LOWER EXTREMITY DEFORMITIES

- Hip, knee, and ankle radiographs for planning corrective osteotomies
- Indications for operative intervention include progressive deformity, pain, ligamentous laxity, and prophylaxis to delay the onset of osteoarthritis.
- Corrective osteotomies commonly include:
  - □ Proximal femoral
  - □ femoral
  - □ Proximal tibial
  - □ Supramalleolar osteotomies
- Operative goals:
  - □ Correct overall limb alignment
  - □ Obtain joint surfaces that are horizontal to the floor
- Lower extremity deformities often recur due to severe ligament laxity.

HIP JOINT DEFORMITIES

- Subluxation, hinged abduction, or lateral extrusion of the hip joint may occur secondary to delayed ossification of the femoral epiphyses.
- Intraoperative arthrography and dynamic fluoroscopic evaluation of the affected hip help to evaluate articular deformity and joint stability.
- Operative intervention, consisting of proximal femoral osteotomy with or without pelvic augmentation, is based upon the fluoroscopic findings.

DIASTROPHIC DYSPLASIA

PATHOGENESIS

- Rare disorder resulting in short limb dwarfism
- Autosomal recessive condition secondary to a mutation occurring in the diastrophic dysplasia sulfate transporter (DTDST) gene.
- This gene is found on chromosome 5 and is believed to regulate the intracellular concentration of sulfate.
- Proteoglycans, a major constituent of cartilage extracellular matrix, contribute to the flow-dependent viscoelastic properties of cartilaginous tissues.
- Mutation of DTDST gene impairs the sulfation of proteoglycans, decreasing their net negative charge and lowering their affinity for water, which impairs the flow-dependent viscoelastic properties of cartilage, ultimately decreasing the ability of cartilage to function successfully as a shock absorber and predisposing the cartilaginous precursors of bone to deformity and precocious osteoarthritis.

DIAGNOSIS

PHYSICAL EXAMINATION AND HISTORY

Clinical Features (Fig. 27-4)

- Rhizomelic shortened stature
- Flattened nasal bridge

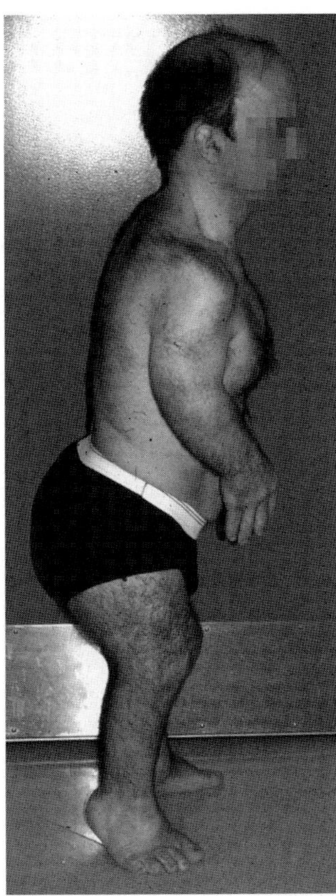

Figure 27-4 Clinical appearance in diastrophic dwarfism.

- High incidence of cleft palate deformities
- Hitchhiker thumb deformity (short, proximally based, and abducted)
- Characteristic cauliflower ear appearance
- *Not* associated with an increased risk of atlantoaxial instability
- Subluxated shoulders and radial heads
- Ankylosis of the proximal interphalangeal joints of the index, middle, and ring fingers
- Clinodactyly
- Lower extremity deformities:
  - Severe hip and knee flexion contractures
  - Genu valgum
  - Dislocated patella
  - Complex deformities of the ankles and feet

Early childhood screenings in the form of comprehensive neurologic examinations and a lateral cervical spine radiograph for the presence or progression of cervical kyphosis are warranted.

Radiographic Features

Cervical spina bifida and kyphosis, midthoracic kyphoscoliosis, and lumbar lordosis are frequently present.

TREATMENTS

CERVICAL KYPHOSIS

- Occurs in over 30% of affected patients
- Associated with quadriplegia and even death
- Kyphosis angle greater than 60 degrees or a round or triangular-shaped, posteriorly displaced, apical vertebrae suggests progressive nature.
- Anteroposterior cervical fusion for progressive deformity or cord compression

HIP JOINT DEFORMITY

- Examination often reveals decreased hip range of motion with an increased tendency to subluxate or dislocate.
- These changes further stress the susceptible hyaline cartilage, leading to progressive deformities and epiphyseal flattening.
- Arthrography is indicated to evaluate the proximal femoral epiphysis.
- A contracted hip joint without evidence of epiphyseal deformity is treated with soft tissue releases.
- Conservative treatment is indicated once epiphyseal flattening is identified.
- Precocious arthritis can be treated with custom hip implant arthroplasty.

LOWER EXTREMITY DEFORMITIES

- Talipes equinovarus is the classic foot deformity associated with diastrophic dysplasia.
- However, the most common deformity may be that of tarsal valgus and metatarsal adductus (43% of foot deformities).
- Deformity is rigid and often refractory to treatment.
- A combination of serial casting and soft tissue releases is required to improve the deformity.
- Interventions need to be individualized based on the patient's response to treatment and the surgeon's experience.

MULTIPLE EPIPHYSEAL DYSPLASIA

PATHOGENESIS

- Multiple epiphyseal dysplasia (MED) is a common form of short limb dwarfism.
- Incidence is estimated at 1 per 100,000.
- Several different disorders with similar manifestations.
- Primarily inherited as an autosomal dominant condition, but autosomal recessive transmission has been reported.
- MED1 and MED2 and their corresponding genetic defects have been identified.
  - The genetic mutation associated with MED1 occurs on chromosome 19 and affects the gene coding for COMP.

- COMP is an extracellular matrix protein normally found surrounding chondrocytes in developing bone. However, the specific mechanisms of this genetic disorder remain unclear.
- A similar defect in COMP is associated with pseudoachondroplasia.

- The genetic mutation associated with MED2 affects the α2-polypeptide chain of type IX collagen.
  - Type IX collagen is a trimer found on the surface of type II collagen, where it functions as a stabilizer.
  - Although the exact mechanism is unclear, it is hypothesized that a defect in type IX collagen predisposes hyaline cartilage to early degeneration.

DIAGNOSIS

PHYSICAL EXAMINATION AND HISTORY

Clinical Features

- Manifestations are variable.
- Mild decrease in stature
- Head, face, and spine are normal.
- "Stubby" hands and feet: stunted growth of metacarpals and metatarsals
- Decreased range of motion, pain, and angular deformities of hips, knees, and ankles
- Patients typically present with complaint of lower extremity pain or limp at about age 7.
- The hips and knees, secondary to their weightbearing nature, are the most frequently involved joints.

Radiographic Features

- The principal radiographic findings can be witnessed in the epiphysis of long bones.
- These epiphyseal centers initially demonstrate delayed ossification, and later appear mottled once ossification has begun.
- Eventual flattening and deformation of joint surfaces occurs, leading to precocious arthritis.
- The key to remember is that MED is bilateral with symmetric joint involvement.
- A symptomatic hip may be mistakenly diagnosed as Perthes disease.
- Plain radiographs revealing symmetric hip, knee, and ankle joint involvement suggest the diagnosis of MED over Perthes disease.

TREATMENT

HIP AND LOWER EXTREMITY DEFORMITIES

- Primary indications for surgical intervention are pain and deformity.
- Corrective osteotomies to restore normal joint alignment with respect to the ground
- Precocious arthritis often necessitates joint arthroplasty.

SPONDYLOEPIPHYSEAL DYSPLASIA

PATHOGENESIS

ETIOLOGY

- Spondyloepiphyseal dysplasia (SED) is several different disorders with similar manifestations.
- Two distinct forms are recognized: SED congenita and SED tarda.
  - SED congenita is an autosomal dominant condition.
    - Most cases arise from spontaneous mutations.
    - Estimated incidence of 3 or 4 cases per million
- SED tarda is an X-linked recessive condition.
- The SED genetic defect occurs in the α-1 chain of type II collagen.

DIAGNOSIS

PHYSICAL EXAMINATION AND HISTORY

Clinical Features

- SED congenita
  - Motor milestones are often delayed secondary to mild hypotonia.
  - Most affected individuals are ambulatory by 2 years of age.
  - Short trunk and limb dwarfism
  - Normal intelligence
  - Odontoid hypoplasia
  - Thoracic kyphoscoliosis
  - Pectus carinatum
  - Lumbar lordosis
  - Coxa vara
  - Hip flexion contractures
  - Equinovarus foot deformity
  - Ocular ailments: retinal detachment, cataracts, myopia, and glaucoma
- SED tarda (Fig. 27-5)
  - Normal at birth, mild symptoms develop in childhood
  - Mildly decreased stature
  - Back pain
  - Lower extremity pain
  - Odontoid hypoplasia, scoliosis, and coxa magna may occur

Radiographic Features

- Plain radiographs may reveal odontoid hypoplasia.
- Flexion–extension views of the cervical spine.
  - Evaluate for atlantoaxial instability (Fig. 27-6).
- Lateral spine radiographs reveal the characteristic biconcave vertebral end plates and flattened vertebral bodies (platyspondyly).
- MRI in flexion and extension may reveal spinal cord encroachment.

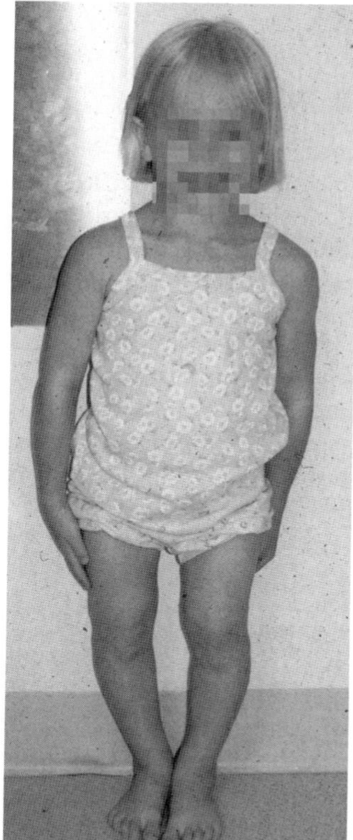

Figure 27-5 Clinical appearance in spondyloepiphyseal dysplasia tarda.

TREATMENT

ODONTOID HYPOPLASIA

- Monitor regularly for the development of instability or myelopathy.
- Myelopathy develops in up to 35% of children.
- Atlantoaxial arthrodesis with or without decompression is indicated for progression of myelopathy or when instability exceeds 8 mm on flexion–extension radiographs.

THORACIC KYPHOSCOLIOSIS

- Bracing when curves are less than 40 degrees
- Posterior spinal fusion plus or minus anterior release/fusion is indicated for severe curves or progressive deformity.

LOWER EXTREMITY DEFORMITIES

- Corrective osteotomies are indicated for deformities and pain.
- Unfortunately, progressive deformities and precocious arthritis are common.
- Foot deformities may be responsive to stretching and serial casting.

OCULAR AILMENTS

- Regular ophthalmologic examinations are encouraged.

SPONDYLOEPIPHYSEAL DYSPLASIA TARDA

- Scoliosis is usually mild and can be managed with bracing.
- Surgery is indicated for curves greater than fifty degrees or continued progression.
- Valgus osteotomy of the proximal femur may improve hip joint congruity and delay the onset of degenerative arthritis.

MORQUIO SYNDROME

PATHOGENESIS

- The mucopolysaccharidoses (MPS) are a group of inherited lysosomal storage disorders resulting from specific lysosomal enzyme deficiencies.

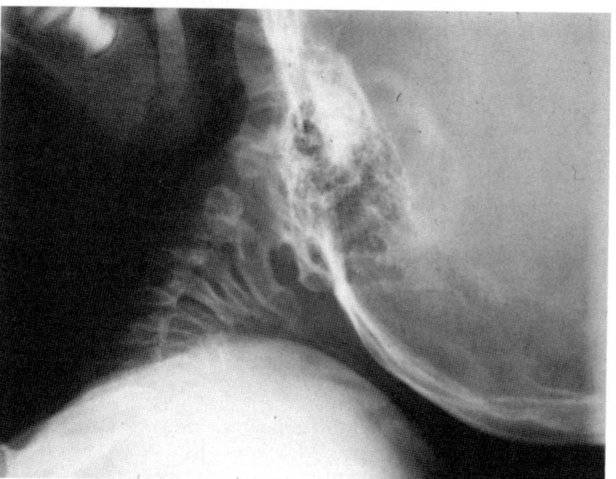

A

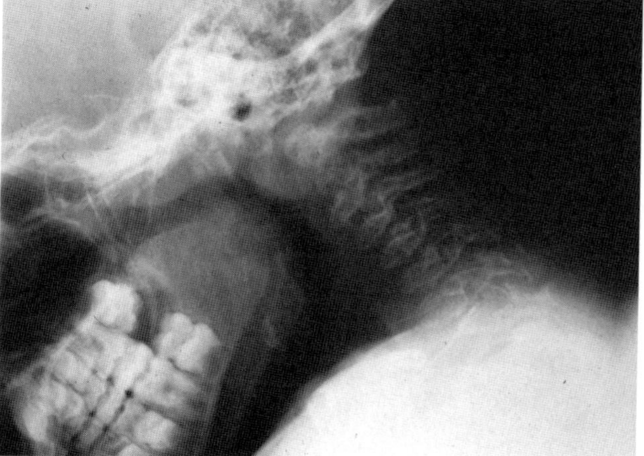

B

Figure 27.6 Flexion (A) and extension (B) radiographs of the cervical spine demonstrating atlantoaxial instability.

- At least 12 types have been identified.
- Morquio syndrome (type IV) is the most common of these disorders.
  - Estimated incidence of 3 per 1 million
  - Three different subtypes of Morquio syndrome are now recognized.
  - All are autosomal recessive conditions characterized by an inability to metabolize keratan sulfate, which accumulates in cell lysosome, altering the metabolic activities of lysosomes and ultimately leading to defective cartilage and connective tissue formation and function.

DIAGNOSIS

PHYSICAL EXAMINATION AND HISTORY

Clinical Features (Fig. 27-7; Table 27-2)

- Normal at birth
- Normal intelligence
- Short trunk dwarfism is appreciated within 2 to 3 years of life
- Odontoid hypoplasia
- Pectus carinatum
- Thoracolumbar kyphosis with platyspondyly
- Hip, ankle, and wrist laxity leading to subluxation and degenerative changes
- Genu valgum
- Cloudy corneas
- Hearing loss
- Coarsened facial characteristics

Radiographic Features

- Plain radiographs may reveal odontoid hypoplasia.

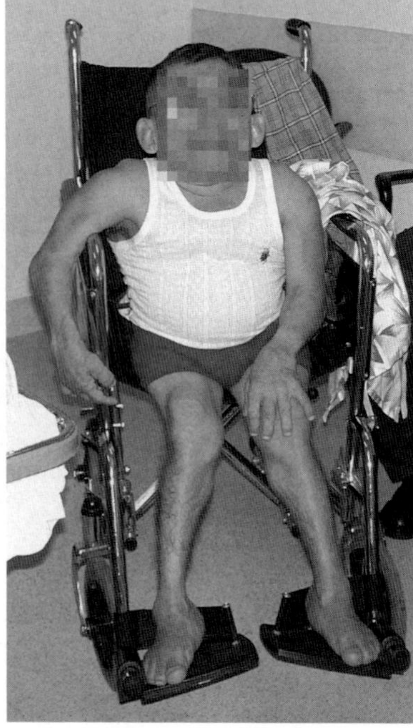

Figure 27-7 Clinical appearance in Morquio syndrome.

TREATMENT

ATLANTOAXIAL INSTABILITY

- Atlantoaxial instability is found in nearly all patients with Morquio syndrome and is the result of odontoid hypoplasia and increased joint laxity.
- Children typically present with decreased endurance, hyperreflexia, clonus, and up-going Babinski sign at about 6 years of age.
- Evaluation with flexion–extension cervical radiographs is helpful but may be misleading.
- Further evaluation using flexion–extension MRI often reveals the accumulation of extradural soft tissue limiting the space available for the cervical spinal cord.
- Posterior spinal fusion with or without decompression of surrounding soft tissue is indicated when myelopathy is apparent.

ORTHOPAEDIC MANIFESTATIONS

- Generally managed with bracing or observation
- Genu valgum: corrective osteotomies once atlantoaxial instability is stabilized
- Thoracolumbar kyphosis is best observed.

SUGGESTED READING

Aldegheri R. Distraction osteogenesis for lengthening of the tibia in patients who have limb-length discrepancy or short stature. J Bone Joint Surg Am 1999;81:624–634.

Bassett GS. Lower extremity abnormalities in dwarfing conditions. Instr Course Lect 1991;39:389–397.

Bassett GS. Orthopedic aspects of skeletal dysplasias. AAOS Instr Course Lect 1991;39:381–387.

Bethem D, Winter RB, Lutter L. Disorders of the spine in diastrophic dwarfism. A discussion of nine patients and review of the literature. J Bone Joint Surg (Am) 1980;62:529–536.

Crossan JF, Wynne-Davis R, Fulford GE. Bilateral failure of the capital femoral epiphysis: bilateral Perthes' disease, multiple epiphyseal dysplasia, pseudoachondroplasia, and spondyloepiphyseal dysplasia congenita and tarda. J Pediatr Orthop 1983;3:297–301.

Dietz FR, Murray JC. Update on the basis of disorders with orthopaedic manifestations. In: Buckwalter JA, Einhorn TA, Simon SR, ed. Orthopaedic basic science. Biology and biomechanics of the musculoskeletal system. Rosemont, IL: American Academy of Orthopaedic Surgeons, 2000:111–131.

Kopits SE. Orthopedic complications of dwarfism. Clin Orthop 1976;114:153–179.

Mankin HJ, Mow VC, Buckwalter JA, et al. Articular cartilage structure, composition, and function. In: Buckwalter JA ET, Simon SR, ed. Orthopaedic basic science. Biology and biomechanics of the musculoskeletal system. Rosemont, IL: American Academy of Orthopaedic Surgeons, 2000:443–470.

McKusick VA. Heritable disorders of connective tissue. St. Louis: Mosby, 1972.

Mikles M, Stanton RP. A review of Morquio syndrome. Am J Orthop 1997;26:533–540.

Poussa M, Merikanto J, Ryoppy S, et al. The spine in diastrophic dysplasias. Spine 1991;16:881–887.

Scott CI. Achondroplasia and hypochondroplastic dwarfism. Clin Orthop 1976;114:18–30.

Sponsellor PD. The skeletal dysplasias. In: Morrissey RT, ed. Lovell and Winter's pediatric orthopaedics, 4th ed. Vol 1. Philadelphia: Lippincott Williams & Wilkins, 2001:244–285.

Tolo VT. Spinal deformity in short-stature syndromes. AAOS Instr Course Lect 1990;39:399–405.

UPPER EXTREMITY

28.1 BRACHIAL PLEXUS INJURIES

CRAIG S. PHILLIPS ■ SOVARINTH TUN

Brachial plexus birth palsy remains a significant problem despite improved obstetric techniques. Predicting a spontaneous recovery requires identification of the level and severity of the brachial plexus injury. Up to 92% of injured infants have a complete recovery by 3 months of age. Infants who do not show recovery, especially biceps function, by 3 months of age have an increased risk of long-term disability and may benefit from neural microsurgery. Upper extremity contracture and weakness may benefit surgical reconstructions that include rotational osteotomies, tendon releases, and tendon transfers.

RELEVANT ANATOMY

- The brachial plexus is the amalgamation of ventral nerve roots arising from C5 to T1 (Fig. 28.1-1).
- After the nerve roots exit their respective neural foramina, they combine to form three well-defined trunks—upper (C5, C6), middle (C7), and lower (C8, T1).
- The trunks divide into anterior and posterior divisions, forming a posterior, medial, and lateral cord; named with reference to subclavian artery proximity.
- The cords terminate in numerous branches, each supplying individual myotomes, and dermatomes.
- The clavicle is an important landmark separating the brachial plexus into proximal (roots, trunks, and divisions) and distal (cords and branches) portions.
- The plexus lies in close proximity to the subclavian and axillary vessels.
- The sympathetic chain lies adjacent to the nerve roots at the neural foramina of C8 and T1.

PATHOGENESIS

Etiology

Obstetric brachial plexus injuries are the result of traction on the brachial plexus, most commonly the upper trunk (C5 and C6) (Fig. 28.1-1). Traction usually occurs during the late phase of delivery when the head is pulled laterally away from the shoulder. Risk factors for an obstetric brachial plexus injury include the following:

- High birthweight
- Prolonged labor
- Breech presentation
- Shoulder dystocia
- Multiparous pregnancy

Epidemiology

- The incidence of brachial plexus injuries is reported to be 0.87 to 2.5 per 1,000 live births.
- No association with race, gender, or maternal age has been described.

Pathophysiology

Knowledge of the anatomy of the brachial plexus is essential in understanding the effects of an injury. The prognosis of an injury deteriorates when the nerve roots are avulsed from the spinal cord (preganglionic lesions). Indications of a preganglionic lesion include Horner syndrome, phrenic nerve palsy, and scapula winging resulting from long thoracic nerve palsy.

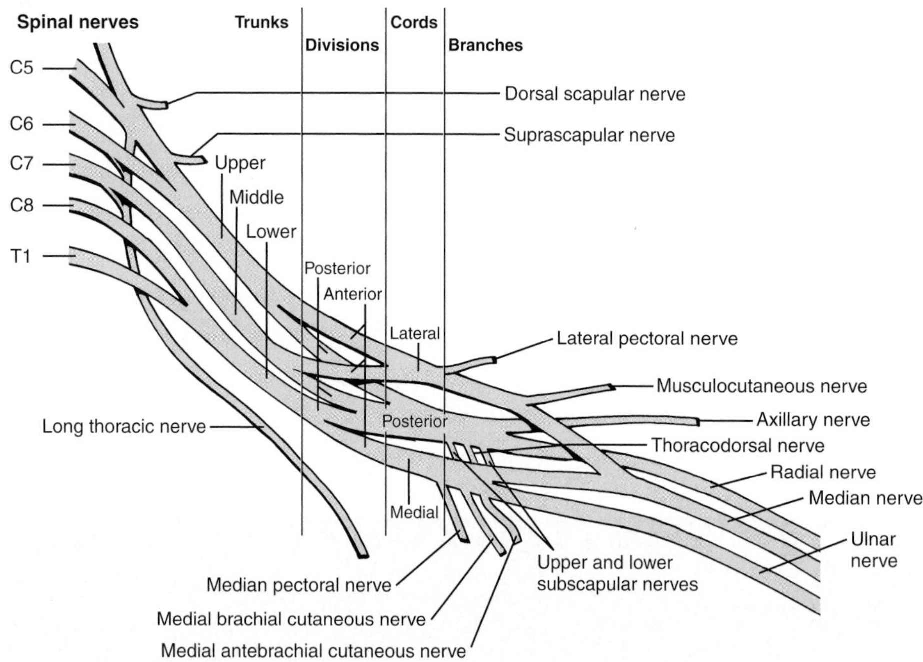

Figure 28.1-1 Structures of the brachial plexus. (Adapted from Waters PM. Obstetric brachial plexus injuries: evaluation and management. J Am Acad Surg 1997;5:206.)

Upper trunk lesions typically involve C5 and C6 which contribute to the suprascapular, axillary, and musculocutaneous nerves. These nerves innervate the rotator cuff, deltoid, biceps, and brachialis muscles. Therefore, weakness is present in shoulder abduction and external rotation as well as elbow flexion. If C7 is also involved, triceps elbow extension is weak. Hand function is more affected by lower trunk lesions that involve C8 and T1, which are usually preganglionic injuries (proximal).

Classification

An anatomic classification for the different categories of brachial plexus injuries includes the following:

- Upper plexus palsy (Erb): C5, C6, and sometimes C7
- Intermediate plexus palsy: C7 and sometimes C8, T1
- Lower plexus palsy (Klumpke): C8 and T1
- Total plexus palsy

The most common palsy involves the upper trunk and is usually a postganglionic injury, unless the delivery is breech, which is associated with a preganglionic injury. An entire plexus injury is less frequent and intermediate or lower plexus palsies are rarely seen.

A modification of the Mallet classification system is used in young children to assess upper trunk function and includes five categories: global shoulder abduction, external rotation, hand to neck, hand on spine, and hand to mouth. Each category is graded 0 to 5 with grade 0 being no muscle contraction and grade 5 being normal voluntary muscle contractions. Fig. 28.1-2 diagrams the intermediate grades II to IV. Muscle strength grading is similar to that used for adults.

DIAGNOSIS

Physical Examination and History

A history of the pregnancy, labor, and early postnatal period must be obtained from the parents. This information should include complications during pregnancy, such as diabetes and toxemia. The duration of the labor, method of delivery, and ease of delivery should also be noted. An early postnatal history of respiratory distress, clavicle or humerus fractures, Horner syndrome, and paralysis is also helpful.

Clinical Features

- Spontaneous movements of the shoulder, elbow, wrist, and finger are the best methods used to define the severity of the neural injury.
  - Performing neonatal reflexes, such as the Moro and asymmetric tonic neck reflexes, assists in providing this information.
- Movements with and against gravity are important for grading muscle strength and can be performed by placing the infant in gravity-eliminated positions and stimulating specific arm movements with toys.
- The "cookie test" is helpful in testing elbow flexion at 9 months.
  - During the test, the child is encouraged to place a cookie into the mouth with the affected shoulder adducted.
  - "The reverse cookie test" is similar and requires the child to remove the cookie from the mouth with the uninvolved extremity restrained.
- Erb palsy typically presents with the shoulder adducted and internally rotated, with the elbow extended, the

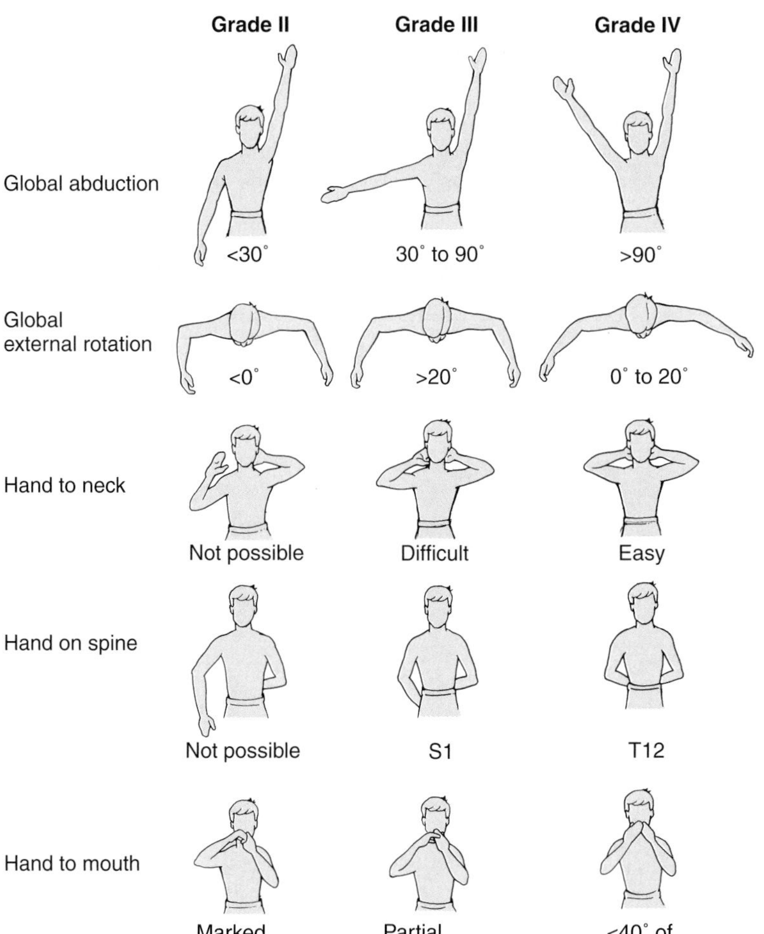

Figure 28.1-2 Modification of the Mallet classification for assessing upper trunk function in young children. Grade I is no function and grade V is normal function. Grades II, III, and IV are depicted for each category. (Adapted from Waters PM. Obstetric brachial plexus injuries: evaluation and management. J Am Acad Surg 1997;5:207.)

forearm pronated, and the wrist and fingers flexed ("waiter tip deformity").

- Total plexopathy presents with a flail and insensate upper extremity.
- Flexion of the fingers should not be mistaken for active motion since this usually occurs as a result of the tenodesis effect, whereby tension on the digital flexors is increased with wrist extension leading to finger flexion.
- In Klumpke palsy, hand paralysis is present, but shoulder and elbow function are maintained.
- Infants with a brachial plexus injury have a tendency to turn their head away from the involved arm.
- Horner syndrome: characterized by ipsilateral facial ptosis, enophthalmos, anhidrosis, and myosis (TEAM)—usually indicates an avulsion injury of the lower trunk as the sympathetic chain lies adjacent to the C8 and T1 nerve roots.
- Phrenic nerve paralysis should be excluded preoperatively by observing abdominal motion and confirmed on fluoroscopy (flattened hemidiaphragm and no motion with respiration) or chest radiographs.
- Plication of the diaphragm may be necessary prior to surgery.
- Other diagnoses should be ruled out by a careful physical examination.
  - Pseudoparalysis can be a result of compression on the brachial plexus by fractures of the clavicles, humeri, and ribs.
  - Shoulder dislocations have also been reported to cause brachial plexus palsies.

Radiologic Features

Myelography, computed tomography (CT) with myelography (CT–myelogram), and magnetic resonance imaging (MRI) are often used preoperatively in adult plexopathies to identify pseudomeningoceles and nerve root avulsions. True-positive rates of 84% for myelography and 94% for CT–myelography have been reported. MRI has the advantage of being noninvasive and allowing for imaging of the entire plexus, while having a true-positive rate similar to CT–myelography. While some experts have found preoperative imaging helpful, many others question the value. The treating physician must justify the potential information gained from these tests as they are often invasive and require general anesthesia in the pediatric population.

Glenohumeral dislocations can be difficult to diagnose on radiographs in infants since the glenoid and humeral head have not yet ossified. A CT, MRI, or arthrogram is sometimes necessary for diagnosing a glenohumeral dislocation and can help identify deformities of the glenoid or humeral head.

Electrodiagnostic Testing

Electromyography and nerve conduction studies to determine neural injury severity and location have provided unreliable results. Denervation is uncommon in infants despite brachial plexus ruptures and avulsions. In addition, sensation in a specific dermatome is also hard to assess in infants. Therefore, many surgeons do not routinely perform electrodiagnostic testing, although others claim potential benefits in determining prognosis.

Diagnostic Workup

The goal of management in caring for a patient with a brachial plexus injury is to maximize upper-extremity function. Treatment begins shortly after diagnosis with physical therapy. The role of therapy is to limit further joint contracture and increase passive motion, to ensure effective muscle function after reinnervation. Physical therapy takes the form of passive joint stretching, stretch casting, and nighttime splints. Recent interest has focused on the use of botulin toxin to limit muscle imbalances.

The goal of treatment is aimed toward obtaining at least the following results:

- Hand: sensation in the hand and fingers
- Elbow: flexion greater than grade III (ability to independently feed)
- Shoulder: stability and abduction with external rotation greater than grade III.

Algorithm 28.1-1 concerns treating children with obstetric brachial palsy injury.

TREATMENT

Microsurgery

Extraforaminal ruptures can be repaired with nerve grafting between the torn nerve ends. Preganglionic root avul-

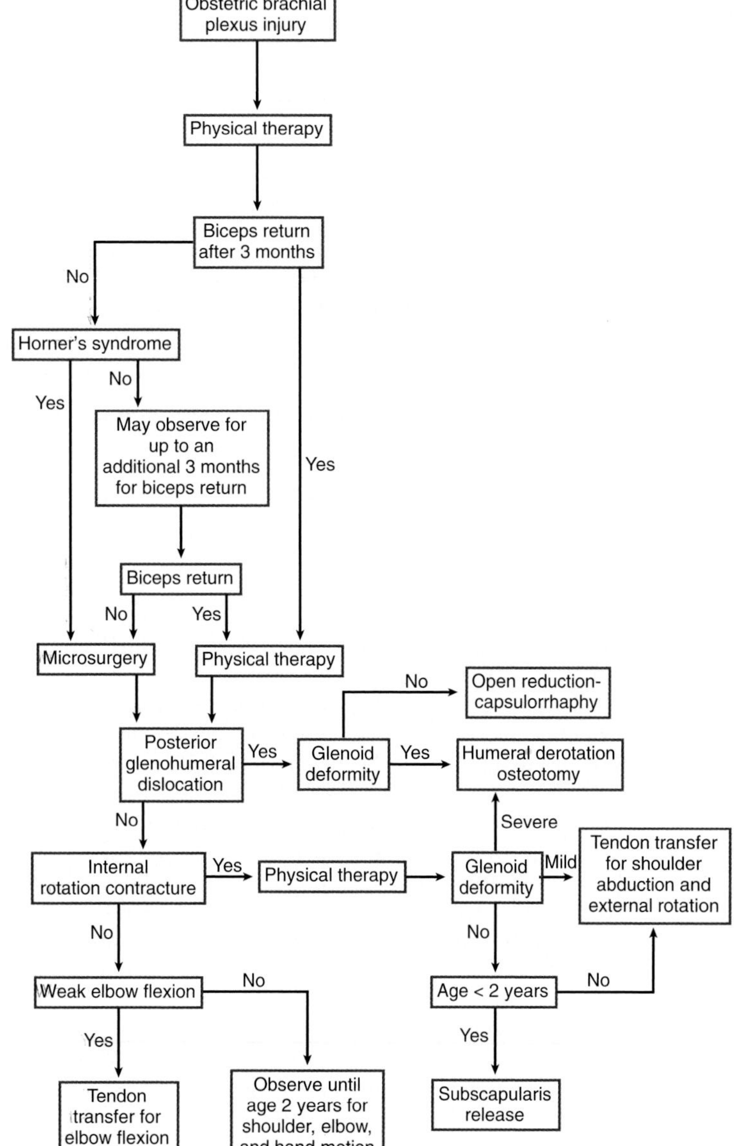

Algorithm 28.1-1 Algorithm for the management of obstetric brachial plexus injuries.

sions, however, are irreparable and require nerve transfers, neurotization, or tendon transfers. Current surgical recommendations are as follows:

- Extraforaminal ruptures
  - Neuroma resection, and sural nerve grafting
- Upper trunk ruptures
  - Sural nerve grafts from C5 and C6 roots to the suprascapular nerve and musculocutaneous nerve or lateral cord
  - Nerve grafts from the upper-trunk posterior division to the posterior cord to ensure elbow extension (triceps) and deltoid function, respectively
- Upper root avulsions
  - Nerve transfers from a branch of the spinal accessory nerve to the suprascapular nerve
  - Reestablish continuity of the musculocutaneous nerve, lateral cord, and the posterior cord using thoracic intercostal nerve transfers or grafts
- Total plexopathy avulsions
  - Surgical options depend on the number of roots not avulsed and therefore amenable to nerve grafting
  - If possible, nerve grafts from the C5 and C6 roots to the median nerve and ulnar component of the medial cord to restore hand sensation and function
  - Spinal accessory and intercostal nerve transfers to the suprascapular nerve and the posterior and lateral cords.

Indications for Microsurgery

- Total plexus palsy with flail arm after 1 month and Horner syndrome
- C5, C6 palsy after a breech delivery showing no signs of recovery by 3 months

Surgical neural reconstruction is usually not performed prior to 3 months of age for anesthesia safety reasons. The literature suggests microsurgical techniques prior to 6 months of age to ensure optimal results.

Shoulder Reconstruction

Open Reduction for Posterior Glenohumeral Dislocation

Glenohumeral dislocations should be suspected when external rotation is limited, and the humeral head is palpable posteriorly. Dislocations can occur in infancy and may require an arthrogram, ultrasound, CT, or MRI to confirm this diagnosis as the humeral head is not yet ossified, and therefore poorly visualized with radiographs.

- Open reduction and capsulorrhaphy are necessary when a glenohumeral dislocation is present.
- An anterior release and posterior capsulorrhaphy are performed through combined anterior and posterior approaches.
- The shoulder is then immobilized in a spica cast for 4 weeks.

Subscapularis Release

Upper trunk brachial plexus palsies cause a muscle imbalance of the shoulder resulting in weak abduction and external rotation while maintaining adduction and internal rotation. Subluxation of the glenohumeral joint eventually occurs, which leads to internal rotation contractures, and glenohumeral deformities.

- A subscapularis release at 1 year of age should be considered when the child has failed physical therapy stretching and external rotation is less than 30 degrees when the shoulder is adducted.
- The subscapularis is released from its origin as shoulder instability can result if detached from the humeral insertion.

Tendon Transfers for Shoulder External Rotation and Abduction

Tendon transfers are successful in restoring partial function to patients with incomplete brachial plexus recovery in early childhood, and are usually performed between 2 and 5 years of age. Important principles that must be adhered to whenever performing tendon transfers include the following:

- Passive functional range of motion of the joint must be obtained preoperatively with physical therapy and dynamic splinting.
- The joint must be reduced and congruent, which may require arthrogram, CT, or MRI confirmation.
- Donor muscle strength must be at least a grade 4 or 5 and not previously paralyzed, as the muscle grade will diminish by one grade with tendon transfer.
- The donor muscle should have adequate excursion to perform the necessary function.
- Each muscle should perform only one function.

For patients with severe shoulder contractures, including external rotation and abduction weakness, an anterior release of the pectoralis major with transfer of the latissimus dorsi and teres major muscles to the rotator cuff is helpful.

- Anteriorly, the pectoralis major tendon is lengthened at its humeral insertion.
- Posteriorly, the latissimus dorsi and teres major tendon insertion is transferred to the greater tuberosity.
- This procedure is best performed between the ages of 2 to 7 years.

Other tendon transfers have been described to obtain shoulder abduction, incurred as a result of deltoid weakness. Techniques include transferring the pectoralis major to the deltoid, transferring the trapezius to the deltoid insertion, and transferring the short head of the biceps and long head of the triceps to the acromion. These methods have been shown to be helpful, but results are limited.

Humeral Derotation Osteotomy

- If severe glenohumeral deformity with fixed internal rotation is present in an adolescent, a humeral derotation osteotomy is preferred.
- A humeral osteotomy is made proximal to the deltoid insertion with the distal humerus placed in 30 degrees of external rotation.

Arthrodesis

Glenohumeral arthrodesis is a reasonable option to treat pain, instability, articular deformity, and arthritis that cannot be addressed with the above procedures. Functional scapular muscles and scapular stability are required for shoulder arthrodesis. Prerequisites for a glenohumeral arthrodesis include a sensate and functional arm and hand.

Forearm Reconstruction

Tendon Transfers for Elbow Flexion

Involvement of the musculocutaneous nerve from an upper trunk brachial plexus palsy leads to weak elbow flexion. Many procedures have been described to restore partial elbow flexion function. One of the earliest transfers described included a transfer of the origin of the flexor–pronator muscle group proximally. Although simple to perform, this procedure may exacerbate a pronation deformity. Results of this procedure allow elbow flexion of 3 to 5 lbs with a range of motion between 30 and 100 degrees.

Surgeons have found good results with bipolar transpositions of the pectoralis major or the latissimus dorsi. The procedure is technically demanding and requires transferring both the origin and insertion of the muscle. Other procedures described in the past, which are rarely performed today, include an anterior transfer of the triceps insertion and a transfer of the sternocleidomastoid muscle through a fascia lata graft.

Tendon Transfer for Forearm Supination

Patients with lower trunk brachial plexus palsy commonly have paralysis of the pronators with a supination contracture of the forearm.

- Transfer of the biceps tendon insertion to the radial aspect of the radial neck can be done to provide pronation.
- If the forearm cannot be passively pronated, a release of the interosseous membrane is necessary.
- An elbow capsuloplasty can be performed to reduce a subluxated or dislocated radial head.
- The elbow is placed in a long arm cast with flexion at 90 degrees and pronation at 20 degrees for 4 to 6 weeks.

Forearm Osteotomy

Since only half of the patients with a biceps rerouting procedure maintain their correction, many surgeons now perform an osteoclasis of the radius and ulna with intramedullary fixation. The osteotomy can also be performed with a biceps tendon transfer to decrease the recurrence rate.

Results and Outcomes

- Most newborns with a brachial plexus injury will do well without surgical intervention and have a complete spontaneous recovery.
- For patients who do not show recovery by 3 to 6 months, microsurgery has been shown to be beneficial.
- Patients who undergo microsurgery are more likely to obtain a higher level of function than similar patients treated nonoperatively.
- Children who undergo nerve grafting appear to have improved outcomes after secondary reconstructive procedures.
- Secondary reconstructions (e.g., tendon transfers and osteotomies) are clearly beneficial to patients with contractures and deformities, allowing improved range of motion to place the arm in a functional position and provide muscle strength of grades III or IV.
  - Patients are able to achieve improved function of their shoulder, elbow, and hand.
  - Function may not be completely normal even with microsurgery and secondary reconstruction procedures.

SUGGESTED READING

Bennett JB, Allan CH. Tendon transfers about the shoulder and elbow in obstetrical brachial plexus palsy. J Bone Joint Surg (Am) 1999; 81:1612–1626.

Clarke HM, Curtis CG. An approach to obstetrical brachial plexus injuries. Hand Clin 1995;11:563–581.

Gilbert A. Long-term evaluation of brachial plexus surgery in obstetrical palsy. Hand Clin 1995;11:583–595.

Greenwald AG, Schute PC, Shively JL. Brachial plexus birth palsy: a 10-year report on the incidence and prognosis. J Pediatr Orthop 1984;4:689–692.

Waters, PM. Obstetric brachial plexus injuries: evaluation and management. J Am Acad Orthop Surg 1997;5:205–214.

28.2 CONGENITAL DEFORMITIES

RODERICK BIRNIE

Throughout the embryologic process, the potential for error is great but malformations are fortunately rare. Amelia (complete absence of a limb), phocomelia (almost complete absence), or ectromelia (partial absence) can occur and defects may involve the whole width of the limb (transverse defect), or the pre- or postaxial border (longitudinal defect). There may be no parts distal to the defective portion (terminal defect) or the middle portion of a series of limb segments may be defective (intercalary defect).

PATHOGENESIS

Etiology

- Most congenital deformities of the upper extremity occur in the embryonic period from the third to the seventh weeks of gestation.
- Many limb abnormalities are isolated lesions that occur sporadically; and rarely, multiple family members have the same limb abnormalities.
- Limb defects also can be associated with non-limb malformation or be part of a genetically based multiple malformation syndrome.
- When transverse terminal defects are present, the origin is most likely vascular.

Epidemiology

- Limb deficiency defects occur in 4.80 to 5.97 per 10,000 live births.
- Upper extremity involvement is significantly more common than lower extremity involvement.
- Unilateral defects occur in 75% to 80% and are more often right-sided, especially in the radius.
- Associated anomalies are found in up to 53% (musculoskeletal defects most frequent).
- Other abnormalities, including defects of the head and neck, cardiovascular system, gastrointestinal tract, and genitourinary tract are present in one-third of all cases.
- Associated abnormalities are seen most frequently with radial defects but are not commonly found with ulnar and transverse terminal lesions.

Pathophysiology

- An abnormal limb may be the result of malformation, deformation, disruption, or dysplasia.
- Malformations are the result of poor formation of tissue that initiates a chain of additional abnormalities. Affected structures seldom revert to normal and surgery is usually required.
- Deformations occur as a result of mechanical forces applied to a normal embryo or fetus and generally occur in the third trimester.
  - Deformities involving the upper extremity have a good prognosis since delivery ends the intrauterine molding.
  - Most 6 to 8 months after birth and surgery is uncommon (10%).
- Disruptions are structural defects that result from destruction of a part that has differentiated normally, such as congenital constriction ring syndrome.
- Dysplasia describes conditions that arise from the abnormal arrangements of cells into tissues (e.g., hamartoma).

Classification

The classification of upper extremity anomalies continues to be based on the gross morphologic presentation and it is not possible to precisely classify all malformations.

TABLE 28.2-1 CLASSIFICATION OF UPPER EXTREMITY ANOMALIES

Category	Description
I	Failure of formation of parts (arrest of development)
II	Failure of differentiation (separation) of parts
III	Duplication
IV	Overgrowth or gigantism
V	Undergrowth or hypoplasia
VI	Congenital constriction band syndrome
VII	Generalized skeletal abnormalities

Adapted from Swanson AB, Swanson GD, Tada K. A classification for congenital limb malformation. J Hand Surg 1983;8:693–702.

The seven categories established in 1968 by Swanson and colleagues remain the backbone of the classification (Table 28.2-1).

DIAGNOSIS

- The initial evaluation should include a careful history about the pregnancy, the child's prenatal course, and family history of similar disorders.
- The history may disclose fetal exposure to drugs, medications, infectious agents, or maternal metabolic imbalances that increase the risks of birth defects.
- Examination should include the general appearance of the child with attention to stature, proportion, head and facial symmetry and contralateral limb, leaving the affected limb to be examined last.
  - Look at the chest for affects in pectoralis major development (Poland syndrome) and the back for any obvious deformity.
  - Infants with positional deformations of the upper limbs should be evaluated for neurologic conditions and possible associated abnormalities in the cervical spine.
- Radial dysplasia, triphalangeal thumb, and hemihypertrophy are potentially associated with life-threatening cardiac, hematopoietic, or tumorous conditions.
- Close communication with the child's pediatrician is important, particularly if surgery is planned.
- To date, most heritable upper extremity defects have not been linked to a specific gene locus and cannot be diagnosed *in utero* using molecular technology.

Clinical Features

Fingers and Thumb

Symbrachydactyly

- Most frequently affects one upper extremity with usual obvious digital anomalies
- Short coalesced digits
- Four types:
  - Short finger type—short fingers normal thumb
  - Oligodactylic type—normal thumb and small finger

- ☐ Monodactylic—aplasia of fingers normal thumb
- ☐ Peromelic—transverse absence of all digits at metacarpal level

Syndactyly
- Fusion of adjacent digits
- One of the most common congenital hand deformities
- Males affected twice as frequently as females
- 10% to 40% familial
- Forms:
  - ☐ Simple syndactyly—skin alone
  - ☐ Complex syndactyly—skin and bone
  - ☐ Complete syndactyly—whole web space
  - ☐ Incomplete syndactyly—partial web space
- Associated with polydactyly, clefting, symbrachydactyly, or ring constrictions
- Apert syndrome
  - ☐ Rare (1 in 45,000)
  - ☐ Craniosynostosis and severe complex syndactyly involving hands and feet
  - ☐ Usually arises by new mutation
  - ☐ Most patients have normal intelligence
  - ☐ Much can be done with the hands to enhance both function and appearance
- Poland syndrome
  - ☐ Small or absent pectoralis major and syndactyly

Polydactyly
- Radial (thumb duplication), ulna, or central
- Most common congenital hand anomaly in African Americans (10.7 per 1,000)
- Twice as common in males
- Ulnar polydactyly 10 times more common in African Americans than in Caucasians
- Radial polydactyly occurs with equal racial frequency
- Central polydactyly is extremely rare
- Ulnar polydactyly varies from skin tag to duplicated finger

Duplicated Thumb
- Occurs more frequently in males
- Right more commonly than left

TABLE 28.2-2 CLASSIFICATION OF DUPLICATED THUMB

Type	Description
I	Bifid distal phalanx
II	Complete duplication of distal phalanx
III	Duplicated distal phalanx with bifid proximal phalanx
IV	Complete duplication of proximal and distal phalanx (most common)
V	Bifid first metacarpal
VI	Complete duplication of thumb including metacarpal (least common)
VII	Elements of a triphalangeal thumb

Adapted from Wassel HD. The results of surgery for polydactyly of the thumb. Clin Orthop 1969;64:175–93.

- Duplication associated with a triphalangeal thumb may be associated with certain syndromes
- Wassel's classification of seven categories is based on the level of skeletal division (Table 28.2-2).

Triphalangeal Thumb
- One in 25,000 births
- 65% of children with bilateral deficiency have a positive family history
- Most unilateral cases have a positive inheritance
- Most frequent association is with thumb duplication
- Less frequently seen with typical cleft hands, radial dysplasias, congenital heart disease, ear anomalies, blood dyscrasias, cardiovascular and gastrointestinal tract anomalies

Macrodactyly
- Condition in which one or more digits are larger than normal.
- May occur as an isolated anomaly (pseudomacrodactyly or true macrodactyly) or as part of a congenital syndrome.
  - ☐ True macrodactyly is noted at birth or soon after and its growth may be static or progressive.
  - ☐ Pseudomacrodactyly is usually due to soft tissue involvement (not bony).
- Macrodactyly is present in several congenital syndromes such as neurofibromatosis, Ollier disease, Maffucci syndrome, and congenital lymphedema.

Symphalangism
- Absent proximal interphalangeal (PIP) joints with normal length of all phalanges
- Often bilateral with radial digits more severely affected
- Rare autosomal dominant inherited condition
- No finger creases over PIP joints

Camptodactyly
- A nontraumatic flexion deformity of the PIP joint of one or several fingers
- Familial cases have an autosomal dominant pattern
- Frequently associated with Marfan, Holt-Oram, and Poland syndromes
- Small finger most commonly affected
- Increasing contracture during growth spurts
- Differential diagnosis: boutonniere deformity, triggering (palpable nodule in the palm), congenital absence of extensor mechanism
- Anomalous lumbricals, a consistent feature
- Results of splintage variable
- Surgery continues to evolve, and surgery before deformity is established probably offers best results.

Clinodactyly
- Digital angulation in the radioulnar plane
- A physical sign, not a disease
- Arises from a disordered growth of bone for a variety of reasons
- Four categories
  - ☐ Familial
  - ☐ Associated with other congenital abnormalities

- Following injury to growth plate
- Triphalangeal thumb
- Splinting alone does not correct.
- Usually no functional loss
- Beware of surgical correction complications.

Kirner Deformity

- Radial and volar curvature of the distal phalanx of the small finger
- May not become apparent until puberty, progressive curvature
- Radiographic diagnosis, majority need no treatment
- Familial with autosomal dominant inheritance, frequent sporadic cases
- Can be associated with a number of syndromes including Down and Turner

Delta Phalanx

- A triangular bone with a continuous physis or epiphysis along the shorter side that links the proximal and distal epiphysis.
- The shape can be triangular, trapezoidal, or almost round.
- Sporadic, inherited, or associated with many syndromes.
- The last bone to develop a primary ossification center shows the greatest disposition toward the anomaly (middle phalanx of the small finger).
- Delta phalanx does not always produce clinodactyly and clinodactyly is not always the result of delta phalanx.
- Mild deformity (10 degrees) can be ignored in the older child.
- Treatment depends on the type of phalanx, the contribution it makes to the length and deformity, the age at presentation, and the family's wishes and expectations.
- Treatment options:
  - Physiolysis (Langenskiöld procedure) to remove the tether on the short side and prevent its reformation with a fat graft
  - Corrective osteotomy
  - Closing is the simplest option, but leads to shortening
  - Opening osteotomy decreases the loss of length
- Excision of abnormal phalanx if small

Amniotic Band Syndrome

- Attributed to the formation of amniotic bands *in utero*
- Precise etiology is unknown but the primary event appears to be rupture of the amniotic membrane so that part of or all of the fetus lies outside the amnion.
- The accepted method of correcting the circular constriction is to excise the deep part of the constriction and break the line of the circular scar with Z-plasties.

Anomalies of Tendons

- Absence, hypoplasia, duplication, and abnormal attachment of tendons are all recognized.
- The most commonly encountered functional tendon anomalies involve the thumb.
- Trigger digits:
  - Clicking or snapping is experienced as the digit moves from flexion to extension. The nodule on the flexor tendon pops in and out through the annular pulley.
  - Can be present at birth, occurs most commonly in the thumb.
  - May develop during childhood, most commonly in the first year
- Triggering rarely seen, usually parents notice that the child does not extend the interphalangeal joint of the thumb
- Possibility of spontaneous resolution during the first year of life and no fixed joint changes for 1 to 3 years
- Consider release at the end of the first year.

Congenital Clasped Thumb

- Absence or hypoplasia of extensor pollicis brevis.
- Characterized by flexion of the metacarpal phalangeal (MP) joint and adduction of the first metacarpal so the thumb lies across the palm.
  - This is the normal posture for the first 3 months, so the diagnosis can only be made after 3 months when this is noted to be persistent.
- Can be an isolated abnormality but more frequently part of a more complex disorder such as a windblown hand.
- Main differential diagnosis is trigger thumb.
- Splinting and passive stretching is usually effective by the end of the first year—if not, surgery is indicated.

Hypoplastic Thumb

- Blauth's classification is given in Table 28.2-3.
- Treatment depends on the type and ranges from no treatment necessary to pollicization.

Hand

Cleft Hand

- Incidence is 0.4 per 10,000 live births.
- Cases occur sporadically but may be familial, autosomal dominant.

TABLE 28.2-3 CLASSIFICATION OF HYPOPLASTIC THUMB

Type	Description
I	Minor hypoplasia; thumb is small but functions normally
II	Thumb is smaller and less stable than normal, with 3 elements: ■ Adduction contracture of the first web space ■ Lack of thenar muscles ■ Laxity of ulnar collateral ligament of the MP joint
III	Type II plus: ■ Skeletal hypoplasia in which the carpometacarpal joint is vestigial ■ Intrinsics are absent ■ Extrinsics are rudimentary
IV	Floating thumb (*pouce flottant*)
V	Total absence

Adapted from Blauth W. Der Hypoplastische Daumen. Arch Orthop Unfall-Chip 1967;62:225–46.

- Clefting can occur without absence of a digit, however most cases have absence of one or more digits and may have varying degrees of polydactyly and syndactyly.
- Often the middle finger alone is missing and the defect may extend to produce a deep V-shaped cleft with absence of the metacarpal.
- Frequent synostosis between capitate and hamate.
- Often bilateral and associated with comparable foot deformities.
- If untreated, these patients or these "hands" develop remarkable hand function.
- The deformity is unsightly and surgery can improve cosmesis while maintaining function.

Wrist, Forearm, and Elbow

Longitudinal Radial Deficiency: Radial Club Hand

- Spectrum varies from a slightly hypoplastic radius or minor degree of thumb hypoplasia to a total absence of the radius, thumb, first metacarpal, scaphoid, and trapezium.
- The entire forearm may be shortened with the ulna thickened and bowed radially.
- The wrist becomes unstable with decreased range of motion.
- Range of motion of the fingers may be decreased.
- Overall hand function can be severely limited.
- Often associated with other congenital defects or syndromes:
  - Blood dyscrasias (e.g., Fanconi, TAR [thrombocytopenia-absent radius syndrome])
  - Congenital heart anomalies, (e.g., Holt-Oram),
  - Craniofacial defects (e.g., Nager)
  - Vertebral anomalies (e.g., VATER [vertebral anomalies, anal atresia, tracheoesophageal fistula, renal and radial anomalies])
- The most common nonsyndromic associated anomalies are listed in Box 28.2-1.
- Prevalence estimated at 1 per 55,000 to 1 per 100,000.
- In unilateral cases, right is greater than left and opposite thumb is often hypoplastic or defective.

BOX 28.2-1 MOST COMMON NONSYNDROMIC ASSOCIATED ANOMALIES

- Triphalangeal thumb
- Radioulnar synostosis
- Syndactyly
- Scoliosis
- Sprengel deformity
- Club foot
- Congenital dislocation of the hip
- Vetriculoseptal defect
- Lung abnormalities
- Cleft lip and palate
- Tracheoesophageal fistula
- Anal atresia
- Patent ductus arteriosus
- Hydrocephalus
- Deafness
- Genitourinary tract anomalies

TABLE 28.2-4 CLASSIFICATION OF LONGITUDINAL RADIAL DEFICIENCY

Type	Description
I	Short radius
II	Hypoplastic radius: distal and proximal epiphysis present
III	Partial absence: proximal, middle, or distal part of radius absent
IV	Total absence

Adapted from Bayne LG, Klug MS. Long term review of the surgical treatment of radial deficiencies. J Hand Surg (Am) 1987;12:169–79.

- Complete absence of the radius is more frequent than partial or hypoplasia.
- Bayne and Klug's classification is described in Table 28.2-4.
- Etiology still uncertain—probably multifactorial
- Hereditary tendencies not common
- Treatment options:
  - No treatment
    - Mild anomalies of the arm
    - Severe associated anomalies or syndromes
    - Older patients who have adjusted
    - Limited elbow flexion in which a straightened hand will not reach the mouth or perineum
    - Severe soft tissue contracture that involves the neurovascular structures
  - Splinting and stretching
    - Type I and II deficiencies with mild radial deviation of the hand and a stable wrist may require only stretching and maintenance until skeletal maturity.
  - Surgery
    - Severe type II, III, and IV with the hand severely displaced and deviated
    - Absent or hypoplastic thumbs and those with soft tissue contractures that cannot be reduced by manipulation and splints
    - Ideal time for surgery is age 6 months to 1 year
    - Enables soft tissue stretching in the first 6 months

Longitudinal Ulnar Deficiency: Ulnar Club Hand

- Incidence is 1 in 100,000 (1:10 ratio with radial deficiency).
- Many variations and the upper arm elbow, forearm, wrist, and hand can be involved.
- The elbow is frequently affected and because of the variable clinical picture, a standard treatment plan is difficult.
- Associated anomalies mainly affect the musculoskeletal system and the syndromes associated with radial club hand are exceptional.
- Indication for surgery is not clear.
- Debate continues about the need to excise the fibrocartilage anlage.
- Despite the appearance, children adapt well to the functional challenges.

- Operations on the forearm are difficult and controversial but improving function of the hand is usually straightforward and rewarding.

Synostosis

- Hand: phalangeal and metacarpal synostosis.
- Wrist: triquetrum to lunate and capitate to hamate most common.
- Elbow: humeroradial and humeroulnar.
- Forearm: radioulnar synostosis (most common).
- Cleary and Omer's classification is given in Table 28.2-5.
- Bilateral in 60%
- Normal pronation and supination within the carpus increases with congenital loss of forearm rotation.
- Compensation for fixed supination deformity is easier to overcome than fixed pronation deformity.
- Operative treatment (derotation osteotomy) at the fusion site probably indicated for excessively pronated forearm greater than 60 degrees
- Mobilization of the synostosis is difficult to maintain because of re-ankylosis.

Congenital Dislocation of the Radial Head

- Most common congenital anomaly of the elbow joint but still uncommon
- Can occur as an isolated entity or as part of a more generalized skeletal malformation syndrome
- Other skeletal disorders occur in 60% of cases.
- Invariably bilateral
- If unilateral, difficult to distinguish from traumatic origin
    - Bowing of the ulna suggests possibility of a traumatic dislocation.
    - Arthrography revealing the radial head outside the elbow capsule also suggests a traumatic dislocation.
- Dislocation can be anterior, posterior, or lateral, with variable reports as to the most common.
- The most characteristic feature radiologically is hypoplasia of the capitellum and a dome-shaped radial head.
- In most cases, the dislocation causes virtually no noticeable disability in childhood.
- Treatment is seldom indicated because of the lack of symptoms and normal function.
- In adolescence and adult life, pain may occur as a consequence of degenerative changes.

TABLE 28.2-5 CLASSIFICATION OF SYNOSTOSIS

Type	Description
I	Clinically radioulnar fusion with normal x-ray
II	Bony fusion; normal radial head
III	Bony fusion; hypoplastic, posteriorly dislocated radial head
IV	Bony fusion; mushroom-shaped radial head dislocated anteriorly

Adapted from Cleary JE, Omer GE Jr. Congenital proximal radio-ulnae synostosis. Natural history and functional assessment. J Bone Joint Surg 1985;67A:539–45.

TABLE 28.2-6 CLASSIFICATION OF SPRENGEL UNDESCENDED SCAPULA

Grade	Description
1	Very mild with no visible deformity when dressed
2	Mild with visible lump in the neck
3	Moderate with raised shoulder joint
4	Severe with scapula near the occiput

Adapted from Cavendish ME. Congential elevation of the scapula. J Bone Joint Surg 1972;54:395–408.

- Radial head excision is best avoided in the growing child as it may lead to instability of the elbow, cubitus valgus deformity, shortening of the forearm, and secondary subluxation of the distal radioulnar joint.

Shoulder

Sprengel Undescended Scapula

- Failure of descent of the scapula from the level of the embryonic limb bud opposite the fifth cervical vertebrae to its thoracic position
- The failure of descent has been attributed to tethering scapulovertebral articulations and defective musculature unable to draw the scapula caudally.
- Most affected individuals have associated anomalies of the clavicle, ribs, vertebrae, and shoulder musculature.
    - Present for evaluation of a webbed neck or loss of shoulder motion or both
- The Cavendish classification given in Table 28.2-6 aids in determining treatment.
    - Grades 1 and 2: can consider resection of the bony prominence and omovertebral bar
    - Grades 3 and 4: require the above for improved cosmesis and derotation and relocation of the scapula if shoulder abduction is less than 120 degrees

Poland Syndrome

- Represents the disruption of the normal sequence of development of the pectoralis major associated with abnormal development of the hand.
- Most patients with Poland syndrome have a spectrum of disorders that includes hypoplasia or aplasia of the pectoralis major, pectoralis minor, serratus anterior, and latissimus dorsi; rib and costal cartilage defects; absence or hypoplasia of the nipple or breast, axillary bands or webs in association with brachydactyly, syndactyly or hypoplasia or aplasia of the carpus or forearm, or all of these.

TREATMENT

Upper limb anomalies can be diagnosed as early as 14 weeks of gestation by ultrasound. Early in gestation, fetal cutaneous wounds heal without scar formation. There is exciting potential for correcting some abnormalities *in utero* and new endoscopic techniques are under development; however, many problems still prevent nonlethal fetal conditions from being managed in this way.

The major treatment considerations are to improve function, prevent increasing deformity, improve appearance, and do no further harm.

Timing

- Immunity to infection develops over time (the infant maintains passive immunity conferred by the mother for the first 5 weeks of life). Active immunity matures by 5 months. Therefore, avoid surgery between 5 weeks and 5 months.
- Early surgery prevents the emotional scarring associated with the child's awareness of the deformity.
- Hand length nearly doubles during the first 2 years of life. A digit tethered to another that fails to grow can produce a major deformity during the early growth spurt.
- Joint surfaces can remodel with growth if treated in the first year.
- Grasp and pinch are established by 1 year and accuracy of prehension and refinement of coordination continue until 3 years. Therefore, abnormal grasp patterns as in cleft hand and thumb aplasia or hypoplasia should be corrected before this time.
- Do not separate children under 5 years of age from parents.
- Plans for surgical reconstruction should be designed to be completed by school age.
- Children more than 2 years old should not have bilateral hands splinted at the same time.

Indications for Immediate Treatment

- Severe constriction band syndrome with distal edema
- Many deformities can be arrested or even partially corrected by early splinting and therapy.
- Decision to use a prosthesis in proximal transverse deficiency. Early use enables the child to incorporate it into normal function. If implemented later, the child will ignore it.

Indications for Treatment Within the First Year

- Early correction required because of rapid growth:
  - ☐ Syndactyly between digits of unequal length (border digits). (Common long to ring finger syndactyly can wait until 1 year of age.)
  - ☐ Syndactyly with bone bridges between terminal phalanges
  - ☐ Acrosyndactyly with partial aplasia of the adjacent digit
  - ☐ Longitudinal radial deficiency (before fixed soft tissue contractures occur).
- Early correction required because of functional concerns:
  - ☐ Early splinting for congenital clasped thumb may result in good outcome (if not improved by 6 months, do tendon transfer)
  - ☐ Cleft hand surgery
  - ☐ Thumb aplasia-pollicization
  - ☐ Duplicated thumb correction (particularly proximal)
- Excision of extra digits

Indications for Treatment After the First Year

- Surgery should be completed before school age.
- Conditions such as trigger thumb and minor clinodactyly may never require surgery.
- If rehabilitation after surgery requires cooperation, the procedure should be delayed until 5 to 6 years of age.
- Anomalies associated with life-threatening problems may need to be delayed until the patient is stable.

Anomalies That Should Not Be Treated

- Lack of elbow flexion in radial clubhand
- Unilateral radioulnar synostoses
- Other synostoses in the wrist and hand rarely need treatment
- In older children a functional pattern may have already been established.

Planning Principles

- Apert syndrome
  - ☐ First surgery at 6 months; plan completion of releases by 3 years.
  - ☐ Surgeries 6 months apart to be sure of digit viability.
  - ☐ Do not release adjacent webs simultaneously.
- Radial aplasia
  - ☐ Start with night splints and passive stretching.
  - ☐ Surgery at 6 months and pollicization 6 weeks later.
  - ☐ If bilateral, do first side at 6 months, other side at 9 months with pollicization completed by 15 months.
  - ☐ Splint full time until 6 years of age and then night splints until skeletally mature.
- Brachydactyly
  - ☐ Minimal requirement is to achieve a mobile thumb to oppose against an ulnar post by age 2 to 3 years.
  - ☐ Transferred toe phalanges with intact periosteum must be done in first year.
- Windblown hand
  - ☐ Splint and manipulate while awaiting surgery.
  - ☐ Treat before 2 years of age (over 5 years results are poor).

Problem Management

- Physical abnormalities may be more difficult for families to cope with than hidden congenital problems.
- Beware of unrealistic expectations.
- Genetic counseling should play a major role in the comprehensive medical management of a child with a hand malformation and information about support groups is particularly helpful.

SUGGESTED READING

Flatt AE, ed. The care of congenital hand anomalies, 2nd ed. St. Louis: Quality Medical Publishing, 1994.

Green D, Hotchkiss R, Pederson W, eds. Green's operative hand surgery, 4th ed. Vol 1. New York: Churchill Livingstone, 1999: 325–551.

Mih AE, ed. Congenital hand disorders. Hand Clin 1998;14:1.

Smith R, ed. Congenital deformities of the hand. Hand Clin 1985;1:3.

Swanson AB, Swanson GD, Tada K. A classification for congenital limb malformation. J Hand Surg 1983;8:693–702.

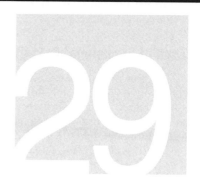

THE PHYSIS

ARABELLA I. LEET
GAIL S. CHORNEY

The growth plate is a unique complex cartilaginous structure that is responsible for bone growth in all long bones. The growth plate consists of columns of chondrocytes that are separated by fibrous septae. The integrity of this architecture is essential for continued growth. The cells in each column undergo a precise proliferation and maturation pattern. Calcification does not occur until the last layer at the border of the metaphysis. Calcification earlier in the process would result in premature closure of the growth plate. The process of bone growth and calcification is strictly regulated. Control is mainly hormonal, but there are mechanical influences on the physis that can both inhibit or promote growth. Closure of the physis occurs around age 13 in girls and age 16 in boys. Infection, injury, or disease can result in growth disturbances, which can be angular, if only part of the physis closes, or result in shortening of the entire bone if the majority of the physis is involved.

STRUCTURE OF THE PHYSIS

The physis is made up of distinctive zones, starting from the secondary ossification center and moving toward the metaphysis:

- Resting or reserve zone
- Zone of proliferation
- Zone of maturation
- Zone of hypertrophy
- Zone of provisional calcification

Resting Zone

- The reserve or resting zone remains a region of mystery in terms of its exact function, although matrix production is very active in this zone.
- The reserve zone is characterized histologically by the irregular distribution of cells within the matrix in contrast to the stacked orderly cell layers in the zones above.
  - Cell proliferation is sporadic although most of the cells in the resting layer are actively making proteins as evidenced by an abundance of intracellular endoplasmic reticulum.
  - Blood vessels pass through the reserve zone en route to the proliferative zone without oxygenating the reserve zone where the oxygen tension is low.
  - The matrix surrounding the cells contains irregular fibrils of collagen rich in type 2 collagen.
    - The reserve zone contains more matrix collagen than any other zone of the physis.
    - The proteoglycans in the matrix are in an aggregate form that prohibits the mineralization of the matrix.

Zone of Proliferation/Maturation

- The zone of proliferation contains the first columnar cells as well as a single germinal cell layer.
  - If this single layer of cells is damaged during trauma, arrest of the entire physis can occur.
  - These stem cells undergo clonal expansion when stimulated.
- The cells are regularly arranged but much flatter-appearing than the cells in the hypertrophic zone.
- Cells are undergoing differentiation and maturation.
- Oxygen tension is high, as are glycogen stores.
- Aerobic glycolysis supports rapid proteoglycan synthesis.
- The growth from a particular physis is determined by the number of cell divisions in the proliferative zone.
- The matrix remains disorganized.

Zone of Hypertrophy

- The cells in the zone of hypertrophy gain height compared to the cells in the proliferative zone.
  - The amount of cell hypertrophy correlates to the growth rate.
- The cells in the zone of hypertrophy align parallel to the diaphyseal shaft of the bone.
- Cells in the zone of hypertrophy actively synthesize matrix proteins, alkaline phosphatase, and type X collagen.
- The cells have a low intracellular conversion of adenosine triphosphate (ATP) to adenosine diphosphate (ADP) compared with the cells in other zones.

- Oxygen tension is low and anaerobic glycolysis is used for energy production.

Zone of Provisional Calcification

- The growth-plate chondrocytes control matrix mineralization through intracellular calcium transport using specialized mitochondria that transport calcium.
- Factors that control matrix mineralization include:
  - Hormones [parathyroid hormone (PTH,) calcitonin, insulin-like growth factor 1 (IGF-1)]
  - Intracellular calcium stores
  - Extracellular matrix
  - Local environment

HORMONAL SIGNALING

Hormonal signaling occurs as an endocrine function in which hormones travel from other areas of the body to exert an effect on the growth plate. Examples of such hormones include growth hormone, thyroid hormone, or vitamin D. Other signaling occurs locally from within the growth center (paracrine) or from the cell itself (autocrine). Examples of locally acting molecules include IGF-1, fibroblast growth factors (FGFs), bone morphogenic proteins, transforming growth factor-β (TGF-β), and parathyroid-related protein (PTHrP).

Growth Hormone

- Peptide hormone produced by the pituitary
- Acts on all zones of the growth plate, but the mechanism by which growth hormone (GH) exerts an effect is not completely known
  - GH may cause chondrocytes to produce IGF-1.
  - GH also regulates the IGF receptors on the target cells.
- Effects chondrocytes in the zone of proliferation

Thyroid Hormone

- The thyroid secretes thyroxine (T_4), which is then deionized in the liver or kidney to form the more potent form, triiodothyronine (T_3).
- Thyroid hormones act to increase DNA synthesis in the cells in the zone of proliferation.
- These hormones also function to stimulate cell maturation.
- Thyroid hormone interacts with other hormones such as IGF-1.

Parathyroid Hormone

- This protein is produced in the parathyroid glands.
- Acts at the zone of hypertrophy
  - Stimulates chondrocyte proliferation and causes an increase in synthesis of proteoglycans
  - Shares a common receptor with PTHrP
  - Through the receptors PTH and PTHrP, PTH causes maturation of cells and transformation to the hypertropic phenotype

Vitamin D

- Two active forms of vitamin D with different mechanisms of action on growth-plate chondrocytes.
  - $25(OH)_1D_3$ is deiodinized in the liver.
  - $1,25(OH)_2D_3$ and $24,25(OH)_2D_3$ are deiodinized for a second time in the kidney.
- The absence of vitamin D causes the elongation of cells in the hypertrophic zone and a decrease in mineralization.
  - Vitamin D metabolites cause a decrease in systemic calcium and phosphorus leading to a decrease in mineralization of growth-plate matrix.
- $24,25(OH)_2D_3$ has a direct effect of increasing DNA synthesis, while $1,25(OH)_2D_3$ inhibits proteoglycan production.

Insulin Growth Factors

- Previously called somatomedins
- Stimulate cellular production of RNA and DNA as well sulfated proteoglycans

Fibroblast Growth Factors

- A family of more than 10 heparin-binding polypeptides
  - Which specific FGF exerts an effect depends on the age of the host.
  - FGF-2 causes development of neonatal chondrocytes, while FGF-1 acts on older growth plates.
- The effects may be potentiated by interaction with IGF-1 as well as autocrine or paracrine modulation in response to GH.
- The FGFs stimulate chondrocytes in mitogenesis, receptor regulation, and protease production.

Transforming Growth Factor-β

- Superfamily includes the bone morphogenic proteins.
- These growth factors tend to up-regulate production of matrix elements.
- TGF-β may both suppress and stimulate chondrocytes depending on the local effect of other hormones.

MECHANICAL STIMULATION

- The physis responds to loads placed across it.
- The Heuter-Volkman law explains this phenomenon and, in general, describes the observation that compressive forces across the physis decrease growth while growth of the bone is enhanced by distraction-type forces.
- There are exceptions to the Heuter-Volkman law as excessive distraction seems to impede growth as much as compressive force.

- Compressive forces:
  - Example: stapling of the physis is thought to stop growth across the physis by compression (applied either to one side of the physis to correct angular deformities occurring in Blount disease or placed on both sides of the physis to stop the growth of the limb (staple epiphysiodesis).
  - Deformity in the staples can be measured and demonstrates the large mechanical load the physis can produce estimated at 1 to 5 MPa.
- Distraction forces:
  - Distraction across a limb.
    - Clinical observations have shown decrease in predicted growth after lengthening.
    - In an animal model of distraction, osteogenesis lengthening of greater than 30% of the limb resulted in decreased growth of the limb that seemed to affect the overall amount of lengthening more than the rate of lengthening.
  - Direct distraction across the physis.
    - Has become a less popular technique, as continued growth of the physis is unpredictable after attempts to lengthen across the physis.
- The physis has different mechanical properties depending on location within the physis and based on the structure of the growth plate.
  - The periphery of the growth plate is more compliant and less permeable than the center of the growth plate.
  - In animal models of the physis subjected to strain, the thicker the physis, the weaker the physis at resisting the forces placed across it.

TRAUMA

- The physis withstands stress or tensile forces better than compression or crushing type forces.
  - Shear loading causes separation of the physis at the zone of hypertrophy, often leaving the resting zone intact.

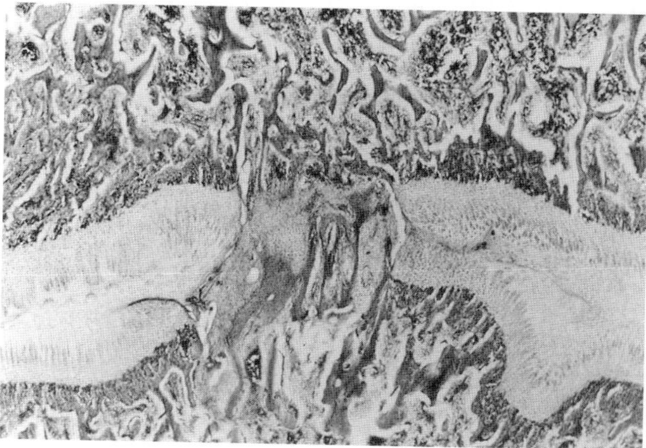

Figure 29-1 Experimental physeal bar created in a pig model of hip dysplasia after pelvic osteotomy. (From Leet AI, Mackenzie WG, Szoke G, et al. Injury to the growth plate after Pemberton osteotomy. J Bone Joint Surg [Am] 1999;81:169–176.)

  - The fate of the physis ultimately rests in the fate of the single cell stromal layer in the proliferating zone (Fig. 29-1).
- Classification system (Table 29-1 and Figs. 29-2 and 29-3):
  - In general, the larger the number, regardless of which schema, the more likely the chance of a physeal closure.
  - Prognosis of a physeal closure is also based on:
    - Patient age
    - Severity of the fracture
      - Skin integrity
      - Amount of comminution
      - Amount of fracture displacement
    - Location of the physis
      - The physes about the knee (distal femur and proximal tibia) contribute most to longitudinal growth (greater than 1 cm/year).

TABLE 29-1 CLASSIFICATION OF PHYSEAL INJURIES[a]

System		
Peterson	Salter	Description
I	—	The fracture is primarily in the metaphysis but extends into the physis
II	II	The fracture goes across the physis and into the metaphysis (Thurston-Holland fragment)
III	I	The fracture line goes along the physis, a shear injury
IV	III	The fracture extends from the physis into the joint (through the epiphysis)
V	IV	The fracture involves the metaphysis, physis, and epiphysis
VI		Loss of tissue: fragment missing
—	V	Crush injury to physis

[a]See also Figures 29-2 and 29-3.

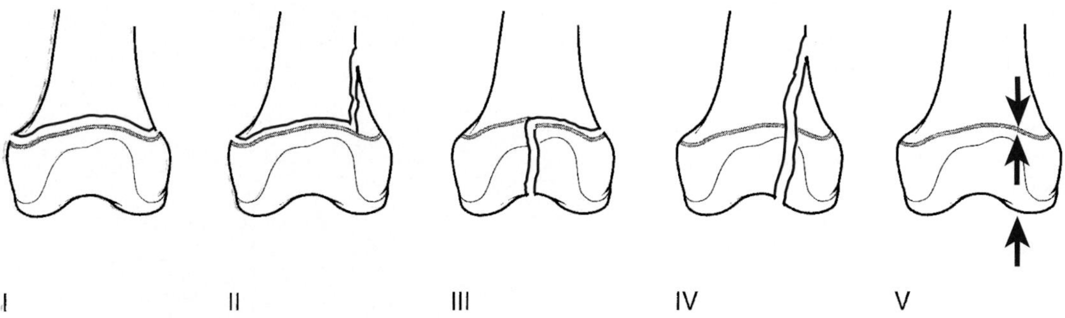

Figure 29-2 Salter and Harris classification of physeal fractures (1963). (Adapted from Peterson HA. Physeal fractures. Part 3: classification. J Pediatr Orthop 1994;14:439–448.)

- If the entire physis closes, there is loss of overall length of the bone; if only part of the physis closes, there can be significant angular deformity.
  - □ The physis closes in trauma as new healing bone forms across the growth plate forming a bone bridge or bar.
  - □ Impending physeal closure is not possible to make an initial diagnosis either clinically or radiographically.
    - □ Often, 6 months or more must elapse before there is an obvious change in the alignment of the bone or there is evidence of bone bridging on radiographic images.
    - □ Extensive bars can be seen on plain films, other more subtle growth-plate disturbances require computed tomography, magnetic resonance imaging, or tomograms.
- Treatment of a premature physeal closure:
  - □ For bars of less than 50% of the entire physis, excision of the bar with placement of an interpositional material (cranioplast or fat).
  - □ Bars not suitable for excision may require complete physeal closure to stop angular deformities from developing.
  - □ If the physis has closed, choices for treatment include closure of the identical physis on the opposite limb, or treatment of the limb length discrepancy with either a shoe lift or a lengthening procedure (depending on the amount of predicted limb length discrepancy at skeletal maturity).

INFECTION

- Infection in children occurs first in the metaphyseal region of the bone where the capillaries form sinusoidal loops.
  - □ The growth plate tends to block infection from spreading into the epiphysis, but significant infection can cause destruction of the physis leading to angular deformity or growth arrest.
  - □ Since infections can occur very early in life the amount of limb length discrepancy can be substantial.
    - □ Treatment is often with distraction osteogenesis.
- Infection tends to spread from the metaphysis (osteomyelitis) to the periosteum (subperiosteal abscess) and finally into the joint space (septic joint).
  - □ Bones in which the metaphysis is intracapsular are at higher risk for a septic arthritis and include the proximal humerus and femur, the radial head, and the distal fibula.
- Common organisms responsible for infection in childhood are listed in Box 29-1.

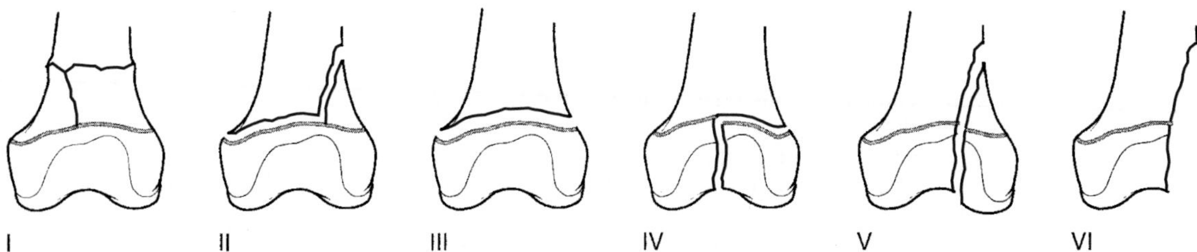

Figure 29-3 Peterson classification of physeal fractures (1994). (Adapted from Peterson HA. Physeal fractures. Part 3: classification. J Pediatr Orthop 1994;14:439–448.)

BOX 29-1 COMMON INFECTIOUS ORGANISMS THAT INFECT BONE

Newborn
- Staphylococcus aureus
- Group B *Streptococcus*
- Enterobacteriacae
- *Neisseria gonorrhoeae*

Children
- *S. aureus*
- *Streptococcus pyrogenes*
- *Streptococcus pneumoniae*
- *Haemophilus influenzae* (all but irradicated in children who have been vaccinated)

Adolescents
- *S. aureus*
- Streptococci
- *N. gonorrhoeae*

Adults
- *S. aureus*

Special Cases
- Sickle cell disease
  Salmonella
- Immunosuppressed
  S. aureus
  Staphylococcus epidermidis
  Pseudomonas aeruginosa

DISEASES OF THE GROWTH PLATE

Diseases of Cellular Proliferation

- Achondroplasia is the most common genetic skeletal dysplasia.
- Rhizomelia, seen in achondroplasia, results from decreased growth involving the proximal long bones.
- Achondroplasia results from a point mutation of the fibroblast growth factor receptor 3 (FGFr-3).
  - FGFs are a family of heparin-binding polypeptides that are potent mitogens of growth-plate chondrocytes whose actions are controlled by receptors (FGFr-1 through 4) on the cell surface.
  - FGFs interact with receptors on the cell surface to cause transphosphorylation and cellular signal transduction.
  - Other genetic mutations of the FGF receptors can result in skeletal dysplasias.
  - Periosteal bone formation continues normally, causing the radiographic feature of widened metaphyses occurring from the uncoupling of longitudinal and latitudinal growth.
- Presentation
  - Shortening of the limbs.
  - Bowing deformities.
  - Developmental delay.
  - Spinal deformity.
    - Kyphosis prior to walking.
    - Spinal stenosis in adulthood.
- Treatment
  - Multidisciplinary approach to address specific problems

Diseases of Abnormal Mechanical Loads

Blount Disease

- Tibia vara, congenital or late onset
- Risk factors
  - Early walking
  - Obesity
- Pathology
  - Biopsy specimens show loss of columnar arrangement of the cells throughout the physis.
  - More pathology is seen on the medial side than on the lateral side.
  - Bone bars (see "Trauma" section earlier in the chapter) have also been identified.
- Presentation
  - Painless
  - Bowing deformity of the involved lower extremity
- Treatment
  - Bracing in young children with three-point fixation and a locked knee hinge
  - Surgical correction in older children or after failure of bracing
  - For recurrence of deformity, identification and resection of a physeal bar using interpositional material or revision osteotomy to restore mechanical alignment

Coxa Vara

- Defined as a decrease in the neck shaft angle (can be congenital or acquired)
- Biopsy specimens taken from the growth plate show:
  - Derangement of the cells in the resting zone
  - Loss of columnar organization in the proliferative and hypertrophic zones
  - Absence or poor formation of the zone of provisional calcification
  - Pathology similar to that seen in Blount disease.
- Presentation
  - Acquired, idiopathic form develops around age 6
  - Usually painless with a limp noted by the family
  - If unilateral, a limb length discrepancy may occur
  - Waddling gait (weakness of hip abductor muscles)
  - Limited range of motion in abduction and internal rotation of the hip
- Treatment
  - Corrective osteotomy to restore normal hip joint mechanics

Slipped Capital Femoral Epiphysis

- The perichondral ring protects the physis against shear forces, with subsequent physeal separation through the hypertrophic zone.

- In slipped capital femoral epiphysis (SCFE), the physis is composed of multiple layers of both dense fibrotic tissue and loosely packed cells.
- In SCFE, there is loss of integrity to the perichondral ring.
  - If the disruption is slow and consists of plastic deformation the patient presents with limp and hip pain of long-standing duration; if the ring fails acutely the presentation can be similar to a fracture with loss of ability to bear weight.
- Risk factors
  - Increased body weight which applies more load to the physis
  - Change in orientation of the physis in adolescents from a more horizontal to vertical direction, leading to more shear stress across the growth center
  - Endocrine disorders, such as hyperparathyroidism and renal failure
- Presentation
  - Pain in the lateral thigh, groin, or knee area
  - Inability to bear weight (by definition an unstable slip)
  - Limp
  - Obligate external rotation of the hip
- Treatment
  - *In situ* pinning of the head
  - Corrective osteotomy for residual deformity

Diseases of Mineralization of Matrix

- Causes can be nutritional (rickets), or resulting from matrix defects in chondrocytes (mucopolysaccharidosis) or osteoblast dysfunction (osteogenesis imperfecta).

Rickets

- Vitamin D derangement occurring from nutritional deficiencies or from cellular resistance to vitamin D
- Lack of vitamin D results in impaired calcification at the zone of provisional calcification.
- Clinical features
  - Bowing of limbs
  - Lower than predicted height for age
  - Radiographs show pathognomonic cupping of the growth plates with growth plate widening.
- Treatment consists of maximizing medical management which often corrects limb deformity. Surgical correction is the choice of last resort.

Mucopolysaccharidosis

- Genetic defects in enzymes that mediate proteoglycan metabolisms resulting in accumulation of fat in the cells
- Clinical presentation varies depending on particular condition but can include mental retardation, stunted growth, facial dysmorphism, and orthopaedic problems such as hip dysplasia, coxa vara, Madelung deformity
- Treatment
  - Bone marrow transplantation

Osteogenesis Imperfecta

- Caused by a mutation of either the *COL1A1* or *COL1A2* gene, both of which have a direct effect on the triple helical pattern of collagen.
- Presents with frequent fractures, blue sclera, and poor dentition.
- Treatment
  - Recently, medical treatment with bisphosphonates has shown some promise in decreasing the rate of fracture.
  - Rodding procedures are also often required.

SUGGESTED READING

Bruder SP, Caplan AI. Cellular and molecular events during embryonic bone development. Connect Tissue Res 1989; 20:65–71.

Buckwalter JA, Einhorn TA, Simon SR, eds. Orthopedic basic science, 2nd ed. Rosemont, IL: American Academy of Orthopedic Surgeons, 2000.

Buckwalter JA, Erlich MG, Sandell LJ, et al, eds. Skeletal growth and development: clinical issues and basic science advances. Rosemont, IL: American Academy of Orthopedic Surgeons, 1998.

Bylski-Aaustrow DI, Wall EJ, Rupert MP, et al. Growth plate forces in the adolescent human knee: a radiographic and mechanical study of epiphyseal staples. J Pediatr Orthop 2001;21:817–823.

Cohen B, Chorney GS, Phillips DP, et al. The microstructural tensile properties and biochemical composition of the bovine distal femoral growth plate. J Orthop Res 1992;10:263–275.

Cohen B, Chorney GS, Phillips DP, et al. Compressive stress-relaxation behavior of bovine growth plate may be described by the nonlinear biphasic theory. J Orthop Res 1994;12:804–813.

Floyd WE III, Zaleske DJ, Schiller AL, et al. Vascular events associated with the appearance of the secondary center of ossification in the murine distal femoral epiphysis. J Bone Joint Surg 1987; 185–189.

Lee SH, Szoke G, Simpson H. Response of the physis to leg lengthening. J Pediatr Orthop 2001;10:339–343.

Peterson HA. Physeal injuries and growth arrest. In: Beaty JH, Kasser JR, eds. Rockwood and Wilkins' fractures in children, 5th ed. Philadelphia: Lippincott Williams & Wilkins, 2001:92–138.

Williams JL, Do PD, Eick JD, et al. Tensile properties of the physis vary with anatomic location, thickness, strain rate and ag e. J Orthop Res 2001;19:1043–1048.

GENETICS

SEVAN HOPYAN
BENJAMIN A. ALMAN

The etiology of any biologic disorder is a combination of genetic predisposition and environmental factors. As such, most musculoskeletal conditions have, in whole or in part, a genetic basis. This chapter reviews basic principles of inheritance and summarizes a number of pediatric orthopaedic disorders with a genetic basis.

Patients with genetic disorders frequently present to orthopaedists, and it is not uncommon for an orthopaedist to be the first to entertain a genetic diagnosis for a given patient. For this reason, it is necessary for the orthopaedists to have at least background knowledge in genetics. When a patient is suspected to have a genetic disorder, appropriate consultation with clinical genetics should be made. In addition, information about genetic disorders is moving at a rapid pace, making it difficult for traditional textbooks to keep up with newest information. An excellent source for up- to-date information is the Online Mendelian Inheritance in Man (OMIM), which is maintained by the National Center for Biotechnology Information, and is located at http://www.ncbi.nlm.nih.gov:80/entrez/query.fcgi?db=OMIM.

GENES

A *gene* is a sequence of DNA (deoxyribonucleic acid) that is required for the production of a protein. Within the nuclei of human cells, there are about 30,000 genes, composed of just four nucleic acids (adenosine, cytosine, thiamine, and guanine). Most cells are diploid, meaning they contain two copies, or *alleles*, of every gene contained within the autosomal and X chromosomes in females, and within the autosomal chromosomes in males (males, of course, have one X and one Y chromosome). Each gene has a region of DNA adjacent to it, which regulates how the gene is activated. The gene itself is arranged into *exon* and *intron* regions. The exons are transcribed and spliced together to form RNA (ribonucleic acid), which then permits translation of the code for amino acid assembly. Many proteins undergo extensive posttranslational processing. A mutation is an irreversible change in DNA sequence, which may be a deletion, an insertion or a substitution of DNA, and can vary in length from a single nucleic acid to large portions of chromosomes. Mutations may exist in all cells, and are termed *germline mutations*, or in only some cells, in which case they are termed *somatic mutations*. Each time a cell divides, it makes a copy of its DNA, a process during which new mutations can develop. Chromosomal abnormalities (trisomies or translocations) occur when large-scale changes occur, causing major errors.

Patterns of Single-Gene Inheritance

A single-gene trait may be new or inherited, and inheritance may be *Mendelian* (classic) or *non-Mendelian* (non-classic). In Mendelian inheritance, single-gene traits segregate within families, and usually occur in fixed proportions among children. *Autosomal* and *X-linked* are terms used to note the chromosomal location of the involved gene, and *dominant* and *recessive* are terms that signify how a specific gene causes its phenotype.

AUTOSOMAL INHERITANCE

Autosomal dominance is the most common pattern of single-gene inheritance. With autosomal dominant inheritance, only one of the two copies of the gene needs to be abnormal to cause disease, and every affected individual has an affected parent. Children of affected individuals have a 50% chance of inheriting an autosomal dominant trait, and phenotypically normal family members do not transmit the phenotype to their children. Males and females are equally likely to transmit the phenotype to children of either sex.

Autosomal recessive inheritance requires both copies of the gene to be abnormal to cause disease. The phenotype is seen in children, but not in parents. The recurrence risk for each sibling of an individual with a disease is 1 in 4. Because of the rarity in the population of many alleles responsible for autosomal recessive conditions, the parents of an affected child may in some cases be consanguineous. Males and females are equally likely to be affected.

X-Linked Inheritance

Because males have one copy of the X chromosome, they are more susceptible to recessive diseases inherited from a gene on this chromosome than women, who have two copies. Most of one of the two X chromosomes in every female cell is inactive. *Inactivation* (*lyonization*) takes place within the first week of development, and is random in any one cell. However, once established, all clonal descendants of a given cell have the same inactive X chromosome. Females therefore have some distribution of two cell populations and are thus *mosaic* with regard to their X-linked alleles. The variability of this mosaicism will affect the degree of manifestation of an X-linked phenotype. Distinction of X-linked dominant and recessive patterns of inheritance may be complicated by mosaicism.

X-linked recessive traits are much more common in males than in females. A responsible allele is transmitted from an affected father through all his daughters who become unaffected carriers. Any of this man's daughters' sons has a 1 in 2 chance of inheriting that allele. The allele is never transmitted from father to son, and affected males in a kindred are related through females. Homozygosity in females is rare, but will lead to an equal chance of being affected or of being a carrier. Sometimes, due to unfavorable mosaicism, heterozygous females may express an X-linked condition with variable severity.

For a condition that is inherited in an X-linked dominant fashion, affected males with non-affected mates will have no affected sons and no unaffected daughters. Both female and male offspring of female carriers have a 1 in 2 risk of inheriting the phenotype, as is the case with an autosomal dominant phenotype. For rare phenotypes, affected females are about twice as common as affected males, but affected females typically have milder expression of the phenotype.

PENETRANCE AND EXPRESSIVITY

Sometimes, the phenotype caused by a mutation may vary with different individuals, even from within the same family. This may be caused by factors altering gene expression, or by modifying genes. *Penetrance* of a phenotype is reduced if it does not affect everyone who carries the appropriate genotype in an all-or-none fashion. This phenomenon can lead to apparent skipping of generations in autosomal dominant conditions. Variable *expressivity* exists when the manifestation of a phenotype differs in individuals with the same genotype. Pedigrees of autosomal dominant conditions may show *anticipation*, the apparent worsening of a condition in successive generations due to variable expressivity.

NON-MENDELIAN PATTERNS OF INHERITANCE

In recent years it was discovered that diseases can be inherited in non-Mendelian manners. Examples of such mechanisms include *unstable segments of DNA*, *uniparental disomy*, *imprinting*, and *mitochondrial DNA inheritance*.

Mitochondria have their own circular chromosome. There are several copies of this chromosome per mitochondrion, and thousands per cell. Mitochondrial DNA (mtDNA) encodes for transfer RNAs and for polypeptides that are subunits of enzymes of oxidative phosphorylation. Some neuromuscular diseases are due to mutations in mtDNA. A unique feature of these disorders is their maternal inheritance, due to the abundance of mitochondria in ova and the lack of them in sperm. A mother will transmit her mtDNA to all her offspring, but only her daughters will transmit that mtDNA in their turn, whereas her sons will not.

Regions in DNA, usually composed of trinucleotide repeats, can become unstable in length with subsequent generations. When the length of a repeat reaches a certain critical threshold it causes disease. Conditions such as fragile X syndrome are caused by unstable DNA repeats.

Imprinting occurs when the gene from one parent influences the expression of the gene from the other parent. When this occurs, the affected individual inherits a genetic abnormality from one parent, which does not cause disease in the parent. However, in the affected individual, the same defect causes disease, for instance by inactivating the normal gene from the other parent.

Uniparental disomy refers to the inheritance of two chromosomes of a given kind from only one parent. This situation can result in the unusual clinical observations of inheritance of an autosomal recessive disorder from only one documented carrier parent, and transmission of an X-linked disorder from father to son, or expression in homozygous form in females.

MOSAICISM

Mosaicism (a mutation occurring in only some cells of the body) is responsible for some unusual observations. A mutation occurring during embryonic development may be present in some fraction of either somatic or germline cells, or both, depending on the stage of development and the anatomic location in which the mutations occur. Somatic mosaicism of a mutation may manifest as a segmental or patchy abnormality. Germline mosaicism may result in the unusual finding of a *new* autosomal dominant phenotype in more than one member of a sibship.

The gene abnormalities responsible for many of the conditions of interest to the orthopaedist are now known. Based on this information, these disorders can be grouped broadly based on the function of the causative gene into five categories:

1. Structural (e.g., collagen)
2. Tumor and cell regulatory (e.g., neurofibromatosis)
3. Developmental (e.g., fibroblast growth factor receptor in achondroplasia)
4. Important in nerve or muscle function
5. Protein processing (enzymes).

In addition, some disorders are caused by large chromosomal abnormalities in which thousands of genes may be involved. Disorders in each of these categories share similarities in their clinical manifestations, treatment, prognosis, and inheritance pattern. A few examples of disorders in these classes are outlined in the remainder of this chapter.

CHROMOSOMAL ABNORMALITIES

Down Syndrome (Trisomy 21)

Down syndrome is the most common chromosomal disorder. It occurs in about 1 in 5,000 births in women under 30, and 1 in 250 births in women over 35. Complete trisomies (due to chromosomal nondisjunction) account for 95% of cases, while mosaicism, translocations, and partial trisomies account for the remainder.

Individuals with Down syndrome have distinctive, easily recognizable physical findings:

- Patients are short in stature.
- They have a characteristic face, with upward slanting palpebral fissures, epicanthal folds, a flattened nasal bridge, low-set ears and a protruding, furrowed tongue.
- The hands are short and broad, often with a single transverse palmar crease and clinodactyly.

Other Down syndrome-associated findings:

- It is the single most common cause of moderate mental retardation.
- Congenital heart disease occurs in about one-third of patients, and other malformations such as duodenal atresia and tracheoesophageal fistula may also occur.
- Auditory loss can occur.
- There is a 15 times higher risk of developing leukemia.
- The incidence of endocrinopathy, particularly, hypothyroidism, is high.
- Infections are common, although the reason for this is unclear.
- Individuals exhibit premature aging and an early development of mental deterioration similar to that in Alzheimer disease.

Nevertheless, with appropriate management of the cardiac, endocrine, and gastrointestinal abnormalities, most affected individuals live to adulthood.

One in five individuals with Down syndrome has a musculoskeletal problem related primarily to joint instability. Changes in joint shape and sites of ligament insertions may contribute to the apparent instability. The results of surgery for joint instability are not as good as for unaffected individuals.

An increased atlantoaxial distance on cervical spine films is found in about 10% of individuals with Down syndrome. In most cases, it is not associated with symptoms. Although the natural history of the cervical spine in these individuals is not fully known, studies following asymptomatic patients with an increased atlantoaxial distance have not identified any acute episodes of spinal cord compromise. The reported complication rate for atlantoaxial arthrodesis in Down syndrome is high. For these reasons, the surgical management of the atlantoaxial articulation focuses on symptoms rather than on radiographic findings. Symptoms can be difficult to identify, and patients may present with subtle findings, such as a change in gait pattern.

Scoliosis and spondylolisthesis can occur in Down syndrome, probably at a higher incidence than in the unaffected population.

Children with Down syndrome can develop hip dysplasia, which often occurs after the first few years of life. Although it is suggested that hip instability leads to functional problems later in life, it is unclear whether operative intervention improves outcome. Children may be habitual dislocators, and there is a high failure rate when hip surgery is undertaken in these patients. Brace treatment for children under 6 years has been advocated, although only small series of children have been reported. Slipped capital femoral epiphysis occurs in children with the syndrome and is associated with a high incidence of avascular necrosis. Knee dislocations are often asymptomatic, rarely requiring surgical intervention. The feet of Down patients develop planovalgus and hallux valgus deformities, which can be managed with shoe wear modification in most cases.

Turner Syndrome (45,XO)

This syndrome is caused by the absence of an X chromosome in females, and has an incidence of 1 in 2,500 births.

- Affected girls have a webbed neck, low hairline, short stature, and sexual infantilism.
- Because of a lack of sex steroid hormones, puberty does not occur and exogenous hormone replacement is usually administered.
- Although its use remains controversial, growth hormone may be administered in these patients, resulting in a modest increase in height.
- Scoliosis is common and patients must be monitored frequently if growth hormone is being used since it may accelerate curve progression.
- Valgus of the elbow and of the knee are common, but rarely causes disability.
- Most individuals have low bone density, probably related to the lack of sex steroid hormones and to altered renal vitamin D metabolism.
- Intelligence and life expectancy are normal.

DISORDERS CAUSED BY TUMOR-RELATED GENES

Neurofibromatosis

Neurofibromatosis type 1 (NF-1) is a common autosomal dominant disorder, occurring in about 1 in 3,000 newborns. Penetrance of the disorder is complete, though expressivity is highly variable. Half of affected patients carry a new, rather than an inherited mutation. Although there are several forms of neurofibromatosis, orthopaedic problems occur primarily in NF-1. A diagnosis of NF-1 requires two or more of the following:

- ≥6 café-au-lait spots whose greatest diameter is 5 mm in prepubertal and 15 mm in postpubertal patients
- ≥2 neurofibromas of any type or one plexiform neurofibroma
- Axillary freckles
- Optic glioma
- ≥2 Lisch nodules (hamartoma of the iris)
- Distinctive osseous lesion
- First-degree relative with NF-1

Most of these findings are absent in the newborn but develop over time. NF-1 is caused by a mutation in the gene encoding neurofibrillin (NF-1) which plays a role in the Ras signaling pathway. Mutant neurofibrillin causes excessive Ras signaling, which leads to increased cell division in patients. Patients have one mutant copy of *NF1*, but loss or mutation of the second copy of *NF1* further dysregulates Ras signaling, and can give rise to malignancy. Affected individuals may have a normal life span, but have a higher risk of malignancy and hypertension (due to renal artery stenosis).

Scoliosis is common and occurs in two patterns. Most curves resemble an *idiopathic* pattern, and can be managed in a manner identical to curves in idiopathic scoliosis. Other curves have a *dystrophic* pattern, involving a short segment (four to six levels), with distortion of the vertebrae and ribs.

- Curves that present in children under the age of 7 have a very high chance of being dystrophic.
- The presence of rib penciling can aid in predicting which curves will become dystrophic.
- Dystrophic curves are refractory to brace treatment, relentlessly progress, and, especially in cases associated with kyphosis, can lead to paralysis.
- They are best managed with early anterior and posterior surgical stabilization.
- Pseudoarthrosis of long bones is typical, with the tibia being the most common location.
  - An anterolateral bow in the tibia is a precursor to a pseudoarthrosis and should be managed with a total contact orthosis to prevent fracture.
  - Intramedullary fixation works well as the initial treatment for the established pseudoarthrosis.
  - Salvage procedures include vascularized bone grafting, distraction osteogenesis techniques, and amputation.
- A variety of neoplastic processes can occur in neurofibromatosis.
  - Most are benign and do not require surgical intervention.
  - Plexiform neurofibromas are difficult to manage due to their vascularity and infiltrative nature.
  - It is difficult to distinguish neurofibromas from neurofibrosarcomas.
  - Lesions that rapidly change in size or become symptomatic should be managed as a potential sarcoma.
  - Children with neurofibromatosis have a propensity to develop other malignancies.

Multiple Hereditary Exostosis

This disorder is characterized by the presence of multiple osteochondromas (exostoses). It is inherited in an autosomal dominant manner, and is caused by a mutation in one of the three *EXT* genes, whose protein products regulate how the hedgehog ligand, which plays an important role in growth-plate function, diffuses through extracellular matrix.

- Clinical problems include pain or cosmetic problems from the bump, limb length inequality, angular bony deformity, dislocation of an adjacent joint, and malignant change.
- Only symptomatic osteochondromas require excision.
- Limb inequality and deformity can be managed using usual techniques.
- Most deformities of the upper extremity do not cause symptoms, and the rarely require operative intervention.
- Malignant change is a rare occurrence, but should be suspected in lesions that grow or become symptomatic after skeletal maturity.

Enchondromatosis

Enchondromas are common benign cartilage tumors of bone. They can occur as solitary lesions or as multiple lesions in enchondromatosis (Ollier and Maffucci diseases). Maffucci disease is also associated with soft tissue vascular malformations.

- Clinical problems caused by enchondromas include skeletal deformity and the potential for malignant change to chondrosarcoma.
- The extent of skeletal involvement is variable in enchondromatosis and may include dysplasia that is not directly attributable to enchondromas.
- Standard techniques are used for the treatment of limb deformity and limb length inequality.
- Changes in symptoms or size of a lesion, especially in skeletally mature individuals, raise the concern about malignant transformation, which occurs in a higher frequency in Maffucci disease.
- Enchondromatosis can be caused by a mutation in the parathyroid hormone-related protein receptor, which dysregulates the same Hedgehog protein that is dysregulated in osteochondromatosis.

DISORDERS CAUSED BY GENES IMPORTANT IN DEVELOPMENT

Achondroplasia

Achondroplasia is an autosomal dominant disorder caused by a mutation in fibroblast growth factor receptor type 3 (FGFR3). Eighty percent of cases are due to new mutations with increased paternal age as a risk factor. FGFr-3 influences chondrocyte maturation in the growth plate, resulting in the chondroepiphysis developing abnormally. There is a greater effect seen in regions of greater endochondral growth, giving rise to the characteristic rhizomelic pattern of shortening (worse shortening of proximal segments) seen in the disorder.

- Children with achondroplasia are identified at birth by the presence of characteristic facial features (frontal bossing and mid-face hypoplasia) and short humerii and femurs.
- The most severe problems in achondroplasia are related to the spine.
- Kyphosis of the lumbar spine develops in infants, but usually resolves on its own in early childhood, when better trunk control develops.
- The rare progressive case that persists past early childhood requires operative intervention.
- In the lumbar spine, the distance between the pedicles narrows, rather than increases, as one proceeds caudally.
- Patients may have more symptoms later in life when degenerative changes are superimposed on the congenital stenosis.
- With respect to the lower extremities in achondroplasia, genu varum occurs but is usually mild.
- Osteotomies can be performed in the patient with severe deformity and symptoms.
- Distraction osteogenesis and the use of growth hormones to increase stature are controversial treatments for these individuals.

Cleidocranial Dysplasia

Cleidocranial dysplasia is an autosomal dominant condition caused by a mutation in the *CBFA1* gene, which encodes a transcription factor that regulates osteoblast differentiation. Heterozygous loss of function of *CBFA1* is sufficient to produce the disorder.

- Characteristic features of cleidocranial dysplasia include midline and other bony defects, such as hypoplasia/aplasia of clavicles, patent fontanelles, supernumerary teeth, short stature, midline pelvic defects, and delayed skeletal development.
- The absence of clavicles may allow patients to adduct their shoulders far enough to touch them together anteriorly.
- Hips can develop coxa vara, which may require treatment with an osteotomy.

DISORDERS CAUSED BY GENES ENCODING ENZYMES

The *mucopolysaccharidoses* are a group of disorders each caused by abnormal function of a particular lysosomal enzyme that degrades a sulfonated glycosaminoglycan. Incomplete degradation products secondarily accumulate in lysosomes. There are a variety of subtypes, most of which are inherited in an autosomal recessive manner, as listed in Table 30-1.

- Features common to these disorders include corneal clouding, organomegaly, epiphyseal deformation, contractures, cardiac disease, and deafness.
- The diagnosis can be made using urine analysis for the specific glycosaminoglycan involved.
- Hurler syndrome is the most common and one of the more severe forms of disease, as patients live only into their second decade.
- Hunter syndrome is less severe, with patients having a normal life span.
  - ☐ Children with Hunter syndrome have upper cervical instability, kyphosis of any region of the spine, hip deformity, and malalignment of the lower limbs.
  - ☐ Bone marrow transplant has been used in severe cases to arrest progression.

DISORDERS CAUSED BY GENES ENCODING STRUCTURAL PROTEINS

Spondyloepiphyseal dysplasia is a short-trunk form of dwarfism with abnormalities of the physes and spine. It can broadly be classified into *congenita* and *tarda* forms.

TABLE 30-1 MUCOPOLYSACCHARIDOSES

Type	Name	Inheritance	Stored Substance and Enzyme Defect
I	Hurler/Scheie	AR	HS + DS; α-L-iduronidase
II	Hunter	XR	HS + DS; iduronidase-2-sulfatase
III	Sanfilippo	AR	HS; four subtypes with different enzymes affected
IV	Morquio	AR	KS, CS; three subtypes: 1. *N*-acetylgalactosamine-6-sulfatase, 2. β-D-galactosidase, 3. unknown
V	(formerly Scheie)		
VI	Moroteux-Lamy	AR	DS + CS; arylsulfatase B, *N*-acetylgalactosamine-4-sulfatase
VII	Sly	AR	CS + HS + DS; *N*-β-D-glucuronidase
VIII		AR	CS + HS; glucuronate-2-sulphatase

AR, autosomal recessive; CS, chondroitin sulfate; DS, dermatan sulfate; HS, heparan sulfate; KS, keratan sulfate; XR, X-linked recessive.

The congenita form presents at birth, and is inherited in an autosomal dominant fashion. It is caused by mutations in type II collagen. Type II collagen is the major form of collagen present in cartilage. The tarda form is milder, with most patients developing manifestations at about 4 years of age, although some do not present until adolescence. The tarda form is an X-linked condition, caused by a mutation in the *SEDL* gene, which plays a role in regulating intracellular protein trafficking. The exact mechanism by which the *SEDL* mutation causes abnormal chondroepiphyseal formation has yet to be elucidated.

- Affected individuals have short limbs and a short trunk.
- In the congenita form one finds coxa vara, valgus alignment of the knees, scoliosis, kyphosis, and increased lumbar lordosis.
  - The hands are normal.
  - Severe myopia, retinal detachment, and sensorineural hearing loss can occur.
- The tarda form is less severe and often presents with hip pain or stiffness (generally in the second decade), flattened vertebrae (platyspondyly), and in many cases, scoliosis.
  - There is failure or delay of ossification of the proximal femoral physis, os pubis, distal femoral physis, talus, and calcaneus.
  - The hips show coxa valga and radiographic changes similar to Perthes disease.
- Odontoid hypoplasia in spondyloepiphyseal dysplasia can predispose to upper cervical instability, and can cause myelopathy.
- Flexion–extension views of the C-spine should be obtained before anesthesia is administered.
- Scoliosis and kyphosis are treated using standard methods and principles for these spinal deformities.
- Lower extremity malalignment may be treated with osteotomies.

GENETIC TESTING

Diagnostic confirmation of a genetic condition, although not always necessary, is definitively ascertained by demonstration of a causal mutation in the patient. In broad terms, mutations are either alterations on a large chromosomal scale or on a small base-pair scale, and a genetic test is chosen largely based on the resolution required to identify the abnormality. A karyotype analysis will identify an excess or absence of an entire chromosome, as in Down and Turner syndromes, or of a large part thereof. Cytogenetic methods combining karyotyping and labeling by hybridizing probes to DNA, as in fluorescent *in situ* hybridization, allow visualization of the presence and number of specific sequences as well as their location in the genome. These methods are useful also in identifying amplification or deletion of genes (e.g., in cancers).

When identification of a small-scale DNA alteration is necessary, a number of tests are possible, depending on whether the number of causal mutations in a given gene are limited and recurring. For recurring mutations, resultant dysfunctional proteins or enzymes can sometimes be identified by biochemical tests, without the need to resort to genetic tests. The presence, absence, and relative abundance of a single gene product can be identified by immunohistochemistry (for protein) or by Northern blot or polymerase chain reaction (PCR) for messenger RNA. Known DNA sequence alterations and translocations that are recurring can be sought rather simply by attempting to amplify the abnormal sequence by PCR, using mutation-specific primers. If the mutations in a given gene vary significantly or have not all been identified, then sequencing the gene either manually or using an automated sequencer becomes necessary. Correlation of a newly identified mutation with pathogenesis may then be required to establish a causal relationship of the mutation.

Southern, Northern, and Western blotting are similar techniques for the visualization, detection, and quantification of genetic material. Southern blotting is used for DNA, Northern for RNA, and Western for proteins. Basically, the technique consists of denaturing the substance to be studied, "blotting" the fragments onto a membrane, and then treating them with a specific labeled probe that allows them to be visualized. Southern blotting was named for its inventor, E.M. Southern. The names Northern and Western blotting were chosen as a bit of a joke, when the technique proved useful for substances other than DNA.

Polymerase Chain Reaction (PCR) is an automated technique used to "amplify" a small amount of DNA into a larger one. It utilizes a heat stable polymerase (the enzymes that replicate DNA) to reproduce short segments of DNA, that are pre-heated to denature them. The process, which is relatively quick and simple, is repeated 25–75 times to produce a useful quantity of DNA.

SUGGESTED READING

Alman BA. A classification for genetic disorders of interest to orthopaedists. Clin Orthop 2002;401:17–26.

Thompson MW, McInnes RR, Willard HF. Thompson & Thompson: genetics in medicine, 5th ed. Philadelphia: WB Saunders, 1991.

EMBRYOLOGY

WILLIAM A. PHILLIPS
SUSAN A. SCHERL

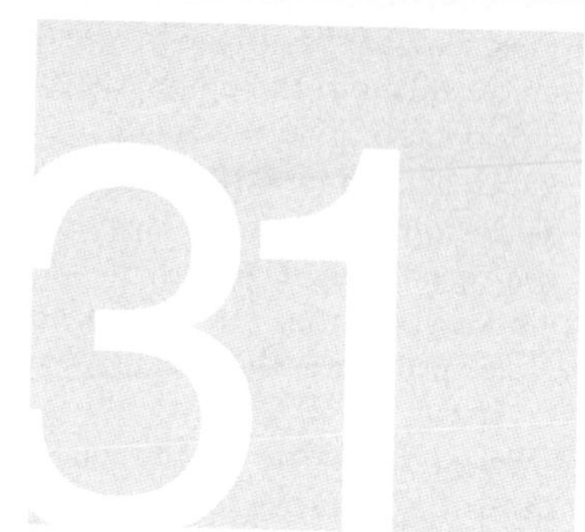

Knowledge of basic embryology, particularly that of the musculoskeletal and nervous systems, is necessary in the practice of pediatric orthopaedics. Many congenital pediatric orthopaedic conditions are a direct result of problems in early fetal development. The birth of a fully formed child 9 months after conception is the culmination of an intricate series of interactions exquisitely choreographed by the expression of many genes at different times and places, beginning with the fertilized ovum. The events of greatest interest to orthopaedists—the development of the musculoskeletal system—occur primarily during the embryonic period, that is, the third through eighth weeks after conception.

Ultimate control of embryonic development is through the expression of the genes contained on the chromosomes. Some of the mechanisms used in development include cell proliferation, cell differentiation, cell migration, and cell death. These cellular events occur not only within cells but also take place as interactions between adjacent cells and tissues. The location of cells in the embryo and their interactions with their local environment play a major role in development. Cells can express genes that up- or down-regulate the expression of other genes. This can occur by direct cell-to-cell contact or by messenger molecules.

DEFINITIONS

- *Zygote*: a fertilized egg and sperm
- *Morula*: a solid ball of cells formed by division of the zygote
- *Blastocyst*: the morula develops a fluid-filled cyst, and becomes a blastocyst
- *Germ layers*: the three germ layers—*ectoderm*, *mesoderm*, and *endoderm*—give rise to all the structures of the embryo.
- *Ectoderm*:
  - Central nervous system
  - Peripheral nervous system
  - Sensory epithelia of eye, ear, and nose
  - Epidermis, hair, and nails
  - Mammary glands
  - Pituitary gland
  - Tooth enamel
  - Neural crest cells
    - Spinal, cranial, and autonomic ganglia
    - Ensheathing cells of the peripheral nervous system
    - Pigment cells of the dermis
    - Tissues of branchial arch origin
    - Adrenal medulla
    - Leptomeninges
- *Mesoderm*:
  - Cartilage, bone, and connective tissue
  - Smooth and striated muscle
  - Heart
  - Blood and lymph vessels and cells
  - Gonads
  - Pericardium, pleura, and peritoneum
  - Adrenal cortex
  - Spleen
- *Endoderm*:
  - Gastrointestinal, respiratory, genitourinary, and auditory epithelium
  - Tonsils
  - Thyroid and parathyroids
  - Thymus and pancreas
  - Liver
- *Mesenchyme:* mesodermal embryonic connective tissue
  - Can differentiate into fibroblasts, chondroblasts, or osteoblasts
- *Intramembranous ossification:* direct transformation of mesenchyme into bone
  - Mesenchymal cells condense and differentiate into osteoblasts, which lay down osteoid to become mineralized into bone.
  - Occurs in the skull and face
- *Endochondral ossification:* ossification of a preexisting cartilaginous bone precursor (anlage)
  - A primary ossification center forms in the diaphyseal region of the anlage, and a secondary center forms in the epiphysis.
  - Mesenchymal cells condense and differentiate into chondroblasts, which secrete collagen and ground substance to form the extracellular matrix.
  - Cartilage begins to appear in the fifth week.

- A primary ossification center forms in the diaphyseal region of the anlage by week 12, and a secondary center forms in the epiphysis, at various times after birth, depending on the bone.
- Occurs in long bones.

- *Notochord:* embryonic structure around which the vertebral column develops
  - Also induces the overlying ectoderm to form the neural plate, the precursor to the central nervous system
- *Neural tube:* the neural plate invaginates centrally to form the neural groove, bounded on either side by the neural folds
  - The folds fuse to form the neural tube.
  - The cranial end of the neural tube becomes the brain, the remainder becomes the spinal cord, and the lumen becomes the ventricles of the brain and central canal of the spinal cord (Fig. 31-1).
  - The neural tube is induced to form different regions along its length by *retinoic acid*.
  - Retinoids activate genes in the *Hox (homeobox)* family.
  - Inhibition of *bone morphogenic proteins* also appears to play an important role in this process.
- *Somites:* paired cuboidal bodies derived from the mesoderm running paraxially alongside the neural tube
  - Give rise to the axial skeleton, trunk musculature, and dermis
  - Each somite differentiates into a ventromedial *sclerotome*, which will form the vertebrae and ribs, and a dorsolateral *dermomyotome*, which separates into the *myotome*, which will form the muscles and the *dermatome*, which will form the skin.
  - Some of the molecular events associated with somite formation include the expression of *Notch pathway* and *Hox* genes.

EARLY FETAL DEVELOPMENT

- Day 1: fertilization, formation of zygote
- Day 2: morula stage
- Day 4: blastocyst stage
- Day 6 to 10: uterine implantation
- Day 11: placental circulation established
- Day 15: first period missed
- Day 16 to 18: notochord and neural plate form
- Day 20: somites form

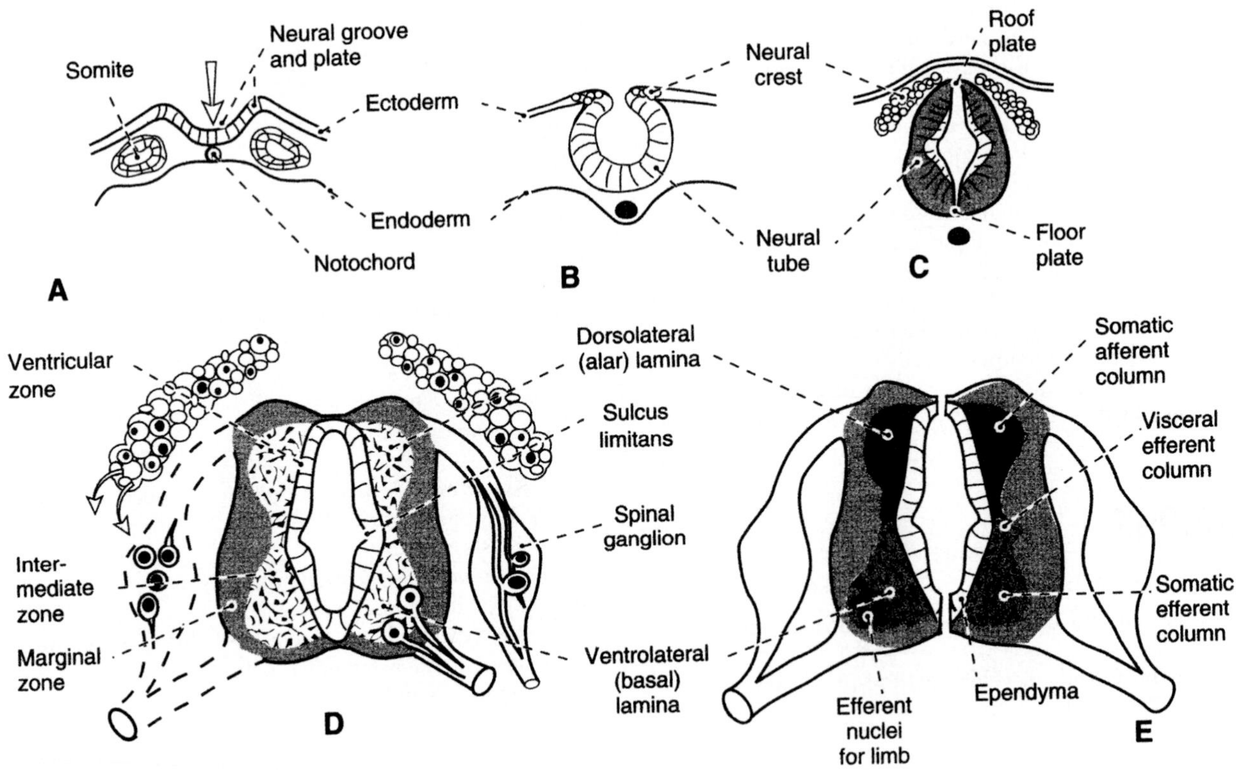

Figure 31-1 Development of the spinal cord. (**A–C**) Formation of the neural tube and neural crest in early somite embryos. (**D**) Cellular differentiation within the cord. (**E**) Development of cell columns in the alar and basal laminae shown on one side for a segment that innervates the limbs and on the other for a segment that contains the visceral efferent column. (From Rosse C, Gaddum-Rosse P. The vertebral canal, spinal cord, spinal nerves, and segmental innervation. In: Hollinshead's textbook of anatomy, 5th ed. Philadelphia: Lippincott-Raven, 1997:152.)

- Early in the third week, formation of the *primitive streak* orients the embryo in all three planes—longitudinal (cranial–caudal), sagittal (dorsal–ventral), and coronal (left–right).
- Cells migrating from the deep surface of the primitive streak move between the dorsally placed ectoderm and ventrally placed endoderm to become the mesoderm.

- Week 4: neural tube forms, heart beats, arm and leg buds appear
- Week 5: mouth, eyes, and hands develop
- Week 6: feet and fingers develop
- Week 7: toes develop

In general, if there is a congenital abnormality in one organ system, it is imperative to rule out abnormalities in all organ systems developing at the same time. For example, since the elements of the spine and heart develop simultaneously, children with congenital scoliosis must be evaluated for heart defects.

ARTICULAR AND SKELETAL DEVELOPMENT

- The skeleton derives from mesodermal mesenchyme.
- Regulators of bone development include bone morphogenic proteins (BMP), transforming growth factor-β (TGF-β), and *homeobox (Hox)* genes.
- In long bones, the mesenchyme develops into a cartilaginous anlage, which undergoes endochondral ossification to form bone.
- In the skull, the mesenchyme transforms directly into bone through intramembranous ossification.
- The vertebrae and ribs develop from the fusion of the upper and lower halves of adjacent somites.
- Joints develop from the interzonal mesenchyme between the bony anlage. Interzonal mesenchyme can differentiate into fibrous or cartilaginous tissue to form a joint, and cavitates to form synovial spaces.
- Malformations of the axial skeleton:
  - Klippel-Feil syndrome: failure of segmentation of cervical vertebrae
  - Spina bifida occulta: failure of fusion of the halves of the vertebral arch
  - Hemivertebrae: failure of appearance of one of the two ossification centers forming a vertebral body, leading to failure of formation of half of the vertebra
  - Rachischisis: failure of fusion of the neural folds
  - Achondroplasia: disruption of endochondral ossification.

LIMB DEVELOPMENT

- Limb buds appear at the end of the fourth week of gestation.
- The upper limb buds develop slightly ahead of the lower.
- The limb buds are formed from somatic mesoderm and ectoderm.
- Limb buds start forming on the ventrolateral surface of the body wall.
- Mesenchymal cells in the lateral mesoderm are activated beneath a thickened band of ectoderm.
  - This thickening is the *apical ectodermal ridge* (AER).
  - The AER interacts with limb bud mesenchyme to promote growth of the limb from proximal to distal.
  - *Fibroblast growth factors* are expressed in the AER.
  - At the posterior margin of the limb bud, mesenchymal cells form the *zone of polarizing activity*, which controls limb development in the anteroposterior axis (first vs. fifth digit sides of limb) through the expression of the *sonic hedgehog (Shh)* gene.
  - The dorsoventral axis (flexor vs. extensor sides of the limb) is determined by *Wnt7* from the dorsal epidermis and *engrailed-1 (EN-1)* from the ventral side.
- *Homeobox (Hox)* genes play an important role in limb development.
  - This gene family was first described in the fruit fly (*Drosophila*). *Hox* genes are highly conserved and regulate vertebra development in a similar manner as they do in *Drosophila*.
  - They code for *transcription factors* that regulate DNA transcription of other genes. In a sense, Hox genes are the switches by which other genes are activated during embryogenesis.
  - The order of *Hox* genes along the chromosome determines the order in which they are expressed. Genes at the 3′ end of a sequence are expressed earlier and more anteriorly on the body.
- At the beginning of the seventh week, the limbs extend ventrally with the palmar surface of the hands and the plantar surface of the feet facing each other. The thumbs and great toes are both on the cephalad, preaxial border of their respective limbs.
- During the eighth week, the upper limbs rotate laterally, pointing the elbows caudally. The elbows flex so the hands meet across the chest. The forearm flexor muscles now lie on the medial side of the arm and the extensors lie laterally. At the same time, the lower limbs rotate medially. This places the soles of the feet in a plantar position. The leg flexor muscles lie dorsally and the extensors lie ventrally.
- Limb development is complete by the eighth week of gestation (Fig. 31-2). By the end of the sixth week, the rays of the hands have formed, followed in a few days by the foot rays. By the eighth week the mesenchyme between the rays breaks down, separating the digits. This occurs through *apoptosis* (programmed cell death) and is regulated by *bone morphogenic proteins*.
- Limb malformations are usually genetic, but environmental and teratogenic factors have also been implicated in some cases, and causation may be multifactorial.
- Often, limb malformations are relatively minor in and of themselves, but they may be associated with other more serious congenital problems or syndromes.
- Limb malformations:
  - Cleft hand and foot—failure of formation of central ray

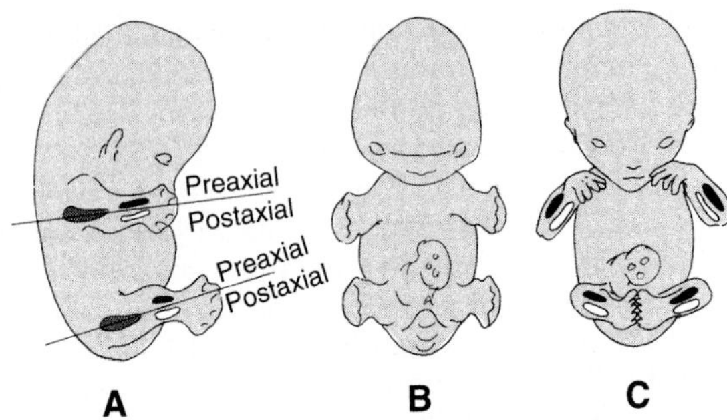

Figure 31-2 (A) Development of the bones in the free limbs in relation to the limb axis. The bone primordium of the proximal segment is dark gray, the preaxial bone of the intermediate segment is black, and the postaxial bone is white. **(B and C)** Successive stages of limb development from a ventral view before the limbs undergo rotation. The position of the preaxial and postaxial bone in the upper and lower limbs is still symmetric. (From Rosse C, Gaddum-Rosse P. Basic structural plan of the limbs. In: Hollinshead's textbook of anatomy, 5th ed. Philadelphia: Lippincott-Raven, 1997:183.)

- Radial club hand—partial or complete absence of the radius. May present with thrombocytopenia (TAR (thrombocytopenia-absent radius] syndrome) or as part of VATER syndrome (vertebral anomalies, anal atresia, tracheoesophageal fistula, renal and radial anomalies)
- Brachydactyly—short fingers or toes, often inherited.
- Polydactyly—extra fingers or toes
  - Postaxial (medial on the upper extremity, lateral on the lower) polydactyly is autosomal dominant
  - Preaxial is rarer and more likely to be a sporadic event.
- Amelia—complete absence of the limbs, caused by early suppression of limb development. Thalidomide, an anti-nausea drug used during pregnancies between 1957 and 1962, can cause amelia.
- Meromelia—partial absence of the limbs, caused by suppression of limb development later in gestation

MUSCLE DEVELOPMENT

- Most skeletal muscle is derived from the ventral dermomyotomal portion of the somites.
- Head and neck muscle is derived from branchial arch mesoderm.
- Limb muscles develop from mesenchyme derived from somatic mesoderm.
- Muscle development is initiated by *Shh* from the notochord and *Wnts* from the neural tube, inducing *Pax-3* and *Myf-5* in the somites.
- *Pax-3* in turn regulates *c-met* expression, which directs migration of the myogenic precursor cells into the limb bud.
- In each limb the cells condense into two masses, dorsal and ventral to the axial mesenchyme.
  - The dorsal muscle mass becomes most of the extensors and supinators of the upper limb and the extensors and abductors of the lower limb.
  - The ventral muscle mass becomes the flexors and pronators of the upper limb and the flexors and adductors of the lower limb.
- Cardiac and smooth muscles develop from splanchnic mesoderm.
- There is wide developmental variation in musculature.
- Absences or variations is size, shape, and position of muscles is common, and generally not of clinical significance.
- The most common significant congenital muscle lesion is torticollis, an intrauterine scarring and fibrosis of the sternocleidomastoid muscle, which causes a fixed rotation and tilting of the head.

NERVOUS SYSTEM DEVELOPMENT

- In the peripheral nervous system, all sensory cells are derived from the neural crest.
  - Neural crest cells in the region of the brain form the sensory ganglia of cranial nerves V and VII through X.
  - The autonomic ganglia are also derived from the neural crest.
  - Motor nerve fibers develop from cells in the fetal spinal cord.
  - Growing limb buds are supplied with segmental motor and sensory innervation, which grow into the mesenchyme.
  - The central nervous system derives from ectodermal tissue on the dorsal aspect of the fetus known as the neural plate.
  - The neural plate infolds to form the neural groove and neural folds.
  - The neural folds fuse to form the neural tube.
  - The neural crest is a layer of cells between the neural tube and the surface ectoderm.
  - The cranial end of the neural tube becomes the brain and the remainder becomes the spinal cord, while the lumen becomes the ventricles of the brain and central canal of the spinal cord.
- Problems during this process are common, and lead to various congenital brain and spinal cord abnormalities, including spina bifida and anencephaly.
- Since this process occurs very early in gestation (at about 3 weeks), typically before a woman knows she is pregnant, preventive measures such as adequate (400 to 800 μg) intake of folate should begin prior to attempts at conception.

SUGGESTED READING

Buckwalter JA, Einhorn TA Simon, SR. Orthopaedic basic science, 2nd ed. Rosemont, IL: American Academy of Orthopaedic Surgeons, 2000.

Dietz FR, Morcuende JA. Embryology and development of the musculoskeletal system. In: Morrissey RT, Weinstein SL, eds. Lovell and Winter's pediatric orthopaedics, 5th ed. Philadelphia: Lippincott Williams & Wilkins, 2001.
Larsen WJ. Human embryology, 2nd ed. New York: Churchill Livingstone, 1997.
Moore KL. The developing human, 3rd ed. Philadelphia: WB Saunders, 1982.
Moore KL, Persaud TVN. The developing human, 7th ed. Philadelphia: Elsevier, 2003.
O'Rahilly RO, Müller F. Human embryology and teratology, 2nd ed. New York: Wiley-Liss, 1996.
Shapiro F. Pediatric orthopedic deformities. San Diego: Academic Press, 2001.
Sweeney LJ. Basic concepts in embryology. New York: McGraw-Hill, 1998.

RADIOLOGY AND IMAGING

EVAN GELLER
BARBARA J. WOLFSON

Children are not small adults, and nowhere is this statement more apparent than in the bones. A child's skeletal system is constantly growing and remodeling. The choice of imaging modality to evaluate the pediatric skeleton is influenced by a child's age, site of clinical concern, and the type of information needed. The femoral head of an infant, for example, is entirely cartilaginous and therefore cannot be visualized on plain radiography. It is best examined by ultrasound, a modality that is capable of imaging cartilage while providing the additional benefit of a dynamic evaluation of hip stability. After the head ossifies (between 4 and 6 months of age), plain radiography is preferred.

Imaging plays a major role in the diagnosis and management of orthopaedic diseases. The mainstay remains plain radiography but in recent years other imaging modalities such as computed tomography (CT), magnetic resonance imaging (MRI), nuclear medicine, and ultrasound have made significant contributions to orthopaedic care. This chapter is intended to provide an introduction and overview of the various available imaging modalities and to give the orthopaedic resident some useful guidelines in choosing the most appropriate modality. It is not intended as an exhaustive review of imaging technology. It is good practice to remember that the radiologist is the imaging expert and should be consulted when imaging questions arise. It is difficult enough for a radiologist to stay current with all the new modalities and applications and a busy orthopaedist caring for patients cannot possibly know as much about imaging as the radiologist.

IMAGING METHODS

Plain Radiography

Since its discovery in 1895, radiography has been known to be an excellent modality for the visualization of bones. For decades it was the only imaging modality available and many important observations about trauma, tumor, dysplasia, and metabolic bone disease were made by radiology pioneers.

- Plain radiographs, or conventional x-rays, provide information about the bony skeleton and, to a more limited extent, the joint spaces and soft tissues.
- X-rays are generated by bombarding a tungsten target with an electron beam.
  - As x-rays pass through a body part, they are absorbed to varying degrees prior to striking a fluorescent film-screen system.
  - It is this differential absorption of x-ray photons that accounts for the differences in the appearance of bone and soft tissue structure.
  - Film technique differences (e.g., KvP and mAs) can be changed to highlight either bone or soft tissue.
- There are five basic radiographic densities seen on plain film.
  - From most lucent to most dense these are air, fat, soft tissue (water), bone (calcium), and metal (Fig. 32-1).
  - Evaluating the density of a structure can help in formulating a differential diagnosis.

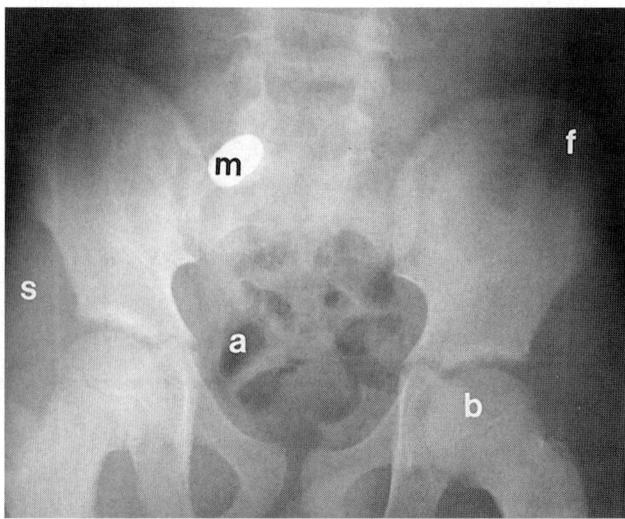

Figure 32-1 Plain radiograph of the pelvis demonstrates the five basic radiographic densities: *a,* air (in bowel); *f,* fat (properitoneal fat stripe); *s,* soft tissue (muscle); *b,* bone (femur); *m,* metal (bullet).

Computed Tomography

- CT is a modality that uses x-rays to look at the body in slices.
  - A series of thin x-ray beams pass through the body as the x-ray tube moves around the body.
  - Detectors placed on the opposite side of the patient receive the x-ray beam.
  - The computer then processes the information obtained and assigns a density to each *pixel* (or picture element).
- Water has been arbitrarily assigned a value of zero.
  - Any substance that is of greater density than water will exhibit a positive value and any substance of lesser density (such as fat or air) will have a negative value.
  - These densities are expressed in Hounsfield units, named for Sir Godfrey Hounsfield who was one of the pioneers of CT imaging.
- CT has the capability of distinguishing differences of density that cannot be distinguished by plain radiography.
- Images are acquired in the axial plane, but modern helical and multidetector scanners can reconstruct the image in multiple planes, which can be useful when evaluating skeletal abnormalities in children (Fig. 32-2).
- Advantages of CT include excellent resolution of bony structures and a fast acquisition time, minimizing the need for sedation.
- Disadvantages of CT imaging include a high radiation dose, high cost, and limited soft tissue delineation.

Magnetic Resonance Imaging

- MRI uses magnets and radio waves to generate an image.
- The routine MRI technique depends upon the mobile hydrogen concentration of tissues.
  - Cortical bone has a low mobile hydrogen content and is therefore virtually devoid of MRI signal.
  - MRI excels in the evaluation of bone marrow, cartilage, and soft tissues.
  - It has become the modality of choice in diseases involving these structures (Fig. 32-3).
- Advantages of MRI over CT include a lack of ionizing radiation, and multiplanar capability.
- Disadvantages include the need for sedation in young children (because of the lengthy nature of the study), high cost, and an inability to evaluate cortical bone.
  - Because strong magnets are used, patients with metal rods or plates, or patients with pacemakers may not be suitable candidates for MRI.

Nuclear Medicine

- Bone scintigraphy is performed by administering a radioisotope intravenously followed by imaging of the musculoskeletal compartment with a gamma camera.
  - The most commonly used agents for bone scintigraphy are the technetium-labeled phosphate analogs that become incorporated into the bone.
- In children, a typical bone scan demonstrates increased isotope activity within the growth plates of the long bones because of the high level of metabolic

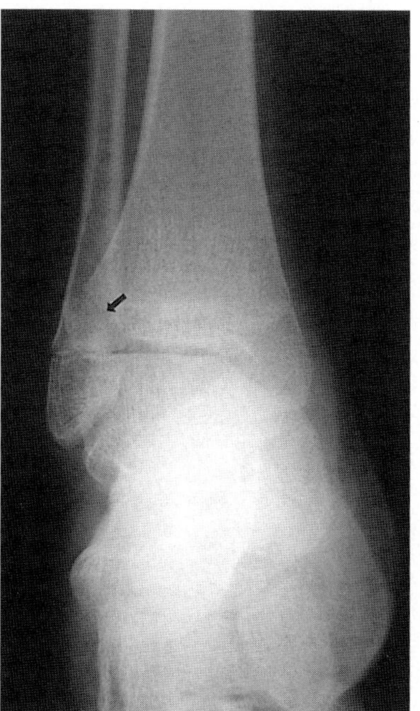

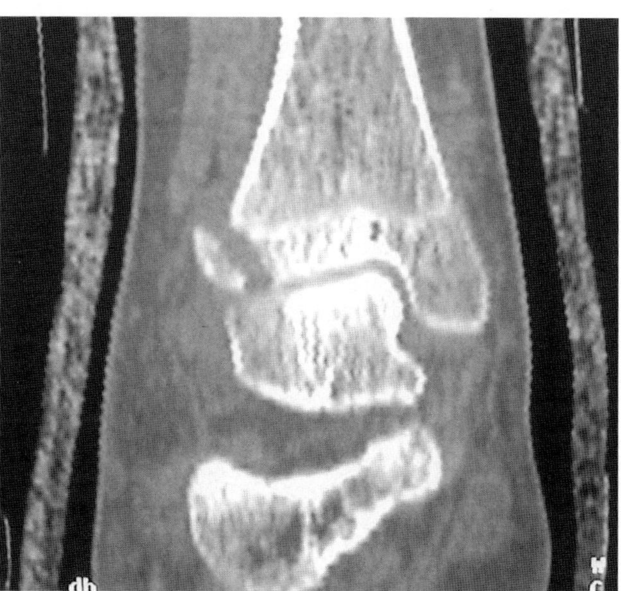

Figure 32-2 Tibial fracture seen better on computed tomography (CT) with three-dimensional reconstruction than on plain film. (**A**) Plain film showing the fracture fragment hidden behind the fibula. (**B**) CT with reconstruction in the coronal plane showing the fracture clearly. Note that there is an overlying cast but the cast does not interfere with CT imaging.

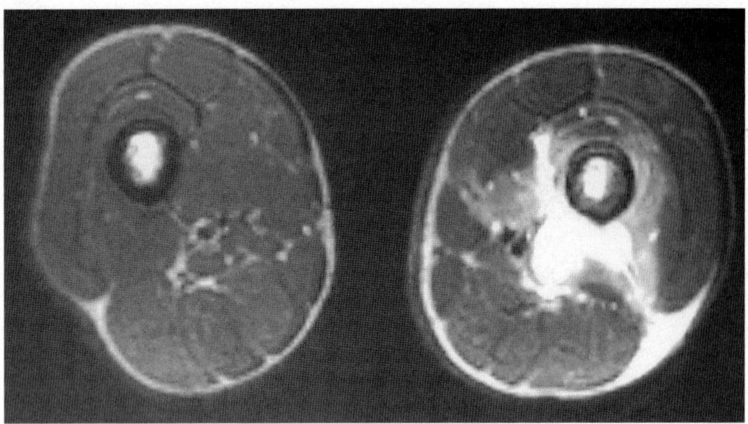

Figure 32-3 Pyomyositis of the left thigh. Magnetic resonance T2-weighted imaging of both thighs in the axial plane demonstrating location and extent of involvement in this 16-year-old boy with sickle cell disease. Note the high-signal intensity consistent with edema of the soft tissues.

activity when compared with other long bone sections (Fig. 32-4).

- Causes of abnormally increased isotope activity include increased blood flow and bone turnover.
- Causes of abnormally diminished or absent uptake include bone infarction, aggressive infection, or high intracapsular pressures due to large joint effusions.
- A *SPECT scan* (single photon emission computed tomography) differs from routine two-dimensional planar images in that it allows improved image contrast by removing overlying structures that may interfere with image interpretation.
  - As with conventional cross-sectional imaging modalities such as CT and MRI, images are presented as "slices" in axial, coronal and sagittal planes, or as a three-dimensional (3D) rotating image.
  - SPECT studies are especially useful in the evaluation of suspected vertebral or rib abnormalities.

Ultrasound

- Ultrasound technology was developed from "sonar" used by the U.S. Navy to detect submarines during World War II.
- An ultrasound transducer is both a transmitter and receiver of sound waves. It sends sound waves out, the sound waves bounce off interfaces, and then return to the transducer.
  - Ultrasound waves cannot go through air or bone.
  - Their natural medium is water and therefore they are most useful when looking at fluid-filled structures or structures with a high water content, such as cartilage.
- Ultrasound is useful in assessing certain cartilaginous structures such as the newborn hip and in identifying joint effusions, fluid collections, and radiolucent foreign bodies in soft tissue (Fig. 32-5).

Bone Densitometry

- A DEXA scan (dual energy x-ray absorptiometry) is useful in the evaluation of bone mineral density and fracture risk assessment.

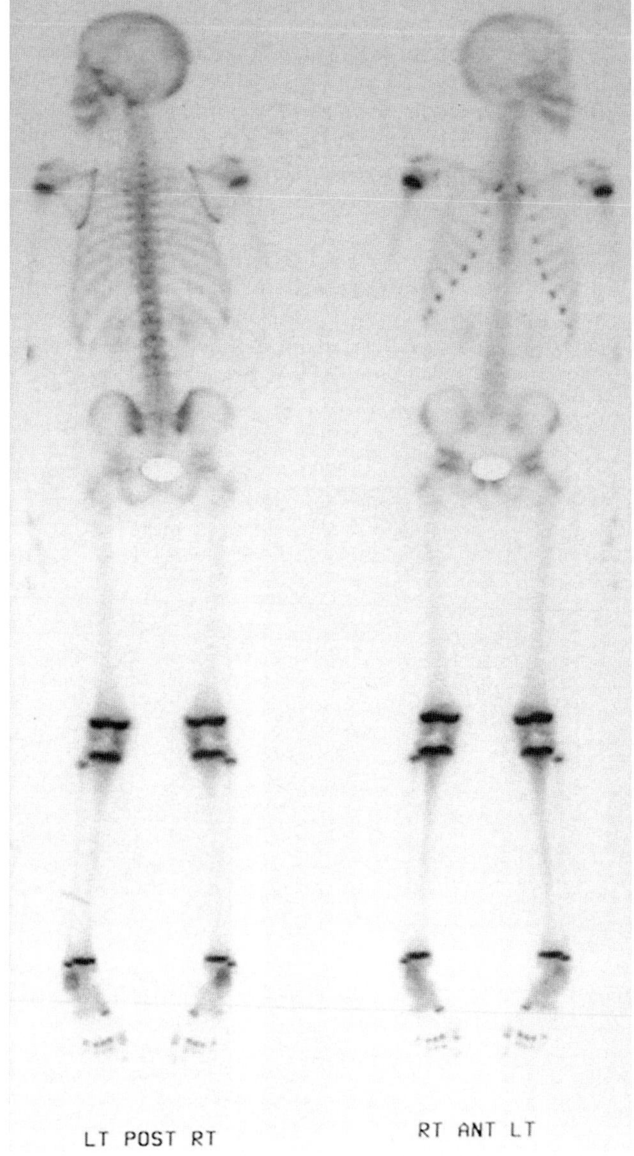

Figure 32-4 Normal radionuclide bone scan of the whole body. Note the increased uptake of isotope at the growth plates that can mask subtle abnormalities.

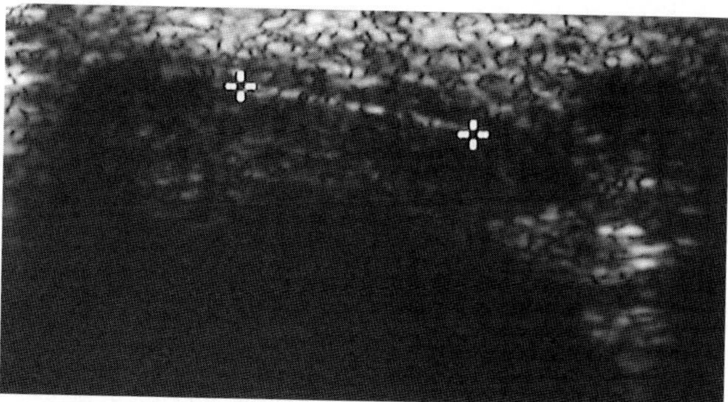

Figure 32-5 Ultrasound of the plantar surface of the foot demonstrating a wooden splinter (*cursors*). This splinter could not be seen on plain film. Ultrasound guidance was used in the operating room to assist in removal of the foreign body.

- It uses low-dose x-rays to evaluate the whole body or selected regions including the lumbar spine or femoral neck.
- It takes approximately 10 minutes to perform so sedation is rarely required.
- In the pediatric age group, results are compared to age-matched controls and are expressed as a "Z score."
  - Greater than 2 standard deviations indicates increased risk for osteoporotic fractures.

CHOICE OF IMAGING METHOD

Diagnostic imaging algorithms have evolved with the development and refinement of imaging technology (Algorithms 32-1 to 32-3). MRI, multidetector CT, and SPECT imaging have revolutionized our approach to certain musculoskeletal disorders and have added considerably to diagnostic accuracy.

Infection

- The imaging workup of musculoskeletal infection begins with the plain radiograph.
  - Osteomyelitis will produce localized and deep soft tissue swelling within 48 to 72 hours.
  - This is followed by osteopenia, bone destruction (osteolysis), and periosteal reaction at 7 to 14 days (Fig. 32-6B).
  - Most cases of long-bone osteomyelitis are metaphyseal in origin, but may spread to the epiphysis in young infants and may involve the adjacent joint if the metaphysis is intracapsular.
  - Osteomyelitis limited to the epiphyses or epiphyseal equivalents (patella, greater trochanter) is less common but does occur.
- MRI and bone scintigraphy provide a much more sensitive means of osteomyelitis detection, especially during the first few days, when the radiograph may still be normal (see Fig. 32-6A).
  - These studies often turn positive within the first 24 hours of infection. MRI demonstrates altered signal intensity consistent with marrow edema.
- A "triple-phase" bone scan is the standard for scintigraphic imaging in infection.
  - The first phase is the "perfusion" or "angiographic" phase that highlights the vascularity of a lesion and is performed by rapid sequence imaging immediately following intravenously administered isotope.
  - The second phase, the "blood pool" phase, is an intermediate phase and is obtained approximately 15 to 20

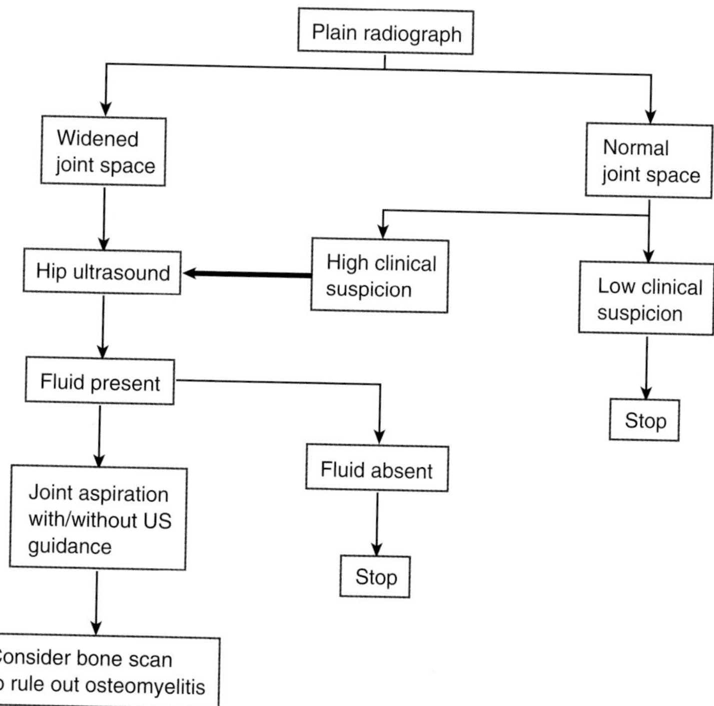

Algorithm 32-1 Workup of joint effusion.

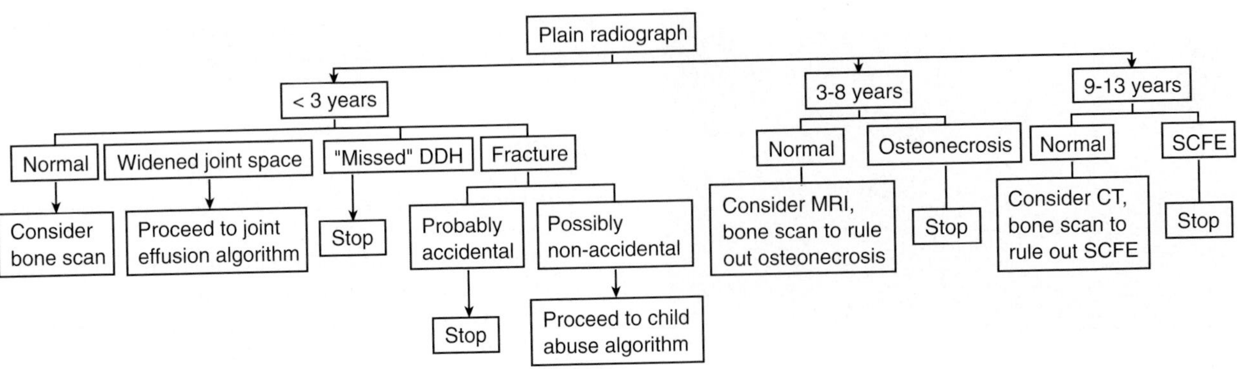

Algorithm 32-2 Workup of hip pain or limp.

minutes following isotope administration. It examines patterns of soft tissue activity.

- The final or "delayed" phase of a triple-phase bone scan is performed 2 to 3 hours after isotope administration and reveals the patterns of isotope localization to the cortical bone.
- The single, largest advantage of a triple-phase scan is its ability to differentiate cellulitis from osteomyelitis.
  - In cellulitis, there is increased activity on the two initial phases *only* (perfusion and blood pool).
  - In osteomyelitis, there is increased activity on all three phases with localization of isotope to the infected bone on the delayed phase.
  - The differential diagnosis of increased uptake on all three phases includes acute trauma and vascular tumor.
  - Absence of uptake may indicate a very aggressive pattern of bone destruction with vascular compromise.

- Scintigraphy is unreliable in the diagnosis of osteomyelitis in the neonatal period.
- The most sensitive imaging modalities in the diagnosis of joint fluid is ultrasound or MRI (Fig. 32-7).
  - Ultrasound is the imaging modality of choice in excluding a septic joint in that it offers the advantage of speed and portability, as well as the ability for real-time–guided needle aspiration of joint fluid.
  - MRI may reveal an associated osteomyelitis, if present, although similar information may be obtained with bone scintigraphy following an initial ultrasound.

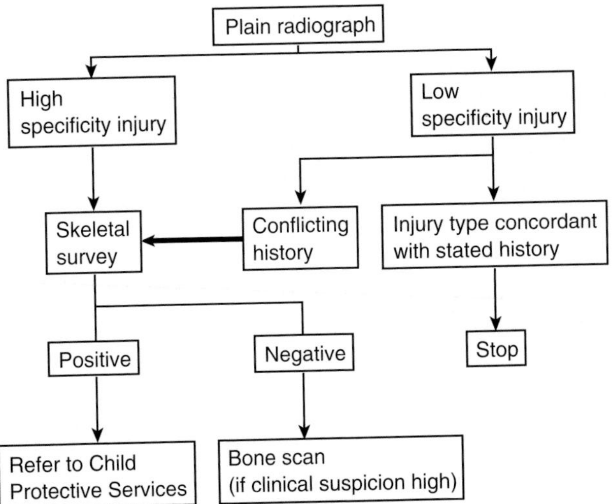

Algorithm 32-3 Workup of suspected child abuse injuries.

Trauma

- Plain radiography is the initial imaging modality for all forms of musculoskeletal trauma, since it shows most fractures and their manner of displacement or angulation.
  - It will also demonstrate the relationship of the fracture line to the growth plate (Salter-Harris classification), a finding that may have prognostic significance.
- CT with 3D reconstruction is useful in defining the exact relationship of fracture fragments in complex injuries and provides a roadmap for surgical reduction (Fig. 32-2).
- MRI may be useful in evaluating osteocartilaginous injury.

Nonaccidental injury deserves special mention.

- The evaluation of a physically abused child includes diagnostic imaging.
- A skeletal survey is the modality of choice in the imaging workup of nonaccidental injury and must be performed correctly to maximize detection of injuries.
- A "babygram," a single image of the entire skeleton, is not acceptable.
- In our institution, a skeletal survey for child abuse includes frontal and lateral views of the axial skeleton and frontal views of the extremities.
- Lesions of high specificity include:
  - Fractures in different stages of healing
  - Metaphyseal "corner" or "bucket-handle" fractures (Fig. 32-8)
  - Posterior rib fractures
  - Fractures of bones that are difficult to fracture including the spinous processes, sternum, and scapulae ("three S's")

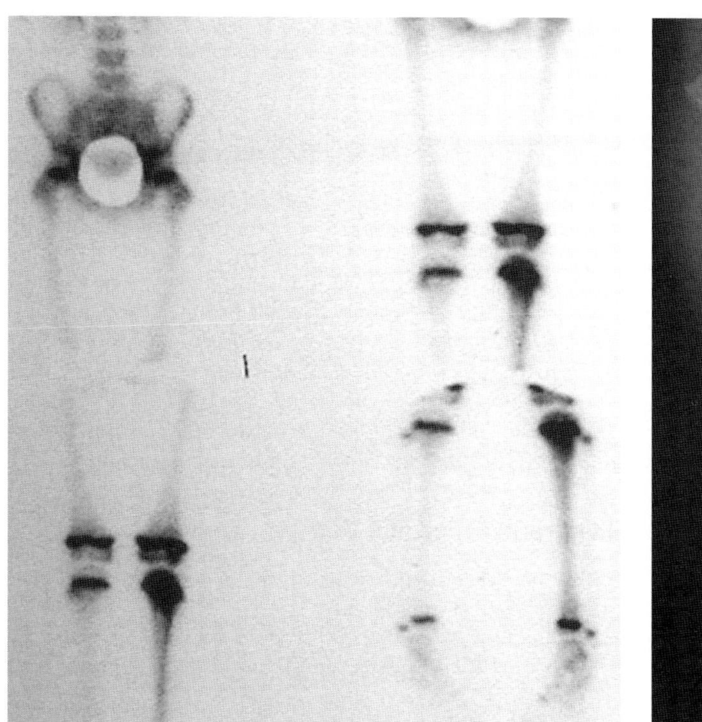
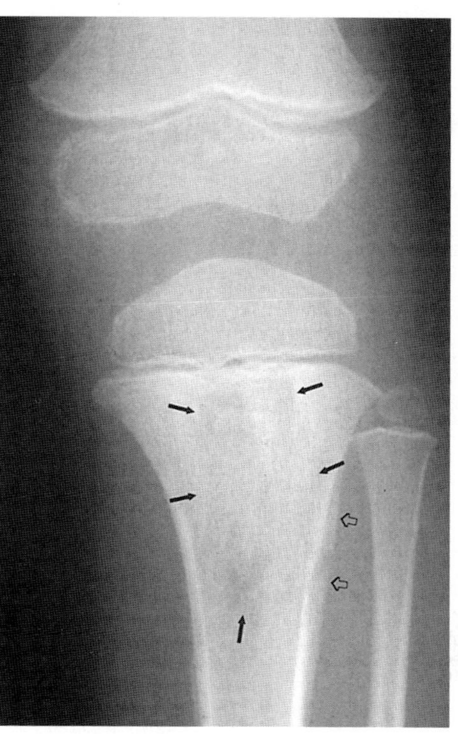

Figure 32-6 Osteomyelitis of the proximal left tibia. (**A**) Bone scan showing increased isotope uptake within the metaphysis. Plain film at this time was normal. (**B**) Plain film obtained 2 weeks later reveals bone destruction (*solid arrows*) and periosteal new bone formation (*open arrows*).

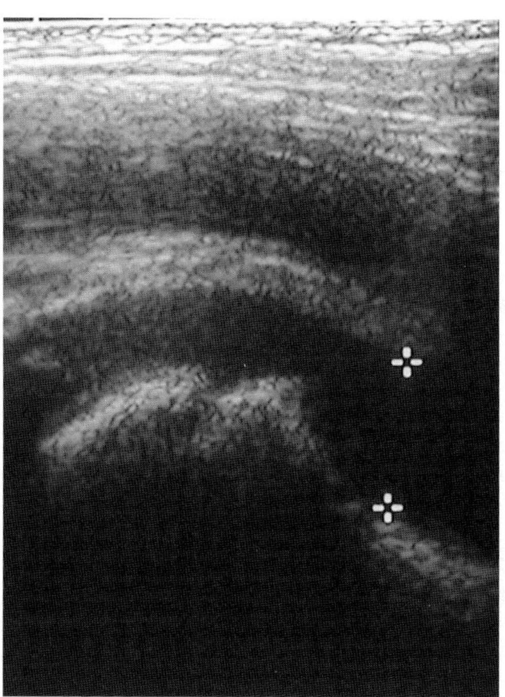
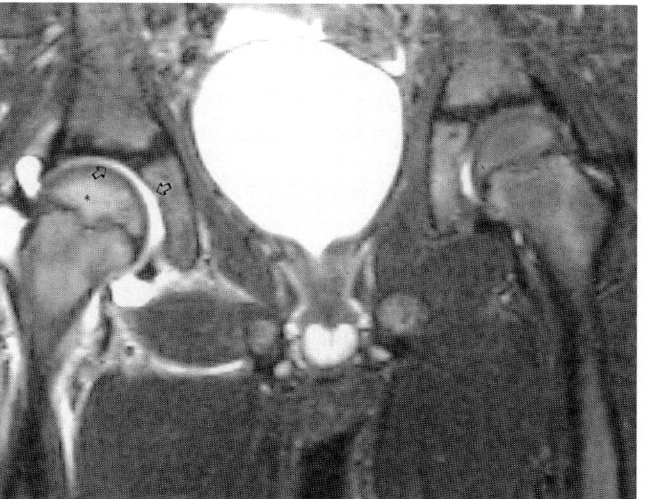

Figure 32-7 Hip effusion. (**A**) Ultrasound. The capsule of the hip joint normally hugs the neck of the femur but when a joint effusion is present, the joint capsule is elevated away from the bone by the sonoluccent fluid (*cursors*). (**B**) Magnetic resonance T2-weighted imaging in another patient reveals a high signal-intensity fluid collection surrounding the right hip (*arrows*). Increased marrow signal (*asterisk*) is noted as well, consistent with edema.

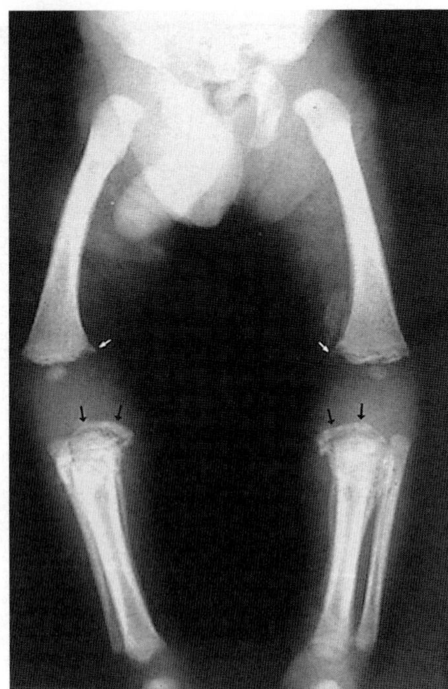

Figure 32-8 Child abuse. Frontal views of both legs show fractures in different stages of healing. Bucket-handle fractures of the proximal tibiae (*black arrows*) and corner fractures of the distal femurs (*white arrows*). Periosteal new bone is noted along the tibial shafts.

- Bone scintigraphy has been used in the initial evaluation of nonaccidental injury.
  - Its strength lies in the discovery of old, near completely healed rib fractures.
  - The major limitation of bone scintigraphy is its inability to recognize subtle metaphyseal injuries in the presence of normal "hot" growth plates.
- The use of both modalities is complementary and should be considered in situations in which the skeletal survey is normal despite a very high clinical suspicion or when there is a paucity of radiographic findings in general.
- A follow-up skeletal survey is an alternative to performing a bone scan.

Developmental Dysplasia of the Hip

- Ultrasound is recommended as the initial imaging modality in the diagnosis of developmental dysplasia of the hip (DDH).
  - Hip ultrasound may be used in the perinatal period and in early infancy until approximately 4 to 6 months of age.
  - Radiographic examination is recommended thereafter as the appearance of ossific nuclei within the femoral epiphyses limits further sonographic evaluation.
  - The hips should not be evaluated by ultrasound before 72 hours because of a high rate of false-positive examinations owing to ligamentous laxity.
  - Many radiologists prefer to wait until the child is between 2 to 4 weeks of age to perform the initial hip ultrasound.
  - Hip ultrasound, by the method of Harcke, is a dynamic evaluation of the cartilaginous femoral epiphysis and its relationship to the bony acetabulum.
    - Provocative maneuvers (Ortolani, Barlow) are employed during the study to assess hip stability (Fig. 32-9).
    - A static hip ultrasound method, described by Graf, is more commonly used in Europe.
  - Ultrasound is also useful on follow-up examinations to assess proper placement of the hip in a Pavlik harness.
- CT may be helpful in evaluating the position of the femoral heads after a spica cast has been applied.

Legg-Calvé-Perthes Disease

- Idiopathic ischemic necrosis of the hips occurs between the ages of 4 and 8 years.
- Radiographic evaluation is pursued initially with the hips examined in the neutral and frog-leg lateral projections.
  - Findings include increased density of the femoral head, subchondral fissure, and with progression, irregularity and flattening of the head with metaphyseal broadening, trochanteric overgrowth, and metaphyseal cysts (Fig. 32-10).
  - Lateral extrusion of the femoral head may occur as a complication.
  - These radiographic findings represent subacute or late changes of osteonecrosis and, as in other causes of osteonecrosis, MRI and bone scintigraphy are more sensitive in the earliest period of symptoms.
- MRI shows alteration in signal intensity within the femoral head.
- Bone scintigraphy demonstrates photopenia within either a portion or the entire femoral head.

Slipped Capital Femoral Epiphysis

- The diagnostic imaging workup of slipped capital femoral epiphysis (SCFE) consists of radiographic evaluation of the pelvis in the frontal neutral and frog-leg lateral projections.
  - The frog-leg lateral radiograph is more sensitive than the neutral radiograph in the detection of an SCFE (Fig. 32-11).
- Radiographs are used to follow these patients after surgical pinning.
  - Alterations in pin position, chondrolysis, or osteonecrosis are complications to be excluded on follow-up radiographic evaluation.
- CT can also be used to evaluate a SCFE, although generally plain films suffice.

Skeletal Dysplasias

- Plain radiography is the modality of choice in the evaluation of skeletal dysplasias.

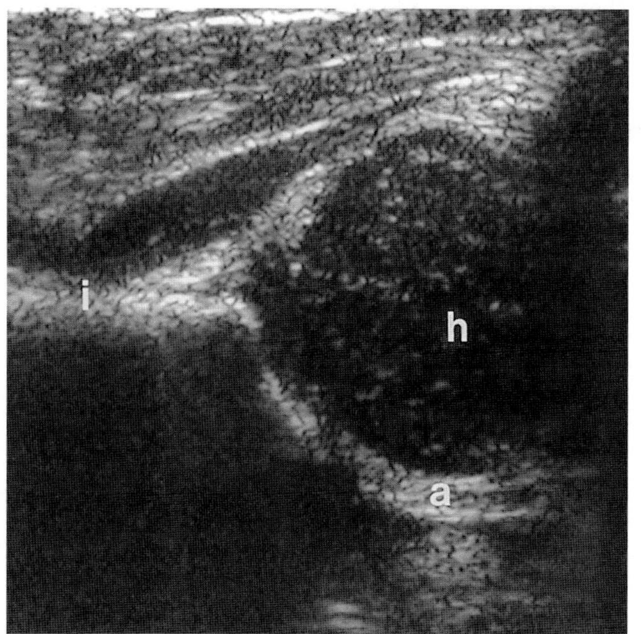

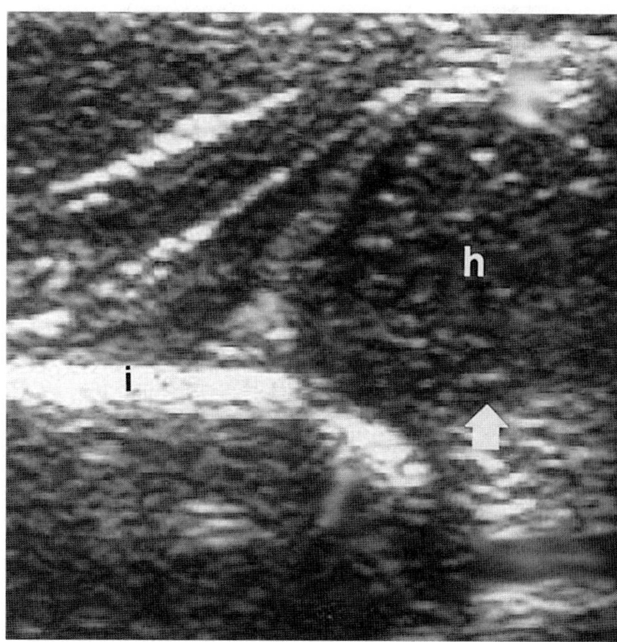

Figure 32-9 Ultrasound of developmental dysplasia of the hip. (**A**) The coronal image of the normal hip shows that the femoral head is seated deeply within the acetabulum. (**B**) The coronal image of the dysplastic hip shows that the acetabulum is shallow and the femoral head is laterally displaced (*arrow*). *h,* cartilaginous femoral head; *i,* ileum; *a,* acetabulum.

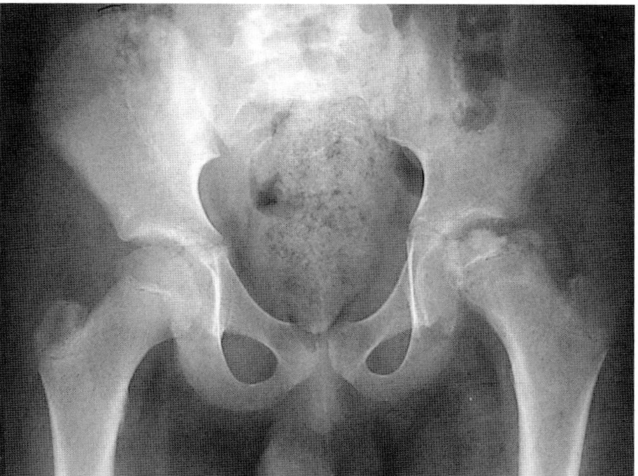

Figure 32-10 Legg-Calvé-Perthes disease. Plain radiograph reveals sclerosis and widening and irregularity of the left femoral head with shortening and broadening of the femoral neck. A widened joint space is also visible.

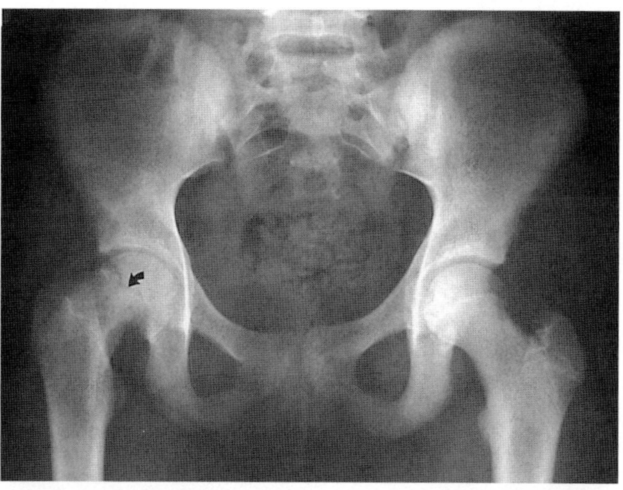

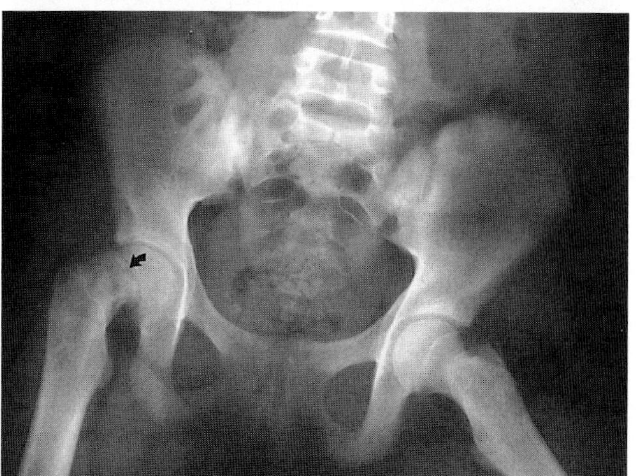

Figure 32-11 Slipped capital femoral epiphysis. (**A**) Frontal view. (**B**) Frog-leg lateral view. The right femoral head has slipped medially on the frontal view and posteriorly on the frog-leg lateral view (*arrows*). A frog-leg lateral is a frontal view of the pelvis but a lateral view of the femur.

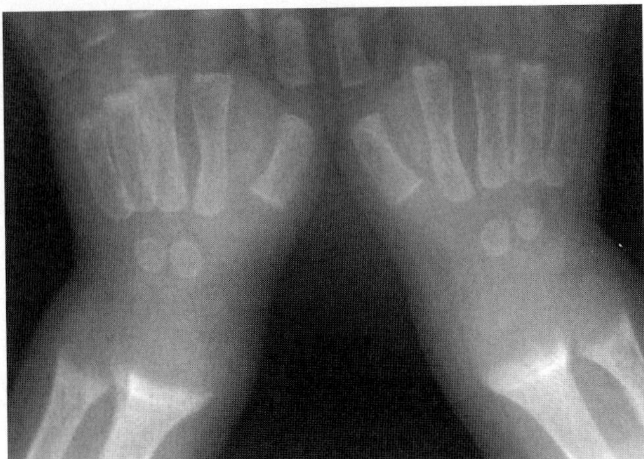

Figure 32-12 Rickets. The hallmark of rickets is loss of the zone of provisional calcification. Note also the cupping and the "paintbrush" appearance of the radial and ulnar metaphyses.

- The workup begins with a skeletal survey, but frequently the findings evolve and repeat examinations may be necessary as the child grows.
- Some common dysplasias such as achondroplasia are easily recognized clinically and radiographically, but skeletal dysplasias are frequently peculiar to a single family and cannot be classified.

Metabolic Bone Disease

- Plain radiography is suitable for imaging of rachitic changes.
  - □ It is best to image the wrists or knees, since these are the fastest growing and most metabolically active regions of the appendicular skeleton.
  - □ Findings include the following (Fig. 32-12):
    - □ Loss of the zone of provisional calcification (ZPC) of the cartilaginous growth plate (white line bordering the metaphysis; earliest finding)
    - □ Metaphyseal fraying, cupping
    - □ Growth-plate widening (deposition of nonmineralized osteoid)
    - □ Bowing deformities
    - □ Rachitic rosary (bulbous overgrowth of costochondral junction)

SUGGESTED READING

Kleinman PK. Diagnostic imaging of child abuse, 2nd ed. St. Louis: Mosby, 1998.

Novelline RA. Squire's fundamentals of radiology, 5th ed. Cambridge, MA: Harvard University Press, 1997.

Ogden JA. Skeletal injury in the child. Philadelphia: Lea & Febiger, 1982.

Resnick D. Diagnosis of bone and joint disorders, 3rd ed. Philadelphia: WB Saunders, 1995.

Silverman FN, Kuhn JP. Caffey's pediatric x-ray diagnosis: an integrated imaging approach, 9th ed. St. Louis: Mosby, 1993.

Taybi H, Lachman RS. Radiology of syndromes, metabolic disorders, and skeletal dysplasias, 4th ed. St. Louis: Mosby, 1996.

PAIN MANAGEMENT

JULIE BUCH

The International Association for the Study of Pain defines pain as "an unpleasant sensory and emotional experience associated with actual or potential tissue damage or described in terms of such damage." Two important points can be taken from this definition. First, pain is subjective and thus, the gold standard for pain measurement is the patient's self-report. In children, one must consider their developmental level when interpreting their pain behavior. Second, there is always an emotional component to pain. Good pain management may include treating anxiety and fear.

Traditionally, pain in children has been undertreated. This can be attributed to a number of factors. These include difficulty in assessing pain, fear about the side effects of narcotics in children, and a fear of addiction. In the 1960s, the medical literature barely refers to pediatric pain and when it does it is only anecdotal. This likely demonstrates a problem with pain assessment.

In 1987, Dr. K. J. Anand began to publish a series of studies showing that infants who did not receive good intraoperative and postoperative pain management had higher incidences of ventilatory dysfunction, acidosis, cardiovascular complications, infections, clotting disorders, and ultimately had higher mortality rates. These articles showed us that not only can pain be treated safely in infants but that there are dangerous consequences of leaving pain untreated.

In the short term, untreated pain causes the release of stress hormones such as glucagon, cortisol, prostaglandins, norepinephrine, and substance P. These in turn promote tissue breakdown and water retention, leading to lactic acidosis and hyperglycemia. This results in a higher heart rate and blood pressure, increased work of breathing, impaired bowel function, impaired immune function, and increased clotting. Together, these factors increase mortality rates in infants who are left with untreated pain.

In the long term, studies indicate that not treating pain in childhood can leave a patient more sensitive to painful stimuli in the future. Since the brain and spinal cord are still forming in infants and children, experiencing painful stimuli can alter the development of these structures. N-methyl-D-aspartate (NMDA) receptors are excitatory amino acid receptors that send messages to the dorsal horn of the spinal cord. They are activated by painful stimuli. If a child receives repeated painful stimuli, this may cause the NMDA receptors to become more plentiful and send an increased message to the dorsal horn resulting in areas of hyperalgesia/exaggerated pain responses in the future. Studies show that undergoing painful procedures, such as circumcision without analgesic therapy can cause sleep disturbances and behavioral changes for prolonged periods of time.

As early as 7 weeks' gestation, cutaneous sensory receptors begin to appear on the fetus. By 20 weeks, all surfaces are covered by sensory receptors. Pain can be transmitted by unmyelinated C fibers and by thinly myelinated A fibers. Myelination occurs between 30 and 37 weeks' gestation. At 42 weeks' postconception, pain pathways are more organized as receptors and transmitters move to positions in the dorsal horn of the spinal cord. Thus, premature infants may not be able to localize their pain but they will still feel it. It can compare to having a "stomachache" in which the pain is diffuse and hard to localize but is still quite uncomfortable.

PAIN ASSESSMENT

To treat pain, we must be able to assess pain. Unfortunately, there is no one precise physical test that can be used to measure pain. A pain assessment scale is a tool used to quantify and monitor pain. In children, one can measure pain subjectively or objectively. The gold standard for pain assessment is the "self-report," a subjective method in which patients tell caregivers how much pain that they feel. This is the subjective method of measuring pain.

To understand how children express their pain, it is helpful to understand the Piagetian cognitive stages of development:

- From birth to 2 years of age, the child is learning to differentiate self from nonself and is incapable of reporting pain in words.
- From 2 to 7 years of age, children can symbolize and pretend. They can differentiate pain but may think of it

as a concrete object. Also, they have egocentrism of thought, that is, they think that everyone is thinking what they are thinking. This may lead children to underreport their pain.

- From 7 to 10 years of age, children become capable of logic and understand cause and effect. They can understand that reporting pain may lead to treatment.
- From 11 to 14 years of age, children begin to understand abstract and hypothetical thought and all the psychosocial aspects of pain come into play.

In some ways, children age 7 to 11 are the easiest patients to assess and treat because they can report their pain in words and can understand why doing this may help them but there aren't as many emotional issues tied to the pain as with preteens and teens.

Many pain scales can be used to quantify pain based upon a child's self-report (subjectively). It may be useful to use the word "hurt" or "owie" instead of pain for some children. A few of the most commonly pain scales include the Visual Analog or 0-to-10 scale, the Oucher scale, and the Wong-Baker FACES scale.

The 0-to-10 scale is a numeric self-reporting pain assessment scale that is often used with adults as well as children. For children to be able to understand how to use this scale, they must be able to count to 10 and understand the concept of greater than and less than. The scale can be used with or without the visual aid of a 0-to-10 diagram. Explain to the patient that if 0 means no pain at all, and 10 is the worst pain (hurt) you can imagine, ask what number the pain would be. The patient may indicate verbally or by pointing to a number on the diagram.

The Oucher scale is a self-reporting scale recommended for children 3 years of age and older. Three versions of the Oucher scale are available (Fig. 33-1). Each has photos showing Hispanic, Caucasian, or African-American children in increasing degrees of pain. One can explain to the patient that the child at the bottom has no pain at all and the child at the top has the biggest hurt that you could imagine. Ask the patient which picture shows how much pain that he or she is feeling right now. Once the child has pointed to a picture, their selection can be converted into a numeric score. This is meant to be a self-reporting tool, so having the caregiver compare the patient's appearance to the pictures on the scale is not an appropriate use of the tool.

The Wong-Baker FACES scale is used similarly and can be used with adults as well as children (Fig. 33-2).

Objective measures of pain use behavioral observations and physiologic changes, rather than self-reporting. Physiologic changes that occur with pain tend to lessen after the body adjusts and can be modulated by coping skills. Generally, these signs are considered less specific and less reliable than patient self-report, but in noncommunicative patients these signs may be all that is available. Physiologic parameters associated with pain include elevated blood pressure, heart rate, respiratory rate, decreased oxygen saturation, sweating, pupil dilation, muscle tension, and nau-

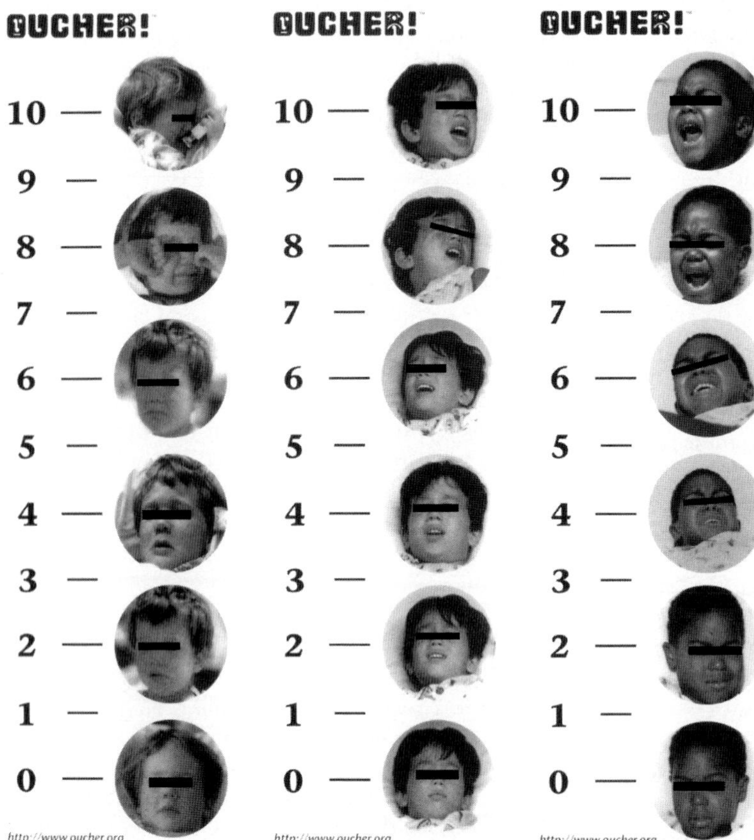

Figure 33-1 Oucher Pain Assessment Scale.

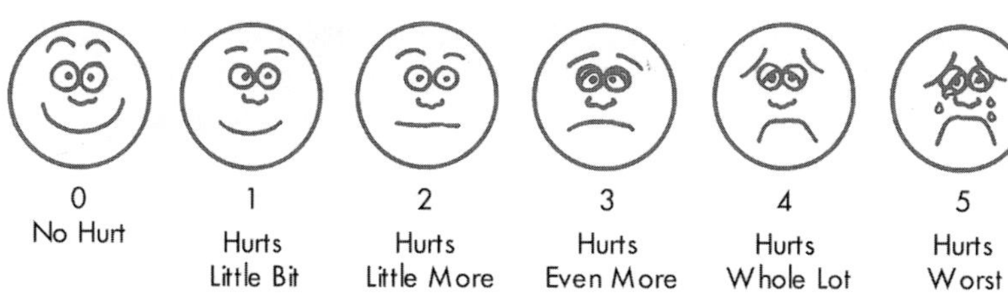

Figure 33-2 Wong-Baker FACES Pain Rating scale. (From Wong DL, Hockenberry-Eaton M, Wilson D, et al. Wong's essentials of pediatric nursing, 6th ed. St. Louis: Mosby, 2001.)

sea. Behavioral observations that may indicate pain include facial grimacing, crying, posturing, guarding, fatigue, difficulty sleeping and eating, and shortened attention span. The CRIES Neonatal Postoperative Pain scale (Table 33-1) is an example of a scale that uses physiologic and behavioral measures. The FLACC Pain scale (Table 33-2) uses only behavioral observations.

TREATMENT

Pain is best treated using a multidisciplinary approach and treatment should be available 24 hours a day. Doctors, nurses, pharmacists, psychologists, and child life specialists working together can provide the most comprehensive treatment. Nurses can be taught to consider pain the fifth vital sign and assess it with every vital sign check. A physician and a clinical nurse specialist can assess the patients once or twice daily and make necessary adjustments in medication (in conjunction with a pharmacist). A child life specialist can provide and teach distraction techniques from pain and input from a psychologist can be valuable. An anesthesiologist can provide neural blockade where helpful.

Whenever opioids are used, certain safety provisions need to be in place. Oxygen, naloxone, suction, and an Ambu bag should be immediately available. A person with airway skills should be in-house 24 hours a day. For all patients using patient-controlled analgesia (PCA), opioid drips or epidurals, continuous pulse oximetry should be considered. Level of consciousness and respiratory rate are monitored regularly.

Patient-Controlled Analgesia

PCA was first developed in adults in the early 1970s by a behaviorist but was not used in children until the late 1980s. PCA is an opioid delivery method that consists of a microprocessor-driven pump with a button that the child presses to self-administer a bolus of pain medicine. The bolus is followed by a preset lockout time interval, and one

TABLE 33-1 "CRIES" SCALE FOR NEONATAL POSTOPERATIVE PAIN ASSESSMENT

Parameter	Finding	Points[a]
Crying	No	0
	Crying but not high pitched	0
	High pitched but infant consolable	1
	Inconsolable	2
Requires oxygen	No	0
	≤30% supplemental oxygen required to keep oxygen saturation >95%	1
	>30% supplemental oxygen required to keep oxygen saturation >95%	2
Increased vital signs	Heart rate and mean blood pressure ≤ preoperative values	0
	Heart rate or mean blood pressure increased but ≤20% from preoperative levels	1
	Heart rate or mean blood pressure increased >20% from preoperative levels	2
Expression	None	0
	Grimace	1
	Grimace with grunting	2
Sleepless	No	0
	Wakes at frequent intervals	1
	Constantly awake	2

[a]The higher the score, the greater the subjective expression of pain.
Adapted from Krechel SW, Bildner J. CRIES: a new neonatal postoperative pain measurement score. Initial testing and reliability. Paediatr Anaesth 1995;5:53–61.

TABLE 33-2 FLACC PAIN SCALE

Category	Score 0	1	2
Face	No particular expression or smile, eye contact, or interest in surroundings	Occasional grimace or frown, withdrawn, disinterested, worried look to face, eyebrows lowered, eyes partially closed, cheeks raised, mouth pursed	Frequent to constant frown, clenched jaw, quivering chin, deep furrows on forehead, eyes closed, mouth opened, deep lines around nose/lips
Legs	Normal position or relaxed	Uneasy, restless, tense, increased tone, rigidity, intermittent flexion/extension of limbs	Kicking or legs drawn up, hypertonicity, exaggerated flexion/extension of limbs, tremors
Activity	Lying quietly, normal position, moves easily and freely	Squirming, shifting back and forth, tense, hesitant to move, guarding, pressure on body part	Arched, rigid, or jerking, fixed position, rocking, side-to-side head movement, rubbing of body part
Cry	No cry/moan (awake or asleep)	Moans or whimpers, occasional cries, sighs, occasional complaint	Crying steadily, screams, sobs, moans, grunts, frequent complaints
Consolability	Calm, content, relaxed, does not require consoling	Reassured by occasional touching, hugging, or talking; distractible	Difficult to console or comfort

Adapted from Merkel S, et al. A behavior pain assessment scale. Pediatr Nurse 1997;23:293–297.

can add a small continuous background infusion of opioid to the PCA. By delivering small doses of opioids on demand in the confines of lockout periods, the PCA can better maintain steady levels of pain medication and therefore consistent pain control, and do it safely.

PCA has many advantages:

- The delay associated with delivering as-needed medications is avoided and the patient is able to maintain a more constant concentration of pain medication thus, avoiding oversedation and other narcotic side effects and also painful periods waiting for more medication.
- It empowers the patient and has been shown to improve the satisfaction of the patient and the family.
- The ability to self-administer boluses in anticipation of a painful event (e.g., dressing change, ambulating, rolling) can improve pain control and reduce the total amount of opioid needed during the event.
- Because nurses do not have to check and administer every dose of narcotic, nursing time is conserved.
- When compared with continuous opioid infusion in children after spine surgery, PCA uses less opioid and has fewer side effects than the continuous infusion group.

PCA is safe because when the patient becomes drowsy, he or she will stop pushing the button. As an extra safety precaution, one can also program a maximum dose of opioid that the child can receive in 4 hours called the 4-hour max. Many studies have shown PCA to enjoy good patient acceptance, increased family satisfaction with pain management, and safety. In one large study, patients receiving morphine PCA (with or without continuous infusion) had lower pain scores, less somnolence, and better satisfaction than patients receiving intramuscular morphine injections. In addition, there were no deaths or major adverse outcomes.

Candidates

- To use PCA effectively, a patient must be able to understand the cause-and-effect relationship between pressing the button and receiving pain relief and must be physically able to press the button.
- Children 6 years of age and older generally can operate the PCA pump. Occasionally, though not reliably, a 5-year-old child is capable. We have not had success with children younger than 5 years.

Drug Choice

- Morphine is the most commonly used opioid in PCA. It comes 1 mg per mL, which helps make calculations easier.
- Hydromorphone and fentanyl are also safe and effective for PCA use.
- Studies have shown these three opioids to have similar side-effect profiles though individual patients may tolerate one opioid better than another.
- Demerol is not a good choice for use in PCA. It is broken down to an active metabolite normeperidine, which then must be renally excreted. In large doses or in cases of renal compromise, normeperidine can accumulate and cause seizures. In addition, when compared with morphine PCA, patients using demerol PCA had poorer pain control.

Intravenous Dosing in Children

Studies have shown that hydromorphone is five times more potent than morphine and that fentanyl is approximately 75 times more potent than morphine in children (Table 33-3).

TABLE 33-3 INTRAVENOUS PATIENT-CONTROLLED ANALGESIA IN CHILDREN

Drug	Bolus Dose	Continuous	4-Hour Max
Morphine	10–30 μg/kg	5–10 μg/kg/hr	300 μg/kg
Hydromorphone	2–5 μg/kg	1–2 μg/kg/hr	60 μg/kg
Fentanyl	0.25–0.75 μg/kg	0.25–0.75 μg/kg/hr	4 μg/kg

Continuous Infusion

Adding a background infusion to PCA has been shown to allow patients to have longer periods of uninterrupted sleep. However, it has also been shown to increase the incidence of side effects such as nausea and sedation.

- Use of continuous infusions with PCA is suggested when the surgery is extensive.
- Starting at the lower end of the dose range (5 μg/kg/hour of morphine) is recommended.
- An alternative to using a continuous infusion is the use of Ketoralac every 6 hours.

Weaning

- The first step in weaning a PCA is to stop the continuous infusion (if it is present).
- It is best to wait until the patient can tolerate a fair bit of oral intake before beginning oral pain medications due to concerns over nausea and vomiting.
- One hour after the first dose of oral pain medication is added, the lockout interval on the PCA is increased to 12 to 20 minutes.
- After the third dose of the oral pain medication, the PCA can be discontinued.

Nurse-Controlled Analgesia

Nurse-controlled analgesia is used in many centers for children unable to use the PCA themselves. It has been shown to be effective pain management and conserve nursing time. However, nurses tend to underestimate pain and give lower doses of narcotics than a matched group of patients with PCA gave themselves.

Parent-Controlled Analgesia

In patients unable to use the PCA themselves, allowing the parent to press the button has been attempted. Although there were no deaths or permanent adverse events, 9 children of 212 using this technique required naloxone, a very high rate when compared with standard PCA patients.

- If parent-controlled analgesia is used, a lockout interval greater than 20 minutes is recommended.

Continuous Opioid Infusions

- Continuous intravenous infusions of opioids can provide effective pain relief after surgery.
- Morphine, hydromorphone, and fentanyl are all safe and effective opioid choices.
- Generally, a range is ordered and the nurses can titrate the infusion to the patient's level of pain control (Box 33-1).

Epidural Analgesia

- Epidural analgesia can provide excellent postoperative pain relief in infants and children.
- It can be given as a continuous infusion, single shot, or even as PCEA (patient-controlled epidural analgesia).
- The epidural space can be accessed at many levels. Most often the thoracic (T7-11), lumbar (L3-L4), and caudal (sacrococcygeal ligament) sites are used.
- By placing the analgesics near the nerves as they emerge from the dural sac, one can produce profound analgesia while only using very low doses of medicine.
- Children can ambulate with assistance and undergo physical therapy with an epidural in place.

A recent study of adolescents who underwent posterior spinal fusion compared intravenous PCA and epidural infusions for postoperative pain control. Both methods were safe and effective, but the epidural group tolerated a full diet and was discharged from the hospital significantly earlier than the PCA group. In infants undergoing Nissen fundoplication, those with epidurals had shorter intensive care unit stays and hospitalizations.

Complications and Safety

The incidence of infection/abscess associated with postoperative epidural placement is very low, and large series have reported no cases of permanent sequelae (e.g., nerve injury or death).

Drug Choice

Generally, postoperative epidurals are run as continuous infusions made up of a local anesthetic and an opioid. The most common local anesthetic used is bupivacaine (Box 33-2).

Opioid receptors are concentrated in the dorsal horn of the spinal cord and in the brain. When opioids bind with

BOX 33-1 DRUGS USED FOR CONTINUOUS OPIOID INFUSIONS

- Morphine, 10–40 μg/kg/hr
- Hydromorphone, 2–8 μg/kg/hr
- Fentanyl, 0.5–2 μg/kg/hr

BOX 33-2 BUPIVACAINE FOR EPIDURAL USE

- Infusion rate should not exceed 0.5 mg/kg/h in children >6 mo of age or 0.25 mg/kg/hr in chilren <6 mo of age
- Concentration can vary from 0.125%–0.05%
- 0.0625% usually provides good pain relief without significant numbness or motor blockade

these receptors in the spinal cord, the release of substance P (a neurotransmitter that facilitates transmission of pain impulses from the dorsal horn) is blocked, and the perception of pain is altered. Opioids also cause the brain to release serotonin, a neurotransmitter that inhibits the transmission of pain impulses.

How opioids act in the epidural space is determined largely by their lipid solubility. Fentanyl, hydromorphone, and morphine are all commonly used in the epidural space. Fentanyl is 580 times more lipid-soluble than morphine, while hydromorphone is 1.4 times more lipid-soluble. Increased lipid solubility leads to more rapid absorption of fentanyl into the epidural fat and also into the bloodstream causing it to have a shorter duration of action and a smaller spread through the cerebrospinal fluid.

- Being more hydrophilic allows morphine to spread up and down the spinal cord and thus, produce a wider band of analgesia that spreads across more dermatomes.
- The rostral spread of morphine can be associated with more opioid-related side effects (pruritus, nausea, respiratory depression) than with fentanyl.
- Hydromorphone provides more rostral spread than fentanyl and slightly less than morphine.

For lower extremity surgery, there is no concern about achieving a level of analgesia above the location of the epidural catheter so many solutions may be acceptable. A few common epidural solutions are listed in Box 33-3.

Candidates

- An epidural can provide analgesia for infants and children with surgical pain located below the nipple line.

BOX 33-3 COMMON EPIDURAL SOLUTIONS[a]

- Bupivacaine 0.0625% plus hydromorphone 10–20 µg/mL at 0.1–0.4 mL/kg/hr
- Bupivacaine 0.0625% plus fentanyl, 2–5 µg/mL at 0.15–0.4 mL/kg/hr
- Bupivacaine 0.0625% plus morphine, 25–50 µg/mL at 0.15–0.4 mL/kg/hr
- Neonates: bupivacaine 0.05% plus fentanyl, 1 µg/mL at mL/hr

[a]Clonidine and butorphanol can also be added to epidural solutions as adjunctive medications to improve pain relief and ameliorate side effects.

- Absolute contraindications to placing an epidural include an infection at the site of placement, a systemic infection, a coagulopathy, and family refusal of the technique.
- Relative contraindications include children with preexisting neurologic deficits, spinal abnormalities, prior laminectomies, and increased intracranial pressure.
- The presence of an indentation or dimple near the sacral hiatus may indicate an underlying pilonidal cyst and a caudal should be avoided.

Single-Shot Caudal Blockade

- Caudal epidural blockade provides postoperative pain relief for most any surgical procedure within the distribution of the dermatomes of the L2-S5 dermatomes.
- In children under 8 years of age, the sacral hiatus is incompletely fused.
- With the patient lying on the side, the caudal space can be accessed through the sacral hiatus, which is formed by the nonunion of the S5 vertebral arch. A loss of resistance is felt as the needle crosses the sacrococcygeal ligament and enters the epidural space.
- If the patient is an outpatient, 0.75 to 1.0 mL/kg of 0.125% to 0.25% bupivacaine with or without epinephrine or ropivacaine given caudally in the epidural space can provide hours of pain relief.
- Adding 2 to 4 µg/kg of clonidine to the solution can prolong the duration of the block.
- If the patient is an inpatient, morphine, 50 µg/kg, or Dilaudid, 10 µg/kg, can be added to the solution and pain relief can be expected to last about 12 hours. This technique is especially useful following repair of a clubfoot.

Peripheral Neural Blockade

- The femoral nerve (L2, L3, and L4) supplies sensory innervation to the anterior thigh and the periosteum of the femoral shaft and motor innervation to the quadriceps.
  - This block can help relieve the pain of femoral shaft fractures/osteotomies and lessen quadriceps spasm.
  - One can place 0.6 mL/kg up to a maximum of 30 mL of 0.25% bupivacaine with epinephrine 1:200,000 lateral to the femoral artery pulsation below the inguinal ligament.
- The brachial plexus can be blocked using many approaches.
  - An axillary block is useful for pain in the forearm and the hand.
  - A parascalene approach can be helpful for shoulder and upper arm pain.
  - Often these blocks are performed with the aid of a nerve stimulator as most children need to be asleep and are unable to detect paresthesias during the application of the block.
  - One can use 0.5 mL/kg up to a maximum of 20 mL of 0.25% bupivacaine with epinephrine 1:200,000 for these blocks.

- A digital nerve block can be used for finger or toe postoperative pain.
  - A dose of 0.5 to 1.0 mL of 0.25% bupivacaine *without* epinephrine can be placed in a ring at the metacarpophalangeal junction.
  - Check the digit's blood supply prior to block. Using large volumes of local anesthetic may lead to compartment syndrome.
- The sciatic nerve (L4, L5, and S1-3) supplies sensory innervation to the foot and much of the leg below the knee. It begins branching 5 to 7 cm above the popliteal fossa and thus, if one wants to anesthetize the foot, one must perform many distal nerve blocks or perform a sciatic block more proximal with a nerve stimulator.
  - An ankle block is performed by basically putting a ring of epinephrine-free local anesthetic around the ankle. Because of the multiple injections, this can be an uncomfortable block for the patient.
  - The saphenous nerve supplies sensory innervation to the foot and can be blocked easily as it comes around the medial aspect of the patella.

Adjuvant Pain Medications

- Ketoralac is the only parenteral nonsteroidal anti-inflammatory drug (NSAID) available in the United States.
- It can be given by the intravenous, intramuscular, or oral route.
- The dose is 0.5 mg per kg up to 15 mg if the patient weighs less than 50 kg and 30 mg if the patient weighs more than 50 kg, every 6 hours for not more than 5 days.
- It is not necessary to give a loading dose.
- It is a very potent analgesic (250 times as potent as aspirin, 25 times as potent as naproxen) that has no respiratory depressant effects and can reduce opioid usage.
- NSAIDs however may cause gastrointestinal upset and bleeding, platelet dysfunction, and renal impairment.
- There is also controversy as to whether Ketoralac significantly inhibits osteoblast growth, and some practitioners limit its use where this is a concern.

Oral Pain Medications

As patients heal and prepare to go home, they need to be weaned to oral analgesics. The most commonly prescribed oral analgesic is acetaminophen plus codeine (Box 33-4).

BOX 33-4 ACETAMINOPHEN PLUS CODEINE

- Available as a tablet (Tylenol #3 is 300 mg acetaminophen and 30 mg codeine) or an elixir (1 mL = 24 mg acetaminophen and 2.4 mg codeine)
- Schedule III narcotic—requires no triplicate form and can be called in to a pharmacy
- Dose is based on the codeine and is 1 mg/kg every 4 hr
- Children should not receive >75 mg/kg/day up to 4,000 mg/day of acetaminophen

BOX 33-5 LORTAB

- Acetaminophen/hydrocodone combination
- Schedule III narcotic—requires no triplicate form and can be called in to a pharmacy
- Less nauseating than codeine
- The tablets come in four strengths: Lortab 2.5 mg/500 mg, 5 mg/500 mg, 7.5 mg/500 mg, 10 mg/500 mg and the elixir is 0.5 mg/33.3 mg
- Dose is based on the hydrocodone and is 0.1–0.2 mg/kg every 4 hr

Codeine must be broken down to morphine to have an analgesic effect. Up to 15% of people lack the enzyme that o-demethylates codeine to allow it to become morphine, rendering the codeine ineffective. Also, codeine is associated with a significant incidence of nausea and vomiting. Some pain services prefer Lortab (Box 33-5) over Tylenol #3.

Oxycodone, morphine, and methadone are schedule II narcotics and do not have any Tylenol added to their preparations. They may be considered for patients with pain (most likely patients with chronic pain) not covered by the aforementioned narcotics.

Nonpharmacologic Pain Management

- Pain is best managed by a combination of pharmacologic and nonpharmacologic therapies.
- Nonpharmacologic interventions include acupuncture, art and play, biofeedback, deep breathing, distraction, guided imagery, heat, hypnosis, massage, comfort positioning, and transcutaneous electrical nerve stimulation.
- One must assess the patient and the technique for developmental fit.

Treating Common Side Effects of PCA and Opioid Infusions

- The common side effects of opioids are nausea, pruritus, respiratory depression or oversedation, and inadequately managed pain (Box 33-6).

Treating Common Side Effects of Epidurals

- Nausea, pruritus, and oversedation can be treated with the same drugs and methods mentioned in Box 33-6.
- You can also lower the infusion rate or switch which opioid is used in infusion.
- Urinary retention is common with epidural infusions. Some practitioners place indwelling bladder catheters preemptively, and others wait to see if the patient can void on his or her own.
- With local anesthetics in the infusion, be careful that patients do not get pressure blisters. This can be avoided by using low (less than 0.1%) concentrations of local

BOX 33-6 TREATING SIDE EFFECTS OF PATIENT-CONTROLLED ANALGESIA, OPIOID INFUSIONS, AND EPIDURALS

Nausea
- Ondansetron, 0.15 mg/kg up to 4 mg every 6 hr, *or*
- Metoclopramide, 0.15 mg/kg up to 10 mg every 6 hr

Pruritus
- Diphenhydramine, 0.5–1.0 mg/kg every 6 hr, *or*
- Hydroxyzine, 0.5–1.0 mg/kg intramuscularly every 4 hr, *or*
- Naloxone, 1 μg/kg up to 40 μg every hr
- If the patient is having excellent pain control, consider lowering or discontinuing the continuous infusion or lowering the patient-controlled analgesia bolus dose
- Consider switching opioids, since patients may find one opioid to be less nauseating or to cause less itching than another

Oversedation
- Stop the opioid for a period and restart administration at a lower dose
- If the patient cannot be roused or is experiencing respiratory depression, administer oxygen and ventilate
- Naloxone, started at 2–5 μg/kg and titrated to response

anesthetics and turning the patient's lower extremities every 2 to 4 hours.

- Compartment syndrome is always a concern in lower extremity trauma. By using more dilute concentrations of local anesthetic, you can reduce the risk of masking a compartment syndrome, but a high degree of suspicion should remain.

SUGGESTED READING

Anand KJS, Hickey PR. Pain and its effect on the human neonate and fetus. N Engl J Med 1987;317:1321.

Berde C, Lehn B, Yee J, et al. Patient-controlled analgesia in children and adolescents: a randomized, prospective comparison with intramuscular administration of morphine for postoperative analgesia. J Pediatr 1991;118:460–466.

Collins J, Geake J, Grier H, et al. Patient-controlled analgesia for mucositis pain in children: a three-period crossover study comparing morphine and hydromorphone. J Pediatr 1996;129;722–728.

Finley GA, McGrath PJ, eds. Measurement of pain in infants and children. Seattle: IASP Press, 1998.

Giaufre E, Dalens B, Gombert A. Epidemiology and morbidity of regional anesthesia in children: a one-year prospective survey of the French Language Society of Pediatric Anesthesiologists. Anesth Analg 1996;83:904–912.

Goodarzi M. Comparison of epidural morphine, hydromorphone and fentanyl for postoperative pain control in children undergoing orthopaedic surgery. Paediatr Anaesth 1999;9:419–422.

Strafford MA, Wilder RT, Berde CB. The risk of infection from epidural analgesia in children: a review of 1620 cases. Anesth Analg 1995;80:234–238.

Taddio A, Katz J, Ilersich A, et al. Effect of neonatal circumcision on pain response during subsequent routine vaccination. Lancet 1997;349:599.

Van Boerum DH, Smith JT, Curtin MJ. A comparison of the effects of patient controlled analgesia with intravenous opioids versus epidural analgesia on recovery after surgery for idiopathic scoliosis. Spine 2000;25:2355–2357.

Wong D, Baker C. Comparison of assessment scales. Pediatr Nurs 1988;14:9–17.

ANESTHESIA AND SEDATION

MARIA MARKAKIS ZESTOS

Sedation provides a calm, cooperative patient but is not without risk. Sedation can result in hypoventilation, apnea, airway obstruction, and cardiac arrest. Safe sedation requires first and foremost, a skilled and vigilant person who can provide appropriate patient selection and monitoring.

PATIENT SELECTION, MONITORING, AND DISCHARGE

Patients who are American Society of Anesthesiologist (ASA) class I or II are considered suitable candidates for sedation by non-anesthesiologists (Table 34-1). An independent observer, usually a nurse or another physician, must continuously monitor the patient and periodically observe and record vital signs while the orthopaedist performs the procedure. To avoid adverse events, monitoring, including pulse oximetry, should continue after the procedure. Many disasters have occurred from airway obstruction in unmonitored patients after sedation. Children who receive deep sedation require a level of vigilance equal to that provided for general anesthesia. This includes recording of vital signs every 5 minutes and the presence of at least one individual trained in basic life support. Intravenous (i.v.) access should be readily available. Finally, appropriate discharge criteria must be followed before sending the patient home. The criteria recommended by the American Academy of Pediatrics are as follows:

- Cardiovascular function and airway patency are satisfactory and stable.
- The patient is easily aroused, and protective reflexes are intact.
- The patient can talk (if age-appropriate).
- The patient can sit up unaided (if age-appropriate).
- For a very young or disabled child, incapable of the usual expected responses, the presedation level of responsiveness or a level as close as possible to the normal level for that child should be achieved.
- The state of hydration is adequate.

TABLE 34-1 AMERICAN SOCIETY OF ANESTHESIOLOGISTS' PHYSICAL STATUS CLASSIFICATION

Class	Description
I	Normally healthy patient
II	Patient with mild systemic disease
III	Patient with severe systemic disease
IV	Patient with severe systemic disease that is a constant threat to life
V	Moribund patient who is not expected to survive without the operation

From American Academy of Pediatrics Committee on Drugs. Guidelines for monitoring and management of pediatric patients during and after sedation for diagnostic and therapeutic procedures. Pediatrics 1992;89:1110–1115.

FASTING GUIDELINES

If the procedure is elective, an appropriate time of fasting should be allowed. Most physicians consider a 6-hour fast from solid food acceptable for the majority of children. The intake of clear liquids has been liberalized in recent years, and only a brief clear liquid fast is now required. See Table 34-2 for fasting guidelines.

TABLE 34-2 PRESEDATION FASTING GUIDELINES

	Fasting Time (hr)	
Age	Milk/Solids	Clear Liquids
<6 mo	4	2
6–36 mo	6	3
>36 mo	8	3

Adapted from Coté CJ. Sedation for the pediatric patient: a review. Pediatr Clin North Am 1994;41:31–58.

Even with an adequate fasting interval, aspiration can still occur. Other factors can increase the risk of aspiration, including obesity, gastrointestinal obstruction, and neurologic dysfunction. Suction should be readily available for all cases. In some patients, lighter sedation or no sedation may be desirable to minimize the risk of aspiration. If the procedure is deemed an emergency, the need to proceed must be weighed against the risk of aspiration.

MEDICATIONS

Many medications can be used for sedation, including barbiturates, benzodiazepines, opioids, phencyclidines, and neuroleptic drugs. There can be an exaggerated effect from the administration of drugs to small infants and children. The route of administration will affect both the onset and duration of action of the drug and can extend the time needed for postprocedure observation. Doses of i.v. drugs should be titrated to effect. Combinations of drugs are often discouraged because of the additive or synergistic effects. In general, a smaller dose of each drug is often given if combinations are to be used. See Table 34-3 for the doses of drugs commonly used for sedation.

Benzodiazepines

- Of any sedative, *Midazolam* comes the closest to producing a true state of conscious sedation in children.
  - Water-soluble, short-acting benzodiazepine with a rapid onset.
  - Most popular sedative in the pediatric age group.
  - Most children do not fall asleep even with larger doses, but are calm and compliant.
  - Oral midazolam has a bitter aftertaste that is partially masked by sweeteners.
  - It has a short half-life (106 ± 29 minutes) and can produce antegrade amnesia.
  - Onset of action varies with route of administration. Can be as short as 2 minutes after i.v. administration and as long as 20 minutes after oral administration.
  - Respiratory depression can occur when used in combination with opioids.

TABLE 34-3 DOSES OF DRUGS COMMONLY USED FOR SEDATION

Drug	Route	Dose (mg/kg)
Barbiturates		
Methohexital	Rectal	20–30
	Intramuscular	10
Thiopental	Rectal	20–30
	Intramuscular	10
Benzodiazepines		
Diazepam	Oral	0.1–0.3
	Intravenous	0.1–0.3
	Intramuscular	Not recommended
	Rectal	0.2–0.3
Midazolam	Oral	0.5–0.75
	Intravenous	0.05–0.15
	Intramuscular	0.05–0.15
	Rectal	0.5–0.75
	Nasal	0.2–0.5
	Sublingual	0.2–0.5
Ketamine	Oral	3–10
	Intravenous	1–3
	Intramuscular	2–10
	Rectal	5–10
	Nasal	3–5
	Sublingual	3–5
Opioids		
Morphine	Intravenous	0.1–0.3
	Intramuscular	0.1–0.3
	Rectal	Not recommended
Meperidine	Intravenous	1–3
	Intramuscular	1–3
	Rectal	Not recommended
Fentanyl	Oral transmucosal	0.015–0.020 (15–20 μg/kg)
	Sublingual	0.010–0.015 (10–15 μg/kg)
	Intravenous	0.001–0.005 (1–5 μg/kg in increments of 0.5–1.0 μg/kg)
Chloral hydrate	Oral	20–100 mg/kg (max 1 g)

Adapted from Coté CJ. Sedation for the pediatric patient: a review. Pediatr Clin North Am 1994;41:31–58.

- *Diazepam* has a longer duration of action than midazolam and produces significant pain at the site of i.v. administration, both of which limit its usefulness for procedural sedation.

Opioids

Opioids provide sedation as well as analgesia for painful procedures. Because of major side effects including apnea, pruritis, nausea, vomiting, desaturation, and delayed emergence, opioids are rarely used solely for sedation. Opioids are useful for procedures such as fracture reduction in which postprocedure pain is expected.

- *Morphine* has a prolonged duration of action of 3 to 4 hours and is often reserved for longer procedures or those with significant postprocedure pain.
- *Fentanyl* is a hundred times more potent than morphine. Fentanyl, administered intravenously, has an onset within 1 to 2 minutes and a short duration of action of 0.5 to 1 hour, but respiratory depression may last considerably longer.
  - Fentanyl should be titrated slowly with several minutes between doses.

Phencyclidines

- *Ketamine* provides excellent analgesia, amnesia, and sedation.
  - It can be administered by any route (Table 34-3) and is useful to facilitate the cooperation of combative or delayed patients.
  - Anticholinergic agents are added to dry upper airway secretions.
  - Absolute contraindications to ketamine include elevated intracranial pressure and elevated intraocular pressure.
  - Side effects include tachycardia, hypertension, increased intracranial pressure, and increased intraocular pressure.
  - Reactions such as emergence hallucinations, vivid dreams, or frank delirium can occur in up to 10% of patients. These reactions are less common in children than in adults and can be prevented by pretreatment with a benzodiazepine. Although undesirable, they do not contraindicate the use of ketamine.
- Emergency medicine physicians recommend the administration of ketamine 3 mg/kg intramuscularly (i.m.), midazolam 0.05 mg/kg i.m., and glycopyrrolate 0.005 mg/kg i.m. as a single bolus injection for children 12 months to 7 years of age who require sedation for minor surgical procedures.
  - Onset of action with this cocktail occurs within 6 minutes in most patients, and adequate working conditions last for 30 minutes.

Neuroleptic Drugs

- *Droperidol* is a butyrophenone that acts centrally to produce a dissociative state.
  - The usual dose is 25 to 75 μg/kg.
  - Its duration of action is 6 to 12 hours.
  - It is generally not used except for antiemetic effects.
  - Its use has recently been discouraged because of a significant incidence of arrhythmias.

Chloral Hydrate

- Traditionally used for sedating young infants and children for nonpainful procedures, it remains one of the most popular sedatives used by non-anesthesiologists.
- The peak effect after oral administration can occur as late as 1 hour after administration.
- Although this drug is said to have a minimal effect on respiration, respiratory depression, airway obstruction and even death have occurred, especially when used in combination with other sedatives or narcotics.
- Children should be observed after sedation, particularly for airway patency.

Demerol Phenergan Thorazine

- Often referred to as a "lytic cocktail."
- This mixture of meperidine (25 mg/mL), promethazine (12.5 mg/mL), and chlorpromazine (12.5 mg/mL), is given intramuscularly.
- Sedation lasts about 5 hours, often outlasting many procedures.
- The dose is 0.1 to 0.2 mL/kg in a healthy child. The maximal dose should not exceed 2 mL. Life-threatening seizures have been reported with its use in children.

Propofol

- Sedative hypnotic with a fast onset, a short duration of action, and some antiemetic effect.
- Sedation has been achieved with a continuous infusion titrated to the response of the child (50 to 200 μg/kg/min).
- Propofol is a general anesthetic, and its use is limited to specialists skilled in airway management.

Nonsteroidal Antiinflammatory Drugs

- Provide analgesia while decreasing opioid requirements and side effects.
  - Opioid use has been decreased as much as 25% when these are used.
  - There is no evidence that one nonsteroidal antiinflammatory drug (NSAID) is more efficacious than the others.
- *Ketorolac* is an NSAID that has been studied extensively in the pediatric population.
  - Its i.v. formulation has increased its popularity over other NSAIDs.
  - Its dose varies with route of administration, with a maximum daily dose of 2 mg/kg/day for 5 consecutive days.
  - Its side effects include renal failure, bradycardia, anaphylaxis, gastrointestinal injury, platelet dysfunction, and perioperative bleeding.

TABLE 34-4 MAXIMUM RECOMMENDED DOSE OF COMMONLY USED LOCAL ANESTHETICS

Local Anesthetic	Maximum Dose (mg/kg)
Lidocaine[a]	7.0
Bupivacaine[b]	3.0
Tetracaine	1.5
Procaine	10.0
Mepivacaine	7.0
2-Chloroprocaine	20.0

[a]Lidocaine is short-acting—approximately 90 min.
[b]Bupivacaine is long-acting—approximately 180–600 min.
Adapted from Coté CJ. Sedation for the pediatric patient: a review. Pediatr Clin North Am 1994;41:31–58.

Local Anesthetics

- Useful in the treatment of pain by both subcutaneous injection and by regional blocks.
- Can anesthetize the affected area and reduce or eliminate pain during manipulation.
- Local anesthetic overdose can result in tinnitus, seizures, vasodilation, arrhythmias, and cardiac arrest. Overdose is more likely in smaller patients who communicate poorly and have delayed drug metabolism and elimination.
- The maximum dose of each commonly used local anesthetic is listed in Table 34-4.

GENERAL ANESTHESIA

Many procedures that are routinely performed in sedated adults are performed under general anesthesia in children. There are a few differences in the preoperative preparation in children when compared with adults:

- Preoperative laboratory studies
  - No laboratory studies are routinely obtained in healthy children for elective surgery.
  - When significant blood loss is expected, a starting hematocrit can be obtained after induction of anesthesia.
- Mask inductions
  - Many children are anesthetized with inhalation anesthetic gases, such as sevoflurane, before an i.v. is placed.
- Parental presence
  - Many operating rooms allow parents to stay with their children during induction of mask anesthesia.
  - This is most useful in children ages 1 to 6 years of age when separation anxiety is a major issue.
  - Parental presence is usually not needed if premedication can be given and if an i.v. is present.
- Preoperative medication
  - Many institutions prefer to premedicate children before induction of anesthesia even if parents are allowed to be present for induction.
  - The most common pediatric premedicant used in the majority of children is midazolam 0.5 mg/kg p.o. (maximum single dose of 25 mg).

SUGGESTED READING

American Academy of Pediatrics Committee on Drugs. Guidelines for monitoring and management of pediatric patients during and after sedation for diagnostic and therapeutic procedures. Pediatrics 1992;89:1110–1115.

Bikhazi GB. Review and update on approaches to sedating children. Pediatr Anesth Rep 1998;1:1–12.

Coté CJ. Sedation for the pediatric patient: a review. Pediatr Clin North Am 1994;41:31–58.

Coté CJ, Karl HW, Notterman DA, et al. Adverse sedation events in pediatrics: analysis of medications used for sedation. Pediatrics 2000;106:633–644.

Malviya S, Voepel-Lewis T, Tait AR. Adverse events and risk factors associated with the sedation of children by nonanesthesiologists. Anesth Analg 1997;85:1207–1213.

Peña BM, Krauss B. Adverse events of procedural sedation and analgesia in a pediatric emergency department. Ann Emerg Med 1999; 34:4,483–491.

Pruitt JW, Goldwasser MS, Sabol SR, et al. Intramuscular ketamine, midazolam, and glycopyrrolate for pediatric sedation in the emergency department. J Oral Maxillofac Surg 1995;53:13–17.

GAIT

RICHARD D. BEAUCHAMP

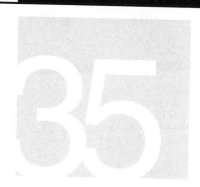

Gait is a term used to describe movement—the translation of the body through space from one point to another. It refers to both walking and running. There are various methods used to describe gait ranging from the very sophisticated three-dimensional computerized gait analyses systems to the simple visual assessment done in either the clinical setting such as the office or orthopaedic outpatient department or the nonclinical setting such as normal observation of someone walking in the community. Pathologic processes can have an effect on a patient's gait. Some conditions in which there can be a profound effect on a patient's gait, such as cerebral palsy, are best studied using the resources of a sophisticated gait lab. However, one should be able to describe a patient's gait even without the availability of a gait lab through direct observation.

GAIT CYCLE

Human locomotion can be divided into two main stages, considering each leg individually: stance phase (when at least one leg is in contact with the ground) and swing phase (when the leg is in the air; Table 35-1). As well as providing forward momentum to the leg, the swing phase also prepares and aligns the foot for heel strike and ensures that the swinging leg clears the floor. Usually, at normal walking velocity, the stance phase occupies approximately 60% of the gait cycle and the swing phase 40% (Fig. 35-1). The faster one walks the shorter the stance phase becomes and the longer the swing phase becomes until the person is running, at which point the stance phase can be as short as 20% and the swing phase as long as 80%. Running is also typified by absence of a double-support phase. In other words, at no time during running are both feet on the ground simultaneously.

Normal walking has several attributes (Box 35-1). The six basic determinants of gait have also been described (Box 35-2). These determinants produce a dampening down of the excessive vertical and side-to-side movement in gait by interacting to create a smooth pathway for the forward displacement of the center of gravity.

Some claim that children's gait does not mature into a heel–toe pattern until at least age 3.5 years, although there is extreme variability in the walking patterns of many children.

TABLE 35-1 TERMINOLOGY IN GAIT ANALYSIS

Term	Definition
Heel strike	The foot position when contact is made with the ground at the beginning of a gait cycle. (In toe-walking, there is no heel strike and *weight acceptance* would be a preferable term.)
Toe-off	The end of the stance phase and the beginning of the swing phase.
Double-support phase	When both feet are on the ground at the same time. It can occur when one is not moving or for short periods in the stance phase of gait.
Stance	When the foot is in contact with the ground.
Swing	When the foot is not in contact with the ground (i.e., is in the air).
Stride	The distance covered from one heel strike to the next ipsilateral heel strike.
Step	The distance from one heel strike to the next contralateral heel strike.

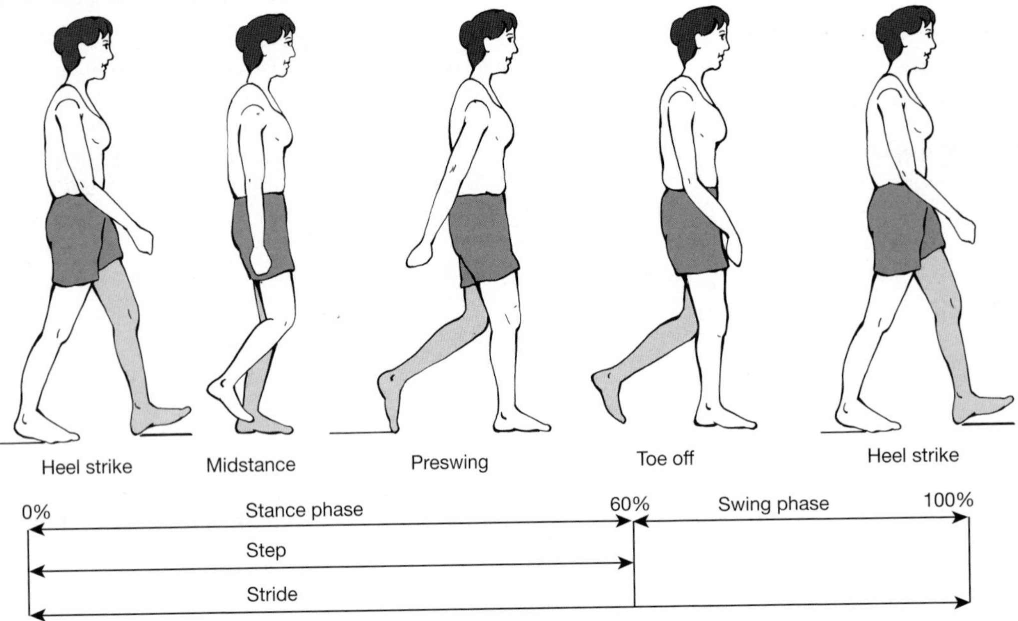

Figure 35-1 The gait cycle.

BOX 35-1 ATTRIBUTES OF GAIT

- Stability in stance
- Sufficient foot clearance during swing
- Appropriate swing phase pre-positioning of the foot
- Adequate step length
- Energy conservation

Adapted from Gage JR. Gait analysis in cerebral palsy. Clin Dev Med 1991;121:101.

BOX 35-2 THE SIX DETERMINANTS OF GAIT

- Pelvic rotation
- Pelvic tilt
- Knee flexion after heel–strike in stance phase
- Foot and ankle motion
- Knee motion
- Lateral displacement of the pelvis

Adapted from Saunders JBM, Inman VT, Eberhart HD. The major determinants in normal and pathological gait. J Bone Joint Surg (Am) 1953;35:558.

OBSERVATIONAL GAIT ANALYSIS

- With the child in shorts or other suitable attire observe him or her both from the frontal plane or front view and the sagittal plane or side view.
- Be aware that gait is occurring on a three-dimensional basis, so be sure to assess rotation or line of progression, which is in the coronal plane or transverse view.
- Watch the position of the child's limbs (upper and lower) and the trunk in double limb stance, before the child begins to walk.
- Ask the child to walk (usually at a "self-selected" pace) toward you and away from you.
- Have the child run. Running can sometimes unmask certain pathologic conditions and exaggerate asymmetry.
- Focus initially on the whole patient and the patient's general movement.
- Look for symmetry and asymmetry. Appreciate trunk sway, arm swing, head and neck position first; then concentrate on a single aspect of the walk, usually localized to one segment of the child's anatomy (Box 35-3).

Many reference tables have been published to describe gait. These scales have the observer assign a numeric value to the patients' walking characteristics. Generally, these reference scales have not been validated but do serve a useful purpose to train the observer to approach observational gait analysis in an orderly fashion. The Physician's Rating

BOX 35-3 OBSERVATIONAL GAIT ANALYSIS

Organized approach: Inspection on coronal and sagittal planes

- Overall impression
  - □ Temporal/spatial characteristics
- Trunk alignment
- Leg positions
  - □ Stance phase
  - □ Swing phase
- Foot position
  - □ Stance
  - □ Heel–toe

TABLE 35-2 PHYSICIAN'S RATING SCALE

Dynamic Function	Score
1. Crouch	
Severe (>20 degrees hip, knee, ankle)	0
Moderate (5–20 degrees hip, knee, ankle)	1
Mild (<5 degrees hip, knee, ankle)	2
None	3
2. Equinus foot	
Constant (fixed contracture)	0
Constant (dynamic contracture)	1
Occasional heel contact	2
Heel-to-toe gait	3
3. Hind foot	
Varus at foot strike	0
Valgus at foot strike	1
Occasional neutral at foot strike	2
Neutral at foot strike	3
4. Knee	
Recurvatum >5 degrees	0
Recurvatum 0–5 degrees	1
Neutral (no recurvatum)	2
5. Speed of gait	
Only slow	0
Variable (slow–fast)	1
6. Gait	
Toe–toe	0
Occasional heel–toe	1
Heel–toe	2
Total	_____

Koman LA, Mooney JF, Smith BP, et al. Management of spasticity in cerebral palsy with botulinum-A toxin: report of a preliminary, randomized, double-blind trial. J Pediatr Orthop 1994;14:300.

Scale has been frequently referred to in articles dealing with gait assessment (Table 35-2).

Temporal Spatial Features

- Appreciate overall symmetry of the patient's gait.
- Assess the stride and step lengths.
- Do the arms swing symmetrically?
- Is walking speed abnormally fast or slow?

Coronal Plane (Front and Back View)

Trunk/Pelvis

- Exaggerated side-to-side trunk sway may represent a compensated Trendelenburg sign. There is normally some degree of trunk sway but it should be noted if excessive.
- The pelvis normally rises a few degrees during single limb stance phase. Exaggerated ipsilateral pelvis elevation during single limb stance is known as a positive Trendelenburg sign and should be noted.
- Consistent asymmetry in pelvic heights (anterior superior iliac spine [ASIS] or posterior superior iliac spine [PSIS]) may indicate a leg length difference.
- Look for any scoliosis and any flank or waist crease asymmetry.

Hip Joint

- Watch for compensatory changes such as circumduction when the hip is "thrown" out into external rotation during swing phase. Some of these maneuvers are compensatory for a leg length discrepancy or weakness.
- Appreciate any abduction contractures of the leg (e.g., as seen in poliomyelitis), and look for adduction in swing and in stance phase ("scissoring") seen in patients with cerebral palsy. Sometimes the thighs are so adducted in stance that it appears the patient requires this for stability.

Knee Joint

- Watch on the frontal plane for excessive knee varus or valgus in stance.
- Lateral or varus thrusting on mid- or terminal stance at the knee may indicate medial or lateral instability from trauma or, in the case of younger children, may be a reflection of the health of the growth plate (e.g., Blount's disease, rickets).

Ankle Joint and Foot

- Static and dynamic knee and foot alignment can include varus and valgus of both the knee and foot.
- Observe the position of the heel or foot at weight acceptance:
  - ☐ Is there excessive calcaneovalgus or calcaneovarus?
  - ☐ Is the foot flat or high arched?
  - ☐ Weight acceptance normally occurs with the lateral border of the heel. The center of force normally then passes distally toward the fifth metatarsal and then proceeds across the metatarsals and exits near the great toe. This represents a pronation then supination attitude to the foot during stance.
  - ☐ The supinated foot prior to toe-off also may be slightly adducted for rigidity and strength (lever arm).

Sagittal Plane (Right and Left Side View)

Trunk/Pelvis

- Appreciate the sagittal alignment of the whole thoracic and lumbar spine.
- Comment on any increased or decreased spinal kyphosis or lordosis.
- Watch for cervical spine and head position.
- Is there an increased anterior pelvic tilt?
  - ☐ This can be partially age-related (common at ages 3 to 7 years).
  - ☐ Increased anterior pelvic tilt and lumbar lordosis can be seen following excessive hamstring lengthening in cerebral palsy.
  - ☐ Hip extensor weakness (spina bifida, muscular dystrophy) can also be associated with anterior tilt.
- Posterior pelvic tilt can be seen with hamstring tightness or spasticity.

Hip Joint

- The hip normally flexes to its maximum range at the end of the swing phase just before the foot strikes the floor. This also assists in achieving toe clearance.

- The hip then goes into extension and remains there throughout the rest of stance and reaches its maximum degree of extension just before toe-off. This produces the proximal portion of a rigid fulcrum or lever for maximum propulsion of the lower leg.

Knee Joint

- The main function of the knee in swing is to raise the foot off the ground to assist in appropriate toe clearance. Only a few millimeters of toe clearance is required for efficient walking.
- The knee therefore has its maximum degree of flexion in mid-swing.
- Initial weight acceptance sees the knee in almost full extension. This is followed by a few degrees of knee flexion before fully extending in terminal stance in preparation of toe-off and propulsion. This adds further strength to the lever arm for lower leg propulsion in conjunction with the hip also in full extension.
- The purpose of knee flexion in initial stance is for a shock-absorbing effect.
- Stiff-legged position at stance and swing would be very tiring and probably lead to increased stresses seen at other joints up the kinetic chain.
- Check for any knee hyperextension or recurvatum that can sometimes occur in mid- to late stance in such conditions as spasticity or equinus contractures.
- Look for persistent knee flexion throughout stance as can be seen in crouch gait.

Ankle Joint and Foot

- The weight acceptance pattern during normal walking is that of heel to toe during stance.
- The ankle position has been described as having three rockers on the sagittal plane (Fig. 35-2):
  - ☐ The first rocker immediately follows heel strike when the ankle plantarflexes for full flat foot weight acceptance.
  - ☐ In mid-stance, the tibia then moves over the talus at the ankle to form the second rocker. This means the foot goes into relative dorsiflexion.
  - ☐ The third rocker then follows as the foot plantarflexes for power generation to propel the patient forward at push-off.
- The foot and ankle are held in dorsiflexion during swing to achieve toe clearance and also to prepare for weight acceptance at heel strike.

Transverse Plane (Top or Bottom View)

Trunk/Pelvis

- There is normally some trunk rotation seen with gait. The ipsilateral leg, when advancing, is associated with internal trunk and pelvis rotation.
- When this normal rotation does not occur, terms such as *pelvic retraction* are used. This can commonly be seen in children with hemiplegia.

Hip Joint

- Circumduction and adduction (coronal plane) can sometimes be confused with rotational changes seen in the hip during swing phase of the gait cycle.
- Transverse plane describes internal and external rotation of the limb during swing and subsequently at weight acceptance.
- Exaggerated femoral anteversion will produce an internally rotated line of progression, whereas femoral retroversion will produce an out-toed gait.
- Sometimes these conditions are exaggerated with running or with fatigue.

Knee Joint

- The transverse plane rotational changes that occur during gait at the knee are so small that they are difficult to appreciate visually.

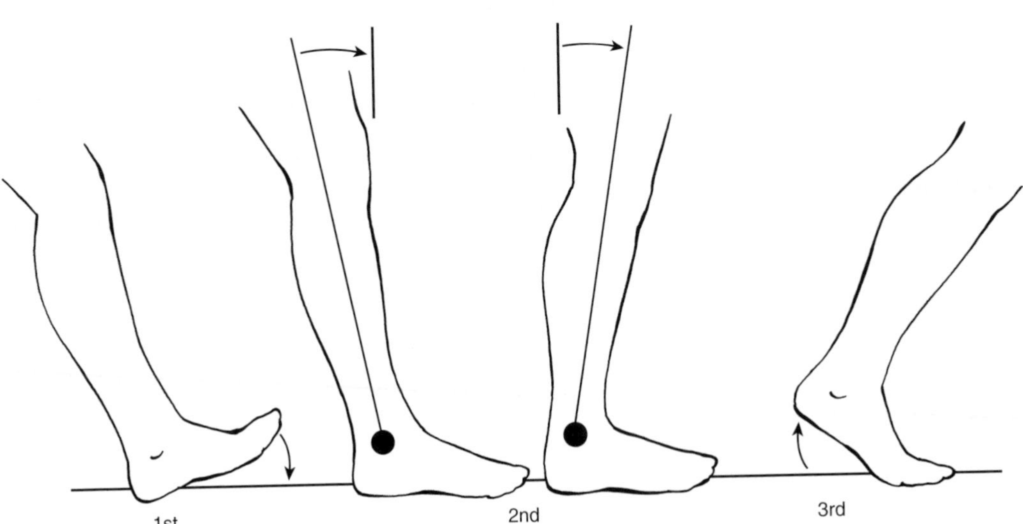

Figure 35-2 The three ankle rockers. (Adapted from Gage JR. Gait analysis in cerebral palsy. Clin Dev Med 1991;121:82.)

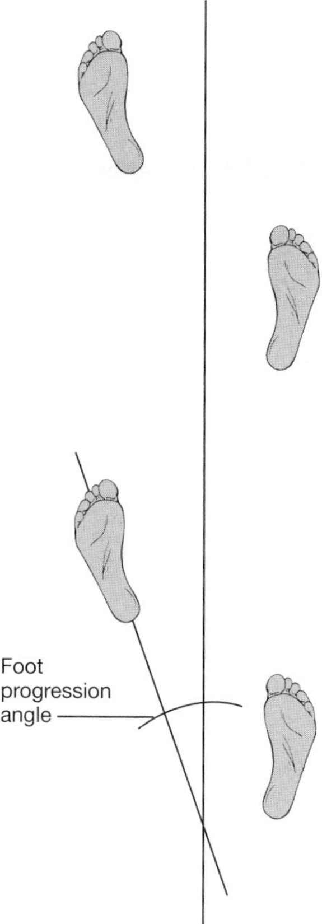

Figure 35-3 The line of progression in gait. In-toeing is expressed as negative degrees and out-toeing as positive.

- There is normally a "screw-home" phenomenon that occurs in terminal stance, serving to lock the knee and provide stability.
- The only way this rotation can be appreciated is when it is increased as in knee instability syndromes. The static rotational changes seen here are a reflection of the developmental internal and external tibial torsion, which also can produce an internally or externally rotated line of progression.

Ankle Joint and Foot

- On the transverse plane, observe the line of progression the foot makes in relation to the trunk and pelvic alignment and comment on in-toeing or out-toeing gait pattern (Fig. 35-3).
- Abnormal foot positions such as metatarsus adductus can be appreciated.
- The foot normally rotates into internal position just prior to toe-off.

THREE-DIMENSIONAL GAIT ANALYSIS

Gait or motion analysis laboratories are becoming an accepted method to critically analyze gait in children and adults with movement disorders. It is especially valuable to assist clinical examination of those patients with complex movement patterns from such conditions as cerebral palsy and spina bifida. Detailed understanding of the intricacies of a gait laboratory is beyond the scope of this chapter; however, the orthopaedic resident or surgeon should be able to understand some of the basic methods of gait analyses and appreciate the results and subsequent treatment recommendations.

Most of the recognized gait lab facilities conducting the test combine visual analysis with video cameras capable of slow motion for review. Kinematics, kinetics, electromyography, plantar pressure profiles, and oxygen cost are also usually performed. The data are collected using three-dimensional analysis: the x, y, and z axes describing the coronal, sagittal, and transverse planes, respectively. The information is gathered after appropriate digitization and usually presented in graphic form. The graphs usually show one stride length, standard deviations, and norms for age or weight.

Kinematics

Kinematics is the term used to describe the relationship of the body and its joints in space. It is a description of motion independent of forces.

- *Temporal spatial characteristics*: these include velocity, cadence, stride, and step lengths. Support times and step widths are also often included.
- *Trunk and pelvic orientations*: for both the right and left strides the rotation, anterior or posterior lean, and elevation or depression are measured and compared with a set of normal for age and weight.
- *Hip, knee, and ankle joint angles*: on the sagittal plane, the degree of flexion and extension is measured through the whole gait cycle (stance and swing phase). The hip has its maximum flexed position at terminal swing whereas the knee has its maximal degree of flexion at mid-swing in order to allow for ground clearance of the swinging limb. Both hip and knee have their maximum extended position in late and terminal stance (Fig. 35-4). The ankle is described as three ankle rockers going from plantarflexion to dorsiflexion and then plantarflexion prior to toe-off (Fig. 35-5).

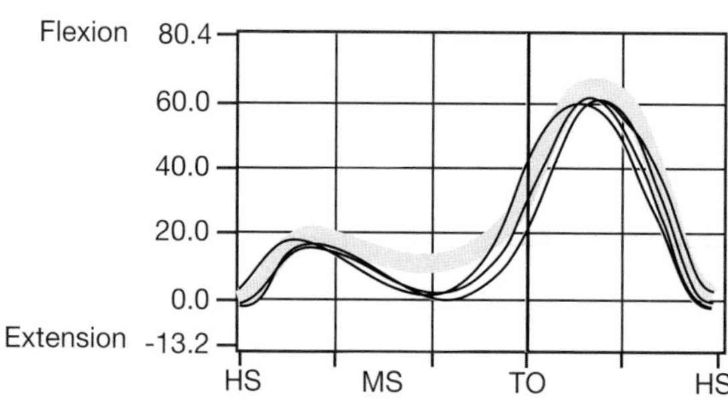

Figure 35-4 Knee joint kinematics. This represents one complete gait cycle from heel-strike to heel-strike. *HS*, heel-strike; *MS*, mid-stance; *TO*, toe-off. (Adapted from Shriners Gait Lab, Sunny Hill Health Centre for Children, Vancouver, BC, Canada.)

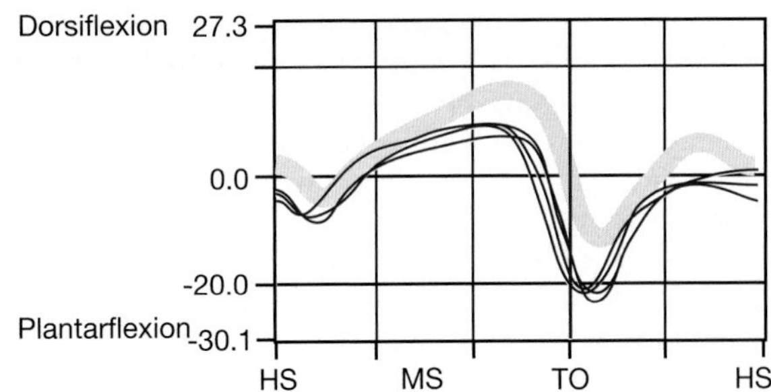

Figure 35-5 Ankle joint kinematics. This represents three separate trials walking in the sagittal plane. *HS,* heel-strike; *MS,* mid-stance; *TO,* toe-off. (Adapted from Shriners Gait Lab, Sunny Hill Health Centre for Children, Vancouver, BC, Canada.)

Kinetics

Kinetics is the term that describes forces that produce movement. They are measured using a specialized force plate concealed in the floor over which the patient walks during the assessment. Data collected include ground reaction forces, joint moments, sagittal joint powers, and forces (Fig. 35-6). Plantar pressure profiles can show the dynamic weight acceptance pattern of the foot and the development of medial and longitudinal foot arches.

Electromyography

To appreciate the muscle function in gait, the timing of the muscle contraction can be measured using ambulatory or dynamic electromyography. This allows the visualization of the muscle contraction during various phases of the gait cycle. Appropriate or inappropriate firing can be appreciated and recommendations made on treatment of these abnormal muscle functions through either muscle or tendon releases or transfers (Fig. 35-7).

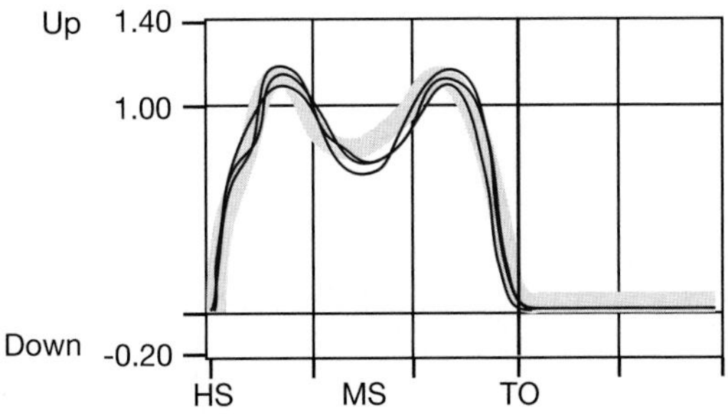

Figure 35-6 Kinetics showing ground reaction forces. This represents stance phase only, as there are no forces when the foot is off the force plate. *HS,* heel-strike; *MS,* mid-stance; *TO,* toe-off. (Adapted from Shriners Gait Lab, Sunny Hill Health Centre for Children, Vancouver, BC, Canada.)

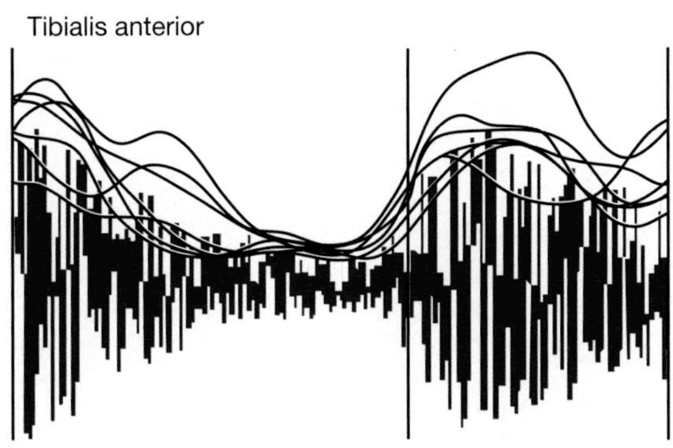

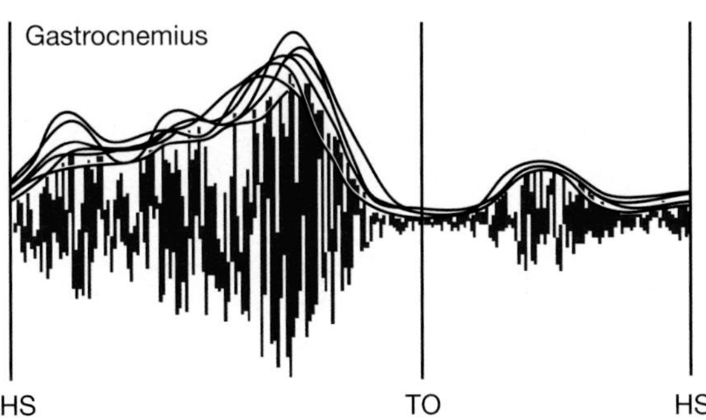

Figure 35-7 Electromyography of tibialis anterior and gastrocnemius muscles. The gastrocnemius muscle fires in the pre-swing phase for toe-off (*TO*) and the tibialis anterior fires in swing to achieve ground clearance and fires again at heel-strike (*HS*) for eccentric deceleration of the foot. (Adapted from Shriners Gait Lab, Sunny Hill Health Centre for Children, Vancouver, BC, Canada.)

SUGGESTED READING

Gage JR. Gait analysis in cerebral palsy. Clin Dev Med 1991;121.

Inman VT, Ralston HJ, Todd F. Human walking. Baltimore: Williams & Wilkins, 1981.

Koman LA, Mooney JF, Smith BP, et al. Management of spasticity in cerebral palsy with botulinum-A toxin: report of a preliminary, randomized, double-blind trial. J Pediatr Orthop 1994;14:299–303.

Perry J. Gait analysis: normal and pathological function. New York: McGraw-Hill, 1992.

Perry J. Kinesiology of lower extremity bracing. Clin Orthop 1974; 102:20–31.

Saunders JBM, Inman VT, Eberhart HD. The major determinants in normal and pathological gait. J Bone Joint Surg (Am) 1953;35:543.

Sussman M. The diplegic child. Shriners Hospital for Crippled Children Symposium. Rosemont, IL: American Academy of Orthopedic Surgeons, 1992.

Sutherland DH, Olsen R, Cooper L, Woo L. The development of mature gait. J Bone Joint Surg (Am) 1980;62:336–353.

INDEX

Note: Numbers followed by "f" indicate figures; those followed by "t" indicate tables; and those followed by "b" indicate boxes.

B

E

G

I

J

K

L

M

S